Ethical Challenges in the Management of Health Information
Second Edition

Laurinda Beebe Harman, PhD, RHIA
Associate Professor and Chair
Department of Health Information Management
College of Health Professions
Temple University
Philadelphia, Pennsylvania

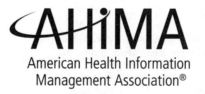

American Health Information
Management Association®

JONES AND BARTLETT PUBLISHERS
Sudbury, Massachusetts
BOSTON   TORONTO   LONDON   SINGAPORE

World Headquarters
Jones and Bartlett Publishers
40 Tall Pine Drive
Sudbury, MA 01776
978-443-5000
info@jbpub.com
www.jbpub.com

Jones and Bartlett Publishers Canada
6339 Ormindale Way
Mississauga, Ontario L5V 1J2
CANADA

Jones and Bartlett Publishers International
Barb House, Barb Mews
London W6 7PA
UK

Jones and Bartlett's books and products are available through most bookstores and online booksellers. To contact Jones and Bartlett Publishers directly, call 800-832-0034, fax 978-443-8000, or visit our website, www.jbpub.com.

Substantial discounts on bulk quantities of Jones and Bartlett's publications are available to corporations, professional associations, and other qualified organizations. For details and specific discount information, contact the special sales department at Jones and Bartlett via the above contact information or send an email to specialsales@jbpub.com.

Library of Congress Cataloging-in-Publication Data
Ethical challenges in the management of health information / edited by
    Laurinda B. Harman. — 2nd ed.
      p. ; cm.
    Includes bibliographical references.
    ISBN 0-7637-4732-7 (casebound)
    1. Health—Information services—Management—Moral and ethical
aspects. 2. Medical care—Information services—Moral and ethical
aspects.   I. Harman, Laurinda B.
    [DNLM: 1. Information Management—ethics. 2. Medical Records
—standards. 3. Confidentiality—ethics. 4. Ethics, Professional.
WX 173 E84 2006]
R118.2.E86 2006
174'.2—dc22
                                    2005023423

6048

Production Credits
Publisher: Michael Brown
Associate Editor: Kylah Goodfellow McNeill
Production Director: Amy Rose
Associate Production Editor: Kate Hennessy
Associate Marketing Manager: Marissa Hederson
Manufacturing Buyer: Therese Connell
Composition: Auburn Associates, Inc.
Cover Design: Timothy Dziewit
Printing and Binding: Malloy, Inc.
Cover Printing: Malloy, Inc.

Printed in the United States of America
10 09 08 07 06   10 9 8 7 6 5 4 3 2 1

I dedicate this book to

my parents and first ethical teachers
Paul William and Gloria Virginia Scott Sugg

my sisters and first ethical friends
Dorette Eirene Welk and Charleen Rene Szabo

TABLE OF CONTENTS

Contributors xvii
Foreword xxi
Preface xxiii
Acknowledgments xxix

PART 1—Professional Ethics 1

Chapter 1—Professional Values and the Code of Ethics 3
        Laurinda B. Harman, PhD, RHIA
        Virginia L. Mullen, RHIA
Learning Objectives 3
Abstract 3
Ethical Dilemmas For The HIM Professional 4
The Health Information System: Then And Now 5
Role of the HIM Professional 8
Professional Code of Ethics 9
Professional Values 10
Building an Ethical Health Information System 15
The Intersection of HIM and Ethics 16
Key Terms 17
Chapter Summary 17
Appendix 1-A: 1957 Code of Ethics for the Practice of Medical Record Science 19
Appendix 1-B: 1977 American Medical Record Association Bylaws and Code of Ethics 20
Appendix 1-C: 1988 American Medical Record Association Code of Ethics and Bylaws 22
Appendix 1-D: 1998 American Health Information Management Association Code of
    Ethics and Bylaws 23
Appendix 1-E: 2004 American Health Information Management Association
    Code of Ethics 25

Chapter 2—Ethical Decision-Making Guidelines and Tools 33
        Jacqueline J. Glover, PhD
Learning Objectives 33
Abstract 33

Scenario 2-A: Documentation and DRG Assignment 34
What Is an Ethical Issue? 34
Why Is it Important to Identify and Address Ethical Issues? .34
But You Can't Teach Ethics, Can You? 35
The Process of Ethical Decision-Making 35
Justification in Ethical Reasoning: How Do You Know What Is Best? 38
Moral Distress 42
Scenario 2-B: Retrospective Documentation to Increase Reimbursement 43
Ethics Resources 43
Conclusion 44
Key Terms 44
Chapter Summary 44
Ethical Decision-Making Matrices:
    -Scenario 2-A: Documentation and DRG Assignment .46
    -Scenario 2-B: Retrospective Documentation to Increase Reimbursement 48
Appendix 2-A: Blank Ethical Decision-Making Matrix 50

Chapter 3—Privacy and Confidentiality **51**
    Laurie A. Rinehart-Thompson, JD, RHIA, CHP
    Laurinda B. Harman, PhD, RHIA
Learning Objectives 51
Abstract 51
Scenario 3-A: Family and Friends: Should I Tell? 52
Privacy and Confidentiality 53
Release of Information 54
The HIPAA Privacy Rule 54
Blanket Authorizations 59
Patient Concerns 60
Professional Concerns 61
Ethical Challenges 61
Conclusion 62
Key Terms 62
Chapter Summary 63
Ethical Decision-Making Matrix
    -Scenario 3-A: Family and Friends: Should I Tell? 64

PART II—Uses of Health Information **67**

Chapter 4—Compliance, Fraud, and Abuse **69**
    Laurie A. Rinehart-Thompson, JD, RHIA, CHP
Learning Objectives 69
Abstract 69
Scenario 4-A: Documentation Does Not Justify Billed Procedure 70
Traditional Regulations that Guide HIM Professionals 71
More Recent Regulations That Guide HIM Professionals 76
HIPAA Administrative Simplification Standards 77
Roles for HIM Professionals 79
Compliance Programs to Prevent Fraudulent Behaviors 79
Dilemmas in Practice 81

Scenario 4-B: Accepting Money for Information 81
    Fraudulent Documentation Practices 82
Scenario 4-C: Retrospective Documentation to Avoid Suspension 82
    Retrospective Medical Record Analysis 83
Scenario 4-D: Coder Assigns Code Without Physician's Documentation 84
    Coding Turnaround Time 84
Conclusion 84
Key Terms 85
Chapter Summary 85
Ethical Decision-Making Matrices:
    -Scenario 4-A: Documentation Does Not Justify Billed Procedure 88
    -Scenario 4-B: Accepting Money for Information 90
    -Scenario 4-C: Retrospective Documentation to Avoid Suspension 92
    -Scenario 4-D: Coder Assigns Code Without Physician's Documentation 94

Chapter 5—Clinical Code Selection and Use **97**
        Lou Ann Schraffenberger, MBA, RHIA, CCS, CCS-P
        Rita A. Scichilone, MHSA, RHIA, CCS, CCS-P, CHC
Learning Objectives 97
Abstract 97
Scenario 5-A: Coding an Inappropriate Level of Service 98
HIPAA and Billing Activities 101
Ethical Approaches to Coding Situations 102
Applying the AHIMA Standards of Ethical Coding 104
Ethical Dilemmas for the Coding Professional 109
Scenario 5-B: Discovering Misrepresentation in Physician Documentation 109
Scenario 5-C: Miscoding to Avoid Conflicts 110
Scenario 5-D: Discovering of Miscoding by Other Staff Members 114
Scenario 5-E: Lacking the Tools to do One's Job 115
Scenario 5-F: Being Required by the Employer to Engage in Negligent Coding Practices 116
Scenario 5-G: Supporting Application Software that Facilitates Questionable Results 118
Professional Practice Solutions 120
The Future of Coding 122
Key Terms 122
Chapter Summary 122
Ethical Decision-Making Matrices
    -Scenario 5-A: Coding an Inappropriate Level of Service 124
    -Scenario 5-B: Discovering Misrepresentation in Physician Documentation 126
    -Scenario 5-C: Miscoding to Avoid Conflicts 128
    -Scenario 5-D: Discovering of Miscoding by Other Staff Members 130
    -Scenario 5-E: Lacking the Tools to Do One's Job 132
    -Scenario 5-F: Being Required by the Employer to Engage in Negligent
     Coding Practices 134
    -Scenario 5-G: Supporting Application Software that Facilitates
Questionable Results 136

Chapter 6—Quality Review **139**
        Patrice L. Spath, BA, RHIT
Learning Objectives 139

Abstract 139
Quality Management 140
Scenario 6-A: Inaccurate Performance Data 142
QM Ethical Issues Facing HIM Professionals 142
Scenario 6-B: Home Health Care and Central-Line Infections 143
Ethical Standards Affecting QM Activities 144
Scenario 6-C: Failure to Check Physician's Licensure Status 146
Scenario 6-D: Hiding Incomplete Medical Records 147
Making Ethical Decisions 148
Scenario 6-E: Audit Results Indicate Inappropriate Health Care 149
QM Situations that Raise Ethical Questions 149
Enabling Ethical Conduct 151
Conclusion 152
Key Terms 153
Chapter Summary 153
Scenarios—Survey Results and Ethical Decision-Making Matrices
        -Scenario 6-A: Inaccurate Performance Data 156
        -Scenario 6-B: Home Health Care and Central-line Infections 158
        -Scenario 6-C: Failure to Check Physician's Licensure Status 162
        -Scenario 6-D: Hiding Incomplete Medical Records 166
        -Scenario 6-E: Audit Results Indicate Inappropriate Health Care 170

Chapter 7—Research and Decision Support **175**
        Merida L. Johns, PhD, RHIA
        J. Michael Hardin, PhD
Learning Objectives 175
Abstract 175
Scenario 7-A: Designing a Survey to Bias the Results 176
Roles of the RS and DSS 177
Ethical Responsibilities of the RS and DSS 181
Conclusion 195
Key Terms 195
Chapter Summary 195
Ethical Decision-Making Matrix
        -Scenario 7-A: Designing a Survey to Bias the Results 198

Chapter 8—Public Health **199**
        Babette J. Neuberger, JD, MPH
Learning Objectives 199
Abstract 199
Scenario 8-A: Reporting HIV Status 200
Public Health: An Overview 201
Ethical Challenges in Public Health 210
Scenario 8-B: When Duty to One's Employer Conflicts with a Duty Owed to the Public 216
The HIM Professional's Role and Responsibility as an Advocate 219
Emerging Issues: Bioterrorism and Global Infections 221
Scenario 8-C: The Terrorism Preparedness Act .222
Conclusion 223
Key Terms 223

Chapter Summary 224
Ethical Decision-Making Matrices
    -Scenario 8-A: Reporting HIV Status 226
    -Scenario 8-B: When Duty to One's Employer Conflicts with a Duty Owed to
    the Public 228

Chapter 9—Managed Care: Lessons of Integration **231**
    Ida Critelli Schick, PhD, MS, FACHE
Learning Objectives 231
Abstract 231
Scenario 9-A: Complexity of Choosing a Managed Care Plan 232
What Is Managed Care? 233
Growth of Managed Care 234
Managed Care Strategies 235
The Role of Information and HIM Professionals in a Managed Care Environment 240
Ethical Dilemmas for HIM Professionals 241
Scenario 9-B: Provision of Information by Physician Practices 243
Scenario 9-C: HIM Professionals in Provider Organizations 245
Policies for Which the HIM Professional Can Advocate 246
Conclusion 247
Key Terms 247
Chapter Summary 247
Ethical Decision-Making Matrices
    -Scenario 9-A: Complexity of Choosing a Managed Care Plan 250
    -Scenario 9-B: Provision of Information by Physician Practices 252
    -Scenario 9-C: HIM Professionals in Provider Organizations 254

Chapter 10—Clinical Care: End of Life **257**
    James F. Tischler, MD
Learning Objectives 257
Abstract 257
Scenario 10-A: Bad News 258
Aging, Frailty, and Information Ethics 258
Evolution of Autonomy 259
Cultural Influences on Autonomy 259
Physician Bias and Equity: A Systems Issue 259
Scenario 10-B: Treatment Choices 260
Information Across a Healthcare Continuum 261
Treatment Goals and Beneficence 261
Scenario 10-C: Advance Care Planning 262
Advance Care Planning: An Opportunity 263
The Meaning of *Terminal* 263
Advance Care Planning and Law 264
Scenario 10-D: Palliative Care 264
Managing Pain 265
Ethics Committees 265
Palliative Care 265
Emerging Issues 266
Key Terms 266

Chapter Summary 266
Ethical Decision-Making Matrices
    -Scenario 10-A: Bad News 268
    -Scenario 10-B: Treatment Choices 270
    -Scenario 10-C: Advance Care Planning 272
    -Scenario 10-D: Palliative Care 274

Part III—Computerized Health Information **277**

Chapter 11—Electronic Health Records **279**
        Mary Alice Hanken, PhD, CHP, RHIA
        Gretchen Murphy, MEd, RHIA, FAHIMA
Learning Objectives 279
Abstract 279
Scenario 11-A: Patient Record Integrity and System Security 280
EHR Systems: Functions and Expected Features 281
EHR Systems in the Twenty-First Century 285
EHR Technology and Ethical Issues 286
Scenario 11-B: Differences when Linking EHR Systems 293
Conclusion 299
Key Terms 299
Chapter Summary 299
Ethical Decision-Making Matrices
    -Scenario 11-A: Patient Record Integrity and System Security 302
    -Scenario 11-B: Differences when Linking EHR Systems 304

Chapter 12—Information Security **307**
        Karen Czirr, MS, RHIA, CHP
        Karen A. Rosendale, MBA, RHIA
        Emily West, RHIA
Learning Objectives 307
Abstract 307
Scenario 12-A: A Curious Human Resource Employee 308
The Healthcare Information Revolution 308
The Role of the ISO 310
Concepts in Information Security 310
Privacy-Related Security 310
Establishing a Security Baseline 312
Scenario 12-B: Failure to Log Off of the System 315
Scenario 12-C: Storing Data on a Laptop Computer 318
Key Terms 319
Chapter Summary 319
Ethical Decision-Making Matrices
    -Scenario 12-A: A Curious Human Resource Employee 322
    -Scenario 12-B: Failure to Log Off of the System 324
    -Scenario 12-C: Storing Data on a Laptop Computer 326

Chapter 13—Software Development and Implementation **329**
        Susan H. Fenton, MBA, RHIA

Learning Objectives 329
Abstract 329
Scenario 13-A: Planning the EHR: Competing Interests 330
Consultant's Approach 330
Information Gathering 331
Conclusion 335
Key Terms 335
Chapter Summary 336
Ethical Decision-Making Matrix
    -Scenario 13-A: Planning the EHR: Competing Interests 338

Chapter 14—Data Resource Management **341**
    Frances Wickham Lee, DBA
    Andrea W. White, PhD
    Karen A. Wager, DBA, RHIA
Learning Objectives 341
Abstract 341
Data Resource Management in Health Care 341
Impact of HIPAA Regulations on Data Resource Management 342
Data Resource Management Tools 342
Scenario 14-A: The Physicians Resist a New Password Policy 346
Ethical Dilemmas for Data Resource Managers 347
Scenario 14-B: Threat to Integrity of the CDR 349
Scenario 14-C: Research Access to Admission/Discharge/Registration Data 350
Conclusion 353
Key Terms 353
Chapter Summary 353
Ethical Decision-Making Matrices
    -Scenario 14-A: The Physicians Resist a New Password Policy 356
    -Scenario 14-B: Threat to Integrity of the CDR 358
    -Scenario 14-C: Research Access to Admission/Discharge/Registration Data 360

Chapter 15—Integrated Delivery Systems **363**
    Brenda Olson, MEd, RHIA, CHP
    Karen Gallagher Grant, RHIA, CHP
Learning Objectives 363
Abstract 363
Scenario 15-A: Scheduling Clerk Has Access to All Clinical Information 364
Privacy and Security Issues 365
Data Quality Issues 368
Scenario 15-B: Inconsistencies in the MPI 372
Required Skills for HIM Professionals 373
Conclusion 373
Key Terms 373
Chapter Summary 374
Ethical Decision-Making Matrices
    -Scenario 15-A: Scheduling Clerk Has Access to All Clinical Information 376
    -Scenario 15-B: Inconsistencies in the MPI 378

Chapter 16—E-Health for Consumers, Patients, and Caregivers 381
    Cynthia Baur, PhD
    Mary Jo Deering, PhD
Learning Objectives 381
Abstract 381
Scenario 16-A: Equity and Privacy 382
E-Health and the Changing Healthcare System 386
E-Health and National Policy 388
E-Health and the HIM Professional 389
Some E-Health Ethical Issues 390
Scenario 16-B: Ensuring Online Quality and Privacy Protections 391
Emerging Issues 393
Conclusion 394
Key Terms 395
Chapter Summary 395
Appendix 16-A: Examples of Guidelines, Policies, and Codes of Conduct for Health Websites .397
Ethical Decision-Making Matrices
       -Scenario 16-A: Equity and Privacy 398
       -Scenario 16-B: Ensuring Online Quality and Privacy Protections 400

Chapter 17—E-HIM: Information Technology and Information Exchange 403
    Meryl Bloomrosen, MBA, RHIA
Learning Objectives 403
Abstract 403
Introduction 404
Scenario 17-A: The HIM Professionals' Role in eHIM 411
Conclusion 412
Key Terms 413
Chapter Summary 414

PART IV Management of Sensitive Health Information 421

Chapter 18—Genetic Information 423
    Barbara P. Fuller, JD, RHIA
    Kathy L. Hudson, PhD
Learning Objectives 423
Abstract 423
Scenario 18-A: Genetic Privacy 424
The Issue of Genetic Information 424
The Relationship Between Genetic Information and Generic Medical Information 426
What Do We Mean by Privacy of Medical Information? 427
Research Records 427
The Misuse of Genetic Information and Discrimination 428
Federal Legislative Protections 429
State Legislative Protections 430
Legislation on Research Record Privacy 431
Ethical Issues for the HIM Professional 433
Conclusion 433
Key Terms 434

Chapter Summary 434
Ethical Decision-Making Matrix
    -Scenario 18-A: Genetic Privacy 436

Chapter 19—Adoption Information **439**
        Martha L. Jones, PhD, LSW
Learning Objectives 439
Abstract 439
Scenario 19-A: Seeking Information Many Years Later 440
Adoption: Historical and Emerging Ethical Issues 442
Who's Who in Adoption: Some Explanations of Terminology 445
Ethical Issues for HIM Professionals 447
Scenario 19-B: An Adoptee Seeks Information on Her Biological Family 448
Scenario 19-C: A Birth Mother Seeks Information on Her Biological Son 450
Future Issues 451
Key Terms 454
Chapter Summary 454
Ethical Decision-Making Matrices
    -Scenario 19-A: Seeking Information Many Years Later 456
    -Scenario 19-B: An Adoptee Seeks Information on Her Biological Family 458
    -Scenario 19-C: A Birth Mother Seeks Information on Her Biological Son 460

Chapter 20—Drug, Alcohol, Sexual, and Behavioral Information **463**
        Sharon J. Randolph, JD, RHIA
        Laurie A. Rinehart-Thompson, JD, RHIA, CHP
Learning Objectives 463
Abstract 463
Scenario 20-A: The Arrest Warrant: Is This Person in Your Facility? 464
Substance Abuse Treatment, Health Information, and the Law 464
Ethical Challenges in Behavioral Health and Substance Abuse Treatment 465
Scenario 20-B: Safety of a Citizen versus Privacy of a Patient 469
Scenario 20-C: Patient Confesses to a Psychiatrist 470
Scenario 20-D: Patient Confesses to the Nurse's Aide 472
Scenario 20-E: Verifying Admission Can Violate Privacy 473
Scenario 20-F: A Prisoner Who May Have AIDS .475
Scenario 20-G: Workers' Compensation Case 476
Scenario 20-H: Children's Protective Services 477
Conclusion 478
Key Terms 478
Chapter Summary 479
Ethical Decision-Making Matrices
    -Scenario 20-A: The Arrest Warrant: Is This Person in Your Facility? 480
    -Scenario 20-B: Safety of a Citizen versus Privacy of a Patient 482
    -Scenario 20-C: Patient Confesses to a Psychiatrist 484
    -Scenario 20-D: Patient Confesses to the Nurse's Aide 486
    -Scenario 20-E: Verifying Admission Can Violate Privacy 488
    -Scenario 20-F: A Prisoner Who May Have AIDS 490

-Scenario 20-G: Workers' Compensation Case 492
-Scenario 20-H: Children's Protective Services 494

PART V Roles **497**

Chapter 21—Management **499**
     Cathy Flite, MEd, RHIA
     Sharon Laquer, MS, RHIA
Learning Objectives 499
Abstract 499
Scenario 21-A: Lateness and Absenteeism 500
Moral Development and Awareness 500
Scenario 21-B: National Convention Misadventures 507
Orientation of New Employees 508
Scenario 21-C: Avoiding the Employee Who Will Be Fired 510
The Code of Ethics is Not Enough 511
When Leadership Fails 511
Scenario 21-D: Failure to Document Poor Work Performance for a Friendly Employee 513
Moral Muteness 514
Conclusion 514
Key Terms 515
Chapter Summary 516
Ethical Decision-Making Matrices
     -Scenario 21-A-1 and A-2: Lateness and Absenteeism 518
     -Scenario 21-B: National Convention Misadventures 522
     -Scenario 21-C: Avoiding the Employee Who Will Be Fired 524
     -Scenario 21-D: Failure to Document Poor Work Performance for a
     Friendly Employee 526

Chapter 22—Entrepreneurship **529**
     Marie Gardenier, MBA, RHIA, CHPS
Learning Objectives 529
Abstract 529
Scenario 22-A: Competing Constituencies 530
Entrepreneurship in Health Information Management .532
Entrepreneur versus Intraprenuer 534
Business Ethics: Concepts and Principles 535
The Intersection of Ethics and HIM Entrepreneurship .540
Scenario 22-B: Negotiating Contracts 549
Scenario 22-C: Unrealistic Client Expectations 550
Scenario 22-D: Discovering Sensitive Information about a Client, Competitor, or Colleague . . .552
Conclusion 555
Key Terms 556
Chapter Summary 556
Ethical Decision-Making Matrices
     -Scenario 22-A: Competing Constituencies 556
     -Scenario 22-B: Negotiating Contracts 560
     -Scenario 22-C: Unrealistic Client Expectations 562
     -Scenario 22-D: Discovering Sensitive Information about a Client, Competitor,
     or Colleague 564

Chapter 23—Vendor Management 567
       Keith Olenik, MA, RHIA, CHP
Learning Objectives 567
Abstract 567
Scenario 23-A: Vendor Request 568
Vendor Relations 568
Scenario 23-B: Vendors as Friends 570
Scenario 23-C: Gifts 570
Scenario 23-D: Preferred Vendors 572
Request for Proposals 573
Scenario 23-E: Negotiating 576
Negotiation 577
Enhancement of Vendor Relationships 579
Ethical Behavior 579
Conclusion 580
Key Terms 580
Chapter Summary 580
Appendix 23-A: Sample Gifts Policy 582
Ethical Decision-Making Matrices
    -Scenario 23-A: Vendor Request 584
    -Scenario 23-B: Vendors as Friends 586
    -Scenario 23-C: Gifts 588
    -Scenario 23-D: Preferred Vendors 590
    -Scenario 23-E: Negotiating 592

Chapter 24—Advocacy 595
       Susan Helbig, MA, RHIA
Learning Objectives 595
Abstract 595
Scenario 24-A: Violating Privacy of a Prominent Citizen 596
Advocacy: The Choice of Ethics in Action 596
Advocating for Patients 596
Scenario 24-B: Compassion in Action for an Alcoholic Peer 600
Advocating for Peers 600
Scenario 24-C: Cockroaches in the HIM Department 602
Advocating for Staff 602
Scenario 24-D: Unfair Treatment of Part-time Workers 603
Scenario 24-E: Small Print on a Consent Form 604
Advocating for the Healthcare Organization 605
Scenario 24-F: The Data Warehouse Wants to Sell Patient Information . . .606
Advocating for the Larger Community and Society 606
Advocating for One's Self 607
Conclusion 607
Key Terms 608
Chapter Summary 608
Appendix 24-A: Example of Organizational Engagement in Societal Advocacy 610
Appendix 24-B: Precepts of Effective HIM Advocacy 611
Ethical Decision-Making Matrices
    -Scenario 24-A: Violating Privacy of a Prominent Citizen 612

-Scenario 24-B: Compassion in Action for an Alcoholic Peer 614
-Scenario 24-C: Cockroaches in the HIM Department 616
-Scenario 24-D: Unfair Treatment of Part-time Workers .618
-Scenario 24-E: Small Print on a Consent Form 620
-Scenario 24-F: The Data Warehouse Wants to Sell Patient Information 622

Glossary **625**

Index **639**

Contributors

Cynthia Baur, PhD
Senior Health Communication and
    e-Health Advisor
Office of Disease Prevention and
    Health Promotion
U.S. Department of Health and
    Human Services
Rockville, Maryland

Meryl Bloomrosen, MBA, RHIA
Vice President and Program Manager
Foundation for eHealth Initiative
eHealth Initiative
Washington, D.C.

Karen Czirr, MS, RHIA, CHP
Manager, Clinical Access and Education
The Children's Hospital of Philadelphia
Philadelphia, Pennsylvania

Mary Jo Deering, PhD
Director for Informatics Dissemination
NCI Center for Bioinformatics
National Cancer Institute
National Institutes of Health, USDHHS
Rockville, Maryland

Susan H. Fenton, MBA, RHIA
Manager, Practice Leadership
American Health Information Management
    Association
Chicago, Illinois

Cathy A. Flite, MEd, RHIA
Assistant Professor, Clinicial Educator
College of Health Professions
Department of Health Information
    Management
Temple University
Philadelphia, Pennsylvania

Barbara P. Fuller, JD, RHIA
Assistant Director for Ethics
National Human Genome Research Institute
National Institutes of Health
Bethesda, Maryland

Marie Gardenier, MBA, RHIA, CHPS
President
G&A Professional Services
Wilmington, Delaware

Jacqueline J. Glover, PhD
Associate Professor
Center for Bioethics and Humanities
University of Colorado Health Sciences
    Center
Denver, Colorado

Karen Gallagher Grant, RHIA, CHP
Corporate Director
Health Information Services
Partners HealthCare System, Inc
Wellesley, Massachusetts

Mary Alice Hanken, PhD, RHIA, CHP
Consultant and Senior Lecturer
    Health Information Administration
School of Public Health and Community
    Medicine
University of Washington
Seattle, Washington

J. Michael Hardin, PhD
Professor of Statistics
Department of Information Systems,
    Statistics, and Management Science
Director of the Institute of Business
    Intelligence
Culverhouse College of Commerce and
    Business Administration
The University of Alabama
Tuscaloosa, Alabama

Laurinda B. Harman, PhD, RHIA
Associate Professor and Chair
Department of Health Information
    Management
College of Health Professions
Temple University
Philadelphia, Pennsylvania

Susan Helbig, MA, RHIA
Director, Health Information Management
VA Puget Sound Health Care System
Seattle and Tacoma, Washington

Kathy L. Hudson, PhD
Director, Genetics and Public Policy Center
Associate Professor, Berman Bioethics
    Institute
Institute of Genetic Medicine
Department of Pediatrics
Johns Hopkins University
Baltimore, Maryland

Merida L. Johns, PhD, RHIA
President
Holistic Training Solutions, LLC
Woodstock, Illinois

Martha L. Jones, PhD, LSW
Common Sense Adoption Services
Mechanicsburg, Pennsylvania

Sharon Laquer, MS, RHIA
Director of Medical Records
Temple University Hospital
Philadelphia, Pennsylvania

Frances Wickham Lee, DBA
Director of Educational Technology
Medical University of South Carolina
College of Health Professions
Charleston, South Carolina

Virginia L. Mullen, RHIA
Director, Service Quality Measurement
Centura Health
Englewood, Colorado

Gretchen Murphy, MEd, RHIA, FAHIMA
Director, Health Information Administration
    Program
School of Public Health and Community
    Medicine
University of Washington
Seattle, Washington

Babette J. Neuberger, JD, MPH
Clinical Associate Professor and
Associate Dean for Academic Affairs
University of Illinois at Chicago
School of Public Health
Chicago, Illinois

Keith Olenik, MA, RHIA, CHP
Principal
The Olenik Consulting Group
Kansas City, Missouri

Brenda S. Olson, MEd, MA, RHIA, CHP
Vice President for Health Information
    Management
Great Plains Health Alliance, Inc.
Topeka, Kansas

Sharon J. Randolph, JD, RHIA
Director, Health Information Management
Methodist Dallas Medical Center
Dallas, Texas

Karen Rosendale, MBA, RHIA
Soarian HIM Product Manager
Malvern, Pennsylvania

Laurie A. Rinehart-Thompson,
  JD, RHIA, CHP
Assistant Professor of Clinical Allied Medicine
Health Information Management & Systems
School of Allied Medical Professions
The Ohio State University
Columbus, Ohio

Ida Critelli Schick, PhD, MS, FACHE
Professor and Chair/Director
Graduate Program in Health Services
  Administration
Xavier University
Cincinnati, Ohio

Lou Ann Schraffenberger, MBA, RHIA,
  CCS, CCS-P
Manager of Clinical Data/Clinical Information
  Services
Advocate Health Care/Oak Brook Support
  Center
Oak Brook, Illinois

Rita A. Scichilone, MHSA, RHIA, CCS,
  CCS-P, CHC
Director, Professional Practice Resources
American Health Information Management
  Association
Chicago, Illinois

Patrice L. Spath, BA, RHIT
Health Care Quality Specialist
Brown-Spath & Associates
Forest Grove, Oregon

James F. Tischler, MD
Board Certified in Internal Medicine
  and Geriatrics
Chief of Staff
Coatesville VA Medical Center
Coatesville, Pennsylvania

Karen A. Wager, DBA, RHIA
Associate Professor
Department of Health Administration
  and Policy
Medical University of South Carolina
Charleston, South Carolina

Emily West, RHIA
Director, Health Information Services
HIA Doylestown Hospital
Doylestown, Pennsylvania

Andrea White, PhD
Director, Master of Health Administration
  Program
Department of Health Administration
  and Policy
College of Health Professions
Medical University of South Carolina
Charleston, South Carolina

FOREWORD

Ethical Challenges in the Management of Health Information was first published at the dawn of a new millennium. This was a time in history when top-rated television shows were featuring health professionals at work; when the race to complete the human genome was rounding its last lap and the proliferation of information technology and biotechnology demonstrated the need to control sensitive healthcare information. Six years have passed since the first publication and in that timeframe the social and ethical concerns confronting society have expanded well beyond what we could have imaged in the past. Information technology appears to be both the answer and potential problem to many ethical challenges facing society today. Concerns about patient privacy are increasing for patients, the healthcare system, and the government.

Mapping of the human genome is complete and a new project is underway—the categorization of all genes that turn healthy cells into cancer. The power of the information generated from the human genome research projects, along with the ability to analyze the DNA of individuals, has both positive and negative consequences. On the positive side, genetic information can be used to develop therapies necessary to keep an individual alive. Conversely, such information may also be used to discriminate against an individual with a known genetic trait or defect. Do we need nondiscrimination genetic information legislation to protect society?

Homeland security, terrorism, bioterrorism, natural disasters, patient safety, medication errors, and increased healthcare costs have contributed to a recent federal mandate to provide electronic health records for all Americans by 2015. One aspect of this mandate is to develop regional health information networks whereby patient information can be accessed by providers as needed. In addition, recent natural disasters such as Hurricanes Katrina and Rita have made us painfully aware how important post-disaster patient tracking systems or central patient repositories can be when needing to treat victims of such disasters. Fundamental concerns relating to how patient confidentiality can be maintained and privacy protected in electronic health record systems are currently being debated.

The societal changes taking place as a result of the above challenges continue to expand the role of health information management (HIM) professionals. The HIM professional was once the guardian or manager of mainly paper-based record systems. Today this guardianship and managerial responsibility covers both paper-based and electronic forms of health information and health information systems. Today's challenges require vigilance concerning the right and wrong uses of patient information and appropriate and inappropriate access to it from a much broader perspective. This vigilance requires the HIM professional to assume the moral responsibility not only to manage, but to protect patient-related data and information resources in whatever form it is contained and at whatever site it may be located. Thus, the HIM professional's scope of ethical responsibilities widens as the demand for healthcare information expands in whatever form it is needed.

Dr. Harman has captured the ethical challenges facing HIM and all healthcare professionals in this rapidly changing environment. She has brought together an excellent cadre of authors who provide an in-depth overview and assessment of these challenges by providing both theoretical and practical discussions of the numerous ethical and moral issues presented by an increasing demand for and use of patient information. Each chapter draws attention to unique ethical problems for integrated delivery systems, managed care, e-health, genetic information systems, quality improvement, and many others. This second edition includes four new chapters related to end-of-life issues, electronic health information management (e-HIM), vendor interactions, and management. Chapters address theories and models of ethical practice, along with detailed practice scenarios related to the practice venues. This book is unique in that there are over 70 case scenarios and an ethical decision-making matrix is provided for each. This resource can guide the practitioner and student to understand the complexity of solving ethical problems.

This second edition of *Ethical Challenges in the Management of Health Information* presents an update and new discussion of core salient topics in one place. As such, it is an excellent resource for students and practitioners alike. Practitioners and students that can be well served by this book include those in the healthcare professions, healthcare administration, public health, information technology, ethicists and, of course, health information management. This book provides standards of conduct and ethical uniformity of practice for the health information profession, thus introducing the student to the basic moral principles and values of HIM practice. For faculty, the book serves as a foundation for debate and discussion that will help weave the moral fiber of tomorrow's practitioners. For the practitioner, it offers a confirmation of the standards of conduct and ethical uniformity of practice that supports the practitioner's resolve to address ethical issues in a proactive, effective manner.

The overall practicality of the book makes it attractive not only to HIM professionals, but to all who are drawn into the professional responsibility of managing health information in a moral, ethical manner. We are fortunate that Dr. Harman and the chapter authors have provided the reader with a moral awareness and solid foundation for ethical practice in the management of health information. I have no doubt that this edition of the book, like its predecessor, will continue to be the major resource when one is confronted with ethical challenges in the management of health information.

Melanie S. Brodnik, PhD, RHIA
Director and Associate Professor
Health Information Management & Systems
The Ohio State University
Columbus, Ohio

PREFACE

Handwritten medical records and electronic health information systems contain many sacred stories—stories that must be protected on behalf of the individual patient and on behalf of the aggregate communities of patients that are served in the healthcare system.

Health information management (HIM) professionals assure the accuracy and timeliness of the information that is collected and released. The protection of privacy and confidential information is the primary ethical obligation of the HIM professional and this obligation is central to the decisions that are made on behalf of patients.

Each contributing chapter author has courageously told the truth about his or her medical records/health information system. As with all ethical situations, telling the truth is often easier said than done. The medical record is a compilation of fact (such as test results) and art through interpretation (such as progress notes and consultations). The medical record is designed to be a communication tool and inherently contains the complexities of all forms of communication. Each author has presented an honest view of the many health information ethical dilemmas that we face in today's healthcare system.

This textbook was written with several audiences in mind: students, healthcare practitioners, ethicists, and others, such as vendors, administrators, public health professionals, patients, and the society-at-large. *Ethical Challenges in the Management of Health Information, Second Edition* reflects a commitment to interdisciplinary collaboration within an ethical decision-making process.

Those who can benefit from reading and discussing the information in this textbook include:

- *Students* enrolled at the associate, baccalaureate, master's, and doctoral degree levels. These students can be enrolled in many different academic programs, including health information management or healthcare programs (physicians, nurses, therapists, public health, healthcare administrators, and the like). These students will increasingly need an understanding of ethical decision-making—particularly given the complexities they will face in their work environments.
- *HIM professionals* who work on behalf of patients to protect privacy and must quickly assess complex situations, such as volatile quality review outcomes, inappropriate requests for information, and fraud and abuse.
- The *healthcare team* who treats the patient and documents the process of the decision making, the actions taken, and the outcomes.

- *Professionals* who work on behalf of patients, such as ethicists, administrators, public, health experts, information technology specialists, and vendors.
- *Patients* since they have many things to learn about the information that is collected about them and given to others who work on their behalf.

Ethical issues do not allow the luxury of the right answer based exclusively on laws, standards, or rules. Ethical criteria need to be added to the list of common healthcare criteria, such as cost, regulation, policy, and the technical feasibility. This textbook describes current ethical issues based on the availability of detailed health/medical information and includes more than 70 case scenarios and a decision-making matrix for each case. Case scenarios provide readers with an opportunity to evaluate and resolve problems based on an understanding of values, obligations, and multidisciplinary perspectives. The matrix facilitates a more expansive view of the problem and the options for an ethical decision.

Ethical Challenges in the Management of Health Information, Second Edition is divided into five parts. **Part I, Professional Ethics,** explores professional values and obligations as guided by the American Health Information Management Association (AHIMA) ethical codes. This section presents ethical decision-making guidelines and tools to be used when faced with an ethical problem. The primary ethical obligation of protecting privacy and confidentiality is explored, including an assessment of the Health Insurance Portability and Accountability Act of 1996 (HIPAA). **Part II, Uses of Health Information,** focuses on the uses of health information for coding, quality review, research and decision support, public health, managed care, and end-of-life clinical decisions. **Part III, Computerized Health Information,** explores the dilemmas created by the electronic health record, information security, software development and implementation, data resource management, integrated delivery systems, and the emerging e-HIM and e-Health systems. **Part IV, Management of Sensitive Health Information,** addresses the issues dealing with the protection of sensitive information including genetic, adoption, drug, alcohol, sexual, and mental health information. **Part V, Roles,** concludes with a review of ethical issues for managers, entrepreneurs, advocates, and those working with vendors.

PROCESS AND STRATEGIES FOR FACULTY, STUDENTS, PRACTITIONERS, AND ADMINISTRATORS

Jacqueline Glover's Chapter 2, *Ethical Decision-Making Guidelines and Tools,* includes an ethical decision-making process, which is presented in the following matrix. All scenarios in this book have been analyzed using this matrix. The matrix is a tool to help organize complex, ethical problems; however, there is no simple fill-in-the-box approach to ethical decision-making. The objective is to follow each step and not move from the question directly to what should be done or how to prevent it next time. If steps are skipped, someone will not fully understand all the values and options for action. Also, the matrices provided in this book are not the only way to examine the problem. An individual or team can make an equally compelling ethical argument for a different decision, as long as all the steps of the matrix are followed.

PROCESS AND STRAGEGY: ETHICAL DECISION-MAKING MATRIX

Steps	Information	
1. What is the ethical question?	QUESTIONS	
2. What are the facts?	KNOWN	TO BE GATHERED
3. What are the values? Examine the shared and competing values, obligations, and interests of the stakeholders (i.e., patient, HIM professional, health-care practitioner(s), administrators, society, and other advocates) involved in order to fully understand the complexity of the ethical problem(s).	STAKEHOLDERS/ADVOCATES Patient, HIM professional, health care practitioner(s), administrators, society and other advocates, appropriate to the issue	OBLIGATIONS/INTERESTS
4. What are my options?	OPTIONS	
5. What should I do?	CORE VALUES	
6. What justifies my choice?	JUSTIFIED	NOT JUSTIFIED
7. How can I prevent this ethical problem?	PREVENTION OPTIONS	

If you are teacher, student, or practitioner, you might ask, "How can I use this book?"

There are three primary ways to use this book; however, teachers and students should feel free to experiment with the analysis of the information and the decision-making matrices as they explore the issues that they are examining.

- Utilize the textbook across the curriculum: the students can use this book in conjunction with all of the courses in the curriculum. Students can be taught the content expertise, such as quality management, coding, the electronic health record, and the other chapter themes in various courses and then discuss the ethical implications of the decisions that must be made. Ethical decision-making can be interwoven in all courses. Students can use this book throughout the academic program and can then keep it as a primary resource as a practitioner.
- Adopt it as a textbook in an existing multidisciplinary ethics course. Many programs already have an ethics course that is taken by students from many disciplines, such as health professions (medicine, nursing, physical therapy, occupational therapy, et. al), religion or ethics programs, public health, computer science, or other disciplines based on the academic programs offered in your institution. These courses deal with clinical ethical

issues, such as "start or stop the treatment, put the patient into the research protocol, or use an experimental drug or procedure?" The adoption of this textbook in these existing courses will allow all students and practitioners who will work within the healthcare system (in both direct and nondirect patient care areas) to be fluent in relevant HIM ethical issues.

- Develop an ethics course for the professional discipline—health information management, healthcare professional, ethics, information technology, healthcare administration, public health, and the like. This allows the student to explore the ethical decision-making process within the context of what they have already learned. This option allows protected time and a focus so that they can fine-tune their ethical decision-making skills, within the context of the healthcare system.

What teaching and evaluation methodologies can be used?

Ethical decision-making cannot be taught or evaluated through multiple-choice examinations or some other exclusively objective mechanism. Knowledge of the definitions in the glossary or some of the lists and steps discussed in the chapters can be evaluated using an objective format but this cannot be the only methodology used to assess ethical decision-making skills.

Small group discussions: Ethical decisions must be analyzed and discussed through qualitative analysis, discussion, and critical thinking documentation. Most ethics classes combine lecture/didactic with small group discussions. If this methodology is used, review the background from the chapter during the lecture and then organize small groups so that they can discuss the issues.

If there are students from multiple academic programs, mix the students up into the various groups so that multiple perspectives (personal and professional) can be heard. Understanding the diversity of obligations and values is essential in the decision-making process. If it is a multidisciplinary course, several faculty members can be used to lead the small group discussions. Also, reach out to alumni and other practitioners in the area to lead these small group discussions. The teacher needs to hear the discussions so that the students can get reinforcement of their use of ethical tools and principles.

Small group or homework assignments: Have the students create the decision-making matrices, making equally compelling counterarguments or a decision that is different than what is presented in the chapter. For example, if the matrix indicates that information should be released, have the students make a counterargument for not releasing the information.

Does the language "make compelling ethical arguments or counterarguments" mean that the people in the small group might end up shouting at each other?

No. When ethicists use the term "argument and counterargument" they want us to be clear about the issue and what facts we know and need to find out. Then identify criteria that we want to use when making the decision (autonomy, beneficence, nonmaleficence, justice, cost, technological feasibility, legal, or accreditation standards) or the like. Then present the case. Those involved in the discussion should be taught to make an argument (complete the matrix) and see if they can convince others. Then they can make the counterargument using the same criteria. The discussion should help the participants to understand what factors might contribute to the intensity with which a particular perspective may be held as more worthwhile than simply turning up the volume. Shouting to make these arguments is not an option and should never be allowed.

I am a practitioner and I want to make ethical decisions, how can I use this textbook?

This textbook can be used as a resource for grand rounds, patient care advocacy groups, small group discussions, book clubs, continuing education, and professional development programs. There can be more than one ethical decision for each case. If an individual or a group can only identify one value or one option for the decision, the analysis of the problem is not complete. Most likely this outcome indicates that the decision-maker is focused on the moral response (this is right, that is wrong) versus the ethical perspective that facilitates an understanding of the values and obligations of all those involved in the case.

SUMMARY

The management of health information increasingly requires decisions that cannot be made by merely applying rules, regulations, or accreditation standards. Regardless of the many roles that support patient care, ethical decisions must be made. The many roles include, but are not limited to, educators, health information managers, healthcare practitioners, information technology experts, vendors and entrepreneurs, ethicists, public health officials, healthcare administrators, and many others. This book is written for students and practitioners who serve patients, employers, the community, and the society-at-large.

Students and practitioners, at all levels of academic preparation, should consistently expand ethical decision-making skills. Understanding the language and tools of ethics, the values embedded in the various professions, and applying knowledge in support of ethical decisions is a rewarding endeavor. Students and practitioners can move from a narrow perspective of what is "right or wrong" to one that is based on an understanding of the ethical decision-making process. If someone learns the language and how to use the decision-making tool, the identification and defense of multiple perspectives and options for ethical decision-making is possible. Decisions can then be made which address the multidisciplinary perspectives of the teams who serve the needs of patients.

Ethical Challenges in the Management of Health Information, Second Edition honors the voice of moral agency for those learning about and working within the healthcare delivery system. These individuals cannot approach the complexities of the electronic health information systems without a solid framework for ethical decision-making. All who work, either directly or indirectly, within the healthcare system must utilize and combine their technical, professional, and ethical expertise.

This book should generate many energized discussions. Ethical decision-making always requires courage. Learn to celebrate the joy and power of courage.

Laurinda Beebe Harman

ACKNOWLEDGMENTS

Two courageous, compassionate, and intelligent teachers guided my learning about health information management and ethics. Louise Huttsell taught me to be passionate about medical records—to always remember the sacredness of the stories I was reading and to be competent and diligent when analyzing, presenting, or releasing health information. Jackie Glover taught me the importance of ethics in my personal and professional life. She is my friend and is always ready to be my mentor. This book could not have been written without her guidance.

I had the opportunity to work with excellent authors who had the courage to describe the ethical issues for their area of expertise. I was honored to work with these authors and thank them for their scholarly and innovative contributions.

In addition to my parents and sisters, I couldn't sustain life without the support of my brother-in-law, Francis Joseph Welk, and my nephews and their partners, Paul Joseph and Courtney, John David and Karen and my Godson, Jeffrey Scott Welk.

Melanie Brodnik and I have been friends and colleagues for many years and she always offers calm and expert advice. I trust the pearls of wisdom of Barbara Fuller and I truly enjoy the sound of her laughter. Sandy Bailey helped me focus on the importance of "telling the truth about medical records". Anita Kristina and Lea Jensen feed my body and my soul. Ann Marie Kiehne is my neighbor, colleague, swim partner, and Galaxy's Godmother. Charlie Seashore is my Mentori and continues to remind me to "think purple!".

The health information management faculty at Temple University—Margaret Foley, Cathy Flite, Lisa Morton, and Karen McBride—and my physical therapy colleagues, Mary Barbe and Ann Barr, all helped me to balance the competing interests of work and play.

Mike Brown, my publisher, was infinitely patient with my questions and suggestions for changes for this second edition.

I want to especially thank Gilbert Lee Hoffer. We share the values of gratitude for the gifts of life, the importance of joy and celebration with family and friends, and most importantly, laughter and love.

PROFESSIONAL ETHICS

Part I covers the importance of ethics and professional expertise in the management of health information. Chapter 1 identifies professional values and obligations of the health information management (HIM) professional by reviewing previous and current HIM Codes of Ethics. Chapter 2 describes ethical theories, principles, and tools that are important when making ethical decisions. This chapter also includes a framework for the ethical decision-making process. Chapter 3 discusses the primary ethical obligation of protecting patient privacy and confidentiality in an era of increasing demands for access to health information.

PROFESSIONAL VALUES AND THE CODE OF ETHICS

Laurinda B. Harman, PhD, RHIA
Virginia L. Mullen, RHIA

Learning Objectives

After completing this chapter, the reader should be able to:

- Describe current ethical dilemmas faced by health information management (HIM) professionals.
- Understand HIM-related ethical dilemmas for those who work on behalf of patients, such as healthcare providers, vendors, information technology experts, researchers, and public health or managed care professionals.
- Identify changes in the healthcare system that have resulted in ethical information management problems.
- Understand the role, values, and ethical obligations of the HIM professional.
- Work toward building an ethical health information system.
- Appreciate the importance of the intersection of HIM and ethical expertise.

Abstract

This chapter describes the importance of ethics for the health information management (HIM) professional, given the complexity of today's healthcare environment. It briefly explores the "then and now" realities of health information systems, which have both manual and electronic components.

Based on a review of several HIM professional codes of ethics, the chapter presents professional values and obligations to the patient, the healthcare team, the employer, the public interest, the peer HIM professional, and the professional associations. A framework for building an ethical health information system is presented. The summary includes a discussion of the importance of the intersection of HIM technical and ethical expertise.

ETHICAL DILEMMAS FOR THE HIM PROFESSIONAL

The current healthcare environment creates many ethical perplexities and ethical decision making does require courage. The environment is complex, constantly changing, and involves many people who have competing interests and values. The busy professional must be able to quickly, yet carefully, assess complex situations. Following are just a few of the types of situations a **health information management (HIM) professional** may encounter:

- The number of delinquent medical records far exceeds the percentage allowed by accreditation standards. The chief executive officer (CEO) has made it very clear that the reported number should not exceed the allowed delinquency rate, and that the continued employment status of the HIM professional is linked with the reported data. How many delinquent records should be reported for the survey? If the actual number is reported, is the HIM professional at risk of unemployment?

- The documentation in the medical record does not support what has been billed. Evidence suggests that the documentation was done retrospectively and is of questionable accuracy. Should the HIM professional allow these practices to continue?

- The physician allows a signature stamp to be used by nurses and others to complete medical records, which is in clear violation of the medical staff rules and regulations. However, timely completion helps with the billing process, and the HIM professional is told to "look the other way." What should the HIM professional do?

- A surgeon begins the dictation of an operative report with "Please type the date of dictation to be the same as the date of the surgery." The surgeon makes this request to ensure compliance with accreditation standards and hospital policy;

however, the report was dictated one week after the operation. Does the transcriptionist tell the truth, typing the actual date of dictation, or does the transcriptionist comply with the surgeon's request? The transcriptionist knows that the surgeon could become extremely angry and create an uncomfortable conflict situation if the correct date of the dictation is included. Would the chief of surgery support truthful documentation or allow the surgeon to insist on an inaccurate dictation date? Would the medical director or the director of the HIM department support the transcriptionist if the true date were typed? Would the CEO support the director? What should be done if the transcription is being outsourced to another country and the surgeon's requests are always followed, regardless of the appropriateness of the request?

- A request for proposal (RFP) will be sent to several vendors in a few months. One of the vendors who will be submitting a proposal offers a gift, such as equipment or resources that are desperately needed by the department and a trip to the corporate headquarters for the HIM director. Is this a conflict of interest? Should the trip and/or gifts be accepted? Will gifts influence the HIM director's decision?

- The insurance company requests patient information that relates to the removal of an appendix. The patient's medical record contains sensitive information related to a psychiatric disorder and alcohol abuse. Should the patient be contacted before the records are released? What happens if the insurance company threatens not to pay the claim if the information is not released? What are the implications of releasing the records, given the Health Insurance Portability and Accountability Act (HIPAA)?

- When reviewing documentation for completeness, the medical record analyst notes that some of the progress notes were written after a problem occurred.

The added progress notes were written as if crucial laboratory information was available, when in fact the physician failed to review the laboratory data during the course of the hospitalization. The analyst knows that these progress notes were written "after the fact," because the patient had been transferred to the intensive care unit, and different identification data are recorded on the subsequent sheets in the medical record. Should the physician be confronted with the discrepancy? Should risk management or legal counsel be contacted?

- Rules for signatures on verbal orders indicate a specific time frame. Repeatedly and consistently, these orders are signed after the designated time limit. HIM professionals are forced to pretend that the orders were signed on time. Should this collusion to hide inaccurate documentation continue? Are other options available?
- A patient's genetic information is released in response to a valid request. The information is then used to discriminate against the patient with regards to employment and health insurance. What is the role of the HIM professional in protecting patient information beyond the primary release? What are the obligations for the redisclosure of private information?
- Dictated histories, physicals, and discharge summaries are being outsourced through telecommunication to a foreign country for transcription. What can be done to ensure technical and language competencies? How will patient privacy be protected?
- A hospital outsources the transcription of medical reports to one vendor who, in turn, contracts with another vendor, who, in turn, contracts with an agency overseas. The hospital finds out about these transactions when an employee from the foreign country calls and says, "I won't release your reports until I get a raise." What should be done?

- A principal investigator (PI) of a major research project is also a practicing physician. This researcher has gained access to clinical patient information that is not part of the research study and wants to place research outcomes in a clinical database. The patients are not being contacted for their authorization in either of these instances. What should be done?
- New software has not been fully tested and is not reliable, yet the chief information officer (CIO) is demanding implementation of the new system. What should be done? Who should be involved in resolving this conflict?
- Negative or unpopular quality-audit outcomes are politically, clinically, and administratively unwanted, and it has been made clear that the job of the HIM professional is in jeopardy if the true outcomes are disclosed. Who can the HIM professional contact?
- A HIM student at a small facility observes the following: Incomplete medical records were placed in a rental truck in the parking lot during an accreditation survey; discharge analysts have a physician stamp for every physician on staff; and a board of trustees member called, asked for, and was given patient information about a local politician. What should the student do?

THE HEALTH INFORMATION SYSTEM: THEN AND NOW

In settings from acute to long-term care, a patient's medical record, whether computerized or handwritten, is the primary communication tool for the healthcare team. Documentation in the record allows those taking care of patients to review what they or others have done or are thinking about doing on behalf of a patient. As a communication tool, it is both a science involving facts (test results or vital signs) and an art involving interpretation and the application of a professional perspective (progress notes or consultations).

The health information system supports the needs of patients, healthcare professionals, administrators, the community, and those involved in research and education. The HIM professional is responsible for the system that supports this communication process. The trust that the healthcare team and the public places in the HIM professional requires careful consideration of both technical and ethical expertise.

Health information systems are in transition. Some consist of handwritten notes; some are designed as highly sophisticated electronic health record (EHR) systems. Most have both handwritten and electronic components. An overview of the health information system—past and present—will help to frame some of the ethical issues faced by HIM professionals today. This section includes historical discussions of the U.S. healthcare system, documentation practices, access and security, coding and reimbursement, and the use of technology.

The Healthcare System

Just a few decades ago, health care was rendered almost exclusively in hospitals, physicians' offices, or nursing homes. Separate medical records were compiled over the span of a patient's life, from birth to death, and were maintained in many locations—physicians' offices, hospitals, ambulatory clinics, and emergency departments. However, these records were not linked in any way. A patient could not be guaranteed that important information would be available from the ambulatory setting when admitted to the hospital in the same community, or vice versa, if care was rendered in a different geographical location.

Also, in the not too distant past, physicians made house calls and lawsuits were extremely rare. Patients were admitted to the hospital even if they were not necessarily ill. A physician could admit a patient for an annual physical examination or other diagnostic workup, such as a series of radiological examinations. A stay in the hospital was routinely several days in length, regardless of the problem.

Today, care is rendered increasingly in nonacute settings, such as psychiatric, substance abuse, and physical rehabilitation units; long-term care facilities; and ambulatory settings, such as urgent care centers, ambulatory surgery centers, and patients' homes. Many patients admitted to the hospital are extremely ill, and the length of stay is carefully monitored by both hospitals and insurance companies involved. Patients increasingly pursue litigation against providers of care, healthcare facilities, and vendors who provide products and services.

Healthcare Documentation

Although the primary purpose of healthcare documentation is patient care, this information is also used for the following purposes (Cofer, 1994):

- Review of the appropriateness, adequacy, and quality of care
- Financial reimbursement for the care provided
- Legal protection for patients, providers of care, and healthcare facilities
- Education of healthcare professionals
- Research
- Public health monitoring
- Planning and marketing of healthcare services

Core health information management issues include what information should be collected, how it should be stored, who should have access to it and under what conditions, and how and why it should be disseminated to others. The protection of patient privacy is central to all of these decisions.

Today, the health information system can be a computerized, interactive, and dynamic documentation and retrieval process that supports patient care and maximizes revenues. Documentation processes must capture the decisions that are made in a timely and efficient manner. Retrospective documentation is viewed as a failure of the system. The quality of the information is key to providing quality health care. Such information also supports strategic planning, marketing, and staffing functions. It also aids in the evaluation of healthcare services.

Access to and Release of Information

In the past, all medical records were handwritten and considered a repository of information. They were rarely accessed by anyone, except for follow-up care. For patients admitted to the hospital, the discharge summary and final diagnoses could be finished several weeks or months after discharge, and the completed record was often put into a "permanent file" in a basement or some other remote storage area and rarely seen again.

The security of medical records in the early years was facilitated by the physical location of the medical records department, which was often in the basement. This location was due to two primary factors: the weight of the records and the live-load limits on higher floors. Another inadvertent security feature was that an individual's medical record could only be accessed by one person at a time, given that it was a paper document.

Patients rarely, if ever, looked at their medical records. In fact, most were unaware of the extent of the documentation that was collected on their behalf. If a patient wanted to review his or her own medical record, the physician authorized the review, and it was done in the presence of the credentialed medical record professional or other healthcare professional.

The criterion for the release of information from a patient's medical record was "need to know." On the basis of a release-of-information request, the medical record was abstracted by a credentialed medical record professional. If surgery had been performed, the HIM professional reviewed the medical record and confirmed the diagnosis, the procedure, and the admission and discharge dates. Insurance companies were given enough information so that they could legitimately pay the bill, but information was never given beyond what was needed or appropriate.

Technological advances introduced duplicating equipment into the release-of-information process—an innovation that radically changed the need-to-know criterion for releasing information. Instead of requiring the credentialed HIM professional to review and abstract a medical record and give the requester what is wanted and appropriate, most healthcare organizations now copy the entire record. It has become routine professional practice to copy the history and physical, discharge summary, operative report, laboratory results, and other documentation. The history and physical includes family and social information (behaviors, risk factors, genetic conditions) that may have nothing to do with the surgery performed or care rendered and may be used in discriminatory ways in employment and insurance. Insurance companies and other requesters now get detailed clinical information that is beyond the need-to-know criterion. That is, they often receive not only information to process a claim, but also additional information that can violate patient privacy.

It is doubtful that anyone envisioned the technological advances that would occur and what would be our reality today with regard to the access of clinical information. The amount of information that is being collected, the number of requesters, and the amount and types of information that are being released all challenge the HIM professional's ability to protect patient privacy. Patients are often unaware that their personal medical information has been released. HIM professionals must serve many different requesters who seek access to health information, and they must constantly balance patients' privacy rights and confidentiality with demands for access. To fulfill their work responsibilities, HIM professionals must demonstrate "behavior that reflects integrity, supports objectivity, and fosters trust in professional activities" (Huffman, 1972, p. 126). See Chapter 3 on privacy and confidentiality to learn more about access to information based on HIPAA legislation.

Today, many stakeholders seek information about patients, and the HIM system is the information hub of the healthcare system. The validity and quality of the health information are under scrutiny by government and insurance agencies. Informed consumers access the Internet for diagnoses, pharmaceutical information, surgical options, and other information that will facilitate their healthcare decision making. Patients place value on the information compiled in their medical records and on their privacy. They routinely get copies of their clinical documentation.

Coding and Reimbursement

In the past, coding of diagnoses, procedures, and providers of care was done primarily for clinical research purposes. Reimbursement was based on the actual cost of care, and there were limited consequences for overspending. Reimbursement was almost exclusively based on fee for service, and hospitals and physicians were reimbursed for what they said it cost them to provide the care; that is, for the usual, customary, and reasonable costs.

Today, coded diagnoses are used as a basis for financial reimbursement, and there is pressure on HIM departments to have coding completed at or within a few days of discharge. Reimbursement is based on the patient's illness and or procedure, his or her co-morbid conditions and other situations that occur during the patient's stay, and on the resources used, not the characteristics of the hospital or the medical staff. The healthcare system consists of a myriad of financing mechanisms, provider types, fee schedules, and reimbursement methodologies. Healthcare funding and reimbursement methodologies are major items on the health policy agenda. The government is also focused on preventing and detecting fraud and abuse. An issue of huge importance is the funding of care for the uninsured, those with high-cost diagnoses, and those with long-term disabilities or chronic conditions—all in the context of diminishing funds for health care (Shi & Singh, 2004).

Technology

For many years, the most advanced "technology" was duplicating machines and microfilm. Today, the HIM system must facilitate simultaneous, multiple access to information for clinical and administrative purposes. Most health information systems have at least some computerization. Although some health information is still handwritten, paper documentation is no longer the primary means of communication. One downside of the reliance on computerized systems is that information can be disseminated directly to some requesters through redisclosure without review by a HIM professional, which would ensure compliance with privacy and confidentiality mandates.

ROLE OF THE HIM PROFESSIONAL

Several characteristics are common to all professionals (Spinello, 1997). First, **professionals** undergo extensive and specific training to master a complex body of knowledge and must have the ability to apply that knowledge. In this respect, HIM professionals are similar to primary and secondary school teachers, occupational and physical therapists, and health services administrators.

Another common characteristic of professionals is the importance of the contribution that they make to society through the services they provide. The value of these services is frequently recognized through licensing, registration, or certification requirements that prohibit entry into the profession unless certain qualifications are met. The services provided by HIM professionals with regard to information stewardship, access oversight, and the maintenance of the security and confidentiality of information are meaningful contributions to society at large and are recognized through a national certification process.

Autonomy over judgment in the work environment is another common characteristic of professionals. Because of their expertise, the opinions and judgments of professionals are highly sought after. Professionals, by their designation, are allowed a significant amount of autonomy in making decisions and exercising judgment.

The HIM profession emerged in the late 1920s when the American College of Surgeons required the review of medical records generated by those seeking admittance to the organization. At that time, medical records were inadequate and could not support the initiatives for standardization and residency approval. The Clinical Congress of the American College of Surgeons devoted their entire session in 1928 to the medical record and invited medical record workers from the United States and Canada to attend the conference. Grace Whiting Myers, librarian emeritus of Massachusetts General Hospital, organized the activities for the conference and was appointed as the first president of the Association of Record Librarians of North America (Huffman, 1963).

Since the early decades of the twentieth century, the medical record professional has been considered the "custodian" and protector of both the physical medical record and the information contained in it. HIM professionals are responsible for designing and maintaining the systems that facilitate the collection, use, and dissemination of health and medical information. They have expertise in the complexity of the healthcare delivery system; clinical medicine; information technology, the electronic health record, and database management; clinical vocabularies, coding and classification systems; policies, rules, and regulations of multiple healthcare delivery sites; quality, financial, and human resource management; and the legal aspects of health information systems, including the laws and regulations governing the release of health information to healthcare providers, researchers, educators, third-party payers, and regulatory and accrediting agencies (American Health Information Management Association [AHIMA], 2000; LaTour & Eichenwald, 2002; Abdelhak, Grostick, Hanken, & Jacobs, 2001).

Technical expertise, though necessary, is an insufficient framework for the complex dilemmas faced by HIM professionals today, which include fraud and abuse, employment and insurance discrimination, and invasions of patient privacy. It is imperative that HIM professionals also understand the ethical principles that must guide their actions.

PROFESSIONAL CODES OF ETHICS

Most professions are regulated by a set of behavioral standards commonly called a code of ethics or *code of conduct*. The HIM profession had its beginnings in 1928 when the American College of Surgeons recognized the importance of quality documentation and the need for professionals to manage these records. As early as 1934, the recently formed American Association of Medical Record Librarians (AAMRL) recorded a pledge that defined a code of conduct. The first official code of ethics was passed in 1957 by the AAMRL House of Delegates. Several revisions to the codes have been approved over the years; five of these codes are included in the appendix so that you can see the changes in language over the years [see Appendixes 1-A (1957), 1-B (1977), 1-C (1988), 1-D (1998), and 1-E (2004)].

Since the profession's inception, HIM professionals have had a clear, definitive ethical obligation to protect patient privacy and have always been a strong ethical voice for the correct course of action as they have assigned the correct diagnostic and procedural codes based on the care that was rendered, released information on behalf of patients, and reliably and accurately reported data secured from the information system. The HIM professional cannot function in today's work environment without a clear understanding of ethical principles within the decision-making context.

The responsibility to protect privacy was clearly defined in the 1934 Pledge of the AAMRL. This pledge was written and read by Grace Whiting Myers at the first annual professional association meeting in Boston:

> I pledge myself to give out no information from any clinical record placed in my charge, or from any other source to any person whatsoever, except upon order from the chief executive officer of the institution which I may be serving. (Huffman, 1972, p.135)

This is a clear obligation: Give nothing to anyone except as authorized. The pledge was expanded in 1935 when the association's emblem was approved, and some statements were added to reinforce the importance of ethical conduct. The amended 1935 pledge incorporated the following standards for conduct (Huffman, 1972, p.136).

> RECOGNIZING that the AMERICAN ASSOCIATION OF MEDICAL RECORD LIBRARIANS seeks to develop and enforce the highest standards of work among its members, I hereby pledge myself, as a condition of membership, to conduct myself in accordance with all its principles and regulations.
>
> IN PARTICULAR, I pledge myself to pursue the practice of my profession in a spirit of unselfishness, and of loyalty to the Association and to the institution which I am called to serve; to bear always in mind a keen realization of my responsibility; to seek constantly a wider knowledge of my profession through serious study, through instruction by competent approved teachers, throughout interchange of opinion among associates, and by attendance at meetings of this and of allied associations; to regard scrupulously the interests and rights

> of my fellow-members, and to seek counsel among them when in doubt of my own judgment.
>
> MOREOVER, I pledge myself to give out no information concerning a patient from any clinical record placed in my charge, or from any other source, to any person whatsoever, except upon order from the chief executive officer of the institution which I may be serving; and to avoid all commercialization of my work.
>
> FINALLY, I pledge myself to cooperate in advancing and extending by every lawful means within my power, the influence of the AMERICAN ASSOCIATION OF MEDICAL RECORD LIBRARIANS.

Source: Pledge reprinted courtesy of American Health Information Management Association, Chicago, Illinois.

PROFESSIONAL VALUES

The American Health Information Management Association (AHIMA) Code of Ethics (AHIMA, 2004), hereafter referred to as the Code, incorporates values, principles, and professional standards that acknowledge the importance of the many parties that are served by the HIM professional: patients and the healthcare team, the public interest, the employer, the professional association, and the individual HIM professional. These values should be revisited often and used when the HIM professional is confronted with difficult ethical choices. How can the values embedded in the Code assist in decision making? A review and comparative analysis of the 1957, 1977, 1988, and 1998 Codes reflect many core values important to the profession (Harman, 2000). The language of the Code has changed somewhat over the years to reflect changes in the healthcare system and the societal vernacular; however, the values and ethical principles of the profession have been embedded in all of the Codes.

Patients and the Healthcare Team

Regardless of the employment site (e.g., acute care hospital, long-term care facility, physician's office, research organization, government agency, law firm, pharmaceutical company, vendor, etc.), the patient must be the focus of the services provided. The HIM professional has the primary responsibility to protect the patient's privacy and confidential information. The values, as identified in the Code over the years, that support this ethical imperative are as follows:

- **Provide service.** The primary role of the HIM professional is to provide service to others with regard to clinical information. Core values include placing service and the honor of the profession before personal advantage and the health and welfare of patients before personal and financial interests. Those served include patients, providers of care, administrators, researchers, insurers and government agencies, vendors, and others who have a legitimate need to access information from the clinical information system. In the early years of the profession, the patient was almost exclusively the focus of the decisions made. Now, of course, many stakeholders have an interest in accessing information, and the competing interests can be in direct conflict with the protection of privacy. In today's work environment, these requesters must be considered, but the HIM professional cannot abdicate the core responsibilities of protecting the patient's privacy and providing service.
- **Protect medical and social information.** It is increasingly apparent that the health information system contains not only health and medical information, but also social information that requires special attention. An individual may not want an employer to know that he or she had a cholecystectomy; however, that information would pale in comparison to some of the social and family history information on such topics as smoking, drinking, hobbies, genetic conditions, or health of family members. Over the years, society has discriminated against those with AIDS, psychiatric diagnoses, genetic risks, and other conditions that have a social component. Protection of social and risk-factor information, including genetic information, requires constant diligence.
- **Promote confidentiality.** The responsibility to protect confidential information includes teaching others about this core principle. It is not sufficient for HIM professionals to value confidentiality. The responsibility transcends personal commitment and requires that others, including the healthcare team and the many stakeholders who gain access to patient information, fully understand "right and wrong" in this arena.
- **Preserve and secure health information.** Privileged health information that is accessed in the capacity of work must be held in absolute confidence. As medical records began to be automated and computerized, it became clear that the protection and preservation of such records had to include electronic security measures. As a result of new technology, there are numerous databases and detailed secondary records and registries that must also be protected.
- **Promote the quality and advancement of health care.** Education of the HIM professional has always included clinical medicine, pharmacology, biostatistics, and quality-improvement methodologies. HIM professionals must be able to read and interpret all clinical information and work with all members of the healthcare team to constantly improve the healthcare system. HIM professionals must support research that will improve quality of care.
- **Report data with integrity and accuracy.** This is extremely important for HIM professionals. Although they cannot

conceal unethical practice and they must report unethical behavior on the part of others, HIM professionals cannot assume the right to make determinations in professional areas outside the scope of HIM practice. The reporting of potential clinical wrongdoing rests with clinical personnel. Such personnel are better able to judge the quality or appropriateness of the care or services rendered. The HIM professional's responsibility is to provide accurate data for review and investigation.

- **Peer review or quality assurance outcomes may result in action against an individual or group, but the HIM professional's responsibility is not to make the clinical judgment but rather to honestly and reliably report the facts and the outcomes of the studies.** The HIM professional is responsible for reporting the data until action is taken consistent with the research or study outcomes. If a physician is found to be incompetent through audit results (documentation of drug abuse, repeated missed diagnoses or misinterpretation of test results, or other similar outcomes), the data must be reported accurately and with integrity. If the information is ignored, the HIM professional should continue to report the findings, sometimes again and again. This responsibility requires engaging core values of truth telling and courage.

- **Promote interdisciplinary cooperation and collaboration.** The HIM professional works with all members of the healthcare and administrative teams. The HIM professional respects and understands the responsibilities of these individuals and facilitates collaboration that will improve care and services that are rendered. This responsibility includes respecting the dignity of all individuals.

Employer

Today, HIM professionals work in various settings in and outside traditional heathcare en-

vironments. The Code's language assures that the HIM professional's values related to an employer help to keep our upstanding professional reputation. Some issues include:

- **Demonstrate loyalty to the employer.** Demonstrating loyalty to the employer by honorably discharging duties and responsibilities is another essential behavior. If it becomes necessary to leave an employer, this responsibility includes giving notice of the impending resignation. HIM professionals change jobs for various and sundry reasons; however, the professional's ethical duty includes telling the employer in advance of the transition. It is unethical to abandon a job given the responsibilities to the many people who depend on the HIM professional. This is more important today than ever, given the mobility of our society and the shortage of HIM professionals.

- **Protect committee deliberations.** Professional medical staff and health service committees are the mechanism by which the problems related to patient care, organizational policies, procedures, and risks are discussed and resolved. Results of these deliberations must be kept as private as a patient's clinical information.

- **Comply with laws, regulations, and policies.** The HIM professional must know and comply with all of the laws, rules, regulations, and other standards that affect the health information system, including state and federal laws, accrediting and licensing standards, and employer policies and procedures. Compliance is a necessary but insufficient guideline for ethical behavior. An action can be legal but not ethical. For example, a small-employer group could ask for a printout of pharmaceutical costs. Although no patient names would be revealed, the employer might be able to quickly determine who has AIDS or cancer or some other major disease. Legally, the employer may be entitled to this information. Ethically, however, this action could violate patient privacy. If the laws, regulations, and policies are not in the best interests of the patients, the HIM professional should become an advocate for changing them.

- **Recognize the authority and power of the HIM position.** Both the authority and the power to protect and secure health information are given to HIM professionals. They must act to prevent inappropriate access to health information that would be detrimental to patients and others. This authority and power must be taken very seriously, and the entrusted duties and responsibilities require conscientious attention.

- **Accept compensation only in relationship to responsibilities.** Monetary compensation in the workplace should be what is customary and lawful for the services rendered. The HIM professional should consider this ethical tenet when confronted with an invitation for unlawful compensation. Some people or organizations may want access to information collected about a patient, a physician, or other healthcare provider. They may even be willing to pay for that information; it would surely be unethical behavior for the HIM professional to receive money in exchange for such information.

Public Interest

HIM professionals must act in the public's best interest. Oftentimes, the public does not know that HIM professionals are on their team, but these professionals must constantly work on the public's behalf. Issues related to the public include the following:

- **Advocate for change.** Today's HIM professional must lead initiatives to change laws, rules, and regulations that do not protect patient privacy and confidentiality. For example, there are rules about time constraints for signing verbal orders. HIM professionals are held accountable for meeting these regulations; however, not every order is signed within the designated time constraint. Those that continue to pursue signatures beyond the specified time are colluding with others to pretend that the orders were signed on time. If the regulation is consistently violated, the HIM professional should either participate in trying to get the rule changed or honestly identify those cases outside the rule. To consistently lie and pretend are not ethical behaviors and could ultimately harm the personal integrity of the practitioner. Advocacy includes actions to protect patients, the healthcare team, the organization, the professional association, peers, and oneself (see Chapter 24 for more information on advocacy).

- **Refuse to participate in or to conceal unethical practices.** The sacred stories involving patients and those who provided the care are embedded in a health information system—the decisions that helped, the decisions that harmed, random consequences, and acts of nature. HIM professionals, given their responsibility to review the documentation for accuracy and completeness, are held accountable to notice the trends and potential problems in relationship to a care provider, a diagnosis, a procedure, or any other similar categorization. HIM professionals must behave in an ethical manner and do what is right, not what is easy; certainly they must not do anything that would harm another. They cannot conceal the illegal, incompetent, or unethical behaviors of individuals or organizations. The Code requires both personal and institutional responsibilities.

- **Report violations of practice standards to the proper authorities.** Once a violation of practice standards has been identified (through quality-assurance audits or other data-collection process), the results must be reported—but only to the proper authorities. Violations can include those related to external standards, employer policies and procedures, or professional practice standards. For example, quality assurance or other audit results may indicate that an individual physician, institution, insurer, or other agency is doing something inappropriate, such as discriminating against employees due to clinical information. The HIM professional's responsibility includes bringing the potential or actual problem to the attention of those responsible for the delivery and assessment of care and services.

Professional Associations and Peers

Another important constituent for any HIM professional is the professional organization—AHIMA. The HIM professional should do the following:

- **Be honest.** Truth and accuracy are core ethical principles. HIM professionals must always be truthful in reporting their credentials, degrees, certifications, and work experiences. Truth and accuracy also include honest disclosure of duality of interests, such as working for a healthcare facility and a vendor. In these two capacities, proprietary information may become available that would place one employer in jeopardy in relationship to the second. Such dualities must be disclosed.
- **Bring honor to oneself, peers, and the profession.** The professional conduct of the HIM professional should bring honor to oneself and those served. The health and welfare of the patients should come before all personal or financial interests.
- **Commit to continuing education and lifelong learning.** HIM professionals are expected to be lifelong learners, ensuring expertise and application of current knowledge. The HIM professional must be committed to maximizing personal competence as well as contributing to the improvement of the quality of the services rendered. It took many years before an official continuing education requirement was specified for HIM professionals, but the intent of continuing education has always been part of the Code. Health information management is a practice-oriented career; degrees and research are required to improve professional contributions. The Code requires action and commitment to degree attainment, continuing education, currency with the professional literature, self-assessment, the design of personal educational programs, and dialogue with peers about solutions to problems. Competency through self-improvement is an important directive that ensures the continuance of the profession.

- **Discharge association duties honorably.** HIM professionals can either volunteer for local, state, or national association positions or be appointed or elected to them. Just as clinical information must be protected, the information that is learned in an official capacity while working on behalf of the professional associations at the local, state, and national levels must also be protected. Sometimes "secrets" are discovered at these levels, and it is important to protect this information.
- **Strengthen professional membership.** All HIM professionals are responsible for recruiting and training the next generation of professionals. Professional practice standards require constant recruitment of new students into the profession so that existing professionals can share their expertise.
- **Represent the profession to the public.** This standard requires education of the public regarding the HIM professional's role and responsibilities. No matter how many times a member of the public asks, "Do you get a degree to file?" the professional must give an answer that reflects the full range of responsibilities. If the public is confused about what HIM

professionals do on their behalf, HIM professionals should accept some responsibility for this confusion. The association's mission, guiding principles, and values must be supported when dealing with the public.

- **Promote and participate in research.** HIM professionals do not have a long-standing tradition of professional practice research; rather, they have mostly assisted other members of the healthcare team with clinical research. As professionals acquire advanced degrees, more specific health information research is being conducted. Like all researchers, HIM professionals should act with integrity and avoid conflicts of interest.

BUILDING AN ETHICAL HEALTH INFORMATION SYSTEM

The following are suggestions for incorporating the values and professional practice standards from the Code into your professional life and work environment:

1. **Further your education.** You should build ethics-related courses into your professional plans for continuing education and when taking on any of the new roles for HIM professionals outlined by AHIMA in its 1999 publication ***Vision 2006,*** which was a far-reaching document of the types of health information management careers available. It is interesting to note that many of the careers listed are ones that are currently being pursued by AHIMA members. In the current climate, professionals must not only understand terms such as DRG, CPT, OASIS, and SQL, but also values and ethical principles as they apply to HIM dilemmas. Begin to learn how these two bodies of knowledge are connected. Include your staff in this initiative. Continue your education, regardless of the degrees or credentials that you currently hold. The acceptance of HIM professionals in the healthcare system is dependent on their continued expertise. Others need to know

that HIM professionals are capable of managing the health information system, and this requires lifelong learning. Education is a gift that you give yourself and to others in return. Include the following questions as part of your self-assessment:

- Are you well informed of the AHIMA Code of Ethics and how it specifically affects your professional area of expertise?
- Do you understand ethical and professional guiding principles as they are related to HIM decision making? Does your decision-making process always include ethical criteria?
- Do you understand your personal values and how these influence HIM decisions, given that values are deeply embedded in the decision-making process?
- Do you understand the need to draw on both technical HIM competency and ethical literacy when making decisions?
- Are you including ethics and the ethical dilemmas that you face as an HIM professional in your plan for further education in your lifelong learning cycle? (Harman, 1999; AHIMA House of Delegates, 2004).

2. **Consult with the ethics committee.** Although facility-wide ethics committees typically deal with clinical bioethical decisions, the members of these committees are experts who are well positioned to help create the arguments and counterarguments for HIM issues such as releasing information, sharing data in relational databases, dealing with fraud and abuse issues, and analyzing issues related to problems with computerized software and security. HIM professionals must take these issues to the ethics committees and to colleagues; they cannot be resolved in isolation. The full clinical team must be involved in resolving such issues; otherwise, the solitary voice of the HIM professional will not be powerful enough to adequately protect patient privacy and confidentiality. Do not just limit the participation of ethicists and the ethics committee to official institutional review board

(IRB) (research-based) problems. If you feel uncomfortable about a decision, it most likely has an ethical component. In that case, you need advice. Go get it.

3. **Change the organizational culture.** Help to change the organizational structure, systems, policies, and procedures if they do not support ethical behavior and ensure patient privacy. Comply with laws, rules, and regulations, but not at the expense of ethical behavior. Organizational integrity is needed to enable HIM practitioners to be ethical. If the system creates the problems, it becomes incredibly difficult to take the correct course of action. If there is a disconnect between what is legal and what is ethical, act with your peers to make the necessary changes in the system. Be an advocate for your patients, their healthcare teams, and those who work on their behalf, either in direct patient care or through administrative agencies. Take your role of protecting patient privacy very seriously. At times, yours will be the only voice of caution at the negotiation table or during committee deliberations. Recognize your power and authority and use your expertise to facilitate the correct action.

4. **Be a role model.** HIM students and practitioners need to understand and use ethical principles and values in their work environment. Clinical experiences are chosen so that students can interact with good role models. It is important to both "talk and walk" ethics. Students learn to incorporate the professional values they observe in others facing difficult decisions. Demonstrate your integrity and be a role model for HIM students by teaching them the complexities of the issues—not only the rules and regulations, but also the range of choices that must be considered. Be honorable at all times. If HIM students see unethical behavior, we will lose them to another profession. Help the next generation of professionals learn to have courage in the face of ethical dilemmas. There is no greater gift to those who represent the future of this profession.

THE INTERSECTION OF HIM AND ETHICS

The ethical dilemmas faced by the HIM professional require action: Should certain information be released? Should software be implemented if privacy cannot be protected? Are computer systems secure? Ethical questions must be asked and answered within the context of the clinical and health information system. The issues currently facing the HIM profession do not allow the luxury of "the right answer" based exclusively on laws, required standards, or rules. In today's arena, HIM professionals must also look to an ethical framework when considering options for the best course of action. Ethical criteria need to be added to the list of common criteria, such as cost, regulation, policy, and technological feasibility (Harman & Mullen, 2004; 2005).

The dilemmas faced by HIM professionals require interdisciplinary ethical collaboration with clinicians, administrators, ethicists, lawyers, policymakers, accreditation agencies, and patients. Regardless of the profession, all providers of care need to understand the implications of documentation, access, and use within an ethical decision-making framework.

HIM professionals are essential teachers in the emerging healthcare system. They need to help the many stakeholders become aware of what happens to the documentation once it is entered into a medical record or computerized database. Instead of hiding behind the scenes, HIM professionals need to become much more public in their role as protectors of privacy and confidentiality.

HIM professionals have always had a strong moral voice for the correct course of action. Visionary leaders launched the HIM profession on the basis of essential ethical values and principles. They recognized the importance of competency, integrity, truth-telling, trust, compassion, dedication to others, and courage in carrying out the responsibilities of an HIM professional. Today, their words still resonate and must be adhered to especially in the context of today's complex health information system, where such values are especially needed.

The HIM professional must act as an organizational change agent, leading initiatives to support systems that guarantee compliance with the laws and principles for privacy and confidentiality. The HIM professional is a leader who must be technically competent, innovative, energetic, and able to envision future scenarios. Ethics must guide the professional's actions.

HIM professionals need to examine and live by the current AHIMA Code of Ethics so that it affords the professional group the necessary decision-making framework. They need to continue to hold themselves accountable with responses and programs that ensure ethical decisions. As the founders of the HIM profession recognized, the profession requires information management expertise, courage, and ethics; this is truer today than ever before. Bioethical decisions always require action. Ethical actions at work always require courage.

Key Terms

- AHIMA Code of Ethics
- Health information management (HIM) professional
- Professional
- *Vision 2006*

Chapter Summary

- HIM professionals must have both technical and ethical expertise due to the complexity of the issues they face. HIM professionals must deal with dilemmas that result from the healthcare environment, documentation requirements, access and release of information requirements, coding and reimbursement systems, and technology.
- HIM professionals have many constituents: patients and the healthcare team, the employer, the public interest, oneself, and professional associations.
- The HIM professional's obligations to patients and the healthcare team are to provide service, to protect medical and social information, to promote confidentiality, to promote the quality and advancement of health care, to stay within the scope of responsibility and refrain from passing clinical judgment, and to promote interdisciplinary cooperation and collaboration.
- The HIM professional's obligations to the employer are to demonstrate loyalty to the employer; to protect committee deliberations; to comply with laws, regulations, and policies; to recognize authority and power; and to accept compensation only in relationship to one's responsibilities.
- The HIM professional's obligations to the public interest are to advocate for change, to refuse to participate in or conceal unethical practices, and to report violations of practice standards to the proper authorities.
- The HIM professional's obligations to him- or herself and to the professional association are to be honest; to bring honor to oneself, one's peers, and the profession; to commit to continuing education and lifelong learning; to discharge association duties honorably; to strengthen professional membership; to represent the profession to the public; and to promote and participate in research.
- Building an ethical health information system requires furthering one's education, consulting with ethics committees, changing the organizational culture to support ethical behaviors, and being a role model for others.

References

Abdelhak, M., Grostick, S., Hanken, M. A., & Jacobs, E. (Eds.). (2001). *Health information: Management of a strategic resource* (2nd ed.). Philadelphia: W. B. Saunders.

American Health Information Management Association [AHIMA]. (1998). *AHIMA code of ethics.* Chicago, IL: Author.

American Health Information Management Association [AHIMA]. (1999). *Vision 2006. Evolving HIM careers: Seven roles for the future.* Chicago, IL: Author.

American Health Information Management Association [AHIMA]. (2000). *RHIA certification examination domains, subdomains, and tasks.* Chicago, IL: Author.

American Health Information Management Association [AHIMA]. (2004). *2004 American Health Information Management Association Code of Ethics.* Chicago, IL: Author.

Cofer, J. (Ed.). (1994). *Health information management* (10th ed.). Chicago, IL: Physicians' Record Company.

Harman, L. B. (1999, October). *HIM and ethics: Confronting difficult decisions.* Paper presented at the National Convention of the American Health Information Management Association, Anaheim, CA.

Harman, L. B. (2000). Confronting ethical dilemmas on the job: An HIM professional's guide. *Journal of the American Health Information Management Association, 71*(5), 45–49.

Harman, L. B. (Ed.). (2001). *Ethical issues in the management of health information.* Gaithersburg, MD: Aspen.

Harman, L. B., & Mullen, V. (2004, September). *Ethics and Health Information Management in the Global Community.* Paper presented at the 14th Congress of International Federation of Health Records Organizations (IFHRO), Washington, DC.

Harman, L. B., & Mullen, V. (2005, October). *Ethics at work: A Case Study.* Paper presented at the American Health Information Management (AHIMA) National Convention, San Diego, CA.

Huffman, E. K. (1963). *Manual for medical record librarians* (5th ed). Berwyn, IL: Physicians' Record Company.

Huffman, E. K. (1972). *Manual for medical record librarians* (6th ed). Chicago: Physicians' Record Company.

LaTour, K. M., & Eichenwald, S. (Eds). (2002). *Health information management: Concepts, principles, and practice.* Chicago: AHIMA.

Shi, L., & Singh, D. A. (2004). *Delivering health care in America: A systems approach* (3rd ed.). Sudbury, MA: Jones and Bartlett.

Spinello, R. A. (1997). *Case studies in information and computer ethics.* Upper Saddle River, NJ: Prentice Hall.

Appendix 1-A: 1957 Code of Ethics for the Practice of Medical Record Science

Note: Gender-neutral language was not used in the 1950s, so the male pronoun should be read as "he or she."]

As a member of one of the paramedical professions he shall:

1. Place service before material gain, the honor of the profession before personal advantage, the health and welfare of patients above all personal and financial interests, and conduct himself in the practice of this profession so as to bring honor to himself, his associates, and to the medical record profession.

2. Preserve and protect the medical records in his custody and hold inviolate the privileged contents of the records and any other information of a confidential nature obtained in his official capacity, taking due account of the applicable statutes and of regulations and policies of his employer.

3. Serve his employer loyally, honorably discharging the duties and responsibilities entrusted to him, and give due consideration to the nature of these responsibilities in giving his employer notice of intent to resign his position.

4. Refuse to participate in or conceal unethical practices or procedures.

5. Report to the proper authorities but disclose to no one else any evidence of conduct or practice revealed in the medical records in his custody that indicates possible violation of established rules and regulations of the employer or of professional practice.

6. Preserve the confidential nature of professional determinations made by the staff committee which he serves.

7. Accept only those fees that are customary and lawful in the area for services rendered in his official capacity.

8. Avoid encroachment on the professional responsibilities of the medical and other paramedical professions, and under no circumstances assume or give the appearance of assuming the right to make determinations in professional areas outside the scope of his assigned responsibilities.

9. Strive to advance the knowledge and practice of medical record science, including continued self-improvement in order to contribute to the best possible medical care.

10. Participate appropriately in developing and strengthening professional manpower and in representing the profession to the public.

11. Discharge honorably the responsibilities of any Association post to which appointed or elected, and preserve the confidentiality of any privileged information made known to him in his official capacity.

12. State truthfully and accurately his credentials, professional education, and experiences in any official transaction with the American Association of Medical Record Librarians and with any employer or prospective employer.

Source: Courtesy of American Health Information Management Association, 1957, Chicago, Illinois.

Appendix 1–B: 1977 American Medical Record Association Bylaws and Code of Ethics

The medical record practitioner is concerned with the development, use, and maintenance of medical and health records for medical care, preventive medicine, quality assurance, professional education, administrative practices and study purposes with due consideration of patients' right to privacy. The American Medical Record Association believes that it is in the best interests of the medical record profession and the public which it serves that the principles of personal and professional accountability be reexamined and redefined to provide members of the Association, as well as medical record practitioners who are credentialed by the Association, with definitive and binding guidelines of conduct. To achieve this goal, the American Medical Record Association has adopted the following restated Code of Ethics:

1. Conduct yourself in the practice of this profession so as to bring honor and dignity to yourself, the medical record profession and the Association.

2. Place service before material gain and strive at all times to provide services consistent with the need for quality health care and treatment of all who are ill and injured.

3. Preserve and secure the medical and health records, the information contained therein, and the appropriate secondary records in your custody in accordance with professional management practices, employer's policies and existing legal provisions.

4. Uphold the doctrine of confidentiality and the individual's right to privacy in the disclosure of personally identifiable medical and social information.

5. Recognize the source of the authority and powers delegated to you and conscientiously discharge the duties and responsibilities thus entrusted.

6. Refuse to participate in or conceal unethical practices or procedures in your relationship with other individuals or organizations.

7. Disclose to no one but proper authorities any evidence of conduct or practice revealed in medical reports or observed that indicates possible violation of established rules and regulations of the employer or professional practice.

8. Safeguard the public and the profession by reporting to the Ethics Committee any breach of this Code of Ethics by fellow members of the profession.

9. Preserve the confidential nature of professional determinations made by official committees of health and health-service organizations.

10. Accept compensation only in accordance with services actually performed or negotiated with the health institution.

11. Cooperate with other health professions and organizations to promote the quality of health programs and advancement of medical care, ensuring respect and consideration for the responsibility and the dignity of medical and other health professions.

12. Strive to increase the profession's body of systematic knowledge and individual competency through continued self-improvement and application of current advancements in the conduct of medical record practices.

13. Participate in developing and strengthening professional manpower and appropriately represent the profession in public.

14. Discharge honorably the responsibilities of any Association position to which appointed or elected.

15. Represent truthfully and accurately professional credentials, education, and experience in any official transaction or notice, including other positions and duality of interests.

Source: Courtesy of American Health Information Management Association, 1977, Chicago, Illinois.

Appendix 1-C: 1988 American Medical Record Association Code of Ethics and Bylaws

The medical record professional abides by a set of ethical principles developed to safeguard the public and to contribute within the scope of the profession to quality and efficiency in health care. This code of ethics, adopted by the members of the American Medical Record Association, defines the standards of behavior which promote ethical conduct.

1. The Medical Record Professional demonstrates behavior that reflects integrity, supports objectivity, and fosters trust in professional activities.

2. The Medical Record Professional respects the dignity of each human being.

3. The Medical Record Professional strives to improve personal competence and quality of services.

4. The Medical Record Professional represents truthfully and accurately professional credentials, education, and experience.

5. The Medical Record Professional refuses to participate in illegal or unethical acts and also refuses to conceal the illegal, incompetent, or unethical acts of others.

6. The Medical Record Professional protects the confidentiality of primary and secondary health records as mandated by law, professional standards, and the employer's policies.

7. The Medical Record Professional promotes to others the tenets of confidentiality.

8. The Medical Record Professional adheres to pertinent laws and regulations while advocating changes which serve the best interest of the public.

9. The Medical Record Professional encourages appropriate use of health record information and advocates policies and systems that advance the management of health records and health information.

10. The Medical Record Professional recognizes and supports the association's mission.

Source: Courtesy of American Health Information Management Association, 1988, Chicago, Illinois.

Appendix 1-D: 1998 American Health Information Management Association Code of Ethics and Bylaws

AHIMA's Mission

The American Health Information Management Association is committed to the quality of health information for the benefit of patients, providers and other users of clinical data. Our professional organization:

- Provides leadership in HIM education and professional development
- Sets and promotes professional practice standards
- Advocates patient privacy rights and confidentiality of health information
- Influences public and private policies including educating the public regarding health information
- Advances health information technologies

Guiding Principles

We are committed to the:

- Creation and utilization of systems and standards to ensure quality health information
- Achievement of member excellence
- Development of a supportive environment and provision of the resources to advance the profession
- Provision of the highest quality service to members and health care information users
- Investigation and application of new technology to advance the management of health information

We value:

- The balance of patients' privacy rights and confidentiality of health information with legitimate uses of data
- The quality of health information as evidenced by its integrity, accuracy, consistency, reliability, and validity
- The quality of health information as evidenced by its impact on the quality of health care delivery

This Code of Ethics sets forth ethical principles for the HIM profession. Members of this profession are responsible for maintaining and promoting ethical practices. This Code of Ethics, adopted by the American Health Information Management Association, shall be binding on health information management professionals who are members of the Association and all individuals who hold an AHIMA credential.

Health information management professionals:

1. Respect the rights and dignity of all individuals.
2. Comply with all laws, regulations, and standards governing the practice of health information management.

3. Strive for professional excellence through self-assessment and continuing education.

4. Truthfully and accurately represent their professional credentials, education, and experience.

5. Adhere to the vision, mission, and values of the Association.

6. Promote and protect the confidentiality and security of health records and health information.

7. Strive to provide accurate and timely information.

8. Promote high standards for health information management practice, education, and research.

9. Act with integrity and avoid conflicts of interest in the performance of their professional and AHIMA responsibilities.

Source: Courtesy of American Health Information Management Association, 1998, Chicago, Illinois.

Appendix 1-E: 2004 American Health Information Management Association

CODE OF ETHICS

Preamble

The ethical obligations of the health information management (HIM) professional include the protection of patient privacy and confidential information; disclosure of information; development, use, and maintenance of health information systems and health records; and the quality of information. Both handwritten and computerized medical records contain many sacred stories—stories that must be protected on behalf of the individual and the aggregate community of persons served in the healthcare system. Healthcare consumers are increasingly concerned about the loss of privacy and the inability to control the dissemination of their protected information. Core health information issues include what information should be collected, how the information should be handled, who should have access to the information, and under what conditions the information should be disclosed.

Ethical obligations are central to the professional's responsibility, regardless of the employment site or the method of collection, storage, and security of health information. Sensitive information (genetic, adoption, drug, alcohol, sexual, and behavioral information) requires special attention to prevent misuse. Entrepreneurial roles require expertise in the protection of the information in the world of business and interactions with consumers.

Professional Values

The mission of the HIM profession is based on core professional values developed since the inception of the Association in 1928. These values and the inherent ethical responsibilities for AHIMA members and credentialed HIM professionals include providing service; protecting medical, social, and financial information; promoting confidentiality; and preserving and securing health information. Values to the healthcare team include promoting the quality and advancement of healthcare, demonstrating HIM expertise and skills, and promoting interdisciplinary cooperation and collaboration. Professional values in relationship to the employer include protecting committee deliberations and complying with laws, regulations, and policies. Professional values related to the public include advocating change, refusing to participate or conceal unethical practices, and reporting violations of practice standards to the proper authorities. Professional values to individual and professional associations include obligations to be honest, bringing honor to self, peers and profession, committing to continuing education and lifelong learning, performing Association duties honorably, strengthening professional membership, representing the profession to the public, and promoting and participating in research.

These professional values will require a complex process of balancing the many conflicts that can result from competing interests and obligations of those who seek access to health information and require an understanding of ethical decision-making.

Purpose of the American Health Information Management Association Code of Ethics

The HIM professional has an obligation to demonstrate actions that reflect values, ethical principles, and ethical guidelines. The American Health Information Management Association

(AHIMA) Code of Ethics sets forth these values and principles to guide conduct. The code is relevant to all AHIMA members and credentialed HIM professionals and students, regardless of their professional functions, the settings in which they work, or the populations they serve.

The AHIMA Code of Ethics serves six purposes:

- Identifies core values on which the HIM mission is based.
- Summarizes broad ethical principles that reflect the profession's core values and establishes a set of ethical principles to be used to guide decision-making and actions.
- Helps HIM professionals identify relevant considerations when professional obligations conflict or ethical uncertainties arise.
- Provides ethical principles by which the general public can hold the HIM professional accountable.
- Socializes practitioners new to the field to HIM's mission, values, and ethical principles.
- Articulates a set of guidelines that the HIM professional can use to assess whether they have engaged in unethical conduct.

The code includes principles and guidelines that are both enforceable and aspirational. The extent to which each principle is enforceable is a matter of professional judgment to be exercised by those responsible for reviewing alleged violations of ethical principles.

The Use of the Code

Violation of principles in this code does not automatically imply legal liability or violation of the law. Such determination can only be made in the context of legal and judicial proceedings. Alleged violations of the code would be subject to a peer review process. Such processes are generally separate from legal or administrative procedures and insulated from legal review or proceedings to allow the profession to counsel and discipline its own members although in some situations, violations of the code would constitute unlawful conduct subject to legal process.

Guidelines for ethical and unethical behavior are provided in this code. The terms "shall and shall not" are used as a basis for setting high standards for behavior. This does not imply that everyone "shall or shall not" do everything that is listed. For example, not everyone participates in the recruitment or mentoring of students. A HIM professional is not being unethical if this is not part of his or her professional activities; however, if students are part of one's professional responsibilities, there is an ethical obligation to follow the guidelines stated in the code. This concept is true for the entire code. If someone does the stated activities, ethical behavior is the standard. The guidelines are not a comprehensive list. For example, the statement "protect all confidential information to include personal, health, financial, genetic and outcome information" can also be interpreted as "shall not fail to protect all confidential information to include personal, health, financial, genetic, and outcome information."

A code of ethics cannot guarantee ethical behavior. Moreover, a code of ethics cannot resolve all ethical issues or disputes or capture the richness and complexity involved in striving to make responsible choices within a moral community. Rather, a code of ethics sets forth values and ethical principles, and offers ethical guidelines to which professionals aspire and by which their actions can be judged. Ethical behaviors result from a personal commitment to engage in ethical practice.

Professional responsibilities often require an individual to move beyond personal values. For example, an individual might demonstrate behaviors that are based on the values of honesty, providing service to others, or demonstrating loyalty. In addition to these, professional values might require promoting confidentiality, facilitating interdisciplinary collaboration, and refusing to participate or conceal unethical practices. Professional values could require a more comprehensive set of values than what an individual needs to be an ethical agent in their personal lives.

The AHIMA Code of Ethics is to be used by AHIMA and individuals, agencies, organizations, and bodies (such as licensing and regulatory boards, insurance providers, courts of law, boards of directors, government agencies, and other professional groups) that choose to adopt it or use it as a frame of reference. The AHIMA Code of Ethics reflects the commitment of all to uphold the profession's values and to act ethically. Individuals of good character who discern moral questions and, in good faith, seek to make reliable ethical judgments must apply ethical principles.

The code does not provide a set of rules that prescribe how to act in all situations. Specific applications of the code must take into account the context in which it is being considered and the possibility of conflicts among the code's values, principles, and guidelines. Ethical responsibilities flow from all human relationships, from the personal and familial to the social and professional. Further, the AHIMA Code of Ethics does not specify which values, principles, and guidelines are the most important and ought to outweigh others in instances when they conflict.

CODE OF ETHICS 2004

Ethical Principles: The following ethical principles are based on the core values of the American Health Information Management Association and apply to all health information management professionals.

Health information management professionals:

I. *Advocate, uphold and defend the individual's right to privacy and the doctrine of confidentiality in the use and disclosure of information.*

II. *Put service and the health and welfare of persons before self-interest and conduct themselves in the practice of the profession so as to bring honor to themselves, their peers, and to the health information management profession.*

III. *Preserve, protect, and secure personal health information in any form or medium and hold in the highest regard the contents of the records and other information of a confidential nature, taking into account the applicable statutes and regulations.*

IV. *Refuse to participate in or conceal unethical practices or procedures.*

V. *Advance health information management knowledge and practice through continuing education, research, publications, and presentations.*

VI. *Recruit and mentor students, peers and colleagues to develop and strengthen professional workforce.*

VII. *Represent the profession accurately to the public.*

VIII. *Perform honorably health information management association responsibilities, either appointed or elected, and preserve the confidentiality of any privileged information made known in any official capacity.*

IX. *State truthfully and accurately their credentials, professional education, and experiences.*

X. *Facilitate interdisciplinary collaboration in situations supporting health information practice.*

XI. *Respect the inherent dignity and worth of every person.*

HOW TO INTERPRET THE CODE OF ETHICS

The following ethical principles are based on the core values of the American Health Information Management Association and apply to all health information management professionals. Guidelines included for each ethical principle are a noninclusive list of behaviors and situations that can help to clarify the principle. They are not to be meant as a comprehensive list of all situations that can occur.

I. Advocate, uphold, and defend the individual's right to privacy and the doctrine of confidentiality in the use and disclosure of information.

Health information management professionals **shall:**

1.1. Protect all confidential information to include personal, health, financial, genetic, and outcome information.

1.2. Engage in social and political action that supports the protection of privacy and confidentiality, and be aware of the impact of the political arena on the health information system. Advocate for changes in policy and legislation to ensure protection of privacy and confidentiality, coding compliance, and other issues that surface as advocacy issues as well as facilitating informed participation by the public on these issues.

1.3. Protect the confidentiality of all information obtained in the course of professional service. Disclose only information that is directly relevant or necessary to achieve the purpose of disclosure. Release information only with valid consent from a patient or a person legally authorized to consent on behalf of a patient or as authorized by federal or state regulations. The need-to-know criterion is essential when releasing health information for initial disclosure and all redisclosure activities.

1.4. Promote the obligation to respect privacy by respecting confidential information shared among colleagues, while responding to requests from the legal profession, the media, or other non-healthcare related individuals, during presentations or teaching and in situations that could cause harm to persons.

II. Put service and the health and welfare of persons before self-interest and conduct themselves in the practice of the profession so as to bring honor to themselves, their peers, and to the health information management profession.

Health information management professionals **shall:**

2.1. Act with integrity, behave in a trustworthy manner, elevate service to others above self-interest, and promote high standards of practice in every setting.

2.2. Be aware of the profession's mission, values, and ethical principles, and practice in a manner consistent with them by acting honestly and responsibly.

2.3. Anticipate, clarify, and avoid any conflict of interest, to all parties concerned, when dealing with consumers, consulting with competitors, or in providing services requiring potentially conflicting roles (for example, finding out information about one facility that would help a competitor). The conflicting roles or responsibilities must be clarified and appropriate action must be taken to minimize any conflict of interest.

2.4. Ensure that the working environment is consistent and encourages compliance with the AHIMA Code of Ethics, taking reasonable steps to eliminate any conditions in their organizations that violate, interfere with, or discourage compliance with the code.

2.5. Take responsibility and credit, including authorship credit, only for work they actually perform or to which they contribute. Honestly acknowledge the work of and the contributions made by others verbally or written, such as in publication.

Health information management professionals **shall not:**

2.6. Permit their private conduct to interfere with their ability to fulfill their professional responsibilities.

2.7. Take unfair advantage of any professional relationship or exploit others to further their personal, religious, political, or business interests.

>   III. *Preserve, protect, and secure personal health information in any form or medium and hold in the highest regards the contents of the records and other information of a confidential nature obtained in the official capacity, taking into account the applicable statutes and regulations.*

Health information management professionals **shall:**

3.1. Protect the confidentiality of patients' written and electronic records and other sensitive information. Take reasonable steps to ensure that patients' records are stored in a secure location and that patients' records are not available to others who are not authorized to have access.

3.2. Take precautions to ensure and maintain the confidentiality of information transmitted, transferred, or disposed of in the event of a termination, incapacitation, or death of a healthcare provider to other parties through the use of any media. Disclosure of identifying information should be avoided whenever possible.

3.3. Inform recipients of the limitations and risks associated with providing services via electronic media (such as computer, telephone, fax, radio, and television).

>   IV. *Refuse to participate in or conceal unethical practices or procedures.*

Health information management professionals **shall:**

4.1. Act in a professional and ethical manner at all times.

4.2. Take adequate measures to discourage, prevent, expose, and correct the unethical conduct of colleagues.

4.3. Be knowledgeable about established policies and procedures for handling concerns about colleagues' unethical behavior. These include policies and procedures created by AHIMA, licensing and regulatory bodies, employers, supervisors, agencies, and other professional organizations.

4.4. Seek resolution if there is a belief that a colleague has acted unethically or if there is a belief of incompetence or impairment by discussing their concerns with the colleague when feasible and when such discussion is likely to be productive. Take action through appropriate formal channels, such as contacting an accreditation or regulatory body and/or the AHIMA Professional Ethics Committee.

4.5. Consult with a colleague when feasible and assist the colleague in taking remedial action when there is direct knowledge of a health information management colleague's incompetence or impairment.

Health information management professionals **shall not:**

4.6. Participate in, condone, or be associated with dishonesty, fraud and abuse, or deception. A noninclusive list of examples includes:

- Allowing patterns of retrospective documentation to avoid suspension or increase reimbursement
- Assigning codes without physician documentation
- Coding when documentation does not justify the procedures that have been billed
- Coding an inappropriate level of service
- Miscoding to avoid conflict with others
- Engaging in negligent coding practices
- Hiding or ignoring review outcomes, such as performance data
- Failing to report licensure status for a physician through the appropriate channels
- Recording inaccurate data for accreditation purposes
- Hiding incomplete medical records
- Allowing inappropriate access to genetic, adoption, or behavioral health information
- Misusing sensitive information about a competitor
- Violating the privacy of individuals

V. Advance health information management knowledge and practice through continuing education, research, publications, and presentations.

Health information management professionals **shall:**

5.1. Develop and enhance continually their professional expertise, knowledge, and skills (including appropriate education, research, training, consultation, and supervision). Contribute to the knowledge base of health information management and share with colleagues their knowledge related to practice, research, and ethics.

5.2. Base practice decisions on recognized knowledge, including empirically based knowledge relevant to health information management and health information management ethics.

5.3. Contribute time and professional expertise to activities that promote respect for the value, integrity, and competence of the health information management profession. These activities may include teaching, research, consultation, service, legislative testimony, presentations in the community, and participation in their professional organizations.

5.4. Engage in evaluation or research that ensures the anonymity or confidentiality of participants and of the data obtained from them by following guidelines developed for the participants in consultation with appropriate institutional review boards. Report evaluation and research findings accurately and take steps to correct any errors later found in published data using standard publication methods.

5.5. Take reasonable steps to provide or arrange for continuing education and staff development, addressing current knowledge and emerging developments related to health information management practice and ethics.

Health information management professionals **shall not:**

5.6. Design or conduct evaluation or research that is in conflict with applicable federal or state laws.

5.7. Participate in, condone, or be associated with fraud or abuse.

VI.   *Recruit and mentor students, peers and colleagues to develop and strengthen professional workforce.*

Health information management professionals **shall:**

6.1. Evaluate students' performance in a manner that is fair and respectful when functioning as educators or clinical internship supervisors.

6.2. Be responsible for setting clear, appropriate, and culturally sensitive boundaries for students.

6.3. Be a mentor for students, peers and new health information management professionals to develop and strengthen skills.

6.4. Provide directed practice opportunities for students.

Health information management professionals **shall not:**

6.5. Engage in any relationship with students in which there is a risk of exploitation or potential harm to the student.

VII.   *Accurately represent the profession to the public.*

Health information management professionals **shall:**

7.1 Be an advocate for the profession in all settings and participate in activities that promote and explain the mission, values, and principles of the profession to the public.

VIII.   *Perform honorably health information management association responsibilities, either appointed or elected, and preserve the confidentiality of any privileged information made known in any official capacity.*

Health information management professionals **shall:**

8.1. Perform responsibly all duties as assigned by the professional association.

8.2. Resign from an Association position if unable to perform the assigned responsibilities with competence.

8.3. Speak on behalf of professional health information management organizations, accurately representing the official and authorized positions of the organizations.

IX.   *State truthfully and accurately their credentials, professional education, and experiences.*

Health information management professionals **shall:**

9.1. Make clear distinctions between statements made and actions engaged in as a private individual and as a representative of the health information management profession, a professional health information organization, or the health information management professional's employer.

9.2. Claim and ensure that their representations to patients, agencies, and the public of professional qualifications, credentials, education, competence, affiliations, services provided, training, certification, consultation received, supervised experience, other relevant professional experience are accurate.

9.3. Claim only those relevant professional credentials actually possessed and correct any inaccuracies occurring regarding credentials.

X. *Facilitate interdisciplinary collaboration in situations supporting health information practice.*

Health information management professionals **shall:**

10.1. Participate in and contribute to decisions that affect the well-being of patients by drawing on the perspectives, values, and experiences of those involved in decisions related to patients. Professional and ethical obligations of the interdisciplinary team as a whole and of its individual members should be clearly established.

XI. *Respect the inherent dignity and worth of every person.*

Health information management professionals **shall:**

11.1. Treat each person in a respectful fashion, being mindful of individual differences and cultural and ethnic diversity.

11.2. Promote the value of self-determination for each individual.

ACKNOWLEDGMENT

Adapted with permission from the Code of Ethics of the National Association of Social Workers.

RESOURCES

National Association of Social Workers. (1999). Code of Ethics. Available at http://www.naswdc. org.
Harman, L. B. (Ed.). (2001). *Ethical challenges in the management of health information.* Gaithersburg, MD: Aspen.
AHIMA Code of Ethics, 1957, 1977, 1988, and 1998.

Revised & adopted by AHIMA House of Delegates—July 1, 2004

2

Ethical Decision-Making Guidelines and Tools

Jacqueline J. Glover, PhD

Learning Objectives

After completing this chapter, the reader should be able to:

- Define ethics.
- Identify the importance of studying ethics for the health information management (HIM) professional.
- Identify ethical concepts, including relevant values, principles, virtues, approaches, and theories.
- Apply a process of ethical decision making to HIM scenarios.

Abstract

Ethics is the formal process of intentionally and critically analyzing, with respect to clarity and consistency, the basis for one's moral judgments. It is important for health information management (HIM) professionals to engage in this process, because they are accountable for their actions as professionals, not just personally as individuals. Ethical reasoning is necessary to resolve the potential conflicts between personal values and professional values and among professional values. This chapter presents a model for ethical decision making and outlines ethical theories and approaches that can help HIM professionals decide on a course of action, justify their choice, and persuade others that their choice is better than other choices.

Scenario 2-A: Documentation and DRG Assignment

You are a health information management (HIM) professional practicing in a 350-bed community hospital. You are analyzing a patient's medical record to determine the appropriate diagnosis-related group (DRG) assignment. The patient complained of shortness of breath and chest pain on admission and received a cardiac catheterization as part of a cardiac workup. The physician determined the final diagnosis to be chronic obstructive pulmonary disease (COPD). The physician documented "possible valvular disorder or endocarditis" on the history and physical. If a cardiac condition is coded, DRG 124 will be assigned, and the hospital will receive over $11,750. If COPD is considered to be the principal diagnosis, DRG 088 will be assigned. The reimbursement for this diagnosis is $7,300, because this DRG does not recognize the catheterization procedure. At this hospital, a cardiac catheterization costs $5,500. You are now facing an ethical issue. What should you do?

WHAT IS AN ETHICAL ISSUE?

An **ethical issue** is one that involves the core values of practice. The case set forth in Scenario 2-A raises ethical issues in that the core values of truth-telling and integrity are in conflict with the values of loyalty and service to the institution. You know you have an ethical issue when such core values are at stake. Oftentimes, your emotions are the first to alert you that something may be wrong. Many people become upset when faced with the potential for lying or perhaps harming their employer.

WHY DO ETHICAL ISSUES NEED TO BE ADDRESSED?

Many people may want to answer questions of professional ethics according to their own personal morality. They may believe that the issue in Scenario 2-A can be easily resolved according to their own personal upbringing and beliefs. They think, "My parents taught me never to lie" or "My parents taught me to be loyal and work hard." But is that type of thinking really sufficient? Notice that the two belief systems are in conflict. How do you resolve the conflict?

Resolving conflict depends on the more formal mechanism of ethics. Personal moral-ity and ethics differ. Most of the time, people do not distinguish between morality and ethics; they just use the words interchangeably. But when a distinction is made, it is often as follows: Morality refers to your own personal moral choices; ethics refers to the formal process of intentionally and critically analyzing the basis for your moral judgments for clarity and consistency. Because of the potential conflict between personal values and professional values, and because of the potential for conflict among professional values, we need ethics to help resolve such conflicts. Ethics provides a formal way to step back from the conflict, search for reasons to support one choice over another, and apply this reasoning in future situations.

This process of stepping back to formally analyze values is important, because you are accountable for your actions as a professional, not just personally. Patients, other professionals, and the general public do not know about your personal moral values. But they do have expectations for your professional conduct. Standards arise from the trust that the public places in you. They expect you to be able to act professionally—even, or perhaps especially, when difficult ethical issues are involved. You have to uphold that trust, and, at the heart of it, that is why you must study ethics.

BUT YOU CAN'T
TEACH ETHICS, CAN YOU?

Two major objections are commonly given to the study of ethics. First, many people claim that their character is already formed, and that the study of ethics is not going to change their behavior if they are inclined not to do the right thing. Second, many people argue that there is no ethical content to teach. There is no knowledge of right and wrong that everyone accepts. Ethics is a matter of opinion, and everyone is entitled to his or her own opinion.

Regarding the first objection, the goal of a course in ethics is not to make you a good person. Rather, it is to enable you to make reliable moral judgments as a professional. Regarding the second argument, as professionals, we expect not just opinions, but judgments backed up by good reasoning. When making medical judgments, healthcare personnel must offer support for their choices and be able to apply that reasoning in similar situations. The same is true when making moral judgments.

An ethics curriculum has three parts:

1. **Knowledge.** The HIM professional needs to be aware of standards of ethical conduct as expressed in the AHIMA Code of Ethics and have knowledge of ethical principles and concepts.
2. **Development.** The moral maturity of the HIM professional needs to be modeled and nurtured. Even if someone's character is formed, it needs reinforcement and application in professional settings. The faculty is responsible for identifying core values and character traits of professionals. This means identifying and reinforcing praiseworthy behavior in practice and applying appropriate sanctions if good character is not guiding appropriate professional conduct.
3. **Skills.** HIM professionals need practice in identifying ethical issues and applying a process of ethical decision making to ethical issues that arise in the practice of HIM.

THE PROCESS OF
ETHICAL DECISION MAKING

Various models for ethical decision making are available in the literature, but all share some of the basic components or steps that are used in this book (Purtilo, 1999; Lo, 1995; Benjamin & Curtis, 1986). You should use an ethical decision-making process to ensure that you make reliable moral judgments in your professional practice. We will demonstrate the decision-making process by applying it to Scenario 2-A. See the end of the chapter for the complete matrix.

The first step of the ethical decision-making process is to ask, "What is the ethical question?" In Scenario 2-A, the ethical question is, "Which DRG code should the HIM professional assign?" In identifying the ethical question, the HIM professional needs to look for the "shoulds." These "shoulds" are the normative questions (i.e., what should or ought to happen according to norms or standards), as opposed to descriptive questions (i.e., what actually does happen).

However, the HIM professional needs to be aware of different kinds of "shoulds." For example, there are the clinical "shoulds": in this case, the DRG code that you should use, according to the content knowledge and judgment of HIM to distinguish cardiac and pulmonary codes from others.

There also are the legal "shoulds" that help you identify what you should do to avoid charges of fraud. Note that the law and ethics differ. First, ethics is more fundamental. We can always ask, from an ethical standpoint: "Is this a good law or should I conscientiously disobey it or work to change the law?" Second, even though the law does have some moral content, it is a kind of minimum. Ethics strives to inspire the best professional behavior; the law demands only a decent minimum. Third, the law can be ambiguous. It is not always clear what the law actually says about a certain question, and the law is often not capable of subtle distinctions. Finally, the law does not address many of the issues that are important in ethics. For example, ethics is concerned not only with what you do, but also with the kind of person you are (virtue or character).

With regard to ethical decision making, we are concerned with the ethical "shoulds." These ethical "shoulds" relate to your duties and obligations as a professional. They involve choosing among the core professional values or between your obligations as a professional and your personal obligations, perhaps even to your family. A key distinguishing feature of the ethical "shoulds" is that they are concerned with the well-being of others and are not self-interested or self-directed.

The second step of the ethical decision-making process involves asking, "What are the facts?" In Scenario 2-A, the facts are as follows:

1. Known facts:
   - Possible cardiac problems documented in the history and physical.
   - Cardiac catheterization performed.
   - Final diagnosis documented: COPD.
2. Facts to be gathered:
   - What is the nature of the patient's cardiac problem?
   - Are there any cardiac comorbidities? (Heart and lung problems often occur together.)
   - What was the patient's source of pain?
   - Would assigning a cardiac DRG code constitute fraud? It is not clear. (Refer to Chapter 4 on fraud and Chapter 5 on coding.)
   - What are the customary practices here? (If you were surveyed, what would the standard be?)
   - What is your supervisor expecting you to do? (If you are the supervisor, what is your boss expecting you to do?)
   - How long have you been at this job? What is your relationship with your supervisor?
   - What is the likely impact of changing jobs on your family?

It is always tempting to avoid a discussion of ethics by claiming that not enough facts are available to make a decision. Although facts are very important—good ethics begins with good facts—the discussion can proceed if you consider why you want to know something and how it will change your analysis. If certain facts are unclear, assume one set of facts for your analysis, and then change the facts to see if your analysis would change.

The third step of the ethical decision-making process is to ask, "What are the values at stake in this scenario?" You must consider the values from various perspectives. Who are the stakeholders? What is their perspective? A **stakeholder** is someone who will be affected by the decision to be made. The following stakeholders are relevant to Scenario 2-A:

- **The patient.** We assume that the patient values an accurate medical record that will be the basis for quality health care. The patient also has an interest in keeping medical costs down so that insurance rates do not increase.
- **The HIM professional.** Assigning the code to maximize reimbursement may compromise the HIM professional's obligation to tell the truth. It could also compromise the values of accuracy and reliability. The HIM professional's integrity is at stake if the professional is willing to violate core values for the sake of reimbursement. Also at stake is the value of fairness—following the rules that have been established for all to follow. All professionals share the ethical obligation to obey the law. However, the values of loyalty to the employer and service to the institution are important as well. The value of avoiding harm (nonmaleficence) is relevant in two different ways. First, less-than-accurate documentation in the medical record may be harmful to the patient. Second, if the institution is not financially viable and has to close, patients and other pro-

fessionals will be harmed. Finally, several personal values are at stake in this scenario. The HIM professional has an obligation to promote the welfare of his or her family members by continuing his or her current employment.

- **Other healthcare professionals.** The other healthcare professionals involved in Scenario 2-A, including the physicians and nurses, also have obligations to promote the patient's welfare. An accurate medical record is essential to continuity of care and the future care of this patient. Other healthcare professionals have truth-telling obligations as well. And fairness—making sure that rules that apply equally to all are followed—is an important value.

- **Hospital administrators.** Hospital administrators have an obligation to promote the welfare of patients and keep them from harm. However, they also have an obligation to promote the welfare of the hospital. Administrators should maximize reimbursement, but not lie to do so. As healthcare professionals, they also have an obligation to tell the truth. Quality-improvement efforts depend on accurate medical records. Just like the patient, the hospital administrators also have an interest in controlling healthcare costs. The value of fairness is also involved. There can be no exception to reimbursement rules that apply equally to all.

- **Society (or at least other members of the same insurance plan).** Some people would argue that everyone in society who pays for health care has an interest in seeing that healthcare costs are controlled. Also, everyone is obligated to promote the just or fair allocation of healthcare resources and to follow the rules of reimbursement that are meant to be applied equally to all participants.

The fourth step of the ethical decision-making process is to ask, "What are the op-

tions in this case?" Specifically, what could you do in this scenario? You could (1) seek out more information, (2) assign the cardiac DRG, or (3) assign the pulmonary DRG.

The fifth step of the ethical decision-making process is to ask, "What should I do?" "What do I think is the best option based on the core values of the profession?" First, you should seek more information. It is important to base your choice on the best available data. If we assume that you have determined that the final diagnosis really is a respiratory problem, that the catheterization was performed to rule out cardiac disease, and that there is no documentation of cardiac disease, then you should assign the pulmonary DRG.

The sixth step of the ethical decision-making process is to ask, "What justifies your choice?" Provide reasons to support your decision based on the values at stake. The decision to assign the pulmonary code is supported by the obligation on everyone's part to tell the truth and to support the accuracy of the medical record. It preserves professional integrity. It is the most fair because it follows the rules that are meant to apply equally to all. This decision also respects the law.

The other choice—to assign the cardiac DRG—is not justified, because it depends on your telling a lie. You would also have to make a special exception to the rules to maximize your institution's reimbursement. That would not be fair to the other institutions that do follow the rules. The whole reimbursement scheme behind the DRG system is based on aggregates, not individual procedures. The reimbursement rate is based on the average cost, and it is meant to even out in the end. It is assumed that other patients with cardiac diagnoses will not have cardiac catheterizations, and that the hospital will still get the higher reimbursement. If everyone altered their coding to maximize reimbursement, it would undermine the whole reimbursement system and cost everyone more in the end. Controlling healthcare costs will ultimately serve everyone's interests.

But what about the other values like loyalty to the institution and being a team player? You have to ask yourself, "What are the institutional values?" Loyal employees can serve values like truth-telling in institutions that have similar values. Should you continue to work for an institution that does not promote professional integrity? An institution that pushes legal boundaries by asking its employees to do the same is probably going to get in trouble eventually. As a professional, you are responsible for your own behavior, and professional standards should be the basis of the values of healthcare institutions, not contrary to them (Griffith, 1993; Worthley, 1997).

The seventh and final step of the ethical decision-making process is to ask, "How could this ethical problem have been prevented?" Are there any systemic changes that could be made to prevent this problem from happening again? The first suggestion would be to learn more about assigning DRGs when expensive procedures, such as cardiac catheterizations, are done to rule out other diseases. You should talk about standards, and the values that support them, with your colleagues. You may have been able to prevent this problem if you had made questions of institutional integrity a part of your interviewing for the job in the first place.

A completed ethical decision-making matrix for Scenario 2-A is included at the end of this chapter. Refer to Appendix 2-A for a blank copy the ethical decision-making matrix that is used throughout this book.

JUSTIFICATION IN ETHICAL REASONING: HOW DO YOU KNOW WHAT IS BEST?

The most difficult aspect of ethics is deciding on the best course of action and providing good reasons to support your choice. There is usually not just one right answer; rather, there is a range of morally acceptable options, with some options being better or worse than others. Some answers are even outside the range of moral acceptability; these should not be chosen.

But how do we know which choices are better or worse? How do you justify your actions? Ethical standards depend on the systematic application of key ethical concepts. Judgments of "better" and "worse" are based on a combination of applying key ethical concepts and your past reflection and experience.

This process of ethical reasoning is very complex. We do not just memorize a few ethical theories and then apply them to problems that arise. What is a theory anyway? Rather than being a kind of special "truth" about the moral life that we can learn and simply apply, **ethical theories** are organizing structures that help us to identify important language and key concepts and provide for systematic reflection and dialogue.

Classic Ethical Theories

Two major types of ethical theories are commonly discussed in the literature: utilitarian and deontological theories (Arras & Steinbock, 1995; Beauchamp, 1982).

■ Utilitarianism

The philosophers Jeremy Bentham (1748–1832) and John Stuart Mill (1806–1873) are credited with the theory of **utilitarianism.** This theory states that actions are right to the extent that they tend to promote happiness and wrong to the extent that they tend to promote the reverse of happiness (Melden, 1967). It is a consequentialist theory in that it judges the rightness and wrongness of an action by its consequences; that is, what will happen if the action is or is not performed. One advantage of this theory is its simplicity. Only one thing needs to be considered—happiness.

Based on this theory, happiness is measurable and comparable. Some objections to this theory are that happiness is not the greatest good, that it is impossible to calculate the probable consequences of every action, and that utilitarianism conflicts with some of our basic moral intuitions (basic ideas that we have been taught). For example, slaves have a claim to be free even if others benefit from continued slavery.

Deontological Theory

Deontological theory is based on the calculation of duties (the Greek word for *duty* is "deon") rather than consequences. Immanuel Kant (1724–1804) is a famous deontological moral theorist (Kant, 1964). If you want to know if a proposed action is morally acceptable, the right question is not, "What are the consequences?" but rather, "Can I, as a rational person, consistently will that everyone in a similar situation should act the same way?" It is a type of universal golden-rule analysis. However, it is not based on individual idiosyncrasies. Rather than "Do unto others as you would have them do unto you," it is really "Do unto others as you would have anyone do unto anyone/everyone else." Another way to put the question is, "By acting this way, am I treating other people as ends in themselves (as people like me with goals and preferences), and not merely as means to my own ends or goals?"

One advantage of deontological theory is that it supports common moral intuitions about the absolute value of persons and not only the instrumental value. Disadvantages include an inability to decide among duties when they conflict and the inability to take some consideration of consequences when they seem to be particularly important. For example, it seems important to break a promise if it is necessary to save someone from severe harm.

Many people analyze the appropriateness of actions according to theology; that is, their particular beliefs about God (*theos*) and their religious traditions. When asked about a certain course of action, they turn to sacred texts that reveal standards of behavior established by God. In our pluralistic society, in which people have different religious beliefs or none at all, it is difficult to base ethical reasoning on appeals to God's word.

However, most major religious traditions support the same kinds of ethical concepts, such as principles, values, and virtues, that are involved in philosophical ethical inquiry. Furthermore, the discussion is enhanced by the rich reflection that is a part of most theological ethics.

Applying Multiple Theories

Philosophers develop and stress ethical theories in their search for an ordered set of ethical standards that can be used to assess what is right and wrong in certain circumstances. In recent years, many philosophers have come to doubt that there can be only one correct theory. They believe that it is a mistake to view the various theories as mutually exclusive claims to moral truth. Arras and Steinbock (1995) suggest that "instead, we should view them as important but partial contributions to a comprehensive, although necessarily fragmented, moral vision" (p. 9).

Ethical theories can be useful if we do not ask them to do too much. They cannot provide us with certain truth, but they can guide and direct our moral reasoning as we strive to make reliable moral judgments. For example, in Scenario 2-A, a utilitarian would examine the consequences. What would happen if I used the cardiac code? The pulmonary code? The cardiac code would maximize reimbursement. But the probable consequence of lying would be the eventual demise of the whole system, which would collapse because it would become unreliable. The closer scrutiny and the penalties for lying that would result would also have to be factored into an analysis of consequences.

A deontological theorist would analyze the duties involved. These would include the duty to tell the truth and to maintain the accuracy and integrity of the medical record. You could not rationally will that everyone alter DRG codes to maximize reimbursement. Eventually, the whole system would collapse under the weight of deception and the lack of overall reliability.

Current Ethical Approaches

Discussions of current healthcare ethics draw not only on the classic ethical theories just discussed, but also on several more current approaches.

▪ Analysis of Principles

Analysis of principles is best exemplified in Beauchamp and Childress' *Principles of Biomedical Ethics* (2001). In this work, the authors identify four core ethical principles: respect for **autonomy** (self-determination); **nonmaleficence** (not harming); **beneficence** (promoting good); and **justice** (fairness). These principles can be very helpful in understanding ethical issues in professional practice and in drafting policies regarding ethical issues. They are not nearly as helpful in clinical applications, where principles may conflict. This approach has also been criticized for its strong reliance on rules and duties and on dealing with patients and others as strangers. It has been characterized as abstract, impartial, and detached.

A principle-based analysis of Scenario 2-A would include the principles of beneficence (promoting good by maximizing the reimbursement) and nonmaleficence (avoiding possible harms that follow from lying and the eventual collapse of the system). The principle of justice supports following the rules that apply equally to all. A choice in favor of the pulmonary code respects more principles. Additionally, some would argue that it is more important to avoid harm than it is to promote good. Notice that two of the principles (beneficence and nonmaleficence) involve consequences and that the other two (respect for autonomy and justice) involve duties. One medical ethicist argues that duty-based principles always should be respected before consequence-based ones (Veatch, 1981).

▪ Analysis of Rights

Much moral discussion, especially in the United States, uses the language of rights (Dworkin, 1977). A *right* is an especially powerful moral claim that others are obligated to respect. In the United States, we speak of such basic human rights as life, liberty (freedom), and the pursuit of happiness. In healthcare ethics, scholars debate a right to die, a right to life, and a right to health care. One advantage of rights-based approaches is that they are fairly simple to apply. There are few basic rights, and they are particularly important; therefore, they automatically trump other moral considerations. However, one disadvantage is that people disagree as to which claims are basic human rights and on what basis they are determined to be so. Another disadvantage is that rights language tends to polarize debate, with one party asserting a certain right (to choice) and the other party asserting an opposing right (to life). If a right is a justified claim about what one person owes another, it may be more fruitful just to analyze the basis for the obligation in the first place. Also, rights language is not readily applicable in all situations. Scenario 2-A, for example, does not lend itself to an **analysis of rights** because there does not appear to be a violation of any basic human right.

▪ Ethics of Care

Proponents of this approach to "doing ethics" emphasize the importance of focusing on the patient and the professional in the context of his or her relationships (Gilligan, 1982; Holmes & Purdy, 1992). An **ethics of care** considers emotional commitment and a willingness of individuals in relationships to act unselfishly for the benefit of others. More than a principle-based approach, an ethics-of-care approach values sympathy, compassion, fidelity, discernment, and love. An ethics of care does not use rights language the way a principle-based approach would. The origins of the ethics-of-care approach are predominantly in theology and in some feminist writings (Larrabee, 1993; Kittay & Meyers, 1987). Although an ethics-of-care approach provides a correction to the too abstract approach of principle-based ethics, its weaknesses include the lack of a well-developed basis for providing justification for courses of action.

An ethics of care would approach Scenario 2-A by exploring the consequences of the action on the relationships between the parties involved: between the HIM professional and his or her colleagues or supervisors, between the HIM professional and the patient, and between the HIM professional and his or her family. What action best supports and nurtures these important relationships? Honesty and truth-telling are important aspects of any relationship. Deception and lack of accuracy have the potential to damage professional relationships. Although it might appear at first that the relationship with the family could depend on the HIM professional doing whatever it took to maintain his or her job, loss of integrity has the potential to backfire and breed resentment.

▪ Virtue-Based Ethics

Closely associated with an ethics of care is a **virtue-based ethics** that emphasizes the agents who perform actions and make choices (MacIntyre, 1981). A *virtue* is a habit of behaving in a good way. With this approach, one would ask, "What would a good HIM professional do?" This approach examines feelings, motivations, and duties. It not only examines actions, but the individual's character as well. For example, as stated in Chapter 1, a good HIM professional should have attitudes of respectfulness, honesty, integrity, courage, compassion, and fairness. A virtuous HIM professional's actions flow from his or her character and attitudes. The HIM professional is in the habit of behaving correctly. Critics of the virtue-based approach note that sometimes virtue is not enough. People of good character who act virtuously can sometimes perform wrong actions.

A virtue-based analysis of Scenario 2-A would ask about the character of the HIM professional involved. What does it say about the HIM professional's character if he or she is willing to lie and compromise the accuracy and integrity of the medical record to maximize reimbursement? Not only is the action wrong, but the HIM professional becomes a liar, and his or her integrity is challenged. The professional's future reputation is at stake.

The Bioethicist's Toolbox

We have reviewed two classic ethical theories and four current approaches to healthcare ethics, outlining the advantages and disadvantages of each and applying them to Scenario 2-A. It should be obvious that no one theory or approach is adequate. But do we simply pick and choose which theories and approaches to use depending on the case? How do we build a clearly reasoned argument to justify our actions?

Eric Juengst (1999) has developed a "bioethicist's toolbox," which we describe here. These tools are very useful for illustrating how we "do ethics" in clinical situations—how we analyze a problem and build a moral justification. Rather than choosing just one ethical theory or approach, aspects of each can be combined in the following ways:

1. Hammers (most powerful):
   - Appeals to shared moral maxims (rules): "Honesty is the best policy."
   - Appeals to shared moral principles: "We should promote nonmaleficence by avoiding the harms associated with deception and should respect justice by following rules equally applied to all."
   - Appeals to shared traditions: "HIM professionals have a rich history and tradition of preserving the accuracy and integrity of the medical record."
   - Appeals to nonmoral goals: "The primary purpose of the medical record (continuity of care for the patient) is enhanced by honesty and accuracy."
2. Clamps:
   - Arguments from precedent: "HIM professionals do not condone other forms of deception like postdated additions to maximize reimbursement."

- Argument by analogy: "Miscoding a diagnosis to maximize reimbursement is like adding extra notes after the fact to maximize reimbursement, which is also wrong."
- Arguments from paradigm cases: "HIM professionals have been taught about cases of fraud where DRG codes have been intentionally miscoded. This case is similar to those types of cases."
- Transcendental arguments: "All reasonable people would agree that deception is wrong if they had all the facts."

3. Wedges:
- Exposing consequences: "Deception will undermine the total system when no information is deemed reliable."
- Exposing implications: "A rationale to justify maximizing reimbursement could justify other deception with direct harm to the patient."
- Exposing inconsistencies: "A cardiac DRG might be inconsistent with medications ordered and other tests."
- Exposing biases: "Reimbursement is only one role of the medical record; putting that role first is a bias that could affect the other roles of the medical record."

4. Duct tape (not very powerful or persuasive):
- Negotiating compromises: "Only this one time."
- Appealing to procedure: "How about voting on it?"
- Passing the buck: "Let the boss decide."

5. Chewing gum (least powerful or persuasive):
- Moral introspection: "That's just the way I feel about it."
- Moral hand-wringing: "This is just awful, and it's just not right."

What if you have been reading along and you disagree with my analysis of the cases and the development of the arguments sup-

porting the choice to assign the pulmonary DRG? This disagreement is not a bad thing. It can improve both of our ethical reasoning skills. You must point out exactly where you disagree with me and tell me why. Disagreement is a necessary part of moral analysis. Confronting counterarguments and responding to them makes an argument stronger. As part of your analysis, you should always make the strongest argument possible for the other choice and then show why your original argument is stronger. If it is not, you should change your mind. What makes an argument stronger? A good argument (1) is based on good information; (2) is supported by respect for the most values, duties, or virtues or by the least infringement of key values, duties, or virtues; or (3) is supported by respect for the most important values, duties, or virtues of the HIM profession.

It is important to identify the possible sources of disagreement. People can disagree about each of the steps in the ethical decision-making process. They can disagree about the facts, the values involved, or the application of moral reasoning. The last type of disagreement is the most difficult to resolve. Resolution requires the skills of respectful attention, patience, and open inquiry.

Although a comprehensive and clear process of moral reasoning usually results in consensus, deep disagreement can still exist. Your responsibility is to be thorough and clear thinking, challenging assumptions, figuring out where disagreements lie, and striving to resolve them. But disagreement is a part of the moral life. People do hold markedly different values, and conscientious objection (withdrawing from participation in a certain situation because of personal moral beliefs) is an essential ethical concept. We must help build moral consensus when possible and respect moral freedom when it is not.

MORAL DISTRESS

Sometimes in professional practice, the ethical issue is not what the right thing to do is, but rather how to do it, given the practice environment. This type of ethical issue has been labeled *moral distress* (Jameton, 1984). For example, consider Scenario 2-B. See the end of the chapter for an ethical decision-making matrix for Scenario 2-B.

There is no question that the practices described in Scenario 2-B are wrong according to the standards of accuracy and integrity. But sometimes HIM professionals believe that by reporting unacceptable practices, they will suffer consequences, such as unsatisfactory reviews, a demotion, or even job loss. This problem is particularly distressing in rural practice, where job opportunities may be severely limited. It takes great moral courage to step up to the challenge of changing the institutional culture and practice. Several practical suggestions follow:

- Talk with trusted colleagues and get advice. Be sure that you approach problems through the proper channels and document your efforts. Confirm discussions with administration by sending memos or letters summarizing meetings. Frame issues for the institution in terms of shared values, using the professional standards that are articulated in the AHIMA Code of Ethics (AHIMA, 2004; Griffith, 1993).
- Appeal to professional sources that are locally available. Many healthcare organizations have institutional mechanisms,

such as organizational ethics committees or compliance officers.
- Don't let the practice go on unaddressed; address it in some way. Remember, you are both ethically and legally liable for the falsification described in Scenario 2-B. Ignoring the problem is not a resolution.
- Make integrity issues part of your job selection in the first place.

ETHICS RESOURCES

HIM professionals who are facing ethical issues in their practice have three main sources of help. Professionals can look in the literature for information about current ethical problems and their resolution. They can also talk with their professional colleagues about the AHIMA Code of Ethics (2004) and its implications in practice. This dialogue should be both with HIM professionals and with colleagues from other professions. Professional meetings also can be a helpful source of ethical dialogue.

As discussed earlier, ethics resources also are available in individual healthcare organizations, including patient care ethics committees. The Joint Commission on the Accreditation of Health Care Organizations (JCAHO) includes standards that require an "ethics mechanism" to help patients, families, and staff address ethical issues in clinical care. HIM professionals can bring issues to the insti-

Scenario 2-B: Retrospective Documentation to Increase Reimbursement

Your job is to analyze medical records for accuracy and completeness. Dr. Jones admits more patients to the hospital than any other surgeon. Repeatedly, you discover that Dr. Jones is adding progress notes after the patient has gone home, because these notes are added while the records are being completed in the department. However, all of the notes are signed and dated as if they were written while the patient was in the hospital. You also know, after reviewing hundreds of medical records, that several physicians add retrospective documentation to the medical record and that some of the retrospective documentation allows these physicians to get more money when they bill for services rendered for hospitalized patients. What are your reporting obligations?

tutional ethics committees for discussion and resolution. It is also helpful to have HIM professionals on ethics committees. Ethics committees are multidisciplinary committees trained in ethical concepts and analysis that help patients, families, and staff address ethical issues. They also educate the staff about ethical issues and write policies that address institutional practices.

JCAHO also requires consideration of the ethical issues that arise in the business practices of healthcare organizations. These standards have prompted healthcare organizations to develop organizational ethics committees in addition to patient care ethics committees (Worthley, 1999).

CONCLUSION

It is important that HIM professionals be able to identify ethical issues and know how to apply the ethical decision-making process to ethical issues that arise in practice and in the development of healthcare policy. Awareness of ethical theories and approaches can be helpful in understanding why some courses of action are better than others. The goal of the study of ethics is to enable HIM professionals to make reliable moral judgments, and thereby uphold the public's trust in the HIM profession.

Key Terms

- Analysis of principles
- Analysis of rights
- Autonomy
- Beneficence
- Deontological theory
- Ethical issue
- Ethical theory
- Ethics
- Ethics of care
- Justice
- Nonmaleficence
- Stakeholder
- Utilitarianism
- Virtue-based ethics

Chapter Summary

- Ethics is the formal process of intentionally and critically analyzing, with respect to clarity and consistency, the basis of one's moral judgments. It is important for HIM professionals to engage in this process, because they are accountable for their actions as professionals, not just personally.
- Ethics is necessary to resolve the potential conflicts between personal values and professional values and among professional values. It provides a formal way to step back from a conflict, search for reasons to support one choice over another, and apply this reasoning in future situations.
- The ethical decision-making process presented in this text has the following steps: (1) identify the ethical question, (2) determine the facts in the case, (3) determine what values are at stake from the perspectives of all stakeholders, (4) identify the available options in the case, (5) determine what you should do, (6) justify your choice, and (7) explore how this ethical problem might have been prevented.
- Two classic theories of ethics are utilitarianism and deontological theory. A utilitarian approach considers the consequences of an action (or failure to take action) in terms of how the action promotes happiness. A deontological approach considers whether it is one's duty to perform or not perform an action. For HIM professionals, such duties would in-

clude professional duties, including duties to the public being served and duties to one's employer or client.

- One current approach to ethics is principle-based analysis. Beauchamp and Childress have identified four core principles of biomedical ethics: respect for autonomy (self-determination), nonmaleficence (not harming), beneficence (promoting good), and justice (fairness).
- Other current approaches are analysis of rights based on consideration of whether an action affirms or violates basic human rights; an ethics of care based on what action best supports the relationships of the parties involved; and a virtue-based ethics that emphasizes how the action expresses and shapes the character of the person who performs it.
- The "bioethicist's toolbox" is a collection of ethical arguments that an HIM professional can draw upon to justify his or her actions and persuade others. According to this classification, the most powerful arguments are appeals to shared moral rules, shared moral principles, shared traditions, and nonmoral goals.
- When confronted with an ethical dilemma, the HIM professional should (1) talk with trusted colleagues and get advice, (2) approach the problem through the proper channels and document your efforts, (3) frame issues for the institution in terms of shared values and the AHIMA Code, (4) appeal to professional sources as necessary, and (5) address the issue in some way rather than letting it go on unaddressed.

References

American Health Information Management Association [AHIMA]. (2004). *AHIMA code of ethics*. Chicago, IL: Author.

Arras, J., & Steinbock, B. (1995). *Ethical issues in modern medicine*. Mountain View, CA: Mayfield.

Beauchamp, T. (1982). *Philosophical ethics: An introduction to moral philosophy*. New York: McGraw-Hill.

Beauchamp, T., & Childress, J. (2001). *Principles of biomedical ethics*. New York: Oxford University Press.

Benjamin, M., & Curtis, J. (1986). *Ethics in nursing*. New York: Oxford University Press.

Dworkin, R. (1977). *Taking rights seriously*. Cambridge, MA: Harvard University Press.

Gilligan, C. (1982). *In a different voice: Psychological theory and women's moral development*. Cambridge, MA: Harvard University Press.

Griffith, J. (1993). *The moral challenges of health care management*. Chicago, IL: Health Administration Press.

Holmes, H., & Purdy, L. (Eds.). (1992). *Feminist perspectives in medical ethics*. Bloomington: Indiana University Press.

Jameton, A. (1984). *Nursing practice: The ethical issues*. Upper Saddle River, NJ: Prentice Hall.

Juengst, E. (1999). The bioethicist's toolbox. *Centerviews: The Newsletter of the Center for Bioethics at Case Western Reserve University, 10*, 5–6.

Kant, I. (1964). *Groundwork of the metaphysic of morals*. Translated by H. J. Paton. New York: Harper & Row.

Kittay, E., & Meyers, D. (Eds.). (1987). *Women and moral theory*. Savage, MD: Rowman & Littlefield.

Larrabee, M. (Ed.). (1993). *An ethic of care: Feminist and interdisciplinary perspectives*. New York: Routledge.

Lo, B. (1995). *Resolving ethical dilemmas: A guide for clinicians*. Baltimore, MD: William & Wilkins.

MacIntyre, A. (1981). *After virtue: A study in moral theory*. Notre Dame, IN: University of Notre Dame Press.

Melden, A. (Ed.). (1967). *Ethical theories: A book of readings*. Upper Saddle River, NJ: Prentice Hall.

Purtilo, R. (1999). *Ethical dimensions in the health professions*. Philadelphia, PA: W.B. Saunders.

Veatch, R. (1981). *A theory of medical ethics*. New York: Basic Books.

Worthley, J. (1997). *The ethics of the ordinary in healthcare: Concepts and cases*. Chicago, IL: Health Administration Press.

Worthley, J. (1999). *Organizational ethics in the compliance context*. Chicago, IL: Health Administration Press.

The ethical decision-making matrix is a tool to help you organize complex, ethical problems; however, there is no simple fill-in-the-box approach to ethical decision making. The objective is to follow each step of the process and not move from the question directly to what should be done or how to prevent it next time. If you skip steps, you will not fully understand all of the values and options for action. Also, the matrix provided for each scenario in this book is not the only way to examine the problem. You can make an equally compelling ethical argument for a different decision—just be sure to follow all the steps of the matrix.

SCENARIO 2-A: DOCUMENTATION AND DRG ASSIGNMENT

Steps	Information	
1. What is the ethical question?	Which DRG code should the HIM professional assign?	
2. What are the facts?	**KNOWN**	**TO BE GATHERED**
	• Possible cardiac problems documented in the history and physical. • Cardiac catheterization performed. • Final diagnosis documented: COPD.	• What is the nature of the patient's cardiac problems? • Are there any cardiac comorbidities? (Heart and lung problems often occur together.) • What was the patient's source of pain? • Would assigning a cardiac DRG code constitute fraud? It is not clear. • What are the customary practices? If you were surveyed, what would your standard be? • What is your supervisor expecting you to do? If you are the supervisor, what is your boss expecting you to do? • How long have you been at this job? What is your relationship with your supervisor/boss? • What is the likely impact of changing jobs on your family?

3. What are the values? Examine the shared and competing values, obligations, and interests of the stakeholders (i.e., patient, HIM professional, healthcare practitioner(s), administrators, society, and other advocates) involved in order to fully understand the complexity of the ethical problem(s).	**Patient:** Values accurate documentation as basis of receiving quality care; interest in keeping costs down. **HIM professional:** Values truth, integrity, accuracy, and reliability (codes accurately and reliably rather than to maximize reimbursement); content knowledge and judgment to code cardiac versus pulmonary; other values include fairness (follow the rules and obey the law); loyalty to employer; avoid harm (inaccurate documentation may harm the patient, closing the facility will harm patients and healthcare workers); personal values (promote welfare of family, avoid loss of job); and obeying the law (fraud and abuse, duty and obligation of HIM professional to assign accurate code; comply with laws, regulations, and policies; refuse to participate or conceal unethical practices). **Healthcare professionals:** Promote welfare of patients through accurate documentation for future care; truth-telling; fairness in following rules equally for all. **Administrators:** Benefit patients and keep from harm; promote welfare of facility; maximize reimbursement without compromising truth-telling; control healthcare costs; fairness in applying rules for all. **Society:** Control costs; promote fair and just allocation of resources; follow rules of reimbursement equally for all.
4. What are my options?	Assign the cardiac DRG *OR* assign the pulmonary DRG.
5. What should I do?	If facts indicate final diagnosis is respiratory COPD and catheterization ruled out cardiac disease, then assign pulmonary DRG.

6. What justifies my choice?	**JUSTIFIED**	**NOT JUSTIFIED**
	• Code pulmonary DRG based on obligation to tell truth. • Support accuracy of the documentation. • Preserve professional integrity. Follow rules equally for all. • Respect the law. • Demonstrate loyalty to employer, unless asked to push legal boundaries.	• Assign cardiac DRG (i.e., tell a lie). • Make special exception to the rules to maximize reimbursement (not fair to others who follow rules). • DRG basis is based on aggregate, not individual cases. • Miscoding undermines the entire reimbursement system (increases costs in the long run).

7. How can I prevent this ethical problem?	• Determine if system changes are needed. • Learn more about the expensive procedures and the impact on reimbursement. • Discuss standards with colleagues and the values that support them. • Evaluate institutional integrity (at job interview and subsequently when ethical problems arise).

The ethical decision-making matrix is a tool to help you organize complex, ethical problems; however, there is no simple fill-in-the-box approach to ethical decision making. The objective is to follow each step of the process and not move from the question directly to what should be done or how to prevent it next time. If you skip steps, you will not fully understand all of the values and options for action. Also, the matrix provided for each scenario in this book is not the only way to examine the problem. You can make an equally compelling ethical argument for a different decision—just be sure to follow all the steps of the matrix.

SCENARIO 2-B: RETROSPECTIVE DOCUMENTATION TO INCREASE REIMBURSEMENT

Steps	Information	
1. What is the ethical question?	Should you try to stop the retrospective documentation?	
2. What are the facts?	**KNOWN**	**TO BE GATHERED**
	Dr. Jones admits more patients to the hospital than any other surgeon. On many occasions, Dr. Jones has added retrospective notes to the patients' records. Several other physicians also add retrospective documentation.	• Would allowing the retrospective documentation be illegal? • Are there ways in which retrospective notations could negatively affect patient treatment? • What are the customary practices in such cases? • What does your supervisor expect you to do? • What is the likely impact on self and family of changing jobs?
3. What are the values? Examine the shared and competing values, obligations, and interests of the stakeholders (i.e., patient, HIM professional, healthcare practitioner(s), administrators, society, and other advocates) involved in order to fully understand the complexity of the ethical problem(s).	**Patient:** Values accuracy of medical record. **HIM professional:** Values truth, integrity, accuracy (does not allow retrospective documentation); fairness (follow the rules and obey the law); loyalty to employer; avoid harm (inaccurate documentation could affect patient treatment and could harm welfare of the facility); personal values (promote welfare of self and family by avoiding loss of job). **Healthcare professionals:** Promote welfare of patients through accurate documentation for future care; truth-telling; fairness in following rules and obeying the law; refuse to participate or conceal unethical practices. **Administrators:** Benefit patients and keep from harm; promote welfare of facility; maximize reimbursement without compromising truth-telling; control healthcare costs; fairness in applying rules for all. **Society:** Control healthcare costs; promote fair and just allocation of resources; follow rules of documentation equally for all.	
4. What are my options?	Allow retrospective documentation to continue *OR* do not allow retrospective documentation to continue.	
5. What should I do?	Do not allow retrospective documentation.	

6. What justifies my choice?	JUSTIFIED	NOT JUSTIFIED
	• Obligation to tell the truth. • Support accuracy of the medical record. • Preserve professional integrity. • Follow rules equally for all. • Respect the law. • Demonstrate loyalty to employer, unless asked to push legal boundaries.	• Allow retrospective documentation to continue. • Make special exception to the rules to maximize reimbursement. • Not fair to others who follow rules. • Retrospective documentation jeopardizes the accuracy of medical records. • Jeopardize professional integrity.
7. How can I prevent this ethical problem?	• Determine if system changes are needed. • Learn more about retrospective documentation and its impact on record validity and reimbursement. • Discuss standards and the values that support them with colleagues. • Evaluate institutional integrity at job interview and subsequently as ethical problems arise.	

The ethical decision-making matrix is a tool to help you organize complex, ethical problems; however, there is no simple fill-in-the-box approach to ethical decision making. The objective is to follow each step of the process and not move from the question directly to what should be done or how to prevent it next time. If you skip steps, you will not fully understand all of the values and options for action. Also, the matrix provided for each scenario in this book is not the only way to examine the problem. You can make an equally compelling ethical argument for a different decision—just be sure to follow all the steps of the matrix.

APPENDIX 2-A: BLANK ETHICAL DECISION-MAKING MATRIX

Steps	Information	
1. What is the ethical question?		
2. What are the facts?	KNOWN	TO BE GATHERED
3. What are the values? Examine the shared and competing values, obligations, and interests of the stakeholders (i.e., patient, HIM professional, healthcare practitioner(s), administrators, society, and other advocates) involved in order to fully understand the complexity of the ethical problem(s).	Patient: HIM professional: Healthcare professionals: Administrators: Society: Other, as appropriate:	
4. What are my options?		
5. What should I do?		
6. What justifies my choice?	JUSTIFIED	NOT JUSTIFIED
7. How can I prevent this ethical problem?		

PRIVACY AND CONFIDENTIALITY

Laurie A. Rinehart-Thompson, JD, RHIA, CHP
Laurinda B. Harman, PhD, RHIA

Learning Objectives

After completing this chapter, the reader should be able to:

- Understand the difference between privacy and confidentiality.
- Understand that the primary ethical obligation of the health information management professional is to protect patient privacy and confidential communication.
- Discuss the practical implications of the Health Insurance Portability and Accountability Act (HIPAA) privacy requirements.
- Know and discuss release-of-information criteria, including the importance of the "need-to-know" criterion and concerns about blanket authorizations.
- Discuss patient and professional concerns about privacy and confidentiality.

Abstract

This chapter explores the primary ethical obligation of the health information management (HIM) professional to protect patient privacy and the confidential information compiled in the health information system. The complexity of balancing the protection of privacy and confidentiality with responding to legitimate requests for information is discussed, particularly in light of the Health Insurance Portability and Accountability Act (HIPAA) privacy rule. Criteria for access to information are identified. The chapter also presents an assessment of the problems with blanket authorizations. Both patient and professional concerns about privacy and confidentiality are identified.

Scenario 3-A: Family and Friends: Should I Tell?

Mary is a health information management (HIM) student completing a clinical practice rotation in an acute care hospital in her community. This week she is learning about the release-of-information process. At the breakfast table, Mary's mother asks her to find out what is wrong with Ruth, their next-door neighbor. Ruth has been admitted to the hospital twice in the last three months, and Mary's mother wants to know why. While processing the requests for release of information that afternoon, Mary comes across one from Ruth's insurance company. Mary learns that Ruth was hospitalized due to physical abuse by her husband. Mary has been in trouble with her mother recently. She knows that if she tells her mother this information, she will score "big points." She is very tempted to tell her mother the information she has learned.

Later that same day, while responding to another request for information, Mary realizes that the medical record she is reviewing belongs to Ron, her best friend's fiancé. Mary learns that Ron has a drug abuse problem and was recently diagnosed with HIV. Mary will be the maid of honor at the wedding of Ron and Patricia two months from now, and she knows that Patricia does not know about Ron's problems. Mary becomes worried and wonders whether she should tell her best friend what she has learned, because Ron's conditions could affect Patricia's health and the quality of her married life.

Questions

1. What should HIM professionals do when family or friends ask them for information about others or when they discover things about people they know during the process of doing their work? Does Mary have the right to reveal this information to others?

2. In the situation regarding Mary's friend Patricia and her fiancé Ron, would Mary be more justified in revealing patient information than in the situation regarding the next-door neighbor? Why or why not?

3. Would Mary be more justified in revealing patient information if Patricia was not her best friend, but her sister? Why or why not?

4. Why are privacy and confidentiality so important to patients who receive care and to those who provide care? Why should they be important to the HIM professionals who are entrusted to protect patient information?

The information contained in a health information system can be the most private information collected about a person. When a patient receives health care, documentation is compiled to support the decisions that are made, the care that is rendered, and the outcomes of the services provided. Telling the truth is vital to the successful delivery of appropriate health care. Yet, this can place the patient in a very vulnerable position. Intimate clinical and behavioral secrets, such as family diseases (e.g., cancer, mental illness), social habits (e.g., smoking, alcohol abuse), or previous medical events (e.g., surgeries, suicide attempts), are revealed by the patient or discovered by the provider as the care is given, as diagnostic test results are reported, and as future options for care are discussed. Information is shared and documented with trust that it will be kept private and protected from unauthorized access. The desire to keep financial information private could pale in comparison to the desire to keep private those intimate details about diseases and habits that are documented in the health information system.

Protecting privacy means that information is kept from those not authorized to access it. Health information management (HIM) students and professionals, as well as other healthcare professionals, gain access to the detailed, confidential information that is documented in every patient's medical record in the course of doing their work. This includes making sure that the medical record is accurate and complete as a legal document, that care and services are coded correctly for clinical studies and reimbursement, that information is released to authorized parties, and that the myriad of other functions that support the complex health information system are performed.

Protecting patient privacy and the confidential information collected in the health information system is the central and defining value and obligation of the HIM professional. HIM professionals would have an absolute ethical obligation to protect health information even if there were no privacy and confidentiality laws. In Scenario 3-A, the HIM student who must make decisions about releasing information requested by family and friends is challenged to stay focused on the responsibility to protect privacy and confidentiality. It can be very tempting to release this information to others, especially when harm might come to family or friends if the information was not revealed.

PRIVACY AND CONFIDENTIALITY

The terms *privacy* and *confidentiality* often are used interchangeably; however, there are im-

portant distinctions. **Privacy** is an important social value that means the right "to be let alone" (Warren & Brandeis, 1890, p.193) and is "the right of individuals to keep information about themselves from being disclosed to others; the claim of individuals to be let alone, from surveillance or interference from other individuals, organizations or the government" (Rognehaugh, 1999, p. 125). Privacy requires the protection of information—the assurance that the information is accurate and that there is no unauthorized use or disclosure of the information. The value of patient authorization is central to privacy and is inherently based on fair and appropriate use of the information.

Although the U.S. Constitution has been interpreted to give fundamental privacy rights in some areas of one's life, such as with regard to marriage or childrearing, protecting those areas to the greatest degree from government intrusion, it has not established a fundamental right of privacy for one's own medical information. Even so, the right of a patient to the protection of his or her privacy has generally been recognized by common law and has been advocated by the health information profession. Now, with the implementation of the federal HIPAA privacy law, which will be discussed at length in this chapter, privacy restrictions are much more clearly defined.

Confidential information results from a clinical relationship between patients and those providing health care. Healthcare providers, institutions, and HIM professionals are obligated to protect the use of the information that is collected. When a patient reveals information to a physician or other provider of care, there is an assumption that this information will be considered confidential and protected as such.

Personal identity is central to **confidentiality** and includes information relating to a person's healthcare history, diagnosis, condition, treatment, or evaluation. Any data or information, whether oral or recorded in any form or medium (e.g., paper, microfilm, or in computer-retrievable form), that identifies or can readily be associated with the identity of a patient and relates to a patient's health care or is obtained in the course of a patient's health care is considered to be confidential (Rognehaugh, 1999, p. 36). If the identity of the patient cannot be ascertained, the information is not confidential. For example, the number of patients with cancer of the prostate would not be considered confidential information.

RELEASE OF INFORMATION

It has been a longstanding essential principle in the health information profession that "an authorization for release of information, signed by the patient or other responsible party, is always necessary when the confidential information is to be released in the absence of any specific law to the contrary" (Huffman, 1972, pp. 395–396). This longstanding health information tenet has been reinforced by the recently enacted federal HIPAA privacy law, which is discussed in the next section. The goal of privacy protection can come into direct conflict with the goal of efficiency and the need for many parties to have access to necessary information (Gostin, 1994). The challenge is to balance the protection of the individual against the needs of a society's agencies and organizations that support healthcare activities and the need for information. As a result, the policies and procedures for the release of information must be established and enforced to ensure that all of these needs are met while protecting the privacy of the patient's information.

Today, both the number of requests for protected health information and the amount of information requested from covered entities are increasing at a phenomenal rate. Many requesters have a legitimate need for information to conduct business, and the healthcare system cannot effectively operate without releasing confidential information. HIPAA governs **requests** for protected health information that are made by individuals and organizations covered by the privacy rule. However, requests are made by covered entities and noncovered individuals and organizations. Requests frequently relate to reimbursement for healthcare services. For example, health insurers want to make sure that their healthcare dollars are being spent wisely; therefore, they have claimed the right to access the patient record—past, present, and future—to verify that medical care actually was provided and to determine the medical necessity of the services rendered. Third-party payers often require access to confidential information as a stipulation of coverage of benefits or for reimbursement. Information is given to administrative personnel, external registries and state agencies, researchers and accrediting and licensing agencies, life insurers, marketing developers, third-party insurance agencies, managed care networks, employers, and other healthcare providers (American Health Information Management Association [AHIMA], 2000).

THE HIPAA PRIVACY RULE

The protection of patient information historically resided with state laws, creating a complex and intriguing patchwork effect: Some states broadly addressed patient confidentiality, others targeted only specific types of records (e.g., HIV/AIDS and mental health) for special protection, and still other states were virtually devoid of patient confidentiality protections.

It wasn't until 1974 that a federal law was passed to protect privacy. However, the federal Privacy Act of 1974 (5 USC sec. 552a) was narrow in that it only applied to information collected by the federal government; further, it was not tailored to the protection of health information. As a result, its impact on the protection of patient information was extremely limited.

Ironically, in years past, although there were fewer laws for the protection of privacy and confidentiality, patients had far greater control over who had access to private health information and over what information was released. Fewer people sought information from a medical record, and the information was reviewed primarily by the providers of care, researchers, or those who supported important review processes, such as quality of care or risk management.

With increasing demands for access to patient information and movement toward an electronic health record, it was logical that public concern about threats to health information privacy would gain momentum and result in federal legislation directed specifically toward patient privacy. Although several bills were unsuccessfully introduced during the 1990s, federal patient privacy legislation was eventually passed by Congress and enacted into law. This was the Health Insurance Portability and Accountability Act of 1996 (HIPAA) (Pub. L. 104-191). The privacy portion of this act was passed because the limited federal patient privacy laws in existence protected only certain types of health information (e.g., drug and alcohol abuse records) or information held by certain entities (e.g., agencies of the federal government). Likewise, state laws are often limited in protecting only certain types of health information. Furthermore, state laws are inconsistent from one state to another, providing varying degrees of protection.

The result of these limited and inconsistent laws was that many types of health information—especially those not deemed to be of a highly sensitive nature—were left unprotected by statute. The only recourse individuals often had if their confidentiality was breached was through the court system, which often is an expensive, time-consuming, and emotionally exhausting experience with no guaranteed outcome. For example, if an individual lived in a state with statutes that protected only information related to behavioral health and HIV, the only recourse for the wrongful disclosure of that individual's highly personal plastic surgery records from a nonfederal healthcare provider was through the court system in that state. HIPAA, conversely, protects all health information equally and is therefore designed to increase patient privacy and confidentiality. As a result, it has caused patient privacy to become a priority as those individuals and organizations affected by it strive to comply with its requirements. It has also created a number of challenges for the healthcare industry and for the HIM profession in particular.

Protection of Patient Information

HIPAA contains five titles, most of which do not specifically address the protection of patient information. Although HIM professionals focus on the patient privacy and security aspects of HIPAA, the broader scope of the act is apparent from its name. Title I protects individuals from losing their health insurance when leaving and/or changing jobs by providing insurance continuity (portability). Titles III, IV, and V contain tax-related provisions relevant to the Internal Revenue Code and requirements for group health plans. The administrative simplification portion of Title II contains the HIPAA privacy rule, but a separate portion of that title increases the federal government's authority over fraud and abuse in the healthcare arena (accountability). Although the HIPAA statute was created and passed by Congress, the U.S. Department of Health and Human Services developed the regulations contained within the HIPAA privacy rule, which delineate the statutory requirements. In 2000, the final HIPAA privacy rule (45 CFR Parts 160 and 164) went into effect, with a compliance date of April 14, 2003.

Because of its complexity and innate relevance to the health information profession's body of knowledge, the many important provisions of the HIPAA privacy rule require additional intensive study by HIM students and professionals. However, some key provisions of the HIPAA privacy rule (hereafter referred to as "HIPAA" or the "HIPAA privacy rule") that relate to discussions in this chapter are described below.

HIPAA applies to **covered entities (CEs)** that conduct certain types of electronic transmissions. CEs include healthcare providers; healthcare clearinghouses, which process transactions between healthcare providers and their payers; and health plans (45 CFR 160.103). HIPAA also applies to **protected health information (PHI),** which is individually identifiable health information relating to an individual's past, present, or future physical or mental health condition; provision of health care; or payment for the provision of health care (45 CFR 160.103). **De-identified information,** which does not identify an individual and for which there is no reasonable basis to believe the information can be used to identify an individual (45 CFR 164.514), is not considered confidential information. For example, the number of patients with Alzheimer's disease would not be considered confidential as long as the identity of each patient could not be ascertained. This basic health information tenet has not been altered by HIPAA, and de-identified information is not protected by the HIPAA privacy rule.

Requirements for Patient Authorization

Protected health information (PHI) may be requested for legal, personal, and myriad other purposes. It is imperative that covered entities be acutely familiar and in compliance with the requirements of the HIPAA privacy rule so that each type of disclosure and use can be sorted out to determine if authorization is required, how much information can be used or disclosed, and how each type of situation should be handled. The HIPAA privacy rule provides specific requirements for patient authorization forms, including those elements that must be included in an authorization for release of information (45 CFR 164.508(c)). Although these required core elements do not differ significantly from the elements historically recommended by AHIMA as professional best practice, they now have the force and effect of federal law because of their inclusion in the HIPAA privacy rule.

- **Description of information.** This description must identify the information to be disclosed in a specific and meaningful fashion. For example, the request should specify what is wanted, such as "the discharge summary and the operative report," rather than asking for "any and all information." Providing the time frame for the information that is to be released (e.g., hospitalization from 9/5/04 to 9/10/04) also provides a more specific description of the desired information.
- **Name or other specific identification of the person(s) authorized to disclose the information.** Identifying information might include demographic data about the disclosing party, such as an address.
- **Recipient of information.** HIPAA requires that the authorization for the release of information include the specific party that is to be given the information, such as the insurance company. This information should be verified by checking the patient demographic information that is collected on admission. If the insurance company information does not match, the patient should be contacted for clarification.
- **Purpose of disclosure.** Although the HIPAA privacy rule requires that this element be present on authorizations, the patient is not required to provide a statement of purpose and "at the request of the individual" is sufficient per the HIPAA privacy rule.
- **Expiration date.** HIPAA requires that an expiration date or expiration event (e.g., at the end of the research study) be included on the authorization.
- **Signature and date.** The patient must sign and date the authorization, and the signature must be verified and compared with the signature elsewhere in the medical record, for example, on the consent-for-treatment form signed upon admission (Huffman, 1972, pp. 392–396). A patient's personal representative may sign the authorization in lieu of the patient provided that a statement is included that describes that person's authority to act for the patient. Although it is best practice for the form to be completed and dated on a date that is later than the date of the service that is being authorized for release, HIPAA does not prohibit predated authorizations as long as the information requested meets HIPAA's specificity requirement (http://www.hhs.gov/ocr/hipaa/).

HIPAA also requires an authorization for the release of PHI to include statements regarding the patient's right to revoke the authorization, the fact that treatment cannot be conditioned upon a signed authorization, and the fact that the released information is subject to redisclosure by the recipient.

Use and Disclosure

With the twin goals of giving individuals greater control over their PHI and restricting access by others, HIPAA affects both the **use and disclosure** of information by CEs. Although HIM professionals often focus on information that is released outside the organization (disclosure), HIPAA is equally concerned with the appropriate degree of access by those within the organization and what they do with that information (use). Covered entities must also comply with HIPAA in their requests for PHI.

For these three functions, HIPAA applies a "need to know" ("minimum necessary") filter on access to a patient's PHI by others (45 CFR 164.502(b)(1)). That is, no one should get or have access to any information unless they are entitled to it, and they should get only the minimal amount of information that is needed to conduct business, such as processing a claim for benefits or an insurance application. There are certain circumstances where the **minimum necessary** requirement does not apply, such as to healthcare providers for treatment; to the individual or his personal representative; pursuant to the individual's authorization; to the Secretary of the Department of Health and Human Services for investigations, compliance review, or enforcement; as required by law; or to meet other HIPAA compliance requirements (45 CFR 164.502(b)(2)).

Treatment, payment, and healthcare operations (45 CFR 164.501), collectively referred to as **TPO,** are functions of a CE that are necessary for the CE to successfully conduct business. It is not the intent of HIPAA to impose onerous rules that hinder a CE's functions. Thus, many HIPAA requirements are relaxed or removed where PHI is needed for purposes of treatment, payment, or healthcare operations.

Patient Authorization Required

Access to protected health information is needed for business decisions, but each request must be considered carefully in the context of privacy, confidentiality, and HIPAA. Not all uses and disclosures are equal; it is therefore vital for HIM professionals to apply their professional ethics and decision-making skills to each potential use and disclosure. It is also important to remember that patients should still have some control over—or at least knowledge of—the disclosures and uses of their health information. Ensuring that patients have such knowledge about their protected health information is one key purpose of the HIPAA-required **Notice of Privacy Practices.**

The HIPAA privacy rule is specific about disclosures that require a patient's authorization and those that do not. The general rule is that, unless it meets an exception where authorization is not required, patient authorization is required for the use and disclosure of PHI. Examples of disclosures that require a patient's authorization include the following:

- Release of information for a patient to obtain life or disability insurance
- Release of information in a civil action for personal injury or malpractice

Patient Authorization Not Required

Although, theoretically, one of the goals of HIPAA is to give patients a great amount of control over their PHI, this is not presently the practical effect. Once the full extent of the HIPAA exceptions is understood, it becomes clear that the breadth of the general rule is not as great as it initially appears. As described above, patient authorization is required for the use and disclosure of PHI unless such use or disclosure meets an exception provided by HIPAA. However, there are a large number of exceptions where HIPAA does not require that an individual be afforded the right to authorize the release of information before it is disclosed (45 CFR 164.502(a)). As a result, detractors of HIPAA argue that the law provides a significant number of loopholes that provide patients with no greater, or even less, control over access to their information by others than they previously possessed. 45 CFR 164.502(a)(1) delineates those circumstances (exceptions) in which a covered entity may use or disclose PHI without an individual's authorization. Keep in mind that other laws (e.g., state laws) may still require a patient's authorization. If that is the case, the more stringent or protective law must be followed and authorization must be obtained. In the situations described below, HIPAA is serving only a permissive function. Below are examples of each of the exceptions:

- Providing information to another healthcare provider where authorization may be waived for disclosures for a "treatment" purpose (as described in Example 1 later in this section) (45 CFR 164.502(a)(1)(ii));
- Releasing health information to secure reimbursement for health care where authorization may be waived for disclosures for a "payment" purpose (as described in Example 2 later in this section) (45 CFR 164.502(a)(1)(ii));
- Internal business audits ("healthcare operations") purpose under 45 CFR 164. 502(a)(1)(ii) or requests for statistical analyses, which may qualify as "healthcare operations" for which patient authorization is waived or which may not be covered under HIPAA because the information has been de-identified. Statistical analyses which qualify as research are subject to an entirely separate set of HIPAA privacy rule mandates (45 CFR sections 164.501; 164.512(i); 164.532);
- Disclosing information to the individual (164.502(a)(1)(i));
- Using or disclosing PHI where the individual had the opportunity to agree or object or, if no such opportunity was available (such as in an emergency situa-

tion), professional judgment is used to determine that such use or disclosure is in the best interest of the individual. Examples include disclosing basic patient information in the facility's directory or providing information to family members involved in the family's care (45 CFR 164.510(a) and (b));
- Disclosing information that is incidental to doing business, such as sign-in sheets at a physician's office, as long as only the minimum necessary information is disclosed (45 CFR 164.502(a)(1)(iii));
- Providing information on behalf of public interest and benefit. This exception encompasses twelve situations: public health activities; reporting victims of abuse, neglect, or domestic violence; disclosures required by law; for specified law enforcement purposes; to comply with state workers' compensation laws; health oversight activities, such as licensing agency requests; judicial and administrative proceedings; specific information about decedents; information relating to cadaveric organ, eye, or tissue donation; research; and situations where serious threats to health or safety exist (45 CFR 164.512). Additionally, given the federal government's homeland security priority, much leeway has been given to governmental entities to access individuals' protected health information for activities that have been deemed to be "specialized or essential government functions," including intelligence, counter-intelligence, and other authorized national security activities (45 CFR 164.512(k)(2)); and
- Releasing limited data sets, where certain identifiers have been removed and certain safeguards have been put into place (45 CFR 164.512(e)).

Patient authorization also is not required for federal investigations of fraud and abuse (45 CFR 164.502(a)(2)). Other situations in which a patient authorization is not required for disclosure involve **business associates,** legally separate organizations or individuals who function for or on behalf of a covered entity and whose activities involve the use or disclosure of **individually identifiable health information** (45 CFR 160.103). Examples include independent transcription companies, a hospital's external legal counsel, or accrediting bodies such as the JCAHO. Although HIPAA does not require a patient's authorization before protected health information is disclosed, a covered entity must have a contract with a business associate, called a *business associate agreement,* in place with each business associate to ensure the confidentiality of information when it is in the hands of that business associate.

Individuals will differ on the wisdom of those exceptions that have been placed into the law. For example, many of HIPAA's protective authorization requirements are relaxed or removed in order to permit a CE to perform the functions of treatment, payment, and operations (45 CFR 164.502(a)(1)). The effect of HIPAA is that it has, in some cases, facilitated the flow of patient information where industry standards previously dictated a tighter control. This has left many CEs feeling uneasy and, as a result, maintaining the stricter standards—where they can—that they established and practiced prior to the implementation of HIPAA. Following are two examples where HIPAA's authorization requirement is more relaxed than the procedures exercised by many HIM professionals.

- **Example 1.** Under the HIPAA privacy rule, a hospital (CE) is not required to procure a patient's authorization before sending records from the patient's hospital stay to a physician who is following up with that patient (treatment purposes). Although many hospitals, in accordance with prior policy, will continue to require an authorization in a situation such as the one described, HIPAA has nonetheless removed that requirement. It is also worth noting that the "minimum necessary requirement" does not apply when PHI is disclosed for treatment purposes, although CEs will want to exercise caution.
- **Example 2.** Under the HIPAA privacy rule, a healthcare provider (CE) is not required to procure a patient's authorization before sending records from a patient's visit to the patient's health insurance company for payment purposes. Again, many providers will continue to require an authorization in accordance with their prior policies; however, it is not required per the HIPAA privacy rule. It is noted that the minimum necessary requirement does apply to disclosures made for payment purposes.

BLANKET AUTHORIZATIONS

Blanket authorizations have traditionally been used by covered entities upon a patient's first visit to a facility or at the outset of each visit. These authorizations, which are referred to by various titles, have sometimes been incorporated into general consent-for-treatment forms. They are often signed by patients prior to the creation of health information and are generally for the release of information to Medicare and other insurers. Blanket authorizations must be given special consideration in light of the specific authorization requirements discussed earlier in the chapter that the HIPAA privacy rule has imposed.

Problems have always accompanied blanket authorizations because of their general nature. First, the circumstances under which patients sign them may be viewed as coercive in nature. Furthermore, patients may unintentionally authorize the release of information about care that was rendered after the authorization date *or* they may not realize, at the time of signing, the significance of what they are signing and what may eventually be released.

A one-time blanket authorization signed by a patient that permits the release of "any and all" information is not permissible under HIPAA because it does not meet the requirement that the authorization be described in a specific and meaningful fashion. Furthermore, although an authorization signed before care is rendered is not a HIPAA violation as long as the form meets the specificity requirements of HIPAA (http://www.hhs.gov/ocr/hipaa/), a covered entity must nonetheless carefully consider that patients cannot truly protect their right to privacy if they approve the release of something about themselves that hasn't occurred yet. For example, a patient may be asked—without violating HIPAA—to sign a blanket authorization upon hospital admission that allows all information from that particular stay to be released to the patient's insurance company. However, a history and physical that are created later during that admission may include documentation about the results of a previous genetic test that has nothing to do with the reason for this admission, but could result in cancellation of the policy if it is disclosed to the insurance company. For this reason, HIM professionals must carefully develop policies so as to be mindful of both the specific requirements and the spirit of the HIPAA privacy rule, as well as their professional ethical obligations.

HIM professionals must also be mindful of the fact that, under HIPAA, not even a blanket authorization is required for the release of information for payment purposes, because TPO is an exception to the patient authorization requirement (45 CFR 164.502 (a)(1)). However, because the "minimum necessary" principle does apply, care should be taken to disclose only that information which is necessary for the covered entity to receive payment. Therefore, policies should be developed accordingly.

PATIENT CONCERNS

In today's electronic environment, protecting privacy has become extremely difficult, and patients are becoming increasingly concerned about the loss of privacy and their inability to control the dissemination of their personal information. "It's not that the laws or ethical codes are being repealed—it's that broad technological, scientific, and economic forces are overpowering the old rules" (Allen, 1998). Patients expect that their information will be kept private and that they alone will decide who has access and what information is revealed; however, they cannot assume that the information in their medical records is private and their own business. Information that is faxed or e-mailed from one healthcare location to another may be left unattended for unauthorized people to see. Although HIPAA includes oral communications within its purview (and such violations are therefore subject to HIPAA's penalties), problems still exist with providers of care discussing cases in hospital elevators, eating areas, and other public venues within a facility. The patients that are being discussed could be (and often are) the friends and families of those within hearing distance of the conversation.

As patients become more aware of the misuses of information, they may become reluctant to share information with their healthcare team. This may, in turn, result in problems with the health care that is provided and the information given to researchers, insurers, the government, and the many other stakeholders who legitimately gain access to the information. Public opinion polls have confirmed these patient fears; although patients feel that providers of care can be trusted, they are concerned about insurers and employers having access to this information, especially if they think that the information will be used for decisions such as demotion, loss of employment, or denial of insurance (Harris-Equifax, 1993; Equifax-Harris, 1995). Whereas, historically, the patient was the least likely to gain access to his or her own information, this fortunately has changed. HIPAA, through one of its guaranteed individual rights, grants patients the right to access their own PHI (45 CFR 164.524). Other HIPAA individual rights include the right to request an amendment to one's records to clarify inaccurate or incomplete documentation (45 CFR 164.526); to request an accounting of disclosures (45 CFR 164.528); to request restrictions of uses and disclosures (45 CFR 164.522(a)); to request confidential communications (45 CFR 164.522(b)); to receive a Notice of Privacy Practices (45 CFR 164.520); and to make complaints regarding perceived HIPAA privacy rule violations (45 CFR 160.306).

Because HIPAA provides a "floor" (i.e., minimum individual rights), state laws that provide patients with even greater control, including access, over their PHI will supersede HIPAA. As patients become more aware of their individual rights, as delineated under HIPAA, they may eventually exercise those rights and use them to make informed choices about the healthcare decisions that must be made and to assess whether the information is accurate. As patients learn more about the information that is collected, analyzed, and disseminated, they will increasingly want access to that information and will seek the assistance of the HIM professional. Evidence of patient awareness is becoming apparent as individuals file complaints with the federal government via the Office of Civil Rights (OCR), Department of Health and Human Services, regarding alleged violations of the HIPAA privacy rule. As of April 2004, per Linda Sanches, a senior advisor on HIPAA privacy at the Department of Health and Human Services' OCR, over 5,000 complaints had been filed with OCR ("Dispelling the HIPAA Myths," AHIMA Audioseminar, April 13, 2004). This reflects a trend toward consumer empowerment with respect to individuals' own health information.

PROFESSIONAL CONCERNS

AHIMA has taken a proactive approach that encouraged support for, and eventual passage of, federal patient privacy legislation. AHIMA supports the HIPAA principles of patient access; restrictions on the collection, use, and disclosure of patient information; notifying patients of information practices; assuring security safeguards; and providing for penalties for violations (AHIMA, 1999).

Proponents for national health privacy policies identify seven issues that collectively make a solid foundation for ensuring that an individual's health record is secure, accessible to that individual, released only by appropriate authorization, and protected from unauthorized use. These components include allowing patients access to their own health record so that they can make informed decisions about the release of their health information; giving patients the

opportunity to decide who, how, and when their health record can be used; notifying individuals of when and how individuals should be notified about how their medical records are used; assuring that HIM professionals have enough guidance when making decisions about releasing information; securing both paper and electronic storage media; protecting patient privacy and providing adequate information to promote the health and safety of humankind; and addressing issues related to access by law enforcement and penalties for violations (Health Privacy Project, 2004).

ETHICAL CHALLENGES

Although the HIPAA privacy rule has spelled out very specific requirements that differentiate lawful uses and disclosures from those that violate the law, situations such as those presented in this chapter's scenario demonstrate that the language of a law can neither anticipate nor address every possible situation. It is within these voids that ethics must prevail and guide our decisions. Even then, personal and professional ethics may conflict with one another. The AHIMA Code of Ethics states that

> "Professional responsibilities often require an individual to move beyond personal values. For example, an individual might demonstrate behaviors that are based on the values of honesty, providing service to others, or demonstrating loyalty. In addition to these, professional values might require promoting confidentiality. . . . Professional values could require a more comprehensive set of values than what an individual needs to be an ethical agent in their personal lives. . . . Ethical responsibilities flow from all human relationships, from the personal and familial to the social and professional. Further, the AHIMA Code of Ethics does not specify which values, principles, and guidelines are the most important and ought to outweigh others in instances when they conflict" (AHIMA, 2004).

The considerations presented in the Code of Ethics, without a specific list of permitted and prohibited behaviors, leads an individual to balance conflicts and obligations internally in order to reach the most appropriate decision in any given situation.

The HIPAA privacy rule has challenged HIM professionals with new ethical issues. While trying to meet HIPAA's mandates to protect patient privacy and give patients the rights they are legally entitled with regard to their PHI, CEs also continue to conduct business as efficiently as possible. Consider the following ethical question:

A CE may ask, "Does a particular activity qualify as a healthcare operation?" If it does, HIPAA's authorization and accounting of disclosure requirements—which can be time-consuming and burdensome—need not be met. For that reason, it is tempting to pigeonhole an activity into such a category. However, it is not ethical to intentionally define an activity as a healthcare operation simply to avoid HIPAA's administrative requirements.

Indeed, HIPAA has caused new ethical issues to emerge. As covered entities and their HIM professionals attempt to develop policies and procedures that balance all of these needs, they will continue to seek advice from the Department of Health and Human Services' Office of Civil Rights in an effort to best comply with HIPAA.

CONCLUSION

The protection of private and confidential information is difficult, but not impossible. The privacy of health information has been an increasingly important national policy initiative over the last several years, culminating in the passage of the HIPAA privacy rule. In addition, many honest, ethical people work every day of their lives to protect information out of a sense of respect and professionalism. The responsibility of the HIM professional is to keep current with mandates in order to protect the entrusted information.

The HIM professional serves as the patient's advocate in the preservation and protection of the information entrusted to the physician and other providers of care. He or she has access to extremely private and confidential information, and other parties who are unfamiliar with the proper disclosure policies for this information may attempt to gain inappropriate access to it. The patient, the healthcare team, and the many parties who seek information from the information system must be able to trust the HIM professional to handle their requests with both technical and ethical expertise.

Responsibility to protect patient privacy and the confidential information in the health information system engages the ethical principles of respect for autonomy (self-determination to decide what information is or is not released), nonmaleficence (not harming or potentially causing discrimination), beneficence (promoting good and providing the necessary information for an appropriate release), and justice (fairness in the appropriate use of the information). If access is inappropriately granted, the action will be in clear violation of ethical principles (beneficence and nonmaleficence), values (need to know, integrity, and courage), and professional responsibilities (reliability). Protecting patient information is an honorable responsibility with evolving complexities.

Key Terms

- Blanket authorization
- Business associate (BA)
- Confidentiality
- Covered entities (CEs)
- De-identified information
- Individually identifiable health information
- Minimum necessary
- Notice of Privacy Practices
- Privacy
- Protected health information (PHI)
- Requests
- Treatment, payment, and healthcare operations (TPO)
- Use and disclosure

Chapter Summary

- Privacy is the right to be let alone or the right to decide what information is released to others.
- Confidential information is compiled during the course of caring for a patient and must be protected by providers of care, HIM professionals, and all others who have legitimate access to information.
- A primary ethical obligation of the HIM professional is to protect patient privacy and the confidential information documented in the health information system.
- There must be a constant balancing between protecting privacy and releasing information, in accordance with federal privacy legislation, to authorized users so that business functions that support health care can be accomplished.
- Several important criteria should be used when evaluating requests for the release of information, including the "need-to-know" (minimum necessary) criterion.
- Patients, HIM professionals, and legislative representatives are concerned about privacy and confidentiality. This concern has provided the impetus for passage of the Health Insurance Portability and Accountability Act of 1996 (HIPAA), which focuses in part on the privacy and security of patient information.

References

Allen, A. (1998). Exposed. *Washington Post,* February 8. Retrieved August 15, 2005, from http://www.washingtonpost.com/wp-srv/national/longterm/exposed.

American Health Information Management Association [AHIMA]. (1999). *Confidentiality of medical records: A situation analysis and AHIMA's position.* Retrieved August 15, 2005, from http:// library.ahima.org/xpedio/groups/public/documents/ ahima/pub_bok2_000623.html.

American Health Information Management Association [AHIMA]. (2000). *Flow of patient health information inside and outside the healthcare industry.* Retrieved August 15, 2005, from http://library.ahima.org/xpedio/groups/public/documents/ahima/bok1_018217.pdf #page%3D1

American Health Information Management Association [AHIMA]. (2004). *AHIMA code of ethics.* Chicago, IL: Author.

American Health Information Management Association [AHIMA]. (2004). *Dispelling the HIPAA myths.* Audioseminar, Linda Sanches, presenter. Office of Civil Rights, Department of Health and Human Services.

Equifax-Harris. (1995). *Equifax-Harris mid-decade consumer privacy survey.* New York: Louis Harris and Associates.

Gostin, L. O. (1994). Health information privacy. *Cornell Law Review, 80*(3), 451–528.

Harman, L. B., DeWald, L. A., & Vollgraff-Rushton, D. (2001). *Privacy and confidentiality in ethical challenges in the management of health information.* Gaithersburg, MD: Aspen.

Harris-Equifax. (1993). *Harris-Equifax health information privacy survey 1993.* Atlanta, GA: Equifax Inc.

Health Privacy Project. (2000). *Key health privacy issues.* Retrieved September 22, 2004, from http://www.healthprivacy.org/usr_doc/Privacy Rights.pdf.

Huffman, E. K. (1972). *Medical record management.* Berwyn, IL: Physicians' Record Company.

Office of Civil Rights, Department of Health and Human Services. (2005). *Medical privacy—national standards to protect the privacy of personal health information.* Retrieved September 22, 2004, from http://www.hhs.gov/ocr/hipaa/.

Rognehaugh, R. (1999). *The health information technology dictionary.* Gaithersburg, MD: Aspen.

Standards for Privacy of Individually Identifiable Health Information. 45 CFR Parts 160 and 164. April 17, 2003.

Warren, S. D., & Brandeis, L. D. (1890). The right to privacy. *Harvard Law Review, 4,* 193.

The ethical decision-making matrix is a tool to help you organize complex, ethical problems; however, there is no simple fill-in-the-box approach to ethical decision-making. The objective is to follow each step of the process and not move from the question directly to what should be done or how to prevent it next time. If you skip steps, you will not fully understand all of the values and options for action. Also, the matrix provided for each scenario in this book is not the only way to examine the problem. You can make an equally compelling ethical argument for a different decision—just be sure to follow all the steps of the matrix.

SCENARIO 3-A: FAMILY AND FRIENDS: SHOULD I TELL?

Steps	Information	
1. What is the ethical question?	Should Mary tell her mother about Ruth being abused? Should Mary tell Patricia about Ron's drug problem and HIV+ status?	
2. What are the facts?	**KNOWN**	**TO BE GATHERED**
	• Ruth is hospitalized because of physical abuse by her husband. • Ron's medical record indicates a drug abuse problem. • Ron has been diagnosed with HIV.	• Would Mary violate confidentiality by telling her mother about Ruth? • May Mary act on her knowledge in any way? • If Mary contacted Ruth directly and discussed the abuse, without acknowledging that she learned this information from Ruth's medical record, would this be acceptable? • Would Mary violate confidentiality by telling Patricia about Ron? • Is it certain that Ron did not contract the HIV disease from Patricia? • Does Patricia already know about Ron's diseases, but she wants to marry him anyway? • What are the customary practices in this situation?
3. What are the values? Examine the shared and competing values, obligations, and interests of the stakeholders (i.e., patient, HIM professional, health-care practitioner(s), administrators, society, and other advocates) involved in order to fully understand the complexity of the ethical problem(s).	**Patient:** Right to privacy and confidentiality of medical and health information; moral obligation to society not to transmit communicable disease. **HIM professional:** Integrity (protect patient's confidentiality); protect information (information learned in the course of professional work cannot be shared with others); avoid harm (could be caused by others not knowing); fairness (follow the rules); legal (obligations regarding privacy and confidentiality); burden of knowledge of information that could affect someone negatively. **Healthcare professionals:** Preservation of confidential information. **Administrators:** Legal obligations regarding protection of privacy and confidentiality. **Society:** Desire to be kept from harm; need for privacy and confidentiality of medical information.	

4. What are my options?	• Refuse to reveal information to family and friends. • Tell the mother about the neighbor's abuse. • Tell the friend about the fiancé's drug addiction and HIV disease. • Approach the neighbor to encourage her to seek help; approach the fiancé to encourage him to seek treatment. • Consult with faculty or clinical supervisor.	
5. What should I do?	Protect information and do not reveal what has been learned to family and friends; maintain patient confidentiality by keeping information about patients private.	
6. What justifies my choice?	**JUSTIFIED**	**NOT JUSTIFIED**
	• Follow rules of patient confidentiality. • Respect patient privacy. • Preserve integrity of the information system. • Avoid possible legal ramifications of breaking confidentiality.	• Tell mother about neighbor's information discovered in the medical record. • Make exception to the rules of confidentiality to get in good favor with mother. • Risk lawsuit due to violation of privacy. • Tell friend about fiancé's drug problem and HIV disease. • Make an exception to the rules of confidentiality.
7. How can I prevent this ethical problem?	• Make sure that educational programs address the special issues related to reviewing health information for family and friends during the course of work. • Change the system so that HIM professionals do not work with the medical records of people they know.	

USES OF HEALTH INFORMATION

Part II explores privacy and confidentiality within the context of the many uses of health information. Chapter 4 reviews the traditional and current regulations, acts, statutes, standards, and penalties related to compliance, fraud, and abuse. Chapter 5 covers ethical dilemmas faced in the process of clinical code selection and use. Professional practice solutions are offered and future ethical issues are presented. Chapter 6 presents quality-management challenges and reviews the importance of patient safety and organizational values. Chapter 7 addresses the importance of research and decision support for data acquisition, access, and reporting and reviews the role of the research specialist, decision support specialist, and institutional review board (IRB). Chapter 8 addresses the management of health information in the field of public health and includes a framework that addresses difficult policy choices when patient information should be reported to government health authorities. The competing interests when trying to meet the needs of society versus the individual's right to privacy are analyzed. Chapter 9 discusses the ethical issues of pricing, access, and quality and the HIM professional's role in the managed care environment, including the importance of advocacy for the patient and the organization and the need for federal legislation. Chapter 10 includes the importance of health information when making clinical care decisions, with a focus on those at the end of life. Chapter 10 reviews ethical issues related to autonomy, beneficence, advance care planning, palliative care, and ethics committees.

Learning Objectives

After completing this chapter, the reader should be able to:

- Discuss the laws and penalties concerning fraud and abuse in health care.
- Identify the responsibilities and liabilities of the health information management (HIM) professional in relation to those laws.
- Identify roles of the HIM professional in establishing compliance programs and meeting the requirements of the Health Insurance Portability and Accountability Act of 1996 (HIPAA).

COMPLIANCE, FRAUD, AND ABUSE

Laurie A. Rinehart-Thompson, JD, RHIA, CHP

Abstract

The health information management (HIM) professional is a key player in the process that begins with the delivery of care to a patient and leads to the submission of a bill for reimbursement for the services provided. One of the HIM professional's major responsibilities is facilitating the collection of the appropriate information needed to properly assign the correct clinical classification codes to the care provided. This process and responsibility sounds straightforward, but either through dishonest motivations to collect more money than properly owed or sloppy procedures and failure to accept responsibility for staying current and informed, the HIM professional can become involved in, and responsible for, submission of a false claim. The penalties are real and expensive and can include prison terms. The HIM professional must have knowledge of the applicable guidelines and an appreciation and understanding of the requisite compliance programs for hospitals, physicians, home health agencies, long-term care facilities, laboratories, and third-party payers. This chapter outlines the laws, penalties, and preventive programs that an HIM professional should be familiar with.

Scenario 4-A: Documentation Does Not Justify Billed Procedure

An active practice of physicians specializing in infertility regularly admits patients to the outpatient surgical department. The practice is a significant source of revenues for the hospital. The physicians perform laparoscopy on many of their patients. This procedure can be performed to determine the extent of endometriosis that is causing the patient pain or to determine the effect of the endometriosis on the patient's current infertile state. Treatment for infertility is not a covered component of the patient's federally reimbursed healthcare plan. Allison, the new HIM director, has come to realize that the physicians' documentation for this procedure always refers only to endometriosis, even when, for example, the nurses' notes repeatedly mention that the patient gives, as the reason for the procedure, to "find out why she is not pregnant."

Questions

1. What should Allison do if she is aware that the documentation in the medical record does not reflect the true underlying reason for a procedure?

2. What should Allison do if the physicians insist that she code only endometriosis, with no reference to infertility? Should she defer to the physicians on this issue, because physician documentation is the only source documentation that coders may code from?

A completed ethical decision-making matrix for the scenario is provided at the end of the chapter.

A critical function in every healthcare provider organization is to ensure that the operation of the HIM department supports ethical and accurate processes to document the care provided to patients, to assign appropriate clinical codes, and to manage health information in a responsible and timely manner. This has always been an important responsibility of the HIM professional, and it is even more important now as government actions to eliminate fraud and abuse have increased.

It is important to understand the distinction between healthcare fraud and healthcare abuse, which are often discussed in tandem, and which most generally relate to federally funded programs. In the healthcare context, **fraud** is defined as knowingly "making false statements or representations of material facts to obtain a benefit or payment for which no entitlement would otherwise exist." **Abuse** is defined as using "practices that are inconsistent with accepted medical practice and directly or indirectly result in unnecessary costs to the Medicare program" (Abdelhak, 2001, p. 636). In 1997, the Office of the Inspector General (OIG) for the U.S. Department of Health and Human Services invited healthcare providers to join the OIG in a national campaign to eliminate fraud and abuse from federal healthcare programs. The agenda included development of compliance guidelines for healthcare sectors, mechanisms to promote self-disclosure of improper conduct, and increased awareness of the sanctions that might be imposed for fraudulent behavior. The goal was to protect the financial integrity of the federal healthcare programs. Three years later, the OIG reported substantial progress toward those objectives (Brown, 2000). The 1999 Accountability Report of the U.S. General Accounting Office (GAO, 1999) stated that more than $2.2 billion was saved during fiscal years 1998 and 1999 from healthcare fraud-related activities. An additional demonstration of the seriousness of the government's intention to combat healthcare fraud was the increase in funding for the number of Federal Bureau of Investigation (FBI) agents assigned to healthcare fraud investigations. In 1992, only 111 agents were assigned to healthcare fraud investigational activities. This number grew to 420 agents in 1998 through increased funding provided as a component of the **Health Insurance Portability and Accountability Act of 1996 (HIPAA).** The effect of these efforts are apparent. In a 2003 joint annual report from the Department of Health and Human Services and the Department of Justice Health Care Fraud and Abuse Control Program, it was cited that federal prosecutors filed criminal indictments in 361 healthcare fraud cases in fiscal year 2002. The struggle by healthcare providers to comply with public and private reimbursement programs can be additionally complicated by physicians' responsibility to consider their commitment to the Hippocratic Oath. Putting the patient's welfare first, while still complying with reimbursement policies, may not always seem possible. One survey of 720 physicians asked if the physicians deceived insurers "sometimes" or more often. Forty percent of the respondents said that they found ways around the rules and regulations of third-party payers to benefit their patients. Terms such as manipulation, fudging, and gaming the system were used to describe the behavior (Prophet, 1997).

HIM professionals, because they manage functions that rely on the documentation and assertions of the physician, are challenged as well. The coding staff's use of the physician's documentation to assign codes used for billing purposes is a key link in the submission of the bill for patient care to the third-party payer.

Given the OIG fraud and abuse campaign, it is essential that HIM professionals

- Ensure that documentation processes capture accurate and timely information
- Code all diagnoses and services accurately
- Refuse to code inaccurately due to pressures to capture more money for the facility
- Manage information in a timely and responsible manner
- Clarify documentation and assertions of the providers if there appear to be inconsistencies
- Maintain awareness of requirements for coding and documentation as set forth by governmental, regulatory, and professional groups

HIM professionals have a crucial role and responsibility in preventing unethical and fraudulent behavior.

TRADITIONAL REGULATIONS THAT GUIDE HIM PROFESSIONALS

A wide range of statutes, regulations, and programs addresses the subject of fraud, abuse, and compliance. The HIM professional must have a general understanding of this subject to fulfill a responsible leadership role in the management of HIM or compliance processes in a healthcare organization.

False Claims Act

Suppose that the owner of a medical clinic and the clinic manager frequently submit claims for reimbursement as if diagnostic tests had been ordered and interpreted by physicians at the clinic, even though they actually have not been ordered or performed. The HIM professional at the clinic is presented with records that appear to be actual visits, the coder in the health information department assigns the appropriate codes for the tests as documented in the records, and Medicare pays over $100,000 for the billings.

The 1986 **False Claims Act** (FCA; 18 U.S.C. §§287 & 1001, 31 U.S.C. §3729; 42 U.S.C. #§1320a-7a) prohibits the presentation of such false or fraudulent claims to the government. Anyone who knowingly makes such a claim may be subject to criminal, civil, or administrative liability. The False Claims Act was enacted during the Civil War to target vendors who supplied the Union with inferior products or cheated the government. The general nature of the statute extends to, and is applied in, the current reimbursement environment of health care. Title 42, section 1320a-7b(a) of the U.S. Code, adds criminal penalties that subject the violator to prison, fines, and mandatory exclusion from federal healthcare programs, including state (Medicaid) programs. In the previous case, the clinic owner and clinic manager, if convicted, could each face a maximum sentence of five years in prison and a $250,000 fine.

The statute qualifies that the submission of false or fraudulent claims must be done "knowingly" to result in a violation (Wagg, 2000). *Knowingly* is defined by *Black's Law Dictionary* (1991) as "With knowledge; consciously; intelligently; willfully; intentionally. An individual acts 'knowingly' when he acts with awareness of the nature of his conduct" (p. 693). This awareness has been described as meaning (1) actual knowledge of the falseness or fraudulence of the claim, (2) deliberate ignorance of the truth, or (3) reckless disregard for the truth (Prophet, 1997).

The Department of Justice (DOJ) has said that intent to defraud is not required for a claim to be considered a false claim. Simply acting in deliberate ignorance of the truth or with reckless disregard for the truth is within the realm of the statute (Wagg, 2000). Although the DOJ has stated that it is not targeting honest billing mistakes or mere negligence (Reno, 1998), ignorance of the law is not considered to be a defense. The DOJ issued guidelines for use of the False Claims Act in 1998. These guidelines outline the conditions for determining whether a false claim exists and whether the provider knowingly submitted the false claims. The DOJ must consider any information bearing on the provider's state of mind in submitting the false claims (U.S. Department of Justice, 1998, p. 459).

The HIM professional has a responsibility to obtain, analyze, and apply the available transmittals from the government regarding documentation and reimbursement guidelines as well as the official coding guidelines, Coding Clinic, published by the American Hospital Association. Failure to accept and apply these responsibilities could fall into the interpretations for "deliberate ignorance or reckless disregard for the truth."

In Scenario 4-A, the clinic manager and owner are guilty of violating the False Claims Act because they have knowingly submitted false claims to a government-sponsored program, Medicare; thus, they have violated the statute. Might the HIM professional also be liable? If the HIM professional did not know that the claims were false, he or she would not be liable. However, the False Claims Act says that acting in deliberate disregard for the truth can be considered to be in violation of the act. If it could be shown that the HIM professional should have known that the tests did not occur—if, for instance, it could be shown that procedures to reconcile records with registration lists were considered a standard practice of HIM departments, and if the HIM professional had no such procedures in place—he or she could indeed be liable.

Qui Tam Statutes

Suppose that an HIM department does not consistently enforce the coding guidelines published for the organization. The coders know that the chief financial officer wants a higher case-mix index to result from the inpatient cases coded and has been known to state that raises may be in order if the case mix, and subsequently reimbursement, improves. Several of the coders have decided that they want to do whatever it takes to get a raise, and they are inappropriately assigning codes that result in a higher DRG for the hospital. One of the other coders knows about this activity and informs the HIM department director. The director says she will look into the situation, but the practice continues. Frustrated that the department director appears to not want to deal with this, the coder initiates a "whistle-blower," or *qui tam,* lawsuit under the False Claims Act.

Qui tam statutes provide a means for private individuals, called *relators,* to bring lawsuits under the False Claims Act alleging that an individual or organization has committed fraudulent behavior against the government. The case brought by the private individual is reviewed by the DOJ. The DOJ then decides whether it will join the case as a co-plaintiff. When the DOJ joins the case, the relator still receives a percentage of the funds recovered. Even if the DOJ declines the case, the individual can proceed on his or her own. Deferral of the case by the DOJ, however, can be a sign that the case is not strong enough to prevail. If the private individual, or "whistle-blower," decides to proceed without the DOJ's participation, then he or she must independently fund the legal actions. Because the legal expenses for a qui tam case can be very costly, it is difficult to proceed without the DOJ's participation. Few cases continue if the DOJ does not join the action.

The number of qui tam suits rose from 17 in 1992 to over 178 in 1996 (Stringer, 1998). The relator can be any person with knowledge of fraudulent behavior. Employees are protected from retribution, and the relator is frequently a disgruntled staff person. In a major civil case brought by the DOJ against Columbia/HCA Healthcare Corporation, a portion of the charges were brought with the assistance of "whistle-blowers," who testified that the company had inappropriately assigned DRGs to cases that were not substantiated by the patient's documented care.

According to the Health and Human Services OIG's semiannual report to Congress in 2004, outlays of $631 million and $840 million by Columbia/HCA Healthcare Corporation represent the largest total recovery for healthcare fraud from any single provider. Again, this case illustrates the role of the HIM professional to establish appropriate coding guidelines and ensure that the coding function submits only those codes that truly reflect the patient's condition or the care provided.

Qui tam suits pose two challenges. The first is the clear responsibility of the HIM professional to manage the health information processes in an accurate, ethical manner and to ensure that compliance with regulations, policies, and procedures occurs. The second challenge is to establish fair, consistent personnel policies to decrease the incidence of disgruntled employees. An unhappy employee who brings a false charge of wrongdoing can rob the HIM professional and institution of time and money that could be better used.

Voluntary Disclosure Protocol

Suppose that a hospital's medical records department changes the patient type on a case from "Inpatient" to "Observation" status after discharge if the patient is discharged in less than 23 hours. The director of the hospital's health information system professional attends a seminar and learns that the decision of the physician to admit the patient as an inpatient cannot be retroactively changed to "observation" if the initial intent was to admit the patient. The fact that the patient stayed less than 23 hours is irrelevant. But the department has been changing patient types like this for over a year.

In October 1998, the OIG implemented a protocol to self-disclose fraudulent conduct that can help HIM professionals who find themselves in situations like this one. This protocol furthers the intent of the OIG to work with the healthcare industry to help identify and resolve irregularities that adversely affect federal healthcare programs as defined in Title 42, section 1320a-7b(f) of the U.S. Code. The goal of the protocol is to remove the disincentives that accompany self-disclosure of wrongdoing. According to then Inspector General June Gibbs Brown,

> In establishing this new guidance, we are renewing our commitment to promote an environment of openness and cooperation. We believe that we must continue to encourage the health care industry to conduct voluntary self-evaluations and provide viable opportunities for self-disclosure. The government alone cannot successfully win the battle against health care fraud; health care providers must be enlisted in this effort. (quoted in OIG, 1998b, p. 2)

Although the protocol does not protect an entity from civil or criminal action under the False Claims Act, it does advise that self-reporting can be considered as a positive mitigating factor when the OIG makes recommendations to prosecuting agencies. By self-reporting, an organization can avoid a full-scale audit, which can be costly and disruptive. Self-reporting also offers the opportunity to negotiate the monetary settlement and to avoid exclusion from further participation in federal healthcare programs. The protocol should be used only for instances involving possible fraudulent behavior where the provider has reason to believe that the fraudulent behavior, either by an employee or the entity, has occurred. Self-reporting usually falls into one of three categories that determine the route of reporting:

1. If the finding is one of an isolated occasional mistake, with no pattern, the provider should simply return the overpayment to the Medicare contractor (regional fiscal intermediary who pays Medicare claims) and there will be no sanction.

2. If there is a pattern of abuse, but with no intent, just ignorance or misinformation, the provider should return the overpayment to the Medicare contractor as a voluntary refund. The contractor, not the OIG, will then review the circumstances. If the contractor determines that the provider knew, had reason to know, or should have suspected fraud, the contractor may decide to refer the case to the OIG (Reinhardt, 2000).

3. If the fraudulent billing was done with actual knowledge of the falseness, deliberate ignorance, or reckless disregard, the self-disclosure should go to the OIG.

Negotiations with the OIG may result in the imposition of a **Corporate Integrity Agreement (CIA).** When such an agreement is reached, the provider must meet certain government-imposed requirements to ensure the provider's ongoing compliance. Typically, the CIA will include an annual audit of billing or other operations by designated auditors. It usually also specifies obligations that must be met by the provider's own compliance plan activities. The majority of audits include review of the documentation maintained in the medical record as a basis for determining the appropriateness of assigned codes directly affecting the amount of reimbursement. CIAs may be imposed only by the OIG, not by the Medicare contractor.

The HIM professional may be involved in these types of audits as a management person who either facilitates arrangements for the audit or conducts the audit. The HIM professional may also serve as an external consultant who comes in to help perform the audit. Knowledge of statistics and sampling techniques is an important skill for the HIM professional as a key player in an audit process. The HIM professional may also be a key player in self-disclosure because, through the course of regular processing of incomplete charts, coding, or performance of ongoing record reviews, it may become obvious that a provider or practitioner is violating regulatory guidelines and benefiting unjustly from reimbursement. The HIM professional has an important responsibility to report the findings to the next level of reporting and to the facility's corporate compliance program as appropriate.

Antikickback Statutes

In one actual case, a physician in Massachusetts received kickbacks from a pharmaceutical company in the following manner. In exchange for receiving free samples from that company of a prescription drug used to combat prostate cancer, the physician switched his prostate cancer patients to that drug. Additionally, the physician billed Medicare for the free samples that he had received. This particular physician was ordered to pay a $5,000 fine for his role in receiving kickbacks from the pharmaceutical company (HHS Office of Inspector General, 2003).

The **antikickback statute** (§1128(b)(7) of the Social Security Act, 42 U.S.C. §1320a-7b) makes it illegal to offer, pay, solicit, or receive anything of value for inducing referrals to a federal healthcare program. These are felony, or criminal, violations for anyone who knowingly and willfully engages in this behavior. Additionally, conviction for these actions results in automatic exclusion from future participation as a provider for federal healthcare programs (OIG Advisory Opinion No. 98-4, April 15, 1998, p. 3, 42 U.S.C. §3120a-7). An exclusion of this type essentially makes it impossible for a healthcare provider to continue to provide services, because a significant percentage of a provider's reimbursement often comes from these programs.

The kickback categories ascribe liability to the parties on both sides of a transaction that violate the statute. In other words, both the person soliciting and receiving anything of value and the person offering or paying it for an impermissible transaction are liable. Even arranging for or recommending these actions is prohibited (OIG Advisory Opinion No. 98-4, April 15, 1998, p. 3, 42 U.S.C. §3120a-7).

Proving antikickback violations also requires the government to prove that the violator possessed intent and engaged in knowing and willful conduct. The criminal standard for burden of proof, "beyond a reasonable doubt," must be met.

Why should the HIM professional be aware of the antikickback statute? Although HIM professionals are seldom likely be in a position to benefit financially from inducing referrals to a federally reimbursed healthcare program, they may be in a position to warn other healthcare providers of the prohibition or to observe such an arrangement. The involvement of HIM professionals in processing healthcare documentation and assigning codes used for billing purposes exposes them to a wide range of knowledge about the activities occurring in the organization. HIM professionals should not ignore what is going on around them as they carry out their professional role and responsibility.

Antireferral Statutes: Stark I and II

Suppose that a physician owns a part of a reference lab that offers specialized laboratory testing. The physician's practice refers a significant portion of its patients to this reference lab for performance of these specialized tests. As an indirect result, the physician benefits through the profits made by the reference laboratory.

The **antireferral statutes** (42 U.S.C. §1395nn), titled the Ethics in Patient Referral Act and enacted as part of the 1989 Omnibus Budget Reconciliation Act (OBRA), prohibit this kind of arrangement. The statutes are commonly referred to as **Stark I and II**, because they were introduced by California Representative Pete Stark. Under Stark, it is unlawful for a physician to make referrals for Medicare-covered services to entities in which the referring physician (or immediate family members) has a financial relationship (Preamble to Stark I Regulations, 1995; 42 U.S.C. §1395nn). The first, early version of the statute (Stark I), passed in 1989, focused on prohibitions against a physician's referral of patients to a clinical lab in which the physician had a financial interest. The second (Stark II), passed in 1995, extended the statute to include referrals to any entity furnishing designated health services. Designated health services are broadly defined to include clinical labs, occupational therapy, physical therapy, orthotics/prosthetics, hospital services, durable medical equipment, parenteral/enteral nutrition services and supplies, radiology, radiation therapy, home health services, and outpatient prescription drugs (Wagg, 2000).

Unlike the federal antikickback statute, the antireferral statute is a civil, not a criminal, statute and carries a lower standard of proof. Only a simple preponderance of evidence, "of greater weight or more convincing than the evidence offered in opposition," or "more likely than not," is needed. Intent need not be shown. In other words, just making the referral puts one in violation of the statute. The penalties for Stark do not involve jail terms, because it is a civil violation. The monetary penalties are high, however. Up to $15,000 per service, in addition to exclusion from future provision of services to federal healthcare programs, can be applied (Withrow, 1997).

As with antikickback regulations, HIM professionals are not likely to be directly involved in the activities that this statute prohibits. But they could be a spouse of a physician, and thus would need to make sure that they are not participating in ownership or financial benefit from an entity that their physician spouse or other immediate family member made referrals to.

"Safe Harbors" and Stark Exceptions

The Stark antireferral statutes specify exceptions (42 C.F.R. §411.350 et seq. and 42 U.S.C. §1395nn), and antikickback statutes designate **"Safe Harbor"** categories (42 C.F.R. §1001.952 & 42 U.S.C. §1320a-7b(b)), defined by the U.S. Department of Health and Human Services, for practices unlikely to bring harm to the federal healthcare programs. These are practices that technically violate either the antireferral or antikickback statutes, but that have been proven to not improperly influence or reward someone. In particular, the federal government has designated exceptions or safe harbors for underserved areas in an effort to promote the accessibility and availability of healthcare providers to residents of such areas. Although antikickback and antireferral violations infrequently turn on the basis of health information documentation and coding activities, the HIM professional should maintain an awareness of these aspects of illegal healthcare arrangements to ensure active participation and support in hospital-wide compliance program activities, as discussed later in this chapter.

Mail and Wire Fraud

Frequently, charges for violations under the preceding statutes will be accompanied by additional charges for violations of mail and wire fraud (18 U.S.C. §1341; 18 U.S.C. §1343). These laws prohibit the use of the U.S. Postal Service or any wire service to execute a scheme related to fraud. Violation of these felony statutes is punishable by a fine of up to $1,000 and imprisonment for up to five years (Wagg, 2000). Because most transmissions of information for reimbursement are by either mail services or wire services, this is another criminal statute, though general in nature, that can be applied in the war against healthcare fraud.

MORE RECENT REGULATIONS THAT GUIDE HIM PROFESSIONALS

In 1996, Congress passed the Health Insurance Portability and Accountability Act (HIPAA; 42 U.S.C. §201 et seq.). Although HIPAA established requirements to ensure the transfer or continuance of insurance benefits when one changes or terminates employment, HIPAA is best known to HIM professionals not only for its standardization of transactions and code sets, but for its national standards that protect the privacy and security of individually identifiable health information. It extends beyond previous statutes discussed earlier in this chapter to include all uses and disclosures of protected health information by healthcare providers, funded by either federal or private payers, who conduct certain healthcare transactions electronically. Although an original intent of the Act was to standardize and simplify electronic transmissions of health information to result in long-term cost savings as a result of efficiencies achieved by switching from paper claims submission to electronic claims submission, the focus of this legislation quickly shifted to compliance efforts in protecting the privacy and security of individuals' health information.

HIPAA Administrative Simplification Standards

HIPAA's Administrative Simplification Standards for covered entities, which consist of health plans, healthcare clearinghouses, and healthcare providers (42 U.S.C. §1320d-2 et seq.), address the situation outlined previously. These standards are aimed at

- Maintaining the integrity and confidentiality of healthcare information
- Protecting against reasonable foreseeable threats to the security and integrity of the information
- Protecting against unauthorized uses or disclosures of the information
- Ensuring compliance by employees
- Standardizing transactions and code sets across the healthcare spectrum

Penalties for violating patient privacy under the administrative simplification section are severe:

- Civil penalties of up to $100 may be applied per violation up to a maximum of $25,000 per year (42 U.S.C. §1320d-5(a)(1)).

- Wrongful disclosure of individually identifiable health information rises to a criminal penalty of a $50,000 fine and/or imprisonment for one year (42 U.S.C. §1320d-6(b)(1)).
- Adding false pretenses to the commission of the crime further increases the penalty to a $100,000 fine and/or imprisonment for five years.
- The highest penalty is $250,000 and/or 10 years in prison, for those who sell, transfer, or use individually identifiable health information for commercial advantage, personal gain, or malicious harm (Tomes, 2000, p. 11).

Security Standards

HIPAA's security standards, which are also part of the Administrative Simplification provisions, apply to any electronic data in a data repository or transmitted over any network. These standards address four main categories:

1. The administrative procedures to guard data integrity, confidentiality, and availability. These must be documented, formal practices.
2. The physical safeguards to guard data integrity, confidentiality, and availability. Again, these must be documented, formal practices.
3. Technical security measures to guard data integrity, confidentiality, and availability. These include the processes that the entity uses to control and monitor information access.
4. Technical security mechanisms to prevent unauthorized access to data that an entity transmits over a communication network.

The HIM professional has a large job to design and document the procedures used to safeguard the data's integrity, confidentiality, and availability. Technical and operational steps will need to be implemented to meet the physical and technical safeguard requirements to protect data and prevent unauthorized access. As one of the main venues for storage, retrieval, and release of medical information, the HIM department is a primary source and keeper of the type of data that HIPAA intends to protect.

Privacy Standards

HIPAA's privacy standards, which are also part of the Administrative Simplification provisions, apply to any individually identifiable health information that is or has been transmitted or maintained in any form by a covered entity that conducts certain healthcare transactions electronically. Health information that has been created by another entity becomes protected health information under HIPAA once it is in the custody of a HIPAA-covered entity. The HIPAA privacy standards generally prohibit the use or disclosure of protected health information without an individual's authorization, although there are many exceptions. Protected health information may be used or disclosed, without individual authorization, for purposes of treatment, payment, and healthcare operations. Use and disclosure may also occur without individual authorization for myriad reasons, including those identified as "public interest and benefit activities." Examples of these activities include public health, research, health oversight, law enforcement purposes, and to coroners or funeral directors (45 CFR 164.512). The chain-of-trust concept requires disclosing entities to ensure that the business partner receiving the information will safeguard the information. The privacy standards also establish basic rights for patients, such as the right to inspect and copy the information; obtain an accounting of certain disclosures; request an amendment or correction of one's own inaccurate or incomplete protected health information; request confidential communications; and request restrictions on the use and disclosure of one's own health information (45 CFR 164.522 through 45 CFR 164.528). For uses

and disclosures that do not require patient authorization, a written notice must be provided to inform patients of these uses and disclosures (45 CFR 164.520(a)).

Enforcement Programs

HIPAA also established four key programs to assist with healthcare fraud enforcement in both the public and private areas of the healthcare industry. The first, the Fraud and Abuse Control Program, was established as a joint effort between the DOJ and the OIG to control healthcare fraud and abuse and to conduct investigations related to the delivery of health care. The second, the Medicare Integrity Program, was established to direct Health and Human Services to enter into agreements with private companies to carry out fraud and abuse protections. The third, the Beneficiary Incentive Program, encourages the reporting of suspected fraud and abuse by Medicare beneficiaries. The fourth, the Healthcare Fraud and Abuse Data Collection Program, was designed to create a national healthcare fraud and abuse database in conjunction with the National Practitioner Data Bank (Wagg, 2000).

False Claims Penalties

HIPAA increased the level of civil monetary penalties from $2,000 per occurrence to $10,000 for each item or service fraudulently billed. The assessment increased from two times the amount of overpayment to three times the amount of overpayment ("treble" damages). Two provider practices affected by this category are

1. Patterns of "upcoding"; that is assigning a code that the person knows or should know will result in greater payments than appropriate
2. Submitting claims for medically unnecessary items or services

The term *pattern* is key to the application of identifying fraudulent acts. A pattern of inappropriate coding must exist, not a random error or difference of opinion (Prophet, 1997).

More substantial criminal penalties are set forth by HIPAA for those who "knowingly and willfully" attempt to defraud any healthcare benefit program or to obtain, by false or fraudulent pretense, money or property owned by, or under the custody of, a healthcare benefit program. Penalties include up to 10 years imprisonment. If a patient suffers serious injury from the violation, the penalties increase to 20 years imprisonment or life if the patient dies (Prophet, 1997).

Roles for HIM Professionals

The components of HIPAA create many opportunities that require the experience and knowledge of the HIM professional. For example, to comply with the privacy standards of HIPAA, an organization must designate a "privacy official" to develop the policies and procedures needed regarding use and disclosure of health information. Extensive education must also be given to all employees and volunteers regarding health information policies and procedures, with ongoing, repeated education at least once every three years. Safeguards such as passwords and door locks must be implemented to comply with the HIPAA security standards. A process to report lack of compliance with the standards must exist. Appropriate sanctions must also be developed (McLeod, 2000). Development of these functions and requirements is a process that the HIM professional can guide and facilitate.

COMPLIANCE PROGRAMS TO PREVENT FRAUDULENT BEHAVIORS

Passage of the Federal Sentencing Guidelines in 1992 established a framework of seven specific elements required for the implementation of **compliance programs** for a broad range of healthcare providers. The OIG has outlined several compliance program guidances in its continued efforts to promote voluntary compliance for the healthcare industry. A compliance program is intended to foster the prevention of fraudulent activities by the development of internal controls. The fundamental intent is to establish a culture that promotes prevention, detection, and resolution of instances of conduct that do not conform with federal, state, and private-payer healthcare program requirements (OIG, 1998a). The OIG first published the **compliance guidance** document for clinical laboratories (62 Fed. Reg. 9435, March 3, 1997). Others published subsequently include guidances for hospitals, home health care, nursing homes, third-party billing companies, and physician practices.

The OIG emphasized that a compliance program must effectively articulate and demonstrate the organization's commitment to compliance. The inclusion of the governing body, upper management, other managers, employees, and physicians should guide the management of the healthcare entity. The OIG recognized that although a compliance program may not entirely eliminate fraud, abuse, and waste from the hospital system, it can significantly reduce the risk of unlawful or improper conduct (OIG, 1998a, p. 4).

The OIG outlined seven essential elements of a compliance program (OIG, 1998a, p. 8), based on the U.S. Sentencing Commission Guidelines (Guidelines Manual, 8A1.2, comment [n3(k)]):

1. **Written standards of conduct and accompanying policies and procedures to promote compliance.** These standards are the basic framework for expressing the organization's values and ethics and the governing body's commitment to corporate compliance. Recent case law suggests that failure of a corporate director to attempt in good faith to institute a compliance program in certain circumstances may be a breach of a director's fiduciary obligation (see, e.g., In re Caremark International Inc. Derivative Litigation, 698

A.2d 959 (Ct. Chanc. Del. 1996)) (OIG, 1998a, p. 3). These standards must be designed to address specific areas of risk for potential fraud, such as claims development, coding, and financial relationships with physicians and others. The OIG Work Plan (1998) outlined known areas of risk that an organization can assess. HIM professionals must carefully document policies and procedures for coding and the associated documentation required to assign the code. Every institution needs coding policies and procedures and accompanying coding compliance plans validating the coding process.

2. **Designation of a chief compliance officer (CCO) and a compliance committee.** This element is to designate the upper-level leadership charged with responsibility of operating and monitoring the compliance program. The CCO reports directly to the CEO and governing body. The scope of the CCO's responsibilities includes general oversight and implementation of the compliance program and regular reports to the governing body, CEO, and compliance committee regarding compliance activities. The CCO ensures that all elements of the compliance plan are carried out.

3. **Development and implementation of regular, effective education programs for all affected employees.** The OIG recommends that ongoing education programs include sessions highlighting the organization's compliance program and that they cover regulations and processes related to compliance such as fraud and abuse laws, coding and documentation requirements, and the claims submission process. The OIG examples include education of upper-level management regarding proper confirmation of diagnoses, alterations to medical records, and proper documentation of services ren-

dered. Providing education on these topics is an area for an active role by HIM professionals in the hospital's compliance program.

4. **Maintenance of an effective method for a line of communication to receive complaints, to protect the anonymity of complainants, and to protect whistle-blowers from retaliation.** The OIG recommends that the compliance officer be accessible to staff. Hotlines and other forms of communication may be established to facilitate this process. The OIG believes that whistle-blowers should be protected from retaliation, as provided for in the qui tam provisions under the False Claims Act. Employees may be forced to file the qui tam actions when there is not a safe, effective method to bring questionable, fraudulent, or abusive situations to the attention of senior officials (OIG, 1998a, p. 38, fn. 45).

5. **Development of a system to enforce standards through well-publicized disciplinary guidelines.** The disciplinary actions for failure to comply with compliance program standards must be established, implemented, and followed. New employees should receive a careful background check. Any criminal conviction or exclusion should be checked carefully against the OIG's recommendations for exclusion from involvement in any federal care program (OIG, 1998a, p. 41).

6. **An ongoing process for auditing and monitoring.** The use of audits or other evaluation to monitor compliance and reduce problem areas is critical to a successful compliance program. The OIG outlines the conduct of regular, periodic compliance audits by internal or external auditors as a program component in the guidance document. Coding and claim development are aspects that should be included in the audit process.

7. **Responding to detected offenses and developing corrective action initiatives.** The appropriate actions must be implemented when offenses are detected. Determining the level of reporting to the correct government authorities must be accomplished. A voluntary self-disclosure action may be invoked as appropriate. In any event, any overpayment must be returned to the government as discovered (OIG, 1998a, pp. 48–51).

The OIG advised that each program be tailored to fit the needs and resources of the hospital. The hospital guidance elements are generally consistent with the instructions found in the OIG guidance documents that are specific to other healthcare entities, such as home health agencies, long-term care facilities, and third-party payer billing companies. Guidance for physician offices also is available. An HIM professional working in one of those specific settings should obtain the guidance document from the OIG for that entity.

The development of compliance program activities in a hospital can benefit significantly from the leadership, participation, and support of HIM professionals. In many instances, HIM professionals have assumed the role of CCO or a significant role in the conduct of aspects of the program, such as auditing and monitoring, education, and reports for the compliance committee or governing board. Obtaining the annual OIG Work Plan is a good starting point to determine the current focus on perceived issues with coding and documentation issues. A corporate compliance plan should discuss coding actions in relation to the seven essential elements of a compliance program that the OIG has outlined.

DILEMMAS IN PRACTICE

HIM professionals are faced on a daily basis with the challenge of finding ways to ensure that health information is documented accurately and efficiently.

Scenario 4-B: Accepting Money for Information

The director of the HIM department serves as the system manager for the department's system that assigns codes to patient accounts. The system downloads patient-identifiable demographics to facilitate the use of the database for facility reporting to analyze physician practice patterns, patient outcomes, and facility utilization. The HIM director's department budget has been cut again this year by 10 percent. The transcription equipment is in need of constant repair, and the fax machine jams on a regular basis.

An entrepreneur starting a service to provide home dialysis visits to patients is trying to decide if there will be enough business to support his new business venture. He also needs to know which patients receive dialysis and which physicians treat patients with this condition. He offers the HIM director a good sum of money for a downloaded listing of information on patients with applicable diagnosis types. The money provided to the HIM director could be used to replace the fax machine and pay for a regular service contract. The business is for a good cause, and the department could really use the money.

Questions

1. Is it acceptable for the HIM director to accept the offer from the new business entrepreneur?

2. Would anyone be harmed if the HIM director released the information to the entrepreneur?

3. Would this violate any HIPAA standard, and, if so, what would the penalty be for this violation?

A completed ethical decision-making matrix for the scenario is provided at the end of the chapter.

Fraudulent Documentation Practices

Let us return to Scenario 4-A. What should an HIM professional do if he or she is aware that documentation in the medical record does not reflect the true underlying reason for a procedure? For both ethical and legal reasons, the HIM professional should not acquiesce to the physician's documentation or insistence. If the physician is committing fraud by signing the final diagnostic statement with information that misrepresents the reason for the patient's treatment, and the HIM professional knows that the information is misrepresented, he or she should report the situation to hospital compliance and legal staff.

With regard to Scenario 4-B, the sale of patient-identifiable information to a business entrepreneur is an unacceptable breach of patients' confidentiality. It is also a violation of HIPAA's Administrative Simplification Standards, which prohibit the sale, transfer, or use of individually identifiable health information for commercial advantage, personal gain, or malicious harm. The HIM director could be in big trouble: a $250,000 fine or 10 years in prison, or both.

Scenario 4-C: Retrospective Documentation to Avoid Suspension

The HIM chart analyst is assessing the medical record of Susan Smith, who was discharged yesterday, and notes that it doesn't have a history and physical on it. The HIM analyst has been told that every medical record needs a history and physical per the standards of the Joint Commission on the Accreditation of Healthcare Organizations (JCAHO). In an effort to "do her job," the analyst flags the doctor to complete a history and physical. At this hospital, if physicians do not complete their medical records, and they subsequently become delinquent, the physicians' admitting privileges are suspended. Dr. Tired goes to the medical record department to complete his incomplete medical records. He gets to the record on Susan Smith and sees the incomplete tag for a history and physical. He knows that Susan was worked up by the consultants on the case, and he assumes that they probably did a history and review of systems when they visited Susan during her stay. Dr. Tired doesn't want to debate the situation with the medical record completion clerk, so he simply reviews the notes from the consultants and fills out the history and physical form. The form is complete now, and he won't get suspended.

Questions

1. Even though the medical record now has a history and physical on it, name as many reasons as you can that this retrospective recording of a history and physical should not have occurred.

2. If this case goes to court, will it represent care as it was truly delivered to the patient? Or, does the history and physical make a difference? Explain your thoughts.

3. What might an HIM professional do to maintain ethical standards of compliance and prevent this kind of problem from occurring?

A completed ethical decision-making matrix for the scenario is provided at the end of the chapter.

Retrospective Medical Record Analysis

It has been a customary practice, after the patient is discharged, to complete whatever medical information has been left uncompleted in the patient's record. But this practice encourages providers to fill in the blanks with dimly recalled, or even unrecalled, information that may be totally erroneous. As such, it may jeopardize the patient's future care—and jeopardize the provider as well. Inadvertent false claims may be filed when a caregiver dictates a report months after a patient's surgery and tries to recall what happened.

More and more healthcare facilities have shifted their focus from retrospective, after-discharge analysis of closed records to completion of documentation concurrently with the delivery of the patient's care (Grabowski, 2000). This "open" record review at the point of care has also become standard practice due to changes in the requirements set forth by the JCAHO. Now the emphasis is on acquiring the documentation at the point of care, when it will benefit the patient the most and when it is fresh in the mind of the caregiver.

HIM professionals can play a major role in this transition. They should request only elements of documentation that were not included in the record at the time of discharge because of transcription or filing delays, because the medical record was not available to the caregiver at the time the care was delivered, or because of an oversight or delay by the practitioner. The focus is on completing or authenticating reports that are dictated or properly completed at discharge, such as a discharge summary, and on ensuring that all documents prepared during the course of the patient's care are properly located and assembled into the patient's record. The JCAHO (2000) maintains that, at a minimum, an organization must establish methods to ensure authentication of the history and physical, operative reports, consultations, and discharge summaries or discharge notes.

Retrospective medical record completion should not promote fabrication of documentation for the sake of "making the medical record complete." For example, if a physician never took a patient's history or conducted a physical exam, then the correct documentation should reflect that no exam was given; documentation should not be created to reflect performance of a history and physical when in fact the patient had no such examination. HIM professionals cannot lose sight of the fact that the real purpose of a history and physical is to provide an overall assessment of the patient's medical condition prior to delivering care, and not just to comply with documentation standards that say there must be one.

Scenario 4-D: Coder Assigns Code Without Physician's Documentation

The HIM director is told by the CFO that her job is on the line if she doesn't get cases coded and billed within 72 hours. Dr. Evans is on vacation again, and he left 20 case records in such an incomplete state that they are uncodable. The HIM director does what it takes to keep her job—and has the coder assign codes as best as he can from what sketchy information is on the chart.

Questions

1. What organizational initiatives should the director take instead of succumbing to the CFO's pressure?

2. What operational actions or interventions could the director have taken to prevent this dilemma from occurring? Name a procedural process change and a governance change that would have helped prevent this dilemma.

A completed ethical decision-making matrix for the scenario is provided at the end of the chapter.

Coding Turnaround Time

It is a challenge for HIM professionals to assemble the proper documentation needed to allow prompt coding of the patient's record so that the claim can be submitted to the third-party payer. Coding standards recommended by the OIG, and frequently required by state law, look for the physician to prepare a final diagnostic statement used for assignment of codes to the patient's claim. If this is not completed accurately to allow coding to proceed, or is not completed in a timely manner, the healthcare entity suffers financially due to unnecessary delay of submission of the bill to the third-party payer. This delay results in an increase in the number of days in accounts receivable, thus delaying receipt of funds owed to the hospital for care already rendered and needed to continue sound financial operations. Regular reports of accounts unable to be billed due to incomplete medical record

coding are routinely created in hospitals and establish one of the challenges to the HIM professional to maintain ethical standards of compliance.

Maintaining standards for coding accuracy and required documentation without compromise must continue despite the simultaneous need to keep the days in accounts receivable as low as possible. This can be done by building strong concurrent documentation systems at the point of care that allow accurate and timely processing by the coders as soon as the care is complete.

CONCLUSION

In the quest to achieve a needed result, whether additional documentation so that the record can be filed in a state of proper completion or timely coding so that the account can be billed, the HIM professional must resist resorting to inappropriate methods. The risk of losing JCAHO accreditation and the cost of delaying billing are strong forces that are present in the daily lives of HIM professionals. Only through competent management of an efficient department that does not get boxed into these dilemmas, and through a well-designed documentation process supported by standards for documentation through the medical staff's rules and regulations, can the HIM professional maintain the required level of performance and resist any intended or unintended violations of regulations posed at preventing fraudulent reimbursement in health care.

Key Terms

- Abuse
- Antikickback statute
- Antireferral statutes
- Compliance guidances
- Compliance program
- Corporate Integrity Agreement (CIA)
- False Claims Act
- Fraud
- Health Insurance Portability and Accountability Act of 1996 (HIPAA)
- Qui tam statutes
- Safe Harbors
- Stark I and II
- Voluntary disclosure protocol

Chapter Summary

- In the late 1990s, the government began stepping up its activities to eliminate fraud and abuse in health care. To ensure institutional compliance—and their own compliance—with the law, HIM professionals must ensure that processes to document the care provided to patients are ethical and accurate, that codes are appropriately assigned, and that health information is managed responsibly.
- The False Claims Act prohibits knowingly presenting false or fraudulent claims to the government. Even if an HIM professional does not know that certain claims processed by the HIM department are false, he or she may be liable if it can be shown that he or she should have instituted standard checking procedures that would have exposed the claims as fraudulent.
- If HIM professionals become aware that past mistakes or abuses have led to erroneous or fraudulent billing of the Medicare program, the facility can follow the OIG's **voluntary disclosure protocol** to report it and return the overpayment to the Medicare contractor. Self-reporting may or may not exempt the provider from sanction, depending on whether there is a pattern of abuse and whether there is intent to defraud or reckless disregard of the truth, but if it does not, it can lighten the penalties. Sometimes it results in the imposition of a Corporate Integrity Agreement (CIA), in which the provider agrees to meet certain government-imposed requirements, such as regular audits of billing or other operations.
- The Health Insurance Portability and Accountability Act of 1996 (HIPAA) established national standards for privacy and security of health information that apply to health care funded by both federal and private payers. These standards penalize the unauthorized uses or disclosures of healthcare information and mandate the implementation of practices to safeguard the integrity, confidentiality, and availability of protected health information. The HIM professional can play an important role in developing policies and procedures, educating staff, and implementing measures to protect patient information in compliance with HIPAA.
- A compliance program is intended to foster the prevention of fraudulent activities in a healthcare organization by the development of internal controls. The OIG has

published several guidances for healthcare organizations attempting to establish a compliance program. Such programs are to include seven elements: written standards of conduct and accompanying policies and procedures; designation of a chief compliance officer (CCO) and compliance committee; regular, effective education programs; maintenance of a hotline to receive complaints and protect anonymity; disciplinary guidelines; an ongoing auditing and monitoring process; and response to detected offenses and development of corrective action initiatives. HIM professionals play an important role in establishing such programs.

References

Abdelhak, M., Grostick, S., Hanken, M. A., & Jacobs, E. (2001). *Health information: Management of a strategic resource.* Philadelphia, PA: W.B. Saunders Company.

Black's Law Dictionary. (1991). Abridged 6th ed. St. Paul, MN: West Publishing.

Brown, J. G. (2000). An open letter to health care providers. Washington, DC: Office of the Inspector General, March 9. Retrieved October 11, 2005, from http://oig.hhs.gov/fraud/docs/openletters/openletter.htm.

Department of Health and Human Services and Department of Justice Health Care Fraud and Abuse Control Program. (2003, September). Annual Report for FY 2002. Retrieved November 19, 2004, from http://www.usdoj.gov/dag/pubdoc/hcfacreport2002.htm.

Grabowski, D. (2000). Simplified deficiency processing brings hospital-wide benefits. *Journal of AHIMA, 71*(3), 58–61.

HHS Office of Inspector General. (2003, March). Kickbacks. Retrieved October 11, 2005, from http://oig.hhs.gov/fraud/enforcement/criminal/03/0303.html#8.

Joint Commission on the Accreditation of Healthcare Organizations [JCAHO]. (2000). CAMH IM standard. *Update* 2, p. 47.

King, E. (1999). In pursuit of health fraud. *Journal of AHIMA, 70*(1), 22–28.

McLeod, L. (2000). Dear Colleagues . . . DHHS proposed rule for privacy standards. *HIM Connection, 2*(7).

Office of the Inspector General, U.S. Department of Health and Human Services. (1998). *The Office of the Inspector General's 1999 work plan.* Washington, DC: Government Printing Office.

Office of the Inspector General, U.S. Department of Health and Human Services. (1998a, February).

Compliance program guidance for hospitals. Retrieved October 11, 2005, from http://www.ahima.org/infocenter/models/oig.pdf.

Office of the Inspector General, U.S. Department of Health and Human Services. (1998b, October 21). OIG issues guidance on voluntary disclosure of health care fraud. Retrieved October 11, 2005, from http://oig.hhs.gov/fraud/docs/complianceguidance/dispress.pdf.

Office of the Inspector General, U.S. Department of Health and Human Services. (2003–2004). Semi-annual report to Congress. Retrieved November 19, 2004, from http://oig.hhs.gov/publications/docs/semiannual/2004/SemiannualSpring04.pdf.

Prophet, S. (1997). Fraud and abuse implications for the HIM professional. *Journal of AHIMA, 68*(4), 52–56.

Reinhardt, C. (2000). MFIS, Transamerica Medicare Administration. RE: Voluntary disclosure protocol. Reply, Friday, April 21; Compliance. HealthLawyers.org.

Reno, J. (1998). Speech presented at the annual meeting of the American Hospital Association, February 2, Washington, DC.

Rogers, J. (1999, November). The OIG's Self-Disclosure Protocol. *Health Care Law Monthly.* Retrieved October 11, 2005, from http://www.mcguirewoods.com/news-resources/publications/health_care/oig.pdf.

Stringer, W. (1998). The 1986 False Claims Act Amendment: An assessment of economic impact. *DOJ Health Care Fraud Report for Fiscal Year 1997.* Washington, DC: Government Printing Office.

Tomes, J. (2000). HIPAA's privacy and security regulations: Administrative complication, not simplification. *Health Law Digest, 28*(1), 14.

U.S. Department of Justice. (1998). False Claims Act guidance. *Bureau of National Affairs. Health Care Fraud Report,* 2(2), 459.

U.S. General Accounting Office [GAO]. (1998). *GAO accountability report for 1999.* Washington, DC: Government Printing Office.

U.S. Sentencing Commission. *Guidelines Manual,* A1.2, comment (n3(k)).

Wagg, D. G. (2000). Learning the laws behind compliance. *Journal of AHIMA,* 71(5), 20–21.

Withrow, S. C. (1997, September 24). Submerged safe harbors against Stark attacks: How to manage the vagaries of anti-kickback and Stark laws. Retrieved October 11, 2005, from http://www.wmolaw.com/stark.htm.

The ethical decision-making matrix is a tool to help you organize complex, ethical problems; however, there is no simple fill-in-the-box approach to ethical decision making. The objective is to follow each step of the process and not move from the question directly to what should be done or how to prevent it next time. If you skip steps, you will not fully understand all of the values and options for action. Also, the matrix provided for each scenario in this book is not the only way to examine the problem. You can make an equally compelling ethical argument for a different decision—just be sure to follow all the steps of the matrix.

SCENARIO 4-A: DOCUMENTATION DOES NOT JUSTIFY BILLED PROCEDURE

Steps	Information	
1. What is the ethical question?	Should Allison insist that the physicians code for infertility?	
2. What are the facts?	**KNOWN**	**TO BE GATHERED**
	• Discrepancy between doctors' notes regarding endometriosis and nurses' notes regarding infertility. • Laparoscopy performed.	• In performing the laparoscopy for infertility, is the extent of endometriosis determined as well? • Is the documentation of endometriosis false documentation? Would billing for endometriosis only constitute fraud? What are the customary practices in such cases? • What is Allison's new boss expecting her to do? • What is the likely impact on Allison's family of changing jobs?
3. What are the values? Examine the shared and competing values, obligations, and interests of the stakeholders (i.e., patient, HIM professional, healthcare practitioner(s), administrators, society, and other advocates) involved in order to fully understand the complexity of the ethical problem(s).	**Patient:** Values accurate documentation as the basis for receiving quality care; interest in keeping costs down. **HIM professional:** Truth, integrity, accuracy, and reliability (code accurately and reliably rather than to maximize reimbursement); fairness (follow rules and obey the law); loyalty to employer; avoid harm (inaccurate documentation may harm the patient; disclosure of inaccurate reporting could close the facility, which would harm patients, doctors, and their families); personal values (promote the welfare of family by avoiding loss of job). **Healthcare professionals:** Promote welfare of patients through accurate documentation for future care; truth-telling; fairness (following rules equally for all); personal values (promote the welfare of family by avoiding legal ramifications). **Administrators:** Benefit patients and keep them from harm; promote welfare of facility; maximize reimbursement without compromising truth-telling; fairness in applying rules for all. **Society:** Control costs; promote fair and just allocation of resources; follow rules of reimbursement equally for all.	

4. What are the options?	• Gather more information. • Comply with physicians' requests to code only endometriosis. • Tell physicians that you will only code what is documented in the medical record.	
5. What should I do?	Code what is documented	
6. What justifies my choice?	**JUSTIFIED**	**NOT JUSTIFIED**
	• Code accurately based on obligation to tell the truth. • Support accuracy of the medical record. • Preserve professional integrity. • Follow rules equally for all. • Respect the law. • Demonstrate loyalty to employer, unless asked to push legal boundaries.	• Continue current practice of coding for endometriosis. • Push legal boundaries. • Make special exception to the rules to maximize reimbursement. • Lack of fairness for others who follow rules. • Miscoding undermines the reimbursement system. • Miscoding increases long-term costs. • Keeping federal monies.
7. How can I prevent this ethical problem?	• Determine if system changes are needed. • Learn more about procedures that are not covered by federal plans. • Discuss standards and the values that support them with colleagues. • Evaluate institutional integrity at job interview and when ethical problems arise.	

The ethical decision-making matrix is a tool to help you organize complex, ethical problems; however, there is no simple fill-in-the-box approach to ethical decision making. The objective is to follow each step of the process and not move from the question directly to what should be done or how to prevent it next time. If you skip steps, you will not fully understand all of the values and options for action. Also, the matrix provided for each scenario in this book is not the only way to examine the problem. You can make an equally compelling ethical argument for a different decision—just be sure to follow all the steps of the matrix.

SCENARIO 4-B: ACCEPTING MONEY FOR INFORMATION

Steps	Information	
1. What is the ethical question?	Should the director take the money and give the entrepreneur the information he requested?	
2. What are the facts?	**KNOWN**	**TO BE GATHERED**
	• HIM professional has access to requested information. • Money is needed to repair office equipment.	• Could entrepreneur make use of the data if it did not include personally identifiable information? • Is there any other way to obtain funding for the office equipment? • What are the customary practices in such cases? • Would selling the information violate doctor and patient privacy and confidentiality? • What does your boss expect you to do? • What is the likely impact on your family of changing jobs?
3. What are the values? Examine the shared and competing values, obligations, and interests of the stakeholders (i.e., patient, HIM professional, healthcare practitioner(s), administrators, society, and other advocates) involved in order to fully understand the complexity of the ethical problem(s).	**Patient:** Has a right to personal privacy and the confidentiality of his/her medical records; could benefit from home dialysis visits; would benefit from efficient operation of the HIM department. **HIM professional:** Integrity (preserve privacy and confidentiality); fairness (follow the rules and obey the law); personal values (promote the welfare of family by avoiding loss of job); would benefit from efficient operation of the HIM department. **Healthcare professionals:** Has professional interest in preservation of personal privacy and confidentiality of medical records; would benefit from efficient operation of the HIM department. **Administrators:** Promote welfare of facility; would benefit from efficient operation of the HIM department. **Society:** Follow rules of privacy and confidentiality equally for all; do not sell health information for money.	

4. What are my options?	• Gather more information. • Sell requested data to entrepreneur. • Sell data that would not include personally identifiable information to entrepreneur. • Do not sell data to entrepreneur.	
5. What should I do?	Do not sell data to entrepreneur.	
6. What justifies my choice?	**JUSTIFIED**	**NOT JUSTIFIED**
	• Obligation to protect doctors' and patients' privacy and confidentiality of medical records. • Preserve professional integrity. • Respect the law. • Demonstrate loyalty to employer, unless asked to push legal boundaries.	• Sell requested information to entrepreneur. • Violate privacy and confidentiality. • Break trust of doctors and patients.
7. How can I prevent this ethical problem?	Determine sources for alternate funding that would not compromise the law/ethics.	

The ethical decision-making matrix is a tool to help you organize complex, ethical problems; however, there is no simple fill-in-the-box approach to ethical decision making. The objective is to follow each step of the process and not move from the question directly to what should be done or how to prevent it next time. If you skip steps, you will not fully understand all of the values and options for action. Also, the matrix provided for each scenario in this book is not the only way to examine the problem. You can make an equally compelling ethical argument for a different decision—just be sure to follow all the steps of the matrix.

SCENARIO 4-C: RETROSPECTIVE DOCUMENTATION TO AVOID SUSPENSION

Steps	Information	
1. What is the ethical question?	Should the HIM medical record analyst report the doctor's retrospective completion of the record?	
2. What are the facts?	**KNOWN**	**TO BE GATHERED**
	• Medical record was not completed at time of patient discharge. • Medical record was completed retrospectively. Doctor completing the medical record did not perform history and physical.	• Were the consultants' notes complete enough to accurately complete the medical record? • Could the patient suffer from possible inaccuracies in her medical record? • Would allowing the doctor to complete charts in this manner constitute a violation of the standards of the JCAHO? • What are the customary practices in such cases? • What does your supervisor expect you to do? • What is the likely impact on your family of changing jobs?
3. What are the values? Examine the shared and competing values, obligations, and interests of the stakeholders (i.e., patient, HIM professional, healthcare practitioner(s), administrators, society, and other advocates) involved in order to fully understand the complexity of the ethical problem(s).	**Patient:** Values accurate documentation as basis of receiving quality care. **HIM professional:** Truth, integrity, accuracy, reliability, and fairness (must comply with JCAHO standards); loyalty to employer; avoid harm (inaccurate documentation may harm the patient; disclosing the indiscretions of the doctor will harm his career and his family); personal values (promote the welfare of family by avoiding loss of job). **Healthcare professionals:** Promote welfare of patients through accurate documentation for future care; compliance with JCAHO standards. **Administrators:** Benefit patients and keep from harm; promote welfare of facility; maximize efficiency without compromising JCAHO standards. **Society:** Compliance with JCAHO standards.	

4. What are my options?	• Allow doctor to complete forms retrospectively and using notes from consultants. • Require that doctor complete the history and physical in a timely fashion and warn about inappropriate retrospective documentation. • Discuss noncompliance with HIM and medical staff leadership.	
5. What should I do?	Require that doctor complete the history and physical and report the problem to superiors.	
6. What justifies my choice?	**JUSTIFIED**	**NOT JUSTIFIED**
	• Obligation to comply with JCAHO standards. • Preserve professional integrity. • Support accuracy of the medical record. • Respect the law. • Demonstrate loyalty to employer, unless asked to push legal boundaries.	• Allow doctor to complete form retrospectively. • Lack of compliance with the law and JCAHO standards. • Not fair to other doctors who follow the rules. • Not fair to patient with potentially inaccurate record.
7. How can I prevent this ethical problem?	• Determine if system changes are needed. • Discuss standards and the values that support them with colleagues.	

The ethical decision-making matrix is a tool to help you organize complex, ethical problems; however, there is no simple fill-in-the-box approach to ethical decision making. The objective is to follow each step of the process and not move from the question directly to what should be done or how to prevent it next time. If you skip steps, you will not fully understand all of the values and options for action. Also, the matrix provided for each scenario in this book is not the only way to examine the problem. You can make an equally compelling ethical argument for a different decision—just be sure to follow all the steps of the matrix.

SCENARIO 4-D: CODER ASSIGNS CODE WITHOUT PHYSICIAN'S DOCUMENTATION

Steps	Information	
1. What is the ethical question?	Should the director comply with the CFO's demands by making use of incomplete information?	
2. What are the facts?	**KNOWN**	**TO BE GATHERED**
	• Medical records are incomplete. • CFO demands 72-hour turn-around.	• Is the CFO aware of legal, financial, and ethical ramifications for inaccurate coding? • Would the HIM director be held liable for inaccurate coding? • What are the customary practices here? • What is the likely impact on HIM director's family of changing jobs?
3. What are the values? Examine the shared and competing values, obligations, and interests of the stakeholders (i.e., patient, HIM professional, healthcare practitioner(s), administrators, society, and other advocates) involved in order to fully understand the complexity of the ethical problem(s).	**Patient:** Values accurate documentation as basis of receiving quality care and reimbursement. **HIM professional:** Truth, integrity, accuracy, and reliability (code accurately and reliably rather than maximize speed); fairness (follow the rules and obey the law); loyalty to employer; avoid harm (inaccurate documentation may harm the patient, closing the facility will harm patient, healthcare workers, and their families); personal values (promote welfare of family by preventing loss of job, preserve personal integrity). **Healthcare professionals:** Promote welfare of patients through accurate documentation for future care. **Administrators:** Benefit patients and keep from harm; promote welfare of facility; maximize speed of reimbursement without compromising accuracy of coding. **Society:** Follow rules of reimbursement equally for all.	

4. What are my options?	• Comply with CFO's directive. • Do not comply with CFO's directive and report the threat/violation to a superior.	
5. What should I do?	Do not comply with CFO's directive and report the threat/violation to a superior.	
6. What justifies my choice?	**JUSTIFIED**	**NOT JUSTIFIED**
	• Preserve professional integrity. • Respect the law. • Demonstrate loyalty to employer, unless asked to push legal boundaries.	• Comply with CFO's directive. • Make special exception to the rules to maximize speed of reimbursement. • Allow doctor to leave incomplete medical records. • Miscoding could compromise patients' future treatment. • Set precedent for future violations.
7. How can I prevent this ethical problem?	• Determine if system changes are needed. • Discuss standards and the values that support them with colleagues. • Evaluate institutional integrity at job interview and when ethical problems arise.	

CLINICAL CODE SELECTION AND USE

Lou Ann Schraffenberger, MBA, RHIA, CCS, CCS-P
Rita A. Scichilone, MHSA, RHIA, CCS, CCS-P, CHC

Learning Objectives

After completing this chapter, the reader should be able to:

- Understand why the assignment or use of diagnosis and procedure codes has ethical implications.
- Understand the American Health Information Management Association (AHIMA) Standards of Ethical Coding.
- Identify a variety of unethical practices related to code selection or use.
- Recognize ethical challenges that coding professionals may face and identify ways to resolve them.
- Identify ways in which ethical practices involving clinical code use can be supported by the larger practice environment.
- Recognize the roles of healthcare providers, clinical service and health information management (HIM) professionals, and business associates in the contribution to code selection and use.

Abstract

The role of the coding function in the processing of health information has changed dramatically over the past two decades. What once was a discipline for data quality is now compromised in some organizations by the relationship of codes to payments. Because of their critical role in data transmission, coders are especially likely to be affected by pressures to participate in or overlook practices that transmit misinformation. This chapter identifies a variety of potentially unethical and/or illegal coding practices. It also explores a variety of ethical dilemmas that coding professionals and clinical data managers may encounter, along with practice standards and guidelines that can be helpful in resolving them.

Scenario 5-A: Coding an Inappropriate Level of Service

As a coding professional, Rose was taught to use information from the medical record to assign codes that reflected the healthcare services rendered so that health plans could pay out benefits according to policy terms. Now she isn't sure anymore that this is what coding is about. She changed physicians, and when she reviewed her own records, she found 16 significant false entries that painted a picture of her own health status that was not true. The documentation described events and examinations that never occurred. When she attended her initial appointment with the new physician, she saw a physician assistant (PA), yet her health plan was billed and paid for a physician visit.

The service in question included a five-minute conversation about her medical history, no examination except for a Pap smear, and very little medical decision making. The visit was assigned a CPT code for a new patient office visit that involves a significant amount of work by the physician. By definition, this code states that a physician provided a comprehensive history, a comprehensive examination, and medical decisions of moderate complexity.

The record reflects all of the key elements to meet the requirements of the code, because the transcription system has a template that fills in all the gaps in the medical history and examination with normal findings. Rose's health plan allows $120 for office visits requiring this level of physician work. Because there is no way for her insurers to know that a physician was not involved in this service, they pay out the benefits for a level of service many reviewers would say may be provided only by a physician. Rose saw the physician for a follow-up for an abnormal Pap smear. When she asked the office staff why a diagnosis code for a routine checkup was used, she was told that Rose's health plan would pay for this service without a copay and they wanted to save her $10. If the office had used a more specific diagnosis code for the abnormal Pap smear, the claim might have been reviewed for medical necessity and may have been subject to different payment rules. The PA might generate $720 an hour for this physician if this practice is extended to all patients.

Questions

1. What implications do the practices of Rose's new physician have for quality of patient care?

2. Suppose that Rose works as a coder for this medical practice and knows that the same things are happening to many of the patients served. What ethical obligations does she have? What ethical principles should she consider?

A completed ethical decision-making matrix for the scenario is provided at the end of the chapter.

This chapter is about fraud and abuse in coding and billing practices, as well as any conduct or behavior regarding clinical coding systems that may create a fraudulent situation or ethical crisis for health information management (HIM) professionals. It will examine the ethical implications of selection and use of codes that represent diagnoses, procedures, and related healthcare services. In addition, it will explore the challenges of code assignments in a system where the codes reported determine the payment for services.

Coding—the transformation of words into numbers—sounds simple enough. Coding professionals read and analyze the medical record, determine what diagnosis was treated and what procedures were performed, and then assign or validate the needed codes for a variety of data uses. The documentation that is used can be found in the paper medical record or in the electronic health record. In any case, the coding professional has nothing to do with what the documentation includes. Coding professionals are charged with linking the documentation to the codes that reflect its meaning. They must take care to avoid embellishment or interpretation that exceeds their role as translators of clinical data. It is important for coders to recognize and promote appropriate documentation practices for optimal code assignment, but they must resist assigning codes for conditions the attending physician has not expressed clearly in diagnostic statements within the record. It is the coders' job to accurately translate what the documentation describes into coded data on claims forms that trigger the payments. How can ethics come into play here? And how can criminal behaviors of fraud and abuse be related to such a seemingly simple process?

The coding function in the processing of health information has changed dramatically in the last two decades and is expected to change significantly in the next five years. What once was primarily a mechanism to index diseases and operations for statistical analyses and to facilitate data retrieval for clinical research has become a mechanism for payment by health insurance plans or the government. According to the author Samuel Butler, "It has been said that the love of money is the root of all evil. The want of money is so quite as truly" (quoted in Augarde, 1992, p. 59).

Coding, once a discipline for data quality, is now compromised in some organizations by the relationship of codes to payments. As more electronic processes are used in managing healthcare transactions and storage, more ethics-based decisions and judgments will be required to protect data integrity and patient privacy, because clinical codes form the basis for electronic data interchange. For many years, coding has been a retrospective, postservice process performed after the patient's episode of care has ended and the documentation completed. As more information capture is moved to "real time," coding professionals are expected to play a larger role in ethical challenges involving initial data capture and data integrity. That requires the coders to look at codes of ethics with a new perspective.

In the early days of health insurance, the third-party payer—whether an insurance company or the government—was primarily interested in identifying the patient as one of its beneficiaries and determining the healthcare provider. Later, the payer required providers to further describe their services by using a procedural coding system, such as CPT, that was linked to an established fee schedule to determine how much money to pay the provider. Next, the payer required the healthcare provider to provide the patient's reason for healthcare services and report this reason as a complete and valid ICD-9-CM diagnosis code. More recently, the payer has developed medical coverage definitions and quality review policies designed to determine if the services should be reimbursed and if acceptable quality of service has occurred and/or optimal outcomes achieved. These initiatives describe what the payer considers to be a medical necessity or a valid reason for a patient to receive services and if the service met expected quality standards. Thus, payers set a number of "rules" for providers to follow in order to be paid.

In this process, coding systems and the individuals that select the codes play a significant role. The coding professional is part of a team of healthcare personnel that serves both the patient and the business interests of the enterprise. The team includes the physician, other healthcare providers, and the business associates who provide the administrative support to run the practice.

The patient seeks health care. The physician or other healthcare provider examines the patient, renders treatment, and documents the situation. Other healthcare providers may become involved with the patient's care and similarly document their interactions. The information is sent in a paper record or in electronic format to the coding professional, who assigns the codes or verifies that an automated system has correctly assigned them. The coded data, which will determine what services can be billed to the payer and at what rates, are transmitted to the billing department, and the claim is produced and submitted to the third-party payer for payment. The claim is paid according to the terms of the health plan. The provider deposits the revenue. Payrolls are met, people are employed, patients receive continued care with limited out-of-pocket costs, capital budgets support new technology and services, and the healthcare provider or facility flourishes.

Problems with this system arise when something goes wrong within the team or within the process used to obtain the reimbursement. Someone does not perform his or her duty appropriately or fails to understand that what he or she does is cheating someone else. For example, the physician bills for services that he or she does not provide or are provided at a lower level of work than the code implies. Ethical problems arise when someone decides not to play by the rules or deliberately avoids learning the rules so that innocence is plausible when he or she is caught. For example, the billing manager does not know what Medicare's noncovered services are. Someone starts to stretch the truth or perhaps completely disregard the truth to protect his or her position or increase his or her income. It may all be unspoken, but everyone on the team discovers how confusing the rules for health plan reimbursement can be, particularly when health plans all follow a slightly different set of rules or contractual obligations are involved. The team members discover that insurance billing is not as simple as it appears.

Because of their critical role in data transmission, individuals who assign or validate codes are especially likely to be affected by pressures to participate in or overlook practices that transmit misinformation. They can end up deeply implicated in practices, such as misrepresenting the diagnosis for a patient to justify the services rendered, that could result in criminal prosecution under some circumstances or loss of employment or professional credentials due to lack of compliance with professional standards. As long as coding directly relates to the payment to be received, human coders and data managers will face ethical dilemmas. Three major areas of concern are upcoding, unbundling, and evading requirements that a service be medically necessary to be reimbursed.

- **Upcoding.** This occurs when a provider bills for a higher level of service than rendered in order to receive a higher reimbursement. Rose, in Scenario 5-A, encountered **upcoding** during her visit to the physician who used a high-level service code when the service was not that complex.

- **Unbundling.** This occurs when a provider bills separately for each component of a procedure instead of using the proper code for the entire procedure. With **unbundling,** the fees for the separate procedures result in a higher reimbursement (King, 1999). Increasingly, health plans want to create disincentives for healthcare providers to pile up hundreds of separate charges for service. Instead, they want to base reimbursement on a system more like a restaurant check. They will pay for what was ordered, but they no longer will pay for use of the silverware, a chef's consultation fee, a rental fee for the use of tablecloths and napkins, and separate charges for each food item and condiment that was made available to the diner during the eating experience. In a healthcare example, health plans reimburse for operative services using "global package" concepts for physicians and "facility fees" for hospitals. Most pay for an operation (expressed as codes) rather than room rent, use of clamps, and so on. For physicians, it is expected that there would be both preoperative and postoperative visits to inform the patient about the process and check on his or her condition before and after the operation. Health plans include these services in the fee for the operation. Getting a health plan to pay for services through code manipulation (changing dates, adding modifiers, etc.) is an example of unethical behavior by a coder when it is done with the intent of securing reimbursement not allowed by a payer.

- **Evading medical necessity requirements.** Coders may be expected to ignore the true (noncovered) reason for a test or service and instead use one of the conditions that is listed in a Medicare national coverage policy as a covered service. They may even be asked to fabricate physician orders with a payable diagnosis and then get a physician signature after the fact.

HIPAA AND BILLING ACTIVITIES

It should be noted that many of the practices just described are potentially fraudulent or abusive billing activities. In 1996, the Health Insurance Portability and Accountability Act (HIPAA) created the Health Care Fraud and Abuse Control Program to combat fraud and abuse in the Medicare and Medicaid programs by providing funds for investigations and the prosecution of offenders and by streamlining data management to make tracking and identification of illegal activities easier. The program is coordinated by the Office of the Inspector General (OIG) and the Department of Justice (DOJ). Other federal and state agencies become involved with fraud and abuse prevention outside of the federal programs (Prophet, 1997). For example, state Medicaid

agencies investigate possible fraud and abuse committed with regard to billing for services rendered to Medicaid beneficiaries.

Resources on fraud schemes and how to recognize and report inappropriate behavior are available at the Centers for Medicare and Medicaid Web site (http://www.cms.hhs.gov/providers/fraud).

According to HIPAA, criminal penalties can be imposed on a healthcare individual who "knowingly and willfully" attempts to defraud a healthcare benefit program of money or property. Such behavior can be punished by criminal penalties, including imprisonment. Civil penalties can cost the individual thousands of dollars in fines and assessments.

Fraud is an intentional deception or misrepresentation that an individual knows to be false or does not believe to be true and that he or she nevertheless makes, knowing that the deception could result in some unauthorized benefit to the person who commits the act. The most frequent kind of fraud arises from a false statement or misrepresentation made, or caused to be made, that is material to entitlement or payment under the Medicare program. The term **abuse** describes incidents or practices of physicians or suppliers of equipment that, although not usually considered fraudulent, are inconsistent with accepted sound medical, business, or fiscal practices (Centers for Medicare and Medicaid, 2004; Wisconsin Physicians Services, 2004).

Providers have the responsibility to stay current with Medicare rules and regulations. It is also the provider's responsibility to ensure that administrative personnel understand Medicare guidelines as they pertain to coding and billing for services provided (Wisconsin Physicians Services, 2004). Can an individual coding professional be prosecuted for a coding error or billing mistake? Yes, those persons who have direct knowledge of and facilitate the process of filing false claims will be held accountable. Innocent errors made without any benefit to the coder (financial gains or other incentives) are generally not considered fraudulent events subject to criminal prosecution, but repeated or significant errors that misrepresent services remain a risk to both the individual and the organization he or she works for.

Members of the team involved with patient care and the subsequent coding and billing of the services (procedure codes) and the reasons they are provided (diagnosis codes) have a duty to establish procedures to prevent mistakes. As with any team, each player has to know the rules and how to perform. Team members, including HIM professionals, must not ignore the rules or be afraid to challenge someone who they know is not following regulatory guidelines. These challenges require ethical behavior, which always requires courage.

ETHICAL APPROACHES TO CODING SITUATIONS

In Chapter 2 of this book, Glover describes two classic ethical theories: utilitarianism and deontological theories. These theories can be used to guide and direct moral reasoning and decision making. Utilitarianism considers the consequences of the action; deontological theories examine the duties that are binding on the person, such as the obligation to abide by the rules and standards of one's profession. Glover reminds us that moral theories do not provide the "answer"— it is still up to the individual to strive to make reliable moral judgments.

Utilitarian Approaches

Utilitarianism is a theory that judges the rightness or wrongness of an action by its consequences and by what will happen if the action is not performed. According to this theory, actions are right in proportion to their tendency to promote happiness and wrong if they tend to promote the reverse.

As applied to coding for healthcare services, a utilitarian approach would examine the consequences of the action. What will happen, for example, if the coder uses one code rather than another code to describe the patient's condition or the treatment rendered so that the insurance company or a government program will pay the bill? The patient will not have to spend money when the insurance company or the government pays, the provider will be happy because money is received, the employer will be happy with the coder's performance, and the coder will be happy because he or she has a good job with a respectable salary due to its association with reimbursement. Won't everybody be happy? Some might be happy with the behavior, but not everyone.

The health benefits plan and the U.S. taxpayer may not be happy when a payment is made for a noncovered service or for a higher level of service than was actually provided. Use of funds in this manner actually adds to the cost of others' legitimate and critically needed healthcare services. Spiraling healthcare costs may cripple the U.S. economy.

Coders who knowingly code from documentation that is intended to defraud, the way the coder for Rose's record did in Scenario 5-A, are potentially harming the patients whose medical records they are coding. For instance, in Scenario 5-A, if Rose's documentation indicates comprehensive exams but she is given only cursory exams, she is being defrauded of the level of care that she is paying premiums for. She is also potentially being placed in jeopardy, because she may have a medical condition that a cursory exam would not uncover or would misdiagnose. If she does have a medical condition, documentation falsely stating that she got a full exam that uncovered nothing important can lull the other providers who deal with her into complacency and make them less observant that something may be wrong (i.e., "Doctor X gave her a full exam and didn't find anything, so I don't have to look closely myself"). A cursory exam could also result in Rose's getting less information about a medical condition and its treatment options than she might receive from a full exam that would allow the provider more time to interact with her. And if her medical records don't mention the abnormal Pap smear, an important part of her medical history that could affect future provider decisions is being obscured. Finally, if Rose is aware of wrongdoing, she may feel coerced into keeping silent because of fears that it will be more difficult for her to get healthcare services in the future. The coder, by going along with this situation, is ethically (and perhaps also legally) implicated in the physician's wrongdoing.

Deontological Approaches

Deontological theories are based on duties rather than consequences. For coding professionals, an important set of duties to be considered in deciding on an ethical course of action is the professional obligations that are outlined in standards and codes of conduct.

The **Standards of Ethical Coding** developed by AHIMA's Coding Policy and Strategy Committee (AHIMA, 2000b) and approved by its board of directors provide a code of conduct that forms the basis for ethical decision making. Although it applies to those individuals with AHIMA credentials, it may also be used by other persons performing the coding function who may not hold either an HIM or a coding certification.

These standards will not provide all the answers for those faced with an ethical decision, because ethics often transcend the normal legalistic view and often involve highly complex situations involving more than just translation of text into numbers according to some rules. However, the fact that fellow coding professionals have declared these standards to be the standards of conduct for an ethical, professional coder can help recommend a course of action.

Core Competencies and Credentials

In addition to the AHIMA Standards of Ethical Coding, credentialed coders may find the established competencies for their certification to be a helpful guide for conduct and practice. For example, AHIMA offers three professional certification examinations: Certified Coding

Associate (CCA), Certified Coding Specialist (CCS), and Certified Coding Specialist—Physician Based (CCS-P) credentials.

The core competencies describe the essential knowledge and skills required for coding professionals. AHIMA validates these competencies by surveying practicing credentialed individuals and asking them what their coding activities and associated tasks include. That is, the credentialed coders agree that the core competencies reflect their daily practice in the workplace. The questions written for these certification examinations are based on these competencies. By passing the examination, candidates demonstrate the prerequisite knowledge and skills described by the competencies. The CCA credential is designed for entry-level coding skill validation. Both the CCS and CCS-P credentials describe competencies related to (1) data identification, (2) coding guidelines, (3) regulatory guidelines, (4) coding, and (5) data quality (AHIMA, 2000a).

Most of the competencies require the individual to "apply knowledge" of a particular function or procedure. However, ethical standards also are included. For example, the CCS coding competencies include the statements "Refuse to fraudulently maximize reimbursement by assigning codes that do not conform to approved coding principles/guidelines" and "Refuse to unfairly maximize reimbursement by unbundling services or codes that do not conform to CPT basic coding principles."

Do these competencies apply only to credentialed coders? The competencies can be used to describe the duties and characteristics of anyone performing coding duties, including physicians and other healthcare providers who assume this function without assistance from an HIM professional. Only certified coders will lose something (the right to use their professional certification) if they fail to abide by these principles; however, all coders can get into legal trouble if they intentionally and purposefully violate these standards for personal gain. When the complexity of competent, ethical coding is not understood, the belief that "coding is simple, just look it up in the index" can result in code assignments that are inaccurate and inappropriate for reimbursement. It behooves the healthcare community to hire coding professionals with these credentials, which substantiate their expertise. The healthcare system, from both clinical and reimbursement perspectives, cannot tolerate inaccurate assignment or use of codes, because this language is what is used in electronic systems to store and transmit clinical facts about healthcare conditions and services.

APPLYING THE AHIMA STANDARDS OF ETHICAL CODING

Code numbers and dollar signs easily can become confused. Team members may lose sight of the informative function of codes and view them only as the means to the end of getting reimbursed. Healthcare providers cannot, or will not, thrive without money, so it is very tempting to use coding to increase payments, even in what many believe are innocent and appropriate methods.

The following potentially unethical coding practices are presented along with the standard from the AHIMA Standards of Ethical Coding that they may violate. The coding professional should not participate in any of the practices mentioned that conflict with the ethical guidelines.

1. Coding professionals are expected to support the importance of accurate, complete, and consistent coding practices for the production of quality healthcare data.

The following are some practices that could conflict with this ethical coding statement:

- Coding incomplete medical records, with the result that incomplete data are produced.
- Selecting a particular code to avoid a billing edit. For example, the billing software includes an edit that does not allow an unspecified code to be used. Instead

of asking the physician for the information, the coder selects another code in the same category just to avoid the edit.
- Assigning the diagnosis codes strictly for those conditions listed on the face sheet or problem list instead of examining the entire medical record. The result is that the coder misses important clinical details that affect the patient's insurance coverage.
- Accepting and coding what the physician provides. For example, the physician consistently only checks off one diagnosis on an encounter form. The coder does not ask the physician for additional diagnoses, even though more are known to exist, because coding goes faster this way and interruptions annoy the physician and delay the billing process.
- Establishing a coding plan with no consideration for quality. For example, the coding supervisor establishes an incentive pay program for coders based on productivity, with no quality standards included. A message is provided here: "A good coder makes the most money possible for each claim."

2. Coding professionals in all healthcare settings should adhere to the ICD-9-CM (International Classification of Diseases, 9th revision, Clinical Modification) coding conventions, official coding guidelines approved by the Cooperating Parties (AHIMA, Centers for Medicare and Medicaid Services, National Center for Health Statistics, and American Hospital Association), the CPT (Current Procedural Terminology) rules established by the American Medical Association, and any other official coding rules and guidelines established for use with mandated standard code sets. Selection and sequencing of diagnoses and procedures must meet the definitions of required

data sets for applicable health-care settings.

The following are some practices that could conflict with this ethical coding statement:

- Ignoring a coding principle and assigning a symptom code for the principal diagnosis when the cause of the symptom is known. Coding the symptom as the principal diagnosis creates a higher-paying DRG.
- Selecting a principal diagnosis so that DRG 468 (Extensive Operating Room procedure, unrelated to Principal Diagnosis) is assigned and a higher reimbursement is received instead of the correct DRG when the more appropriate principal diagnosis is assigned.
- Disregarding the notation of "separate procedure" in the CPT book and assigning multiple CPT codes when one comprehensive code may be more appropriate because, from the coder's point of view, this is a rule that does not apply to the facility's coding.
- Coding "rule-out" conditions as if the condition existed in an attempt to substantiate the need for the outpatient test or service.
- Using an unlisted CPT code for a service that is known to be included in evaluation and management services, such as removal of sutures placed by the same physician.
- Assigning a CPT for an outpatient office visit based on the amount that will be paid for that CPT code, because the physician considers the payments for other codes to be too low.
- Ignoring the Official Advice in *Coding Clinic* concerning V-codes, because the business office director is adamantly against any V-code in the first position on an outpatient claim.

3. Coding professionals should use their skills, their knowledge of the currently mandated coding and classification systems, and official resources to select the appropriate diagnostic and procedural codes.

The following are some practices that could conflict with this ethical coding statement:

- Ignoring Coding Clinic advice about the way a particular condition should be coded because a higher-paying DRG would be assigned if a different diagnosis code were assigned as the principal diagnosis.
- Failing to read or review *National Coverage Decisions* from CMS or the local Carrier or Fiscal Intermediary Medicare bulletins and local medical review policies.
- Failing to subscribe to authoritative references such as the AHA *Coding Clinic* or AMA *CPT Assistant,* because the "coders don't have time to read them anyway."
- Basing code assignments on maximization of insurance reimbursement rather than any other criteria and disciplining coders when code selection does not result in the highest possible payments.

4. Coding professionals should only assign and report codes that are clearly and consistently supported by physician documentation in the health record.

The following are some practices that could conflict with this ethical coding statement:

- Using a CPT code while knowing that it does not accurately describe the procedure, because no other code can be used except an unlisted one.
- Assigning a code that qualifies as a complication in the DRG system based on lab results (e.g., postoperative anemia) that are not mentioned by the physician in the documentation.
- Coding diagnoses supplied by the physician or other healthcare provider for a service that is not supported by documentation within the body of the record.
- Following the advice of a coding consultant who directs the coder to code conditions described in EKG, echocardio-

grams, and laboratory reports regardless of whether the physician has mentioned the same conditions in the record and outlined their clinical significance.

- Coding all cystoscopies performed on patients for "practice" by the residents as substantiated by urinary incontinence.
- Coding all patients seen in the clinic by the end of the day even if the patients' records cannot be located and assigning a standard "fill-in" code of 799.9 (other unknown and unspecified cause of morbidity and mortality) in the absence of the patient's record.
- Assigning the "acute" condition code for all patients treated in the emergency room, even if the physician does not qualify the condition as "acute or subacute."
- Continuing to facilitate the reporting process when it is known that the documentation or health-record entries on which the codes are based is false, because the coder is assured that he or she has no personal liability in the matter.

5. Coding professionals should consult physicians for clarification and additional documentation prior to code assignment when there are conflicting or ambiguous data in the health record.

The following are some practices that could conflict with this ethical coding statement:

- Failing to query the physicians or asking questions to clarify documentation; instead directing coders to code what the physician writes anywhere in the record or what they can assume based on their clinical expertise.
- Failing to wait for a physician to respond to an inquiry about incomplete documentation, because all coding must be completed within three days after discharge.
- Asking questions only of physicians who are "nice" to the coder and avoiding those physicians who are difficult to communicate with.

- Encouraging physicians to add entries to the record to support comorbid conditions or complications that affect DRG assignment that were not important enough to document during the hospital stay; asking physicians to add these into existing progress notes or postdate them so that they appear to have been written during the episode of care.
- Assigning codes to health-record entries created by healthcare workers not authorized by law to diagnose or provide treatment.

6. Coding professionals should not change codes or the narratives of codes on the billing abstract so that the meanings are misrepresented. Diagnoses or procedures should not be inappropriately included or excluded because the payment or insurance policy coverage requirements will be affected. When individual payer policies conflict with official coding rules and guidelines, these policies should be obtained in writing whenever possible. Reasonable efforts should be made to educate the payer on proper coding practices in order to influence a change in the payer's policy.

The following are some practices that could conflict with this ethical coding statement:

- Assigning diagnosis codes based on coverage policies to ensure "reimbursement appropriateness" and minimize denials.
- Locating a "better or payable" diagnosis for an outpatient service after the original reason for service provided by the physician does not reflect medical necessity for the test.
- Coding a record so that the payer or patient will have the lowest possible financial liability. For example, knowing that self-pay patients are billed according to the DRG assigned to a case, a coder

codes a record as a normal delivery because the patient is the coder's niece, even though the delivery had complications. With the lower DRG assigned, the patient will have a lower bill to pay than she would have been responsible for if the record had been coded correctly.

- Eliminating coding of certain conditions. For example, a coder in a long-term care facility leaves off diagnoses that reflect trauma the patient received in a fall in the facility, because the facility administrator is concerned that state surveyors might question the treatment rendered at the facility.

- Modifying the coding of certain conditions. For example, a coder changes a psychiatric diagnosis to a nonspecific medical diagnosis so that a patient can continue to receive treatment from the primary care physician instead of being sent to a psychiatrist, as is the policy of the managed care company.

- Coding for conditions that patients no longer have. For example, a coder is directed to use a code for a condition the patient previously had because it was used the last time the bill was paid.

- Coding for conditions that patients do not have. For example, a coder is directed to use a code for a condition that the patient does not have but that allows a test to be paid for.

- Avoiding the reporting of preexisting conditions that are the focus of treatment when the patient's health plan will not cover the service and instead using a different diagnosis that involves the same therapy.

- Omitting the codes for postoperative complications and nosocomial infections to protect the facility from a negative statistical profile.

7. Coding professionals, as members of the health care team, should assist and educate physicians and other clinicians by advocating proper documentation practices, further specificity, resequencing, or inclusion of diagnoses or procedures when needed to more accurately reflect the acuity, severity, and the occurrence of events.

The following are some practices that could conflict with this ethical coding statement:

- Retyping a progress note that includes additional diagnoses and directing the physician to sign the note for incorporation into the record, knowing that the physician rarely reads what is signed.

- Failing to attempt to provide coding and documentation education to the medical staff, because "they never listen anyway" or "they do not have the time."

- Failing to take action to rectify or report a process that is known to be unethical and to abuse the third-party payer benefit system because of a lack of personal or professional confidence.

- Accepting the notion that the government and the healthcare insurance companies deserve to be cheated, because reimbursement for services never equals the charges made.

- Failing, on the part of the organization, to make physicians accountable for providing diagnoses and procedural information and instead requiring the coders to make do with what is available or to create codes that result in paid claims.

8. Coding professionals should participate in the development of institutional coding policies and should ensure that coding policies complement, not conflict with, official coding rules and guidelines.

The following are some practices that could conflict with this ethical coding statement:

- Developing a coding policy that directs coders to code from encounter forms or one section of the record instead of using the entire medical record.

- Developing an internal coding policy for the coding of respiratory failure as the principal diagnosis, which results in a higher DRG payment, thus conflicting with the official coding guidelines.
- Writing corporate coding policies that direct the coder to code from lab reports and to interpret certain situations as postoperative complications, even if the physician does not support the claim with documentation.
- Purchasing automated encoding software that matches all known payable diagnoses with the associated procedures but does not allow any other code to be reported for that service.

9. Coding professionals should maintain and continually enhance their coding skills, as they have a professional responsibility to stay abreast of changes in codes, coding guidelines, and regulations.

The following are some practices that could conflict with this ethical coding statement:

- Failing to validate the DRG assigned and submitted for payment.
- Requiring that every patient sign an "Advance Beneficiary Notice" prior to receiving services, regardless of the service to be received and the reason for the service. Even if the provider is unaware that blanket waivers are illegal and could subject every claim to a false claims charge, the practice is not acceptable.
- Performing coding accuracy studies only on certain payers; for example, reviewing only Medicare and Medicaid claims for accuracy.
- Failing to attend ongoing continuing education. For example, an organization may not budget or allow coding professionals to use work time to attend conferences, read pertinent professional literature, or receive additional professional development or education. The coding professional may accept this as a

reason for not knowing that a particular coding practice was inappropriate.

10. Coding professionals should strive for the optimal payment to which the facility is legally entitled, remembering that it is unethical and illegal to maximize payment by means that contradict regulatory guidelines.

The following are some practices that could conflict with this ethical coding statement:

- Billing for more services based on time than could reasonably be performed in a business day.
- Failing to rebill the Medicare fiscal intermediary for a particular claim when a coding audit determines that a lower-paying DRG should have been assigned instead of the original DRG assigned.
- Basing a regional corporate coding director's yearly bonuses on the DRG reimbursement received at hospitals in his or her territory even though the coding policies created by the director are in conflict with official coding guidelines.
- Failing to acknowledge that the coding professional has violated coding guidelines that have resulted in significant overpayment for services and failing to bring this to the attention of appropriate persons who are responsible for the claims so that steps may be taken to resolve the issue appropriately.
- Following the advice of a coding consulting practice that advises healthcare organizations in methods to "game the system" and obtain reimbursement under false pretenses.
- Failing to report that a colleague or employer is engaging in fraudulent methods to obtain payment and not using the organization's compliance program out of fear of reprisal.
- Creating a documentation template for a physician to support upcoding by padding the record with normal values and exami-

nation elements that were not part of the work performed during the visit.

- Creating records and coding and billing for services that appear to be completed by a physician when in fact a nonphysician, such as a physician assistant, a nurse practitioner, an office nurse, a medical assistant, a medical student, or a medical resident in a teaching arrangement, rendered the service.
- Submitting codes under a provider number other than the one for the provider who actually provided the service because the rendering provider has yet to be credentialed or enrolled by the health plan or government service responsible for the patient's healthcare costs.
- Recommending or endorsing software that influences the assignment or service documentation based on the health plan requirements without regard to the accuracy of the concepts or services that the code reflects. Failure to point out known accuracy problems or facilitation of falsified health record documentation with an automated coding software program would also be considered a variant

of unethical behavior for a coding professional.

Use of information technology is a concern for government programs so "prudent hospitals will take steps to ensure that they thoroughly assess all new computer systems that impact coding, billing, or the generation or transmission of information . . ." The AHIMA Standards of Ethical Coding application is critically important, because as more processes are automated, the risk of inappropriate reporting of coded data increases.

Standards reprinted here with permission of American Health Information Management Association's Coding Policy and Strategy Committee, Standards of Ethical Coding, *Journal of the American Health Information Management Association,* Vol. 71, No. 3, ©March 2000, American Health Information Management Association.

ETHICAL DILEMMAS FOR THE CODING PROFESSIONAL

The following are some typical ethical dilemmas that the coding professional may encounter.

Scenario 5-B: Discovering Misrepresentation in Physician Documentation

Jim, a coding professional, is employed by a group of urologists who bill Medicare, Medicaid, and all private insurance plans for several laboratory tests that are considered to be screening tests. They also perform cystoscopies in the office and in the hospital where they are on staff. Jim's job involves assignment of the diagnosis code for these services and review of the CPT codes that the physicians have checked. He codes from the encounter form that has been filled out by the physicians, because, typically, several days pass before the dictation and results are available for review, and the physicians want the bills out one day after the date of service. All applicable coding principles are applied, and the encounter forms are reviewed each year for CPT coding changes. When Jim once asked why the individual laboratory tests were reported rather than the disease panel codes, the physician explained that there was a clinical requirement for the individual tests.

Jim enjoys a salary that is $5.00 per hour more than that of his peers at the hospital, and everyone in the office receives a year-end bonus if the practice exceeds a certain revenue target. Recently, he attended a workshop where medical necessity requirements for Medicare patients were discussed. Fraudulent billing practices by physicians for unnecessary services and tests were presented, along with the penalties that could be assessed. Jim realized then that his employer was making much of its income in this fashion. He contacted AHIMA and was told to assign and report only codes that are clearly and consistently supported by physician documentation in the health record. Although Jim's coding is accurate, he knows that the information that it is based on may be false.

Question

1. What is Jim's best course of action?

A completed ethical decision-making matrix for the scenario is provided at the end of the chapter.

Credentialed coding professionals are bound by professional ethics and a standard of conduct. Coders are taught communication methods and data analysis to solve data-quality problems. Table 5–1 shows one course of action that may keep the employer from difficulties with business ethics violations and earn the respect of the physician that employs the coder.

Scenario 5-C: Miscoding to Avoid Conflicts

Gretchen, a registered health information technician (RHIT) and a clinical coding specialist (CCS), has worked for the Headache and Pain Center for over 10 years. Her job responsibilities include diagnosis and procedure coding for the services provided by the Ambulatory Surgical Center (ASC) owned by a group of anesthesiologists. The physicians routinely provide pain management services to Medicare patients, including epidural injections involving cervical, thoracic, and lumbar vertebrae. Claim forms are submitted to Medicare with CPT4 codes.

Several years ago, Gretchen read in a credible professional coding resource that the CPT book's description had changed recently to reflect only procedures performed on the lumbar region and that there was no longer any valid CPT code for an epidural injection of a steroid into the cervical and thoracic vertebrae. Knowing that the physicians sought reimbursement by Medicare for a facility fee when this procedure was performed, she contacted the Medicare provider representative. The representative suggested that she continue to use the CPT for the epidural. She trusted this advice and did not speak to the physicians about her concerns.

Gretchen was somewhat uncomfortable with using a CPT code that did not exactly describe what had been done, but not using the codes would make the physicians very angry, because no facility payment would be made. To avoid any misunderstanding, she changed the description in the billing system with the codes to reflect cervical epidural injection.

continues on page 113

Table 5–1 Business Ethics Action Plan

Action Options	Specific Tasks	Potential Outcome
A. Devise a plan to be approved by the medical director for a complete review of office billing procedures. Present this plan to all physicians.	1. Stop the practice of "insurance only" billing so that the patient appropriately shares in the cost of care and is not "talked into" a cystoscopy because there is no cost.	Physician loses money. Coder's salary or bonuses are frozen or decreased. Other employees lose jobs, including the coder.
	2. Plan an audit of claims (CMS1500 forms) with the associated clinical documentation and encounter form to identify variances between codes submitted and codes supported.	Problems with billing may be discovered.
	3. Decide if the audit is done retrospectively after the bills have been paid or on a pre-billing basis before the claim is submitted.	a. Payment may have to be returned. Doctor may have to prepare for restitution with the payer. b. Claims may have to be amended. Doctor may have to prepare for less reimbursement.
B. Identify resources needed for the audit.	1. Select a sample number of cases for each physician in the highest risk areas; for example, lab tests and cystoscopy performed.	a. Physician liaison may need to be available for clinical advice to staff during review process.
	2. Determine the minimum number of cases to be reviewed per physician.	
	3. Locate record, paid claim, or prepared bill for each case.	
	4. Use health plan medical necessity criteria and/or Medicare's national or local medical review policies.	
	5. Use HCFA-CMS-AMA documentation guidelines for evaluation of visit level appropriateness.	
	6. Use current ICD-9-CM and CPT coding books.	
	7. Design audit worksheets.	
	8. Identify competent staff to conduct review.	
C. Review the findings of the audit.	1. Prepare a summary by doctor of the audit findings.	a. Audit may or may not reveal a pattern of questionable charges.

continues

Table 5–1 continued

Action Options	Specific Tasks	Potential Outcome
	2. Determine how audit findings will be communicated.	b. Sporadic questionable charges may be identified by all physicians or individual physicians. c. Widespread questionable charges may be identified.
D. Determine the impact of the audit findings.	1. Determine that no further study is needed. 2. Determine if more records should be examined. 3. Consider voluntary self-disclosure to the government and other health plans to minimize fines and penalties.	a. No impact on practice. b. External coding and billing professionals may be needed to assess audit findings or conduct a more comprehensive audit. c. Seek legal counsel to proceed with voluntary disclosure activities with the payers.
E. Determine what actions are needed to correct problems identified, especially concerning documentation and billing practices.	1. Inform physicians of the audit findings. 2. Educate physicians on the risk of falsifying records to obtain insurance payment. 3. Emphasize the use of the Advance Beneficiary Notice and full disclosure of the cost of care and the patient's right to refuse. 4. Emphasize the physician's obligation to inform the patient why the test or procedure is necessary.	a. No action needed. b. Change the billing process to require completed documentation before submission of claim and assigning codes based on documentation rather than checking off boxes on an encounter form. c. Facilitate ready access to health plan requirements in a convenient place for physician reference so that appropriate documentation is captured at the time the test is ordered.
F. Make recommendations for ongoing review.	1. Assume that the audit verified suspicious variances and revealed inappropriate and excessive use of tests and cystoscopy to inflate practice income; take steps to correct billing abuses. 2. Implement ongoing and routine review of code assignment with documentation, and monitor billing patterns. 3. Subject questionable audit findings to peer review by a physician inside or outside the practice. Physicians at variance must explain.	a. An ethical business plan is created. b. Remove the incentive for the physician and biller to upcode. c. Provide employment bonuses based on valid job-related performance rather than practice income from health plans.

Scenario 5-C continued

Because the Medicare representative said the coding would be appropriate, she went ahead and billed this way for three years until CPT corrected the problem in 2000. Now, a postpayment review by Medicare has discovered the coding variance and has made the physician return the substantial overpayment for noncovered ASC facility services. The physicians blame Gretchen for miscoding the services and are taking the issue to court.

Questions

1. What ethical and/or compliance issues are evident in this scenario?

2. What could Gretchen have done to avoid this situation? How could everyone involved have prevented the situation?

A completed ethical decision-making matrix for the scenario is provided at the end of the chapter.

As a credentialed coding professional, Gretchen is expected to have at least minimum competency in the management of health information and a mastery level of knowledge concerning coding systems and guidelines. Part of this knowledge includes knowing who and what to trust as the source of coding and billing information. Gretchen made a mistake in relying on "unofficial" and inaccurate advice from an individual person at the insurance company instead of getting a policy in writing. As a result, she used a CPT code that did not accurately describe a procedure, all the while knowing that it did not, because no other code existed other than an unlisted code that could be used. In doing so, she violated standard 4 of AHIMA's Standards of Ethical Coding, which states that "coding professionals should only assign and report codes that are clearly and consistently supported by physician documentation in the patient record." In addition, she was too nervous to approach the physicians and instead took the easy way out. She should have discussed this problem with the physicians and made no changes without their full knowledge and consent.

As it was, her decision created bigger problems in the long run. The physicians who submit claims have their signatures affixed to the claim form, so it is generally not possible for them to escape personal accountability. When things go wrong, people want to affix blame; therefore, the person who assigned the codes may be held responsible.

This kind of situation can be prevented by employing a competent coding professional and by requiring billing staff to be aware of and use official coding guideline resources such as *CPT Assistant* from the American Medical Association and *Coding Clinic for ICD-9-CM* from the American Hospital Association. Physicians must be approachable concerning coding problems encountered, and they must stay involved to make sure the process is accurate or face the consequences. Engaging a qualified coding and billing consultant to periodically assess billing procedures and review claim information with clinical documentation can help prevent costly errors. Once miscoding has been discovered, a complete review should be undertaken to calculate the amount of overpayment from insurance plans that based payment on the wrong code. Business ethics demands that overpayments should be returned to the health plans with an admission of the billing error.

Scenario 5-D: Discovery of Miscoding by Other Staff Members

Right after obtaining her clinical coding specialist, physician-based CCS-P credential, Shirley is hired by a prominent psychiatrist to provide coding and reimbursement assistance for his billing. The policy of this office is to assign codes for a "standard" visit that consists of a 50-minute psychotherapy session unless the physician indicates that a different service has taken place.

Shirley begins to notice that as many as 23 patient claims for a single date of service contain the code for a 50-minute psychotherapy session. She also reviews the requirements of the code for "face-to-face" services and observes that the physician indicates this service when only medical record review, medication adjustment, or instructions to nursing staff at the hospital have been performed. The physician has a long-term employee (his wife's sister), Anne, who prepares and submits all insurance claims. Shirley speaks with Anne regarding her concerns about the 50-minute visits. Anne assures Shirley that there is no need for concern, because Medicare has denied no services and because "extra" services are commonly bundled into psychotherapy services in this region.

Questions

1. What should Shirley's role be in this situation?

2. Suppose that an investigation of this practice's billing irregularities is now under way by the Office of the Inspector General. What steps should Shirley recommend for this practice?

3. How could the threat of a government investigation and a criminal court action have been prevented in the first place?

A completed ethical decision-making matrix for the scenario is provided at the end of the chapter.

Shirley was not a part of the creation of the fraud, but when she accepted the position she took on an ethical obligation to assist the practice in correct use of the coding systems and to facilitate a correction of the problem in a forthright and ethical manner. The psychiatrist's practice is billing for more services than could reasonably be performed in a business day, thereby violating standard 10 of AHIMA's Standards of Ethical Coding, which states that "coding professionals should strive for the optimal payment to which the facility is legally entitled, remembering that it is unethical and illegal to maximize payment by means that contradict regulatory guidelines."

What should be Shirley's role in this situation? The practice is already in the "hot seat," because false claims have been identified, so correction of the coding and billing practices is the first order of business. Shirley should discuss with the physician and the biller the specific services that are included in each code. She should discuss what codes can be used to describe the physician's services and how to recognize when certain physician services cannot be coded and billed.

If things have gone so far that an investigation is under way by the government, Shirley should fully cooperate with the review process and organize a compliance plan to outline corrective measures, including an ongoing coding and billing review process by a neutral outside party. She should educate current billing staff on correct procedures and then monitor their work to ensure that only what is supported by documentation is submitted for reimbursement. She should also provide regulatory requirements to the psychiatrist by showing examples of appropriate billing and sample documentation that supports it.

Practices can avoid the threat of OIG investigation and criminal court action by staffing their business operations with competent, educated professionals who are knowledgeable concerning billing and coding requirements (or by using a qualified billing service). They can also ensure that everyone understands which services are and are not included in a particular code. Further, it should be understood that because each patient is unique, having a "standard" for any specific class of patients for documentation shortcuts is a dangerous practice. No services should be billed for that were not provided at the level stated by the code. Finally, billing review and audits can be conducted to ensure that correct information is being submitted on claim forms for health plan reimbursement (getting the site of service right).

Scenario 5-E: Lacking the Tools to Do One's Job

Charlene, a CCS, works for Healthy Management Association Inc. (HMAI), which contracts with a large university hospital for providing healthcare services for patients in a health maintenance plan administered by HMAI. The arrangement provides that the HMAI will pay the university 114 percent of the DRG base rate for patients served. HMAI does not have a DRG grouper, so when the claims come to Charlene for processing, she uses the DRG that is handwritten in the "remarks" column of the UB-92, the billing claim form. Charlene's job is to review the coding on the claims for accuracy and completeness and serve as the organization's "resident expert" for coding issues. Although Charlene is an excellent coder, she has had very little experience in reimbursement systems, including DRG assignment. She assumes that the university hospital's DRG assignment is valid, because they have professional coders and special software. She is happy with her job—it is one of the easiest jobs she has ever had as a coder.

One afternoon, Charlene is called into a conference room where the CEO, CFO, and board members are having a meeting. They want an accounting of DRG validity, because the university hospital has overcharged the organization by sometimes writing in the wrong DRG assignments.

Question

1. What steps could Charlene have taken to avoid getting into this predicament?

A completed ethical decision-making matrix for the scenario is provided at the end of the chapter.

To some degree, Charlene knew this job was easier than it should have been. Charlene failed to further her education in an area that affected her job responsibilities, thereby violating standard 9 of AHIMA's Standards of Ethical Coding, which states that "coding professionals should maintain and continually enhance their coding skills, as they have a professional responsibility to stay abreast of changes in codes, coding guidelines, and regulations." She has also made the age-old error of assuming too much. Rather than taking the hospital's DRG assignment as gospel, she should have informed administration that she could not attest to the accuracy of DRG assignment without the appropriate grouping software or reference materials. By not pressing this issue, she participated in a process that resulted in inappropriate reimbursement for her organization. She failed in her ethical duty to continue her professional development through additional continuing education. She also failed to recognize that her lack of knowledge (and lack of initiative) put the organization at risk.

Scenario 5-F: Being Required by the Employer to Engage in Negligent Coding Practices

Susan, RHIA, CCS, has been manager of clinical data for Alliance Health Systems for the past 10 years. Recently a new CEO was appointed. This CEO is intent on making sure that the physicians refer more patients to the hospital than the competing health system and that the system establishes its own labs and surgery centers. Susan has always been fastidious about data quality and has insisted that coding and abstracting can be completed only when a completed record is available. But because of a high dollar amount in accounts receivable, the new CEO is demanding that hospital bills be dropped within two days of discharge. This requires the coding staff to work with unassembled and incomplete records without discharge summaries, final diagnostic statements, and operative reports.

To stem the loss of payment for ancillary services ordered by physicians that admit to the hospital, the CEO is instructing that coders assign diagnosis codes according to Local Medical Review Policies to ensure "coverage" and minimize denials. Coders are not to "harass" physicians or their office staffs when no diagnosis is provided at the time of the test but are to code on the basis of test results.

Also, the CEO has stated that the coding staff will now be providing ICD-9-CM codes for claims generated by a clinic serving the city's homeless population. The coders are to assign appropriate diagnosis codes to justify the CPT services indicated on the forms per Medicaid guidelines. No medical record documentation will be provided to the coding staff, only the encounter forms.

Susan is a single parent with two sons in college. She cannot afford to lose her job.

Question

1. What should Susan do?

A completed ethical decision-making matrix for the scenario is provided at the end of the chapter.

Susan is in an ethical quandary; she knows the process outlined by her new CEO is inconsistent with accepted coding practices. The practice of coding incomplete records with the result that incomplete data are produced violates standard 1 of AHIMA's Standards of Ethical Coding, which states that "coding professionals are expected to support the importance of accurate, complete, and consistent coding practices for the production of quality healthcare data." The practice of assigning codes based only on coverage policies to ensure payment and minimize denials violates standard 6, which states "diagnoses or procedures should not be inappropriately included or excluded because the payment or insurance policy coverage requirements will be affected." And the practice of coding from encounter forms rather than the complete medical record violates standard 8, which states that "coding professionals should . . . ensure that coding policies complement, not conflict with, official coding rules and guidelines." Susan is concerned about the billing of services to the homeless, but she is at a loss concerning what her role should be in this situation.

An ethical approach for Susan would first involve gathering information and documenting facts, not opinions; approaching the CEO with concerns about pressures placed on the HIM department; defining the physician role in providing adequate documentation to support hospital services; and, if the CEO continues to refuse to yield to these concerns and continues to demand processes that violate standards of ethical coding and published regulations, approaching the organization's compliance officer.

Some questions that would need to be asked concerning the recommended process changes before Susan pushes the issue are:

1. How has this change in procedure affected coding accuracy? (Ask for quantified data based on coding review by qualified persons.)

2. How many physicians do not provide final diagnosis and procedure information at the time of patient discharge?

3. How many outpatient tests are requested without physician orders and a valid diagnosis (reason for test)? Which physicians and/or groups are the worst offenders?

4. What are the physician penalties for failure to complete records by a specified time, and how are they enforced?

Some questions to research and present concerning documentation standards and record content requirements are:

1. What, if any, state laws affect physician orders?

2. What, if any, payer-specific requirements have been agreed to that involve physician orders?

3. What do JCAHO or other accreditation agencies have to say about incomplete records, time of coding, and order documentation?

4. What are the Medicare Conditions of Participation for record content and completion?

5. What is the risk of HIM staff "creating" orders after the fact for authentication of a test already completed, at a time long after the test was run?

6. Has this new process affected claims acceptance for payment or denial of payment?

7. Is it appropriate to code on the basis of test results rather than the reason for the test for outpatient testing?

Some helpful data that Susan could provide to her organization's compliance officer are:

1. A comparison of DRG assignments based on coding from incomplete records versus those based on coding from completed records, with financial impact recorded.

2. A breakdown by physician of failure to meet record completion requirements or failure to provide written orders for outpatient tests.

3. Any and all information concerning recruitment of homeless patients and why

records are not available as source documents for code selection. Where are the records kept for these people? Who is the physician treating them?

The following review process concerning the appropriateness of the two-day postdischarge DRG assignment/bill drop might persuade the CEO to allow a return to coding only from completed records:

1. Financial analysis showing the DRG impact

2. Risk of fines and penalties from submitting codes that are not reflected in the final diagnostic statements of the physician (possible inadvertent DRG upcoding)

3. Evidence showing that coding early detrimentally affects coding accuracy and that accounts receivable are not affected significantly in the long run, whether the claims go out two or seven days after discharge

Scenario 5-G: Supporting Application Software That Facilitates Questionable Results

Linda is a clinical data specialist and vocabulary manager for Cutting Edge Health Center. This state-of-the-art clinic uses an electronic health record (EHR) system with an embedded reference terminology (SNOMED-CT®). To complete the billing process and populate the data repository required for indexing, research, decision support, and external reporting to health plans, Linda reviews aggregate coding data from codes assigned by the MiracleMap software. MiracleMap translates data elements and clinical findings captured in the reference terminology and links them to the ICD and HCPCS/CPT codes required for claims by HIPAA. Linda keeps abreast of current guidelines and reporting and compliance requirements and watches for variances or problems with the software. Due to the expected accuracy of MiracleMap to translate 99 percent of knee-related orthopedic procedure concepts to the appropriate CPT code, these procedures are reviewed for accuracy (via a statistically valid sample) once every quarter.

When comparing the source documents to the classification system and inpatient procedure codes recommended by MiracleMap, a CPT upcoding "drift" is recognized for an arthroscopic knee service frequently performed in the clinic, so the reimbursement for at least the past three months is 25 percent greater than it would be if the correct procedure code were used in two of their major contracts. Linda reports her concern to the CIO of Cutting Edge. The CIO tells her that the Informatics experts at MiracleMap are more qualified than she is to make a determination about the accuracy of the maps and she must be mistaken about the code assignment.

Question

1. How can Linda resolve this ethical situation in a professional manner?

A completed ethical decision-making matrix for the scenario is provided at the end of the chapter.

New roles in an e-HIM environment require coding professionals to apply the AHIMA Code of Ethics and the Standards of

Ethical Coding to automated systems involving more than diagnosis and procedure codes. As new medical terminology and coding systems are used to meet the demands of a changing industry, HIM professionals are obligated to understand how systems work and take steps to protect the integrity and validity of the transactions and data elements attached to a patient's services.

Linda is obligated by the AHIMA Code of Ethics and the Standards of Ethical Coding to contest the CIO's assessment by taking steps to illustrate her concern by compiling facts that illustrate the compliance risk to the facility by continued use of this software. Table 5-2 shows the options available to Linda.

Although the reimbursement concern exists in specific health plans, inaccurate coding should be corrected even if there is no monetary effect. Patients deserve to have information about their services be reflected accurately and coding professionals have an ethical obligation to do all they can to ensure this occurs.

Table 5–2 Options for Scenario 5-G

Action Options	Specific Tasks	Potential Outcome
Request a physician audit.	Contact the medical director to ask for a case review by orthopedic surgeons to confirm mapping errors in the software.	Medical director would then require action be taken by the CIO with the MiracleMap vendor to fix software problems.
Contact other users of the MiracleMap software product.	Determine if other users have reviewed the coding accuracy for this procedure.	Conduct research and return to the CIO with additional information about other user's assessment of software performance related to this specific concern.
Contact the compliance office for Cutting Edge.	An investigation from the compliance office would be undertaken to confirm the risk to the organization.	The CIO may not be happy with this approach. If the organization has an appropriate compliance plan, Linda should follow the steps verbatim, beginning with the outlined process for voicing compliance concerns.
Do nothing.	Continue to monitor code assignments closely per normal routine.	Compliance risk compounds with each arthroscopic knee procedure performed at Cutting Edge, and now the ethical stakes are much higher. Linda suspected a problem, but failed to take action to resolve it. This makes the behavior inconsistent with AHIMA's Code of Ethics and the Standards of Ethical Coding.

PROFESSIONAL PRACTICE SOLUTIONS

Coding professionals can be supported by various professional practice solutions to ethical situations. Such tools include coding compliance plans, established facility-specific coding guidelines, and established facility-specific methods of responding to potentially fraudulent activity.

Coding Compliance Plans

Developing and implementing a comprehensive coding compliance plan is likely to provide the organization and the coder with numerous benefits, such as

- Meeting coding compliance requirements
- Reducing the need to add additional staff
- Reducing the chance of triple damage penalties
- Reducing billing delays
- Avoiding bill resubmissions
- Reducing the tendency to code defensively
- Improving performance on severity-adjusted provider report cards (Averill, 1999)

The DOJ has stated that it is not its policy to assess fines and penalties for honest billing mistakes (Reno, 1998). However, the DOJ has also stated that hospitals and other healthcare providers must establish adequate internal procedures to ensure the accuracy of claims submission. Failure to establish such procedures represents a disregard for the requirements of the law and can turn an honest billing mistake into a false claim that is subject to penalties. According to the False Claims Act (31 U.S.C. §3729 [1863, amended 1986]), intent to defraud is not required for a claim to be considered a false claim (see Chapter 4).

A coding compliance plan includes an oversight function, policies and procedures, regularly scheduled education, open communication, a disciplinary policy with action statements, and ongoing auditing and monitoring with problem resolution and corrective action (AHIMA, 1999). A well-written and well-implemented plan provides a basis for solid business practices and ethical decision making. The compliance plan can define "how to do things the right way."

AHIMA's Standards of Ethical Coding can serve as the basis of a healthcare organization's code of conduct for a compliance program to ensure corporate integrity.

Established Coding Guidelines

To promote accurate and ethical coding, the coding professional must promote quality documentation and the use of official coding guidelines (AHIMA, 1997). By advocating the use of official coding guidelines, the coding professional can make (and defend, if necessary) consistent and reliable coding assignments.

In addition to guiding assignment of the correct codes, coding guidelines provide more general directives, such as the following:

- Review the entire medical record as part of the coding process in order to assign and report the most appropriate codes.
- Adhere to all official coding guidelines as approved by the Cooperating Parties (AHIMA, Centers for Medicare and Medicaid Services [CMS] National Center for Health Statistics [NCHS], and the American Hospital Association [AHA]).
- Observe sequencing rules identified by the Cooperating Parties.
- Select the principal diagnosis and procedures for hospital inpatients according to the Uniform Hospital Discharge Data Set definitions.
- Assign and report codes, without physician consultation, to diagnoses and procedures not stated in the physician's final diagnosis only if these diagnoses and procedures are specifically documented by the physician in the body of the medical record and this documentation is clear and consistent.
- Use medical record documentation to provide coding specificity without obtain-

ing physician concurrence (e.g., use a radiology report to identify a fracture site).

- Maintain a positive working relationship with physicians through ongoing communication and open dialogue (AHIMA, 1996).

Both the official coding guidelines issued by the Cooperating Parties and facility-specific coding guidelines that are not in conflict with the official guidelines support the coder who is faced with coding dilemmas. The coding professional can use the guidelines to explain to other healthcare individuals why a particular diagnosis can or cannot be the principal diagnosis and why a higher-weighted DRG is not appropriate for a record. Coding guidelines can be used to help a physician accurately describe the patient seen in the office when no diagnosis has been established. One particular challenge in establishing facility-coding guidelines is to resolve conflicts between guidelines issued by different sources. Especially disturbing are situations when health plans or government benefit programs appear to ignore official coding guidelines endorsed by authoritative sources (DeWald, 1999).

Coding professionals should make every effort to resolve conflicts concerning code use as they occur to preserve data integrity and consistency across payer lines. When there are no universally held coding guidelines, a set of ethical standards is very difficult, if not impossible, to enforce or respect. Patients often pressure a healthcare facility, and even a coder at times, to break the rules so that they receive payments that they do not deserve under the terms of their health plan or government program. This creates pressure from the business or financial arm of the institution to compromise coding ethics, because it is clear that if the health plan does not pay, it will be difficult or impossible to collect from the patient.

Responses to Fraudulent Activity

What should a coding professional do when faced with an unethical and possibly fraudulent activity? It is generally a good idea to attempt to resolve the matter internally before involving external agencies or individuals. The coding professional may consider the following:

- Gather all the facts about the matter. Gather documentation that supports the ethical decision.
- Follow the organization's chain of command—meet with the immediate supervisor and department director first. If this is unsuccessful, try communicating with administrative personnel, such as the compliance committee chair, the chief financial officer, the chief operating officer or compliance officer, or corporate office staff.
- Explain the problem and the reason(s) why the coding practice is unacceptable. Discuss the potential risk to the organization.
- Consider using a hotline or another anonymous medium to report questionable or fraudulent conduct without fear of retribution if the initial meeting(s) are not satisfactory and there is no access to other individuals.
- Document each meeting, including your recommendations to promote ethical practices and the response from the person in authority.
- Document your opposition to the coding practice in a memo to the supervisor, director, and administrative personnel if no action is taken and the unethical practice continues. In this memo, describe the issue, your opposition to the coding practice, the reasons for your opposition, and all of your efforts to date to resolve the matter. Cite all official sources backing your position. Although there is no guarantee that this memo will prevent the coding practice from continuing, it will help protect you from future liability and safeguard your reputation.
- Terminate employment in some situations. Under no circumstances should you agree to participate in fraudulent practices.

- Decide to report the provider or facility externally to the local U.S. Attorney or the Office of the Inspector General's investigative field office in extreme situations. This also usually requires you to resign your job if the provider comes under investigation (Prophet, 1998).

Every situation is different. Some ethical dilemmas can be resolved quickly with a reasonable conversation. Other situations can be more involved and can require considerable effort to resolve.

THE FUTURE OF CODING

The coding professional's role is rapidly involving more than assigning diagnosis and procedure codes after review of text and handwritten record entries. EHRs and other technology innovations are automating some of the process previously performed by human coders. Software applications are both saving work and creating additional concerns and vulnerability for data integrity and ethics in health care. Rather than production workers who read documents and assign numbers and then enter them back into a processing system, tomorrow's coders must be knowledge workers. Instead of choosing the codes, they validate accuracy and appropriateness and then direct their use for a number of different information needs and data warehouses. Coding has never been a simple, technical task due to the variety of rules and guidelines involved. Even though computers can do some of the work, it is critical for human coders to apply ethical decision making to the process.

The health record of the future will be a combination of audio, video, and text-based electronic accounts of the care and services provided. The component of the system that supports EHRs probably will involve natural-language processing or some other computer-assisted method that generates diagnosis and procedure or service codes. As new methods and the use of controlled medical vocabulary in the EHR becomes commonplace and automated maps and other automated coding processes are introduced, new ethical challenges will arise for information managers who work with coded data. Sometimes referred to as "knowledge engineers," the coding professionals of the future will continue to be involved in managing and displaying clinical data sets, evaluating clinical trends, and ensuring data quality. The automation itself will not replace the ethical issues of coding and billing. These issues will remain as long as coded elements are tied to payment for health services and the potential for inaccurate or inappropriate translation of the service into codes is possible.

Coding professionals and HIM professionals are charged with leadership in their organizations concerning the appropriate use and dissemination of health information. Reimbursement and compliance issues will require the coding professional to make sound and ethical business decisions. Healthcare providers must rely on HIM professionals to help establish an ethical compliance program. The challenge is defining that role and improving the methods of ensuring that the coded data reported for payment are consistent with the truth.

Key Terms

- Abuse
- Fraud
- Standards of Ethical Coding
- Unbundling
- Upcoding

Chapter Summary

- In our current healthcare system, the diagnostic and procedural codes reported determine the payment for services; therefore, coders are likely to be affected by pressures to participate in or overlook practices that transmit misinformation. They can end up deeply implicated in practices such as misrepresenting a patient's diagnosis to justify the services rendered.

- Three major areas of ethical concern in coding practice are (1) upcoding, (2) unbundling, and (3) evading requirements that a service be medically necessary to be reimbursed.

- Coders face ethical dilemmas when they discover miscoding by others or misrepresentations in physician documentation on which codes are based and when they feel pressured to miscode or to engage in negligent coding practices in order to avoid conflicts with physicians or administrators.

- To resolve ethical dilemmas in coding, or to prevent them from arising in the first place, HIM professionals need to be familiar with current coding requirements and with AHIMA's Standards of Ethical Coding. Also, coding professionals can be supported by various professional practice solutions to ethical situations, including coding compliance plans, established facility-specific coding guidelines, and established facility-specific methods of responding to potentially fraudulent activity.

- In the future, coding professionals will be asked to monitor and evaluate software applications that affect code selection and use. New ethical problems will surface with advances in automation, but the same principles apply to electronic data management as apply to traditional processes.

References

American Health Information Management Association [AHIMA]. (1996, February). Issue: Data quality. Practice Brief. Chicago, IL: Author.

American Health Information Management Association [AHIMA]. (1997). Resolution from the 1997 House of Delegates: Advocating for quality documentation and adherence to official coding guidelines. Chicago, IL: Author.

American Health Information Management Association [AHIMA]. (1999, October). Seven steps to corporate compliance: The HIM role. Practice Brief. Chicago, IL: Author.

American Health Information Management Association [AHIMA]. (2000a). Certification guide. Chicago, IL: Author. Retrieved November 28, 2005, from http://www.ahima.org/certification.

American Health Information Management Association [AHIMA], Coding Policy and Strategy Committee. (2000b). Standards of ethical coding. *Journal of the American Health Information Management Association, 71*(3), [Insert].

American Health Information Management Association [AHIMA]. (2004). *Code of ethics 2004.* Chicago, IL: Author.

Augarde, T. (1992). *The Oxford dictionary of modern quotations.* New York: Oxford University Press.

Averill, R. (1999). Honest mistake or fraud? Meeting the coding compliance challenge. *Journal of the American Health Information Management Association, 70*(5), 16–21.

Centers for Medicare and Medicaid. (2005). *Fighting fraud and abuse.* Retrieved August 8, 2005, from http://www.cms.hhs.gov/providers/fraud.

DeWald, L. (1999). Stumbling blocks to coding compliance. *CodeWrite* (Society for Clinical Coding, AHIMA affiliate), *8*(5), 1–5.

King, E. (1999). Playing a part: The FBI's role in healthcare fraud investigations. *Journal of the American Health Information Management Association, 69*(1), 43.

Prophet, S. (1997). Fraud and abuse implications for the HIM professional. *Journal of the American Health Information Management Association, 68*(4), 52–56.

Prophet, S. (1998). On the line: Professional practice solution. *Journal of the American Health Information Management Association, 69*(1), 45–46.

Reno, J. (1998, February 2). Speech presented at the annual meeting of the American Hospital Association, Washington, DC.

Wisconsin Physicians Services. (2005). Medicare Part B carrier for Illinois, Michigan and Wisconsin. Web Site for Medicare Providers, Special Topics. Retrieved August 8, 2005, from http://www.wpsic.com/misc/fraud.shtml.

The ethical decision-making matrix is a tool to help you organize complex, ethical problems; however, there is no simple fill-in-the-box approach to ethical decision making. The objective is to follow each step of the process and not move from the question directly to what should be done or how to prevent it next time. If you skip steps, you will not fully understand all of the values and options for action. Also, the matrix provided for each scenario in this book is not the only way to examine the problem. You can make an equally compelling ethical argument for a different decision—just be sure to follow all the steps of the matrix.

SCENARIO 5-A: CODING AN INAPPROPRIATE LEVEL OF SERVICE

Steps	Information	
1. What is the ethical question?	Should Rose report the office's false coding practices?	
2. What are the facts?	**KNOWN**	**TO BE GATHERED**
	• The physician's office is intentionally using inaccurate codes. • Rose's medical record contains inaccurate information.	• Who is responsible for the coding practices? Is it an officewide problem? • Does the assignment of inaccurate codes in these instances constitute fraud? • What are the customary practices in such cases? • What would Rose's own supervisor expect her to do? • What is the likely impact of having to change physicians?
3. What are the values? Examine the shared and competing values, obligations, and interests of the stakeholders (i.e., patient, HIM professional, healthcare practitioner(s), administrators, society, and other advocates) involved in order to fully understand the complexity of the ethical problem(s).	**Patient:** Values accurate documentation as basis of receiving quality care; interest in keeping costs down. **HIM professional:** Code accurately and reliably (ensure truth, integrity, accuracy, and reliability, rather than to maximize reimbursement or affect insurance plan coverage by code manipulation); avoid misrepresentation of clinical or service facts in coding, which could result in an investigation that could cause a financial loss for the provider or facility; follow rules of data submission for reimbursement requirements impartially and according to recognized authorities; meet professional obligation to report incidences of fraud. **Healthcare professional:** Promote welfare of patients through accurate documentation for future care; truth-telling; fairness in following rules equally for all; refuse to participate in or conceal unethical practices; report violations of practice standards to the proper authorities. **Administrators:** Benefit patients and keep from harm; promote welfare of practice; maximize reimbursement without compromising truth-telling; fairness in applying rules for all. **Society:** Control costs; promote fair and just allocation of resources; follow rules of reimbursement equally for all.	

4. What are my options?	• Do not report inaccurate coding and find another physician. • Report inaccurate coding. • Do not report inaccurate coding and continue to see physician.	
5. What should I do?	Report, if inaccurate coding constitutes fraud.	
6. What justifies my choice?	**JUSTIFIED**	**NOT JUSTIFIED**
	• Obligation to tell the truth. • Support accuracy of the documentation. • Preserve professional integrity. • Follow rules equally for all. • Respect the law. Assist this physician practice in creation of a compliance program.	• Do not report inaccurate coding and continue to see physician. • Allow practice of making special exceptions to the rules to maximize reimbursement. • Not fair to others who follow rules. • Miscoding undermines the entire reimbursement system. • Miscoding increases costs in the long run. • Knowingly participating in fraudulent behavior.
7. How can I prevent this ethical problem?	• Evaluate integrity of physician's practice before seeing physician and subsequently when ethical problems arise. • Discuss standards and the values that support them with colleagues and other professionals when opportunities arise. • Learn more about office-based procedures and professional fees and their impact on reimbursement.	

The ethical decision-making matrix is a tool to help you organize complex, ethical problems; however, there is no simple fill-in-the-box approach to ethical decision making. The objective is to follow each step of the process and not move from the question directly to what should be done or how to prevent it next time. If you skip steps, you will not fully understand all of the values and options for action. Also, the matrix provided for each scenario in this book is not the only way to examine the problem. You can make an equally compelling ethical argument for a different decision—just be sure to follow all the steps of the matrix.

SCENARIO 5-B: DISCOVERING MISREPRESENTATION IN PHYSICIAN DOCUMENTATION

Steps	Information	
1. What is the ethical question?	Should Jim report potentially inaccurate information in the physician reports?	
2. What are the facts?	**KNOWN**	**TO BE GATHERED**
	• Group performs laboratory tests and cytology examinations. • Individual laboratory tests are reported rather than disease panel codes.	• Does reporting of tests rather than disease panel codes constitute fraud? • Is information in medical records false? • What are the customary practices in such cases? • What does Jim's supervisor expect him to do? • What is the likely impact of changing jobs or of decreased income on Jim's family?
3. What are the values? Examine the shared and competing values, obligations, and interests of the stakeholders (i.e., patient, HIM professional, healthcare practitioner(s), administrators, society, and other advocates) involved in order to fully understand the complexity of the ethical problem(s).	**Patient:** Values accurate documentation as basis of receiving care; interest in keeping costs down. **HIM professional:** Truth, integrity, accuracy, and reliability (code accurately and reliably rather than to maximize reimbursement); fairness (follow the rules and obey the law); avoid harm (inaccurate documentation may harm the patient, loss of income may harm healthcare workers and their families); personal values (promote welfare of self and family by avoiding loss of income or job); refuse to participate or conceal unethical practices, report violations of practice standards to the proper authorities. **Healthcare professionals:** Promote welfare of patients through accurate documentation for future care; truth-telling; fairness in following rules equally for all; loss of income may harm welfare of self and family. **Administrators:** Benefit patients and keep from harm; promote welfare of facility; maximize reimbursement without compromising truth-telling; control healthcare costs; fairness in applying rules for all. **Society:** Control costs; promote fair and just allocation of resources; follow rules of reimbursement equally for all.	

4. What are my options?	• Report inaccurate records to supervisor/discuss with physicians. • Continue to code based on inaccurate records.	
5. What should I do?	Discuss with supervisor and physicians if facts indicate that the medical records and billing are inaccurate.	
6. What justifies my choice?	**JUSTIFIED**	**NOT JUSTIFIED**
	• Obligation to tell the truth. Support accuracy of the medical record. • Preserve professional integrity. • Follow rules equally for all. • Respect the law. • Demonstrate loyalty to employer, unless asked to push legal boundaries.	• Continue to code based on inaccurate reporting procedures. • Tell a lie. • Make special exception to the rules to maximize reimbursement. • Not fair to others who follow rules. • Miscoding undermines the entire reimbursement system. • Miscoding increases costs in the long run.
7. How can I prevent this ethical problem?	• Determine if system changes are needed. • Learn more about expensive tests and examinations and their impact on reimbursement. • Discuss standards and the values that support them with colleagues. • Evaluate practice's integrity at job interview and subsequently when ethical problems arise.	

The ethical decision-making matrix is a tool to help you organize complex, ethical problems; however, there is no simple fill-in-the-box approach to ethical decision making. The objective is to follow each step of the process and not move from the question directly to what should be done or how to prevent it next time. If you skip steps, you will not fully understand all of the values and options for action. Also, the matrix provided for each scenario in this book is not the only way to examine the problem. You can make an equally compelling ethical argument for a different decision—just be sure to follow all the steps of the matrix.

SCENARIO 5-C: MISCODING TO AVOID CONFLICTS

Steps	Information	
1. What is the ethical question?	Should Gretchen admit to wrongdoing?	
2. What are the facts?	**KNOWN**	**TO BE GATHERED**
	• There was no valid CPT code for epidural injections of a steroid into the cervical and thoracic vertebrae. • Gretchen was told by the Medicare provider representative to use the CPT for the epidural. • Medicare has made the physician return the overpayment.	• Will the Medicare representative admit to having told Gretchen to use the CPT for the epidural? • Is there any documentation of the conversation with the Medicare representative? • Should Gretchen have pursued her concerns with others? • What are the customary practices in such cases? • Did Gretchen intentionally commit fraud? • Did Gretchen explain the situation to the physicians at the time of the code change? • Do physicians have a history of insisting on improper coding? • What would Gretchen's supervisor have expected her to do? • Did she seek advice from her supervisor? • Was Gretchen responsible for any previous coding violations? • What is the likely impact of admitting wrongdoing? What is the likely impact of defending the coding practices?

3. What are the values? Examine the shared and competing values, obligations, and interests of the stakeholders (i.e., patient, HIM professional, healthcare practitioner(s), administrators, society, and other advocates) involved in order to fully understand the complexity of the ethical problem(s).	**Patient:** Interest in keeping costs down. **HIM professional:** Truth, integrity, accuracy, and reliability (code accurately and reliably rather than to maximize reimbursement); give an accurate account of the sequence of events; fairness in following the rules and obeying the law. **Healthcare professionals:** Truth-telling; fairness in following rules equally for all; comply with laws, regulations, and policies; recognize authority and power; refuse to participate or conceal unethical practices; be honest; bring honor to self, peers, and profession. **Administrators:** Promote welfare of facility; maximize reimbursement without compromising truth-telling; control healthcare costs. **Society:** Control costs; promote fair and just allocation of resources; follow rules of reimbursement equally for all.
4. What are my options?	• Admit to and take responsibility for knowingly miscoding records. • Do not accept blame for miscoding by citing instructions from Medicare representative and physicians' desire to maximize reimbursement.
5. What should I do?	Admit to and take responsibility for knowingly miscoding records, if there is no documentation to prove that the Medicare representative told Gretchen to miscode and if Gretchen did not discuss the situation with the physicians.

6. What justifies my choice?	**JUSTIFIED**	**NOT JUSTIFIED**
	• Obligation to tell the truth. • Preserve professional integrity by admitting to having relied on unofficial and inaccurate advice. • Respect the law. • Demonstrate loyalty to employer.	• Do not accept blame for miscoding. • Downplay violation of AHIMA standard and official guidelines for code selection and reporting. • Lose professional integrity.
7. How can I prevent this ethical problem?	• Determine if system changes are needed. • Discuss all system changes with physicians. • Be aware of and use official coding guideline resources. • Engage qualified coding and billing consultant. • Be sure to be current with coding policies. • Check with others, if advice is questioned. • When miscoding is discovered, refund overpayments to insurance plans.	

The ethical decision-making matrix is a tool to help you organize complex, ethical problems; however, there is no simple fill-in-the-box approach to ethical decision making. The objective is to follow each step of the process and not move from the question directly to what should be done or how to prevent it next time. If you skip steps, you will not fully understand all of the values and options for action. Also, the matrix provided for each scenario in this book is not the only way to examine the problem. You can make an equally compelling ethical argument for a different decision—just be sure to follow all the steps of the matrix.

SCENARIO 5-D: DISCOVERY OF MISCODING BY OTHER STAFF MEMBERS

Steps	Information	
1. What is the ethical question?	Should Shirley report the inaccurate coding?	
2. What are the facts?	**KNOWN**	**TO BE GATHERED**
	• Some of the codes reported are inaccurate. • The practice has a history of inaccurate coding of which both the physician and long-term employee are aware.	• Does assigning such codes constitute fraud? • What are the customary practices in such cases? • Has the employee been advised by Medicare to code in this manner and, if so, is this in writing from an official source? • What is the likely impact on self and family of Gretchen's changing jobs?
3. What are the values? Examine the shared and competing values, obligations, and interests of the stakeholders (i.e., patient, HIM professional, healthcare practitioner(s), administrators, society, and other advocates) involved in order to fully understand the complexity of the ethical problem(s).	**Patient:** Values accurate documentation as basis of receiving quality care; interest in keeping costs down. **HIM professional:** Truth, integrity, accuracy, and reliability (code accurately and reliably rather than to maximize reimbursement); fairness (follow the rules and obey the law); loyalty to employer; avoid harm (inaccurate documentation may harm the patient, reporting inaccuracies may causes financial loss and could harm healthcare workers and their families); personal values (promote welfare of self and family by avoiding loss of job). **Healthcare professionals:** Promote welfare of patients through accurate documentation for future care; truth-telling; fairness in following rules equally for all; professional integrity. **Society:** Control costs; promote fair and just allocation of resources; follow rules of reimbursement equally for all.	

4. What are my options?	• Allow the inaccurate coding to continue. • Report the inaccurate coding to Medicare	
5. What should I do?	Report the inaccurate coding to Medicare, if Medicare does not authorize the bundling of extra services.	
6. What justifies my choice?	**JUSTIFIED**	**NOT JUSTIFIED**
	• Obligation to tell the truth. • Support accuracy of the medical record. • Preserve professional integrity. • Follow rules equally for all. • Respect the law. • Demonstrate loyalty to employer, unless asked to push legal boundaries.	• Allow the inaccurate coding to continue. • Tell a lie. • Make special exception to the rules to maximize reimbursement. • Not fair to others who follow rules. • Miscoding undermines the entire reimbursement system. • Miscoding increases costs in the long run.
7. How can I prevent this ethical problem?	• Determine if system changes are needed. • Learn more about coding for mental health services. • Discuss standards and the values that support them with colleagues. • Evaluate practice integrity at job interview and subsequently when ethical problems arise.	

The ethical decision-making matrix is a tool to help you organize complex, ethical problems; however, there is no simple fill-in-the-box approach to ethical decision making. The objective is to follow each step of the process and not move from the question directly to what should be done or how to prevent it next time. If you skip steps, you will not fully understand all of the values and options for action. Also, the matrix provided for each scenario in this book is not the only way to examine the problem. You can make an equally compelling ethical argument for a different decision—just be sure to follow all the steps of the matrix.

SCENARIO 5-E: LACKING THE TOOLS TO DO ONE'S JOB

Steps	Information	
1. What is the ethical question?	Did Charlene knowingly violate coding standards and ethics?	
2. What are the facts?	**KNOWN**	**TO BE GATHERED**
	• Charlene lacked the resources to perform her job correctly. • The university hospital has, on occasion, assigned inaccurate DRG codes. • Charlene has little experience with reimbursement systems.	• What are the customary practices here? • How might a more experienced coding professional have handled the situation? • What is the likely impact on self and family of losing job?
3. What are the values? Examine the shared and competing values, obligations, and interests of the stakeholders (i.e., patient, HIM professional, healthcare practitioner(s), administrators, society, and other advocates) involved in order to fully understand the complexity of the ethical problem(s).	**Patient:** Values accurate documentation as basis of receiving quality care; interest in keeping costs down. **HIM professional:** Truth, integrity, accuracy, and reliability (code accurately and reliably using necessary resources); do not take DRG assignments for granted; fairness (follow the rules and obey the law); avoid harm (inaccurate documentation may harm the patient and cause the employer to lose money); personal values (promote welfare of self and family by avoiding loss of job). **Healthcare professionals:** Promote welfare of patients through accurate documentation for future care; truth-telling; fairness in following rules equally for all. **Administrators:** Promote welfare, including financial stability, of facility; control healthcare costs; promote good relationships with clients. **Society:** Control costs; promote fair and just allocation of resources; follow rules of reimbursement equally for all.	

4. What are my options?	• Deny violation of standards and ethics. • Admit violation of standards and ethics.	
5. What should I do?	Admit violation of coding standards and ethics.	
6. What justifies my choice?	**JUSTIFIED**	**NOT JUSTIFIED**
	• Obligation to tell the truth. Support accuracy of the medical record. • Preserve professional integrity. • Respect the law.	• Deny violation of standards and ethics. • Tell a lie. • Undermine standards and ethics of coders. • Lose professional integrity.
7. How can I prevent this ethical problem?	• Further education in areas that affect job responsibilities. • Inform administration when lacking tools to perform job. • Discuss standards and the values that support them with colleagues. • Evaluate personal professional integrity when ethical problems arise.	

The ethical decision-making matrix is a tool to help you organize complex, ethical problems; however, there is no simple fill-in-the-box approach to ethical decision making. The objective is to follow each step of the process and not move from the question directly to what should be done or how to prevent it next time. If you skip steps, you will not fully understand all of the values and options for action. Also, the matrix provided for each scenario in this book is not the only way to examine the problem. You can make an equally compelling ethical argument for a different decision—just be sure to follow all the steps of the matrix.

SCENARIO 5-F: BEING REQUIRED BY THE EMPLOYER TO ENGAGE IN NEGLIGENT CODING PRACTICES

Steps	Information	
1. What is the ethical question?	Should Susan report the coding violations?	
2. What are the facts?	**KNOWN**	**TO BE GATHERED**
	• Coders are not given proper information for accurate coding. • CEO is aware of potential inaccuracies in coding.	• Would assigning codes without full medical records constitute fraud? • What are the customary practices in such cases? • Does the CEO understand the illegality and potential ramifications of inaccurate coding and filing of false claims for reimbursement?
3. What are the values? Examine the shared and competing values, obligations, and interests of the stakeholders (i.e., patient, HIM professional, healthcare practitioner(s), administrators, society, and other advocates) involved in order to fully understand the complexity of the ethical problem(s).	**Patient:** Values accurate documentation as basis of receiving quality care; interest in keeping costs down. **HIM professional:** Truth, integrity, accuracy, and reliability (code accurately and reliably using completed reports); fairness (follow the rules and obey the law); loyalty to employer; avoid harm (inaccurate documentation may harm the patient, financial loss will harm Susan and her family and may harm healthcare workers and their families); personal values (promote the welfare of self and family by avoiding loss of job). **Healthcare professionals:** Promote welfare of patients through accurate and complete documentation for future care; fairness in following rules equally for all. **Administrators:** Benefit patients and keep from harm; promote welfare of facility; maximize reimbursement without compromising truth-telling; control healthcare costs; fairness in applying rules for all. **Society:** Control costs; promote fair and just allocation of resources; follow rules of reimbursement equally for all.	

4. What are my options?	• Continue inaccurate coding practices. • Report coding violations.	
5. What should I do?	Report coding violations, if the CEO is aware of the illegality and potential ramifications of inaccurate coding practices and still insists on them.	
6. What justifies my choice?	**JUSTIFIED**	**NOT JUSTIFIED**
	• Obligation to tell the truth. • Support accuracy and completeness of the medical record. • Preserve professional integrity. • Follow rules equally for all. • Respect the law. • Demonstrate loyalty to employer, unless asked to push legal boundaries.	• Continue inaccurate coding practices. • Make special exception to the rules. • Not fair to others who follow rules. • Miscoding undermines the entire reimbursement system. • Miscoding increases costs in the long run. • Loss of professional integrity. • Participating in illegal or unethical activity to protect personal interests.
7. How can I prevent this ethical problem?	• Determine if system changes are needed. • Learn more about coding standards and ethics. • Discuss standards and the values that support them with colleagues. • Evaluate institutional integrity at job interview and subsequently with the compliance program or equivalent office when ethical problems arise.	

The ethical decision-making matrix is a tool to help you organize complex, ethical problems; however, there is no simple fill-in-the-box approach to ethical decision making. The objective is to follow each step of the process and not move from the question directly to what should be done or how to prevent it next time. If you skip steps, you will not fully understand all of the values and options for action. Also, the matrix provided for each scenario in this book is not the only way to examine the problem. You can make an equally compelling ethical argument for a different decision—just be sure to follow all the steps of the matrix.

SCENARIO 5-G: SUPPORTING APPLICATION SOFTWARE THAT FACILITATES QUESTIONABLE RESULTS

Steps	Information	
1. What is the ethical question?	Should Linda take steps to compile facts that illustrate the compliance risk of the software?	
2. What are the facts?	**KNOWN**	**TO BE GATHERED**
	• Linda is a clinical data specialist and vocabulary manager. • The clinic uses an EHR system with an embedded reference terminology. • A CPT upcoding "drift" is recognized for an arthroscopic knee service, so the reimbursement, for at least the past 3 months, is 25 percent more than it should be. • Linda reports her concern to the CIO of Cutting Edge who tells her that the Informatics experts at MiracleMap are more qualified than she is to make a determination about the accuracy of the maps and she must be mistaken about the code assignment.	• Should Linda contact the medical director and request that the surgeons confirm the mapping errors in the software? • Should other users of the software be contacted to determine their assessment of the software? • Should the compliance officer be contacted to confirm the risk to the organization? • Should Linda continue to monitor code assignments for this condition and others?
3. What are the values? Examine the shared and competing values, obligations, and interests of the stakeholders (i.e., patient, HIM professional, healthcare practitioner(s), administrators, society, and other advocates) involved in order to fully understand the complexity of the ethical problem(s).	**Patient:** Values accuracy in the coding and reimbursement processes; interest in keeping costs down; deserves to have information about services be reflected accurately. **HIM professional:** Truth, integrity, accuracy, and reliability (code accurately and reliably, utilize software applications that result in accurate data outcomes); fairness (follow the rules and obey the law); loyalty to employer. **Healthcare professionals:** Promote welfare of patients through trustworthy computer applications that substantiate the care that has been given; fairness in following rules equally for all. **Administrators:** Benefit patients through use of technological applications; promote welfare of facility; maximize reimbursement without compromising truth-telling; control healthcare costs; fairness in applying rules for all. **Society:** Control costs; promote fair and just allocation of resources; follow rules of reimbursement equally for all; use technology appropriately.	

4. What are my options?	• Continue to use the software so that increased funds can be collected. • Take steps to compile facts that illustrate the compliance risk of the software.	
5. What should I do?	Take steps that illustrate the compliance risk of the software.	
6. What justifies my choice?	**JUSTIFIED**	**NOT JUSTIFIED**
	• Apply the AHIMA Code of Ethics and the Standards of Ethical Coding to automated systems involving diagnosis and procedure codes. • Obligation to protect the integrity and validity of the transactions and data elements attached to a patient's services. • Contest the CIO's assessment by taking steps to illustrate concerns by compiling facts that illustrate the compliance risk to the facility by continued use of this software.	• Fail to follow appropriate codes of ethics. • Avoid conflict with the CIO and allow the potential problem to continue. • Violate values of integrity and validity of data. • Risk compliance problems.
7. How can I prevent this ethical problem?	HIM professional participation in the vendor selection process for all software applications that affect the ability to provide quality services.	

6

QUALITY REVIEW

Patrice L. Spath, BA, RHIT

Abstract

Today's rapidly changing healthcare environment is creating new ethical issues for HIM professionals who have quality and resource management responsibilities. Rising costs, scarce resources, the hierarchical nature of healthcare organizations, and conflicting values are introducing both challenges and opportunities into the workplace. This chapter draws on a survey of members of the American Health Information Association regarding their assessment of five scenarios depicting typical ethical dilemmas faced by HIM professionals involved in **quality management** activities. The scenarios, the answers provided by the survey respondents, and the standards for ethical decision making explored in this chapter are intended to help HIM professionals sort out the ethical issues that they may have to deal with during the performance of quality management activities.

Learning Objectives

After completing this chapter, the reader should be able to:

- Identify the common ethical issues in healthcare quality management (QM).
- Identify the ethical issues confronting health information management (HIM) professionals involved in QM activities.
- Identify the professional and organizational standards of behavior and personal values that influence the ethical decisions of HIM professionals involved in QM activities.
- Identify common responses to ethical issues that may be presented to HIM professionals who are involved in QM activities.

QUALITY MANAGEMENT

HIM professionals have always played an important role in healthcare QM activities (Spath, 2001). In the 1940s, medical record librarians routinely served on hospital medical staff committees charged with reviewing the quality of record documentation (Seltze, 1948). Record librarians helped select cases for morbidity and mortality reviews, analyzed records for completeness, and provided regular reports on the number of incomplete or inadequate records (Hill, 1948). It appears that little was written in the earlier years of the profession about the ethical decisions that may have been required of HIM professionals involved in QM activities; however, in 1946 Eleanor F. Hull, medical record librarian at Fullerton Hospital in Fullerton, California, wrote, "To work with our doctors . . . requires a person who by study and thought keeps herself in touch with changing times; a person of kindness and culture, sympathetic and honest, courteous and honorable" (p. 76).

Continuing education, kindness, honesty, courtesy, and honor are as important today as they ever were; however, since the 1940s a number of healthcare industry milestones have occurred that are challenging the HIM tradition of striving to be "honest and honorable." The passage of Medicare legislation, changes in healthcare configurations and reimbursement systems, increased litigation, and publicly available provider "report cards" have affected QM and have created an environment that is ripe for ethical dilemmas. An ethical dilemma occurs when a person must decide whether to do something that, although beneficial to him- or herself or the organization, may be considered unethical.

Ethical questions surrounding these QM activities have become more difficult as the complexity and competitiveness of health care has increased. This chapter describes the common QM ethical issues that healthcare organizations face today. The professional standards, organizational rules of conduct, and personal values influencing ethical behavior for those involved in QM activities are presented.

With the passage of the Medicare law in 1965, a new source of revenue became immediately available to healthcare organizations. Hospitals and skilled nursing facilities were required to have utilization review (UR) programs to ensure that Medicare dollars were spent only on medically necessary services. By the late 1970s, it became apparent that these UR programs were ineffective in controlling rising costs, largely because there was no financial incentive for organizations to limit the number of services provided to Medicare patients. Although facility leaders were ethically bound to comply with federal regulations, the lack of financial penalties for noncompliance created a "don't ask, don't tell" environment.

In the late 1960s, the courts began to hold healthcare facilities accountable for the actions of practicing physicians, and by the early 1970s, healthcare organizations and individual physicians experienced an increased number of lawsuits and higher monetary awards to plaintiffs. Commonly referred to as the "medical malpractice crisis," the events of the 1970s led to an increase in the secrecy surrounding **peer review** activities. Fear of litigation and the potential for misinterpretation of committee decisions by juries in malpractice cases caused some organizations to limit documentation of quality problems or to fabricate committee minutes.

The 1980s brought yet another crisis to the healthcare industry, this time a financial one. In response to growing concerns about the rising cost of healthcare services, the Medicare prospective payment system was implemented, and private health plans enacted significant cost-control measures. At this same time, the payers and regulators of health care began in earnest to promote comparative measurement initiatives, many of which included public disclosure of the results in report-card-style commentaries. One of the most significant public data releases occurred in 1986, when the Centers for Medicare and

Medicaid Services (CMS) (formerly known as the Health Care Financing Administration) calculated the 1985 raw death rates for hospitalized Medicare patients and allowed this hospital-specific information to be made public. Almost immediately, public releases of other types of provider-specific comparative **performance measurement** data increased, and consumers began to demand access to mortality and complication rates. Groups such as the Joint Commission on the Accreditation of Healthcare Organizations (JCAHO) and the National Committee for Quality Assurance (NCQA) started sharing organization-specific accreditation results with the public. Healthcare organizations were for the first time being asked to provide data that consumers could use to judge an organization's performance.

The Institute of Medicine's report on errors in health care, released in December 1999, rekindled the public's desire for provider-specific performance information (Kohn, Corrigan, & Donaldson, 1999). The report called for the establishment of a nationwide mandatory reporting system to gather information about adverse medical events that resulted in death or serious harm to a patient. All of these new demands for publicly available performance data changed the healthcare environment from "don't ask, don't tell" to "do ask . . . but we're not sure if we want to tell."

Passage of a Medicare reform law in 2003 created new financial pressures intended to increase public access to hospital performance data. Hospitals reporting to CMS the results of 10 quality measures for heart attack, heart failure, and pneumonia will receive a 3.3% increase in their Medicare rates in 2005, an adjustment that reflects the rate of full inflation. Hospitals that do not report their results only receive a 2.9% increase (American Hospital Association, 2004).

The ethical dilemma of truth-telling arises when healthcare organizations are asked to accurately report performance results, reveal accreditation deficiencies, or recount adverse patient events that might cause them to look undesirable when compared to other reporting organizations.

Healthcare organizations have legal, regulatory, and social responsibilities to provide high-quality patient care services. To fulfill these responsibilities, they have implemented a wide range of QM activities that are much more comprehensive than the review functions that HIM professionals helped to support in the 1940s. Today, QM activities encompass a wide variety of functions including, but not necessarily limited to, institution and medical staff performance monitoring and evaluation activities, utilization management, **risk management,** infection control, and **patient safety** improvement.

HIM professionals are employed in QM positions at all levels in healthcare organizations. Sometimes their responsibilities are limited to data collection, but in many instances they are intimately involved in the design and interpretation of patient **outcome** studies and/or physician credentialing and peer review activities. Caregivers rely on the expertise of HIM professionals to assist them in judging the quality of patient care and the competence of people who are providing that care.

In December 1999, I surveyed a random sample of 100 AHIMA members employed in QM positions. The intent of the survey was to determine the types of ethical questions that they might be experiencing. The survey was administered by mail and completed by 34 respondents employed in a cross section of healthcare organizations. The questionnaire covered three general areas of interest: (1) ethical issues and related experiences; (2) organizational policies and practices aimed at improving ethical conduct; and (3) how the respondent would react to actual QM events that might present an ethical dilemma. The key findings of the survey are described throughout this chapter.

Economic tensions, downsizing, competition, and shifting "social values" are placing more demands on healthcare leaders. These forces may influence leaders to ask HIM professionals to compromise their professional or personal ethics in order to get the QM job done. HIM professionals may face pressures to conceal information that could be potentially damaging to the organization, remain silent about quality-of-care concerns, forge documentation, falsify performance data, or under-report adverse patient incident data.

Some of these ethical questions have no easy answers, especially when the HIM professional must choose between continued employment and "standing firm" on ethical standards. The chapter ends with some specific actions that can be taken by HIM professionals to enable ethical conduct in support of the organization's QM activities.

Scenario 6-A: Inaccurate Performance Data

You work as the quality director in the corporate office of a large health maintenance organization (HMO). One day you notice that the HMO's performance data posted on the health plan's Web site are inaccurate. The data make the health plan's performance quality actually look better than it is. You ask the chief executive officer (CEO) about the data, and she says, "I'm aware of the discrepancies, but we don't want the public to lose faith in us. HMOs are getting too much undeserved bad publicity these days!"

Question

1. What is your next course of action?

A completed ethical decision-making matrix for the scenario is provided at the end of the chapter. Table 6–1, also at the end of the chapter, presents the responses from the AHIMA survey respondents.

QM ETHICAL ISSUES FACING HIM PROFESSIONALS

HIM professionals play an important role in healthcare QM activities. The following are the top five tasks performed by the 34 respondents to the QM Section member survey in order of reporting frequency:

1. Create quality/risk management reports for administration or medical staff (74%).
2. Gather data for quality/risk management activities (74%).
3. Attend administrative/medical staff meetings related to quality/risk management (74%).

4. Screen records to identify cases needing further review by physicians or other clinicians (68%).
5. Perform utilization review and/or **case management** activities (53%).

While performing QM tasks, HIM professionals may find themselves pressured to engage in unethical practices. More than 26% (13) of the 34 survey respondents said they had been asked on at least one occasion by administrators, physicians, or other employees to compromise their professional or personal standards of ethical behavior. The 13 respondents who felt persuaded to engage in unethical practices reported that the most common types of misconduct involved hiding accreditation or regulatory deficiencies from surveyors (78%), keeping silent about known quality problems (78%), and falsifying committee minutes or other records dealing with quality of patient care (33%). Other, less common unethical practices that the HIM professionals were asked to do included overlooking/not reporting obvious overutilization problems (15%), falsifying data/other reports sent to accreditation/regulatory agencies (15%), altering patient records to conceal a quality-of-care problem (15%), publicly blaming another provider for an error made at their facility (8%), and using inaccurate/incomplete data sources to report performance measures (8%).

HIM professionals generally lack control over the ethical practices of people in positions of power in the organization. When suggestions made by the organization's leaders or physicians appear to violate ethical professional or business conduct, HIM professionals are placed in a difficult situation. In the area of QM, some of these conflicts can be gut-wrenching because of the potential for patient harm. For example, if the organization's leaders consciously chose to overlook recurrent patient management mistakes made by an incompetent physician, such as repeated infections following surgery or misreading of radiology reports, the HIM professional may be faced with several questions:

- What can the HIM professional do besides repeatedly bringing the physician's mistakes to the attention of administrative and medical staff leadership?
- What is the HIM professional's obligation to protect future patients from the physician's incompetent behavior?
- Is it wrong for the HIM professional to accept the leaders' decision that nothing needs to be done about the problem?

- Will the HIM professional be shunned by colleagues for bringing the physician's behavior to the attention of the organization's compliance officer or risk manager?
- Should the HIM professional risk loss of job or disciplinary action by discussing the issue directly with the organization's governing board chair?
- What if the leaders can provide compelling and logical reasons for not taking any action, such as "This physician is well respected by his patients" or "This physician brings the most revenue to the hospital"?
- If HIM professionals know about a situation that is unsafe for patients, are they bound by professional standards to act, regardless of what the organization's leaders might suggest?

Given the very real threats that may be associated with any action beyond continued collection and reporting of information about the physician's mistakes to the organizations' leaders, the HIM professional could be faced with a profound ethical dilemma.

Of course, there is always the option of leaving the problem behind by changing employers. But this choice does not change the fact that future patients may be unnecessarily injured or killed by an incompetent physician. It is not an appropriate ethical choice to change employers without taking some definitive action to protect patient safety. HIM professionals faced with such "life-or-death" QM ethical situations must consider their professional standards as well as their moral obligation to stop neglect or abuses that threaten the well-being of patients.

Scenario 6-B: Home Health Care and Central-Line Infections

You have been newly hired as the QM in a home health agency. Records show that during the last quarter, four patients developed central-line infections. Your boss asks you not to report these data to the JCAHO in your next data submission. He says that infections like this have never happened before and that reporting them will only make the agency look bad, when it actually provides very high quality patient care.

Question

1. What is your next course of action?

A completed ethical decision-making matrix for the scenario is provided at the end of the chapter. Table 6–2 presents the responses from the AHIMA survey respondents.

ETHICAL STANDARDS AFFECTING QM ACTIVITIES

Standards of conduct that define how HIM professionals should behave are influenced by professional ethics, organizational values, and personal convictions about right and wrong. These principles will not always dictate a single ethically acceptable course of action. In some instances, HIM professionals working in QM roles may be faced with conflicting messages. At times, a person's desire to be honest may clash with the desire for a job. At other times, a person's wish to act for the good of the patient must be balanced against the wishes of other stakeholders. When ethical standards and values conflict, personal choices must be made.

Patient Safety and Professional Ethics

People who provide healthcare services have a legal, professional, and moral duty to ensure the safety of patients—that is, the duty "to protect healthcare recipients from being harmed by the effects of healthcare services" (Spath, 2000, p. 1). People working in health care are bound by legal standards and professional ethical principles to do whatever they can to promote a patient-safe environment. This may include taking action to safeguard patients when their health or welfare may be adversely affected by the incompetent, unethical, illegal, or inappropriate practices of another person.

The legal standards affecting various clinical disciplines are found in state medical licensure laws. **Licensure** is the process by which an agency of government grants permission to persons meeting predetermined qualifications to engage in a given occupation and/or to use a particular title. Licensure is conducted under a state board. Oftentimes, the members of such boards not only are members of the respective profession, but also are proposed by the state professional society for nomination by the governor. The legal precedent for medical licensure was begun by physicians as a way to raise the level of competence of physicians and lessen competition from other health providers (Derbyshire, 1969). Texas was the first state to pass a physician licensure law in 1873, and by the end of the nineteenth century all states had medical licensure laws. The nursing profession soon followed the lead of physicians, and by 1923 every state had a nurse registration act (Lesnik & Anderson, 1947). Since that time, several clinical disciplines have established state licensure requirements. State licensure laws for medical occupations are intended to protect the health, safety, and welfare of the public by ensuring that only competent individuals are permitted to practice within the state. Regulation of medical professionals is viewed as being in the public interest—something that benefits society in general, not just the members of the profession.

State medical licensure laws contain a legal definition of the profession and scope of practice. Although state regulations do not contain ethical codes, the regulations do define what is considered inappropriate professional behavior. For example, the Texas statutes regulating the practice of professional nursing state that a nurse may be subject to denial of license or disciplinary action for "failure to care adequately for a patient or conform to the minimum standards of acceptable nursing practices in a manner that, in the board's opinion, exposes a patient or other person unnecessarily to risk of harm" (Nursing Practice Act, 1999). Similar statements are found in the state licensure laws governing all medical professions. It is clear that people holding a license that allows them to be employed in a medical occupation are expected to act in a manner that does not jeopardize patient safety.

Specific ethical principles that influence the actions of healthcare professionals are found in the code of ethics statements of the associations to which people belong. Perhaps because many of the people working in healthcare QM jobs also hold a professional license, the ethical codes of most healthcare associations representing people involved in QM activities do not explicitly address the subject of patient protection. For example:

- The Code of Ethics for the National Association of Healthcare Quality (NAHQ, 1999) states that QM professionals will inform employers or clients of possible positive and negative outcomes of management decisions in an effort to facilitate informed decision making. The NAHQ Code of Ethics does not mention what QM professionals should do if patients may be harmed by management decisions.
- Members of the American Society for Healthcare Risk Management (ASHRM) are expected to adhere to a code of professional ethics and conduct that states that risk management professionals should enhance the overall quality of life, dignity, safety, and well-being of every individual needing health care (ASHRM, 2001). Risk management professionals are expected to advise em-

ploying organizations and/or colleagues when existing policies, procedures, or behaviors are inconsistent with this goal.

- Healthcare professionals belonging to the American Society for Quality (ASQ) will find little guidance about protecting patients from harm in the ASQ Code of Ethics. This organization represents quality professionals from many industries, and the Code of Ethics focuses on issues more often found in technical than in service industries. For example, members of the ASQ are expected to promote the reliability and safety of all products that come under their jurisdiction and to inform employers or clients of the adverse consequences to be expected if the quality professional's judgment is overruled (ASQ, 2004). Although the intent of these ethical philosophies is honorable, the terminology found in the ASQ Code of Ethics may not apply to the healthcare environment.
- The ethical integrity of American Health Information Management Association (AHIMA) members is guided by the AHIMA Professional Code of Ethics, but this code does not specifically mention the duty to protect patients from harm. The code of conduct does state that HIM professionals should put service and the health and welfare of persons before self-interests, which implies that protecting patients from harm is an ethical principle for AHIMA members (AHIMA, 2004). The AHIMA Code of Ethics does speak to performance measurement activities, indicating that HIM professionals should not hide or ignore review outcomes.
- The National Cancer Registrars' Association (NCRA) has a definitive statement about patient safety in the code of ethics. The NCRA (1995) ethical code states that the cancer registrar shall give "primary consideration in all decisions as to the effect actions may have on a patient's health and welfare."

Scenario 6-C: Failure to Check Physician's Licensure Status

You work as a medical staff coordinator at a 200-bed community hospital. The medical staff president has hired a part-time physician to cover for him during an upcoming vacation. He requests that you expedite the physician's appointment to the medical staff, saying that one way to do this is to forgo checking the physician's current licensure status. He also tells you not to bother checking the National Practitioner Data Bank because "I personally know he hasn't had any lawsuits." He suggests that you indicate on the application that these steps were done even when they were not. The medical staff president assures you that he's worked with this physician before and knows that he is a good practitioner. "Besides," he says, "the physician is only going to be seeing patients at the hospital for four weeks."

Question

1. What is your next course of action?

A completed ethical decision-making matrix for the scenario is provided at the end of the chapter. Table 6–3 presents the responses from the AHIMA survey respondents.

Inconsistencies Among Professional Conduct Codes

A consistent and shared code of ethics does not currently exist for all of the stakeholders in health care (Berwick, Hiatt, Janeway, & Smith, 1997). Seeing the need for some type of worldwide ethical consensus, a multidisciplinary international group of physicians, nurses, executives, ethicists, and other health-care professionals met in London in 1998 to develop a set of ethical principles that would guide healthcare behavior for all those involved in the delivery of health care (i.e., individuals, organizations, insurers, employers, and governments). This group, known as the Tavistock Group, proposed five ethical principles in January 1999 (Exhibit 6–1).

One of the Tavistock principles relates to patient safety, stating, "All individuals and groups involved in health care, whether they provide access or services, have the continuing responsibility to help improve its quality" (Smith, Hiatt, & Berwick, 1999, p. 144). Although quality of patient care is not explicitly mentioned in the ethical standards of associations representing QM professionals, it is certainly implied. However, if an association's ethical code is intended to help members mediate ethical conflicts, then a precise statement about the professional's duty to protect the safety of patients seems necessary. A very tight relationship exists between the code of ethics and a profession's identity. The identity of clinical professionals is clearly spelled out in state licensure regulations. However, many allied health professionals, including certified HIM professionals, are not subject to medical licensure requirements. Thus, it would seem even more important for the ethical codes of allied health associations to include an explicit statement about the members' role in protecting patients from harm. Professional associations whose members are involved in QM activities should assert an ethical commitment to quality patient care by adopting a quality-related professional ethics statement, as suggested by the Tavistock Group.

A completed ethical decision-making matrix for the scenario is provided at the end of

Exhibit 6–1 Ethical Principles Proposed by the Tavistock Group

1. Health care is a human right.
2. The care of individuals is at the center of healthcare delivery but must be viewed and practiced within the overall context of continuing work to generate the greatest possible health gains for groups and populations.
3. The responsibilities of the healthcare delivery system include the prevention of illness and the alleviation of disability.
4. Cooperation with each other and those served is imperative for those working within the healthcare delivery system.
5. All individuals and groups involved in health care, whether they provide access or services, have the continuing responsibility to help improve its quality.

Source: Reprinted with permission from R. Smith, H. Hiatt, D. Berwick, A Shared Statement of Ethical Principles for Those Who Shape and Give Health Care: A Working Draft from the Tavistock Group, *Annals of Internal Medicine,* No. 130, pp. 143–147, © January 19, 1999, American College of Physicians.

the chapter. Table 6-4 presents the responses from the AHIMA survey respondents.

Organizational Values

The HIM professional is bound by professional standards and by employers' values and ethical principles. In many organizations, these values and principles are found in written standards of conduct. In December 1998, the Survey of Georgia CEOs on Business Ethics conducted by the Southern Institute for Business and Professional Ethics (1999) found that approximately three-quarters of large public and private corporations had or planned to implement a formal statement of an ethics policy. The survey findings also revealed that companies in heavily regulated industries (i.e., health care, utilities, financial) were more likely to have a written ethics policy and more likely to provide ethics educational programs to employees. In a 2002 survey conducted by the same group, 25 (14%) of 173 survey respondents were from healthcare and social assistance organizations (Southern Institute for Business and Professional Ethics, 2002). One significant change in 2002 was the degree to which CEOs believed high ethical standards tend to strengthen a company's competitive position—both in the short term and in the long run. When asked to rate the causes of unethical business conduct, the 2002 respon-

Scenario 6-D: Hiding Incomplete Medical Records

You work as the director of the HIM department in a large metropolitan area hospital. The hospital's JCAHO survey will occur in 15 days. Your immediate boss asks you to hide any incomplete records that are more than 30 days old so that the surveyors won't discover them during the visit.

Question

1. What is your next course of action?

dents uniformly agree that misconduct results from a failure of leadership in establishing ethical standards and culture. This topped the list of reasons for misconduct and was rated considerably higher than any other factors.

Of 34 respondents to an ethics survey mailed to AHIMA members, 26 (76%) indicated that their organization had written standards of ethical conduct. Of the eight respondents who said that their organization lacked such standards or they didn't know if such standards existed, six (75%) worked in ambulatory care settings (physicians' clinic, outpatient mental health treatment center) and two worked in small rural hospitals.

Generally, the rules of conduct found in healthcare organizations address ethical issues in care and treatment of patients, marketing, admission, transfer, discharge, billing practices, and relationships with other providers and groups. The ethical value statements of most healthcare facilities include a declaration of the organization's commitment to **quality** and/or patient safety. For example, the code of conduct for HCA-The Healthcare Company (1998, pp. 5–6) states that the organization is committed to providing patients with quality care that is sensitive, compassionate, promptly delivered, and cost effective. The quality statement in some organization's ethical principles is tailored to the needs of the type of patients or clients served. For example, the policy on ethics of the Division of Child Mental Health Services of the State of Delaware Department for Children, Youth and Their Families (State of Delaware, 1997) states that children and youth have the right to competent individualized treatment in the least restrictive environment.

Personal Convictions

Personal moral beliefs also influence ethical decision making during the performance of QM activities. Most people have convictions about what is right and wrong that are based on religious beliefs, cultural roots, family background, and personal experiences.

These personal beliefs influence people's choices when they decide how to act when presented with an ethical question.

Rarely do professional ethical standards and organizational codes of ethics conflict with a person's core beliefs or values. It seems unlikely that a person would choose a profession or work for an employer that had ethical standards in conflict with his or her personal values. However, the ethical principles of a person's chosen profession or employer can change over time, and the HIM professional may be faced with new ethical dilemmas. For example, the QM supervisor in an outpatient clinic may personally disagree with the doctors' decision to perform late-term abortions. If the person's core beliefs or values cause him or her to disagree with the universal ethical principles held by the profession or the employer, it may be time to change occupations.

MAKING ETHICAL DECISIONS

Every action has implications or consequences. When faced with an ethical decision, people have an obligation to consider the implications of their decision. But knowing the implications and being committed to act ethically is not always enough, especially when unnecessary harm to the patient may be one of the consequences. The process of ethical decision making requires that HIM professionals perceive the ethical implications of decisions, evaluate the facts, and then select the best choice without unduly harming other people. In some instances, HIM professionals involved in QM activities have a narrow scope of responsibility, and their authority is limited. However, the ethical person must be concerned with what is right to do, not with what he or she has a right to do.

The AHIMA Code of Ethics implies that HIM professionals have an obligation to protect the health and welfare of patients, although it is not specifically stated. If it is agreed that all people working in health care should adopt the ethical principles proposed by the Tavistock Group, then the HIM professional has a duty to help improve the quality of healthcare services. All healthcare professionals involved in QM activities, regardless of their professional **license** or credential, are morally obligated to apply their knowledge in ways that benefit society. When there are competing values, HIM professionals must ask what impact their decision will have on the quality of care for patients.

A completed ethical decision-making matrix for the scenario is provided at the end of the chapter. Table 6-5 presents the responses from the AHIMA survey respondents.

Scenario 6-E: Audit Results Indicate Inappropriate Health Care

You work as the quality director in a small rural hospital. A new physician joins the staff. Within three months you discover several cases in which this physician's practices appear inappropriate (e.g., unnecessary surgery, failure to perform appropriate diagnostic studies, failure to use generally accepted treatments). A few cases are so obvious that even a layperson would doubt the physician's judgment. Nurses and clinical staff in the hospital are also talking about this physician's questionable behavior. You do two studies to substantiate the problems and give the data to the administrator and the medical staff president. Both times, these people fail to take any action, saying that they don't think the new physician is a problem.

Question

1. What is your next course of action?

QM SITUATIONS THAT RAISE ETHICAL QUESTIONS

The people responding to the 1999 AHIMA member survey reported that they had not experienced a significant increase in pressure to compromise professional ethics or personal values. Less than 12% (4 out of 34) felt that such pressures had increased in the previous five years. Six of the respondents (18%) reported that pressures had actually decreased. Almost three-fourths of the survey respondents felt that nothing had changed in the previous five years. Although it may appear that many HIM professionals involved in QM activities are not facing significant ethical problems, the survey results could be misleading on this point. The healthcare environment is changing rapidly. Organizational pressures to share performance data with the public and maintain high marks on regulatory/accreditation surveys and performance reviews are just beginning to test the discipline's "truth-telling" ethics. Increasing economic constraints and societal issues such as physician-assisted suicide are likely to challenge "patient-protection" ethics. What appeared yesterday to be a clear-cut decision could easily become a situation in which people are being asked to compromise their professional integrity by supporting a leadership decision. People involved in QM activities must be alert to the insidious changes that are occurring in the healthcare environment and society; otherwise, they may not rightfully view some situations as being ethical dilemmas.

It is quite likely that HIM professionals will be facing more "tough calls" in the future. That is why it is important to explore the issue of ethical decision making in the performance of QM activities. To aid in this discussion, the survey distributed to members of AHIMA included five scenarios representing typical QM situations in which the HIM professional might be confronted with an ethical dilemma. For each scenario, respondents were provided with a specified number of actions they could choose from. Each of the alternative actions had a predefined rationale and probable consequences. People were asked to consider the alternative actions, the rationale for each of the actions, and the probable consequences. They were told to select the one action that most closely described how they would proceed, based on the rationale and probable consequences. In some instances, the same action was offered with different rationales, and people had to determine which rationale they would use in selecting an action.

The survey instructions indicated that there was no right answer in any of the situations. A logical argument could be made for each of the alternative actions. The respondents had to consider the rationale, benefits, burdens, and risks of the alternatives and make a judgment about what they would most likely do in each situation. If respondents would have taken an action that was significantly different from any of the alternatives presented, they were allowed to write in their chosen course of action.

This chapter has presented a variety of ethical decision-making scenarios. Completed decision-making matrices for each scenario appear at the end of the chapter. The alternatives, rationale, probable consequences, and choices made by the HIM professionals who answered the AHIMA survey are presented in the Tables 6–1 through 6–5, which also are located at the end of this chapter. Note that people did not provide an answer for every situation. The number of respondents selecting an alternative action for the scenario is shown in the last column on the right. Respondents were allowed to write in an action that was not listed as a choice in the survey. The write-in action choices, if any, are listed below the tables of predefined action choices that were offered to the respondents.

Further analysis of all these situations can be facilitated by the following discussion. Such analysis will help HIM professionals to be more sensitive to their ethical roles in the performance of QM functions. It will also improve decision-making capabilities in the presence of ethical dilemmas and help clarify what someone "ought" to do if confronted with similar situations.

1. What precisely must be decided by the HIM professional in this scenario?
2. Are any of the listed alternatives clearly impractical, illegal, or improper? If so, eliminate the action as a choice.
3. Do any of the listed alternatives require the sacrifice of any ethical principle?
4. Is the full range of ethically justifiable actions listed? If not, add additional actions, with a rationale and with consequences that are likely to occur if the action is taken.
5. Do the consequences of the alternatives appear plausible? Are the consequences likely to occur? What other consequences might happen?
6. Is there a statement in the current AHIMA Code of Ethics that provides some guidance for the decision maker in this situation?
7. Is there a statement in the ethical codes of other quality-related organizations that provides some guidance for the decision maker in this situation?
8. What do you consider the best course of action? After choosing the best course of action, see if you answer "yes" to each of the following questions:
   - If you take this action, are you treating others as you would want to be treated?
   - Would you be comfortable if your reasoning and decision were made public?
   - Are you practicing what is preached by the ethical standards of your profession?

ENABLING ETHICAL CONDUCT

Ethics can sometimes seem very abstract and hypothetical. It may be viewed as something that is nice to think about when time permits, but that may be pretty far down the list when there are important things to be done. Nevertheless, when you cut through all the theory, ethics is really just about what HIM professionals do. The profession must constantly seek out ways of encouraging and enabling its members to follow their good intentions in the complex and sometimes contradictory healthcare environment. Likewise, organizations that employ HIM professionals for QM duties must foster a working environment and culture that enable these excellent and knowledgeable individuals to practice ethically.

Role of the Profession

From the profession's standpoint, the 2004 AHIMA Code of Ethics incorporates some of the beliefs found in the "Shared Statement of Ethical Principles" published by the Tavistock Group (Smith et al., 1999) into day-to-day practices. **Quality improvement** applies to all people who are involved in the delivery of health care, not just licensed clinical professionals. The importance of health information in the improvement of health care is listed as an AHIMA mission. HIM professionals have a duty to improve the quality of patient care and protect the public from physical or emotional harm. For instance:

- The coder is obligated to report patient care practices that vary from accepted **guidelines** when they are discovered during the review of patient records.
- The patient record analyst is responsible for taking action when inaccurate record entries, which could compromise patient outcomes, are found.
- The clinic office manager has an ethical duty to do something when it is discovered that abnormal diagnostic reports are filed in ambulatory patient records

without having been seen by the attending physician.
- The senior executive is responsible for protecting patients from an incompetent practitioner.
- The information specialist who designs an effective billing compliance program can and should help to protect patient safety.

The ethical principles of the Tavistock Group also encourage each professional group involved in healthcare delivery to promote a culture of ethics within its own membership. This culture of ethics must be instilled right from the start, with professionals receiving ethics training in their basic educational preparation. Most business schools now offer special courses in business ethics, and ethics education is a regular part of the training of clinical practitioners. More than 75 percent of nurse executives recently reported that they had received ethics instruction in their basic educational preparation (Riley, 1999). Ethics education is also part of the core curriculum for HIM programs at all academic levels accredited by the Commission on Accreditation for Health Informatics and Information Management Education (CAHIIM).

After the practitioner enters the workplace, professional groups must continue to emphasize the importance of ethical principles. Associations can promote ethics in a number of ways. For instance, the members of the ASQ receive a copy of the ASQ Code of Ethics with their annual membership renewal. The ASQ code is published periodically in society journals, is available on the society's Web site, and is included in every **certification** and recertification package. Details about member expulsions for violations of the code of ethics are made available to the profession as well as the public ("Members Expelled," 1999). The National Society of Professional Engineers (NSPE) regularly publishes case situations that raise ethical questions common to engineering practice and research. The Board of Ethical

Review of the NSPE describes the ethical issues involved in each case and the board offers an opinion on whether the action of the engineer complied with the NSPE Code of Ethics (Online Ethics Center, 1999).

In the healthcare industry, associations representing physicians, nurses, and other clinical professionals routinely support ethics research and training. The healthcare professions also use many of the same techniques used to promote ethics in private industry. For example, during the development of the 2004 AHIMA Code of Ethics, efforts were already under way to create membership awareness and ethics training initiatives. At national and state HIM conferences, AHIMA members are beginning to openly discuss some of the "tough calls" facing HIM professionals. All professional associations whose members are involved in QM activities can, and should, be promoting a culture of ethics and patient care quality within their membership.

Role of the Employer

Professional ethics and personal integrity require explicit attention from the profession as well as the organizations that employ HIM professionals. Twenty-two (65%) of the AHIMA members surveyed indicated that their organization has an ethics officer, ombudsperson, or ethics committee to whom they felt they could turn for advice when confronted with an ethical dilemma. But the survey respondents, as well as other QM professionals, may find that ethics officers and committees prefer to focus on bioethical issues and are reluctant to become involved in organizational ethical questions ("Doing What's Right," 1997). Some respondents said they would contact the organization's compliance officer for advice if faced with a QM ethical dilemma. Yet the compliance officer may not be well versed in how to apply an ethical decision-making framework to QM situations. Generally, compliance officers have healthcare administration, financial auditing, and/or legal backgrounds, according

to the 1999 survey of healthcare compliance officers conducted by Walker Information and Tyler and Company for the Health Care Compliance Association (Health Care Compliance Association, 1999). In handling ethical issues in patient care, most hospital nurses reportedly first discuss the issue with peers or departmental leaders (Fry, Killen, & Robinson, 1996). HIM professionals facing QM ethical dilemmas should use these same tactics. It is advantageous to consult compliance and/or ethics committee members when faced with a particularly difficult or complex decision involving quality of care or patient safety.

CONCLUSION

An ethical dilemma occurs when key factors within a situation lead to different decisions and each of the decisions is equally valid. The five situations presented in the AHIMA membership QM survey represent ethical dilemmas because no one action for any of the cases was chosen by a clear majority of the respondents.

If faced with an ethical dilemma, HIM professionals involved in QM activities must consider the positive and negative consequences connected with each possible action. Consider who will be helped by what you do. Who will be hurt? What kind of benefits and harms are involved? Some "goods" (like preventing patient injuries) are more valuable than others (like a pay raise for good performance). Consider the effect of the actions over the long term as well as short term. Hiding the fact that too many patient records are incomplete may bring short-term gains (continued accreditation), but over the long term, patients may be hurt when up-to-date information is not available to caregivers. Once you have narrowed the list of possible actions down to two or three, it is time to consider the actions themselves. How do they measure up against the ethical principles of the HIM profession and the values of your employer? Do any of the actions "cross the line" in terms of simple decency? If there is a conflict between ethical principles and the rights of patients, what action is least problematic for all stakeholders?

In 1946, Eleanor Hull wrote about how important it was for HIM professionals to be honest and honorable in their dealings with physicians. In the same article, she also wrote about loyalty. According to Ms. Hull, the record librarian "must have the loyalty to see that the rules of the staff and the administrator are carried out, but not the blind loyalty which will not permit her to suggest changes when they are needed" (p. 75). This premise holds true today. HIM professionals are obligated to act when patient safety is threatened by the decisions or actions of an individual or an organization. Saying "It's not my job" is something that Ms. Hull would not have done in 1946, and it should not be our profession's response today.

In the performance of healthcare QM activities, HIM professionals may have to balance economic, professional, and social pressures and select the best alternative. Although there may be several ethical responses to a situation, all are not equal. Making ethical choices is complex because in many circumstances there is a multitude of competing interests and values. Often the decision maker must prioritize competing standards and values and choose the right thing to do.

Because most people's decisions are based on imperfect information and "best guess" predictions, it is inevitable that some ethical choices will be wrong. Occasionally, decisions will fail to produce the intended consequences or will produce unforeseen results. Remember, ethical practice is not just "doing the right thing." It is an ongoing personal effort to develop and strengthen problem-solving and ethical decision-making skills.

Key Terms

- Case management
- Certification
- Guidelines
- License
- Licensure
- Outcome
- Patient safety
- Peer review
- Performance measurement
- Quality
- Quality improvement
- Quality management
- Risk management

Chapter Summary

- Economic tensions, downsizing, competition, and shifting social values that are placing more demands on healthcare leaders may influence those leaders to ask HIM professionals in QM to compromise their professional or personal ethics in order to get the job done. HIM professionals may face pressures to conceal information that could be potentially damaging to the organization, remain silent about quality-of-care concerns, forge documentation, or underreport adverse patient outcome data.
- HIM professionals faced with such ethical dilemmas must consider their professional standards as well as their moral obligation to stop neglect or abuses that threaten the well-being of patients.
- The ethical codes of most healthcare associations representing people involved in QM activities (NAHQ, ASHRM, ASQ, AHIMA) do not explicitly address the subject of patient protection. However, a commitment to quality of patient care is implied in these codes and is directly stated in the ethical principles proposed by the Tavistock

Group for all individuals and organizations involved in the delivery of healthcare services.

- The process of ethical decision making requires that HIM professionals perceive the ethical implications of decisions, evaluate the facts, and then select the best choice without unduly harming other people. When there are competing values, HIM professionals must ask what impact their decision will have on patients' quality of care.

- In some instances, HIM professionals involved in QM activities have a narrow scope of responsibilities, and their authority is limited. However, the ethical person must be concerned with the right thing to do, not with what he or she has a right to do. In all instances in which patient safety is threatened by the decisions or actions of an individual or an organization, the HIM professional is obligated to act.

- Within organizations, ethics officers, ombudspersons, and ethics committees may prefer to focus on bioethical issues and be reluctant to become involved in organizational ethical questions, and compliance officers may be better versed in legal requirements than in ethical decision-making frameworks for QM situations. HIM professionals facing QM ethical dilemmas are advised to consult peers or departmental leaders first and to consult compliance and/or ethics committee members regarding particularly difficult situations involving quality of care or patient safety.

References

American Health Information Management Association [AHIMA]. (2004). *AHIMA Code of Ethics*. Chicago: Author.

American Hospital Association [AHA]. (2004). *Quality advisory: American Society for Healthcare Risk Management*. Chicago: Author.

American Society for Healthcare Risk Management [ASHRM]. (2001). Code of professional ethics and conduct. Retrieved September 2004 from http://www.ashrm.org/ashrm/files/Codeof Conduct.02.doc.

American Society for Quality [ASQ]. (2004). Code of ethics. Retrieved September 2004 from http://www.asq.org/join/about/ethics.html.

Berwick, D., Hiatt, H., Janeway, P., & Smith R. (1997). An ethical code for everybody in health care. *British Medical Journal, 315,* 1633–1634.

Derbyshire, R. (1969). *Medical licensure and discipline in the United States*. Baltimore: Johns Hopkins University Press.

Doing what's right for patients isn't always good business. (1997). *Medical Ethics Advisor, 5*(3), 42–43.

Ethics Resource Center. (1999). 1997 ERC/SHRM business ethics survey. Retrieved October 1999 from http://www.ethics.org/1997surv.html.

Fry, S. T., Killen, A. R., & Robinson, E. M. (1996). Care-based reasoning, caring, and the ethic of care: A need for clarity. *Journal of Clinical Ethics, 7*(1), 41–47.

HCA-The Healthcare Company. (1998, January). One clear voice: Code of conduct. [Brochure]. Nashville, TN: Author.

Health Care Compliance Association, Tyler & Company, Walker Information. (1999, October). *Second annual survey: Profile of health care compliance officers*. Philadelphia: Author.

Hill, F. T. (1948). The professional audit to control efficiency. In A. C. Hayden (Ed.), *Medical record administration* (pp. 233–240). Chicago: American Hospital Association.

Hull, E. F. (1946). Both sides are to blame if M.R.L. spells N.A.G. *Modern Hospital, 67*(12), 75–76.

Kohn, L. T., Corrigan, J. M., & Donaldson, M. S. (Eds.). (1999). *To err is human: Building a safer health system*. Washington, D.C.: National Academy Press.

Lesnik, M., & Anderson, B. (1947). *Legal aspects of nursing*. Philadelphia: J. B. Lippincott.

Members expelled for violating ASQ code of ethics. (1999). *Quality Progress, 32*(9), 51.

National Association for Healthcare Quality [NAHQ]. (1999). NAHQ Code of Ethics and Standards of Practice. Retrieved October 1999 from http://www.nahq.org/about/code.htm.

National Cancer Registrars Association [NCRA]. (1995). Guide to the interpretation of the Code of Ethics. Retrieved April 18, 2000, from http://www.ncra.org.

Nursing Practice Act (Chapter 301). 1999. Texas occupations codes and statutes regulating the practice of professional nursing, as amended 1999. Retrieved April 17, 2000, from http://www.bne.state.tx.us/npatc.htm.

Online Ethics Center. (1999). Engineering ethics cases. Retrieved November 25, 1999, from http://www.onlineethics.org/cases/engcases.html.

QM Section Board. (1990). Quality management defined. *Quality Resource, 8*(3), 1–2.

Riley, J. M. (1999). Nurse executives' response to ethical conflict and choice in the workplace. *Nursing Ethics Network*. Retrieved December 1999 from http://www.bc_edu/bc_org/avp/son/ethics/research.html.

Seltze, W. B. (1948). The role of the hospital superintendent in record room control. In A. C. Hayden (Ed.), *Medical record administration* (pp. 55–65). Chicago: American Hospital Association.

Smith, R., Hiatt, H., & Berwick, D. (1999). A shared statement of ethical principles for those who shape and give health care: A working draft from the Tavistock Group. *Annals of Internal Medicine, 130*, 143–147.

Southern Institute for Business and Professional Ethics. (1999). Second annual survey of Georgia CEOs on business ethics. Retrieved November 1999 from http://www.southerninstitute.org/SI%20Surveyone.htm.

Southern Institute for Business and Professional Ethics. (2002). Survey of Georgia CEOs on business ethics. Retrieved April 2003 from http://www.southerninstitute.org/CEO-Survey-Main.htm.

Spath, P. L. (2000). *Patient safety improvement guidebook*. Forest Grove, OR: Brown-Spath & Associates.

Spath, P. L. (2001). Quality review. In L. B. Harman (Ed.), *Ethical challenges in the management of health information* (pp. 91–112). Gaithersburg, MD: Aspen.

State of Delaware Department for Children, Youth and Their Families, Division of Child Mental Health Services. (1997, October 3). *Policy on ethics*. Wilmington, DE: Author.

SCENARIO 6-A: INACCURATE PERFORMANCE DATA

Table 6–1 Survey Results

Alternative Actions	Rationale for This Action	Probable Consequence(s) of This Action	Survey Results $N = 34$
Do nothing further.	The CEO has the ultimate responsibility for the accuracy. It's not my job.	Taking this action could mean that the data would remain inaccurate or that the CEO would personally decide to post corrected data on the Web site.	21 (64%)
Send corrected data to the health plan's Webmaster and ask that the information on the Web page be updated.	Data will not be corrected if I don't do it myself.	Taking this action might invoke the ill will of the CEO and could lead to disciplinary action.	3 (9%)
Anonymously notify the National Committee for Quality Assurance concerning the inaccurate data.	I feel that the group that accredits the HMO should be aware of the inaccurate data that are being shared with the public.	Taking this action might cause your organization to be sanctioned or lose accreditation.	2 (6%)
Notify the state health insurance commission.	I feel that the state agency that regulates HMOs should be aware of the inaccurate data that are being shared with the public.	Taking this action might cause your organization to be fined or sanctioned by the insurance commission.	2 (6%)

Write-In Actions

Four respondents (12%) indicated that they would talk further with the CEO and, perhaps with the help of the corporate compliance officer, persuade this person to correct the data inaccuracies.

One respondent (3%) indicated that he or she would report the actions of the CEO to the board of directors.

The ethical decision-making matrix is a tool to help you organize complex, ethical problems; however, there is no simple fill-in-the-box approach to ethical decision making. The objective is to follow each step of the process and not move from the question directly to what should be done or how to prevent it next time. If you skip steps, you will not fully understand all of the values and options for action. Also, the matrix provided for each scenario in this book is not the only way to examine the problem. You can make an equally compelling ethical argument for a different decision—just be sure to follow all the steps of the matrix.

SCENARIO 6-A: INACCURATE PERFORMANCE DATA

Steps	Information	
1. What is the ethical question?	Should you report the inaccuracies to the proper parties?	
2. What are the facts?	**KNOWN**	**TO BE GATHERED**
	• The performance data posted on the Web site are inaccurate. • The CEO has advised you to do nothing further.	• Would you be guilty of fraud if you did nothing further? • What are the possible repercussions of attempting to have the data corrected? • What are the customary practices in such cases? • What is the likely impact on self and family of changing jobs?
3. What are the values? Examine the shared and competing values, obligations, and interests of the stakeholders (i.e., patient, HIM professional, healthcare practitioner(s), administrators, society, and other advocates) involved in order to fully understand the complexity of the ethical problem(s).	**Patient:** Values accurate information. **HIM professional:** Truth, integrity, accuracy; promote disclosure of accurate information; fairness; follow the rules and obey the law; protect committee deliberations; refuse to participate or conceal unethical practices; report violations of practice standards to the proper authorities; be honest; personal values (promote welfare of self and family by avoiding loss of job). **Administrators:** Promote welfare of facility; maximize profits without compromising truth-telling. **Society:** Support accuracy of publicly disseminated data.	
4. What are my options?	• Do nothing. • Report the inaccuracies to the proper parties.	
5. What should I do?	Report the inaccuracies to the proper parties (e.g., compliance officer, chair of governing board).	
6. What justifies my choice?	**JUSTIFIED**	**NOT JUSTIFIED**
	• Obligation to tell the truth. • Support accuracy of disseminated data. • Preserve professional integrity. • Respect the law. • Demonstrate loyalty to employer, unless asked to push legal boundaries.	• Do nothing. • Tell a lie. • Not fair to patients who will make decisions based on inaccurate information. • Jeopardize professional integrity.
7. How can I prevent this ethical problem?	• Determine if system changes are needed. • Learn more about the dissemination of performance data. • Discuss standards and the values that support them with colleagues. • Evaluate institutional integrity at job interview and subsequently as ethical problems arise.	

SCENARIO 6-B: HOME HEALTH CARE AND CENTRAL-LINE INFECTIONS

Table 6–2 Survey Results

Alternative Actions	Rationale for This Action	Probable Consequence(s) of This Action	Survey Results $N = 34$
Comply with the request.	I'm new to this job and I don't want to argue with my boss.	Taking this action will mean that the data submitted by the agency to the Joint Commission will be inaccurate. It may also mean that the agency will not investigate further to discover the cause of the infections and take the actions necessary to prevent future infections.	2 (6%)
Comply with the request.	It's been my experience that other organizations don't accurately report all of their complications.	Taking this action will mean that the data submitted by the agency to the Joint Commission will be inaccurate. It may also mean that the agency will not investigate further to discover the cause of the infections and take the actions necessary to prevent future infections.	0
Comply with the request, but also go back into the records to determine if these are not the first central-line infections that have occurred.	If I don't investigate the issue, further problems may never be brought out into the open.	Taking this action could cause conflict between you and your new boss. Such an action also does not ensure that the agency will investigate further to discover the cause of the infections or take the actions necessary to prevent future infections.	11 (33%)
Comply with the request and later anonymously let the Joint Commission know that erroneous data were submitted by the agency.	I feel that the accreditation group that is receiving the information should be aware of the data inaccuracies.	Taking this action might cause your organization to be sanctioned or lose its accreditation. Such an action also does not ensure that the agency will investigate further to discover the cause of the infections or take the actions necessary to prevent future infections.	1 (3%)

Alternative Actions	Rationale for This Action	Probable Consequence(s) of This Action	Survey Results N = 34
Refuse the request.	I don't want to be involved in reporting data that are known to be inaccurate.	Taking this action could cause your boss to take disciplinary action or fire you from your job. Such an action also does not ensure that the agency will investigate further to discover the cause of the infections or take the actions necessary to prevent further infections.	19 (58%)

Write-In Actions

No "write-in" actions.

The ethical decision-making matrix is a tool to help you organize complex, ethical problems; however, there is no simple fill-in-the-box approach to ethical decision making. The objective is to follow each step of the process and not move from the question directly to what should be done or how to prevent it next time. If you skip steps, you will not fully understand all of the values and options for action. Also, the matrix provided for each scenario in this book is not the only way to examine the problem. You can make an equally compelling ethical argument for a different decision—just be sure to follow all the steps of the matrix.

SCENARIO 6-B: HOME HEALTH CARE AND CENTRAL-LINE INFECTIONS

Steps	Information	
1. What is the ethical question?	Should you report the infections?	
2. What are the facts?	**KNOWN**	**TO BE GATHERED**
	• During the last quarter, four patients developed central-line infections. • Your boss has asked you not to report the data to the JCAHO.	• Would not reporting the information constitute fraud? • Is there a systemwide problem that is causing these infections? • What are the customary practices in such cases? • What is the likely impact on self and family of changing jobs?
3. What are the values? Examine the shared and competing values, obligations, and interests of the stakeholders (i.e., patient, HIM professional, healthcare practitioner(s), administrators, society, and other advocates) involved in order to fully understand the complexity of the ethical problem(s).	**Patient:** Values institutional integrity; values high-quality care. **HIM professional:** Truth, integrity, accuracy, and reliability; submit accurate, truthful data to the JCAHO; fairness; follow the rules and obey the law; avoid harm (the infections could be the result of a systemwide problem); personal values (promote welfare of self and family by avoiding loss of job); refuse to participate or conceal unethical practices; report violations of practice standards to the proper authorities; be honest. **Healthcare professionals:** Promote welfare of patients through identification of possible systemwide problems. **Administrators:** Benefit patients and keep from harm; promote welfare of facility without compromising truth-telling. **Society:** Disclose accurate information and adhere to JCAHO standards.	

4. What are my options?	• Report the infections. • Do not report the infections.	
5. What should I do?	Report the infections.	
6. What justifies my choice?	**JUSTIFIED**	**NOT JUSTIFIED**
	• Obligation to tell the truth. • Support accuracy of data. • Preserve professional integrity. • Respect JCAHO standards. • Demonstrate loyalty to employer, unless asked to push legal boundaries.	• Do not report the infections. • Tell a lie. • Make special exception to the rules to protect agency. • Not fair to others who follow rules. • Not fair to patients. • Infections could be the result of a systemwide problem.
7. How can I prevent this ethical problem?	• Determine if system changes are needed. • Learn more about JCAHO disclosure requirements. • Discuss standards and the values that support them with colleagues. • Evaluate institutional integrity at job interview and subsequently when ethical problems arise.	

SCENARIO 6-C: FAILURE TO CHECK PHYSICIAN'S LICENSURE STATUS

Table 6–3 Survey Results

Alternative Actions	Rationale for This Action	Probable Consequence(s) of This Action	Survey Results $N = 34$
Comply with the request.	The medical staff president is personally liable for the actions of any doctor that he hires to work for him. I don't think he would want to risk a lawsuit by hiring a questionable practitioner.	Taking this action would mean that a practitioner whose credentials had not been adequately verified would be caring for patients at your hospital.	0
Comply with the request. Let the hospital risk manager know about the situation.	Even though I'm complying with the request, I want someone else to know about the situation in hopes that they'll do something to prevent me from being put in the situation again.	Taking this action would mean that another member of the organization would be aware of the situation, but it might not ensure that the visiting physician would be properly credentialed before caring for patients at your hospital.	1 (3%)
Obtain approval from the hospital administrator before complying with the request.	Even though I'm complying with the request, I want someone in a position of power to know about the situation in hopes of preventing me from being put in the situation again.	Taking this action would mean that a person in a position of power within the organization would be aware of the situation. However, taking this action might not ensure that the visiting physician would be properly credentialed before caring for patients at your hospital.	4 (12%)
Refuse the request and refer the issue to the hospital administrator.	It's my job to follow the credentialing process established at the hospital. If I'm being asked to change the process, then I want someone higher up to make that decision.	Taking this action would send a message to a person in power in your organization that you felt strongly about not fulfilling the request of the medical staff president. However, taking this action might not ensure that the visiting physician would be properly credentialed before caring for patients at your hospital.	14 (42%)

Alternative Actions	Rationale for This Action	Probable Consequence(s) of This Action	Survey Results N = 34
Refuse the request and refer the issue to the medical staff credentials committee.	It's my job to follow the credentialing process established at the hospital. If I'm asked to change the process, then I want the group responsible for managing the process to make that decision.	Taking this action would send a message to people in power who have professional influence on the medical staff president. It would also show how uncomfortable you are with what the president asked you to do. However, taking this action might not ensure that the visiting physician would be properly credentialed before caring for patients at your hospital.	7 (21%)
Refuse the request. Conduct the necessary inquiries.	It's my job to follow the credentialing process established at the hospital, and I'm going to do it the way I'm supposed to without exception.	Taking this action might slow the visiting physician's application process and would quite likely anger the medical staff president. However, taking this action would ensure that the visiting physician was properly credentialed before caring for patients at your hospital.	7 (21%)

Write-In Actions

No "write-in" actions.

The ethical decision-making matrix is a tool to help you organize complex, ethical problems; however, there is no simple fill-in-the-box approach to ethical decision making. The objective is to follow each step of the process and not move from the question directly to what should be done or how to prevent it next time. If you skip steps, you will not fully understand all of the values and options for action. Also, the matrix provided for each scenario in this book is not the only way to examine the problem. You can make an equally compelling ethical argument for a different decision—just be sure to follow all the steps of the matrix.

SCENARIO 6-C: FAILURE TO CHECK PHYSICIAN'S LICENSURE STATUS

Steps	Information	
1. What is the ethical question?	Should you skip the background checks on the physician?	
2. What are the facts?	**KNOWN**	**TO BE GATHERED**
	• A series of background checks is required to be appointed to the medical staff. • The medical staff president is a friend of the part-time physician. The medical staff president has advised you to forgo the background checks and to indicate that you did conduct them.	• What could be the consequences if the physician has been involved in lawsuits? • What could be the consequences if the physician's license is not current? • Would forgoing the background checks and indicating that you performed them be legal? • What are the customary practices in such cases? • What does your boss expect you to do? • What is the likely impact on self and family of changing jobs?
3. What are the values? Examine the shared and competing values, obligations, and interests of the stakeholders (i.e., patient, HIM professional, healthcare practitioner(s), administrators, society, and other advocates) involved in order to fully understand the complexity of the ethical problem(s).	**Patient:** Values treatment by qualified, licensed professionals. **HIM professional:** Truth, integrity, accuracy, and reliability (perform background checks on all physicians who apply for appointment to the medical staff); fairness; follow the rules and obey the law; loyalty to employer; avoid harm (inaccurate documentation could result in harm to patients and to the facility); personal values (promote welfare of self and family by avoiding loss of job). **Healthcare professionals:** Promote welfare of patients; value maintenance of institutional standards. **Administrators:** Benefit patients and keep from harm; promote welfare of facility; maximize system efficiency without compromising truth-telling; fairness in applying rules for all. **Society:** Allow only licensed, qualified professionals to treat patients.	

4. What are my options?	• Conduct the background check. • Skip the background check.	
5. What should I do?	Conduct the background check.	
6. What justifies my choice?	**JUSTIFIED**	**NOT JUSTIFIED**
	• Obligation to tell the truth. • Obligation to protect welfare of patients and facility. • Support accuracy of the appointment system. • Preserve professional integrity. • Follow rules equally for all. • Respect the law. • Demonstrate loyalty to employer, unless asked to push legal boundaries.	• Skip background checks. • Tell a lie. • Make special exception to the rules as a favor to the medical staff president. • Not fair to others who applied for appointment. • Failure to conduct background checks undermines the entire system. • Place welfare of patients and facility in jeopardy. • Jeopardize professional integrity.
7. How can I prevent this ethical problem?	• Determine if system changes are needed. • Learn more about standard procedures for appointment to medical staff. • Discuss standards and the values that support them with colleagues. • Evaluate institutional integrity at job interview and subsequently as ethical problems arise.	

SCENARIO 6-D: HIDING INCOMPLETE MEDICAL RECORDS

Table 6–4 Survey Results

Alternative Actions	Rationale for This Action	Probable Consequence(s) of This Action	Survey Results $N = 34$
Comply with the request.	I don't think that incomplete records compromise patient care quality, and besides, everyone does it.	Taking this action will improve the likelihood that your organization will pass the accreditation survey and make your immediate boss happy. However, by participating in the falsification of information that is used to make an accreditation decision, you may be violating the AHIMA Code of Ethics. Your professional colleagues may not ever find out about this violation.	1 (3%)
Comply with the request, but accurately report the number of incomplete records to the surveyors.	I'll do what my boss has asked me to do, but I'll also be sure to give the surveyors accurate information about the number of incomplete records.	Taking this action will make your boss happy, as you've done exactly what you were asked to do. However, reporting accurate numbers to the surveyors may cause the Joint Commission to issue a recommendation for improvement. If this occurs, your boss will eventually discover what you've done, and this may lead to ill will or disciplinary action.	0
Comply with the request, but in secret tell the surveyors about the records while they are on site.	I'll do what my boss has asked me to do, but I'll also be sure the surveyors know what I've done and why.	Taking this action will initially make your boss happy, but when the Joint Commission discovers that your organization tried to mislead the surveyors, it is likely that your facility will be put on probation or lose its accreditation. Your boss may eventually discover what you've done, and this may lead to ill will or disciplinary action.	10 (30%)

Alternative Actions	Rationale for This Action	Probable Consequence(s) of This Action	Survey Results *N* = 34
Comply with the request, but after the survey anonymously call the Joint Commission and tell them about the incomplete records.	I'll do what my boss has asked me to do, but after the survey is done I'll alert the Joint Commission to what our organization did to hide incomplete records.	Taking this action will initially make your boss happy, but when the Joint Commission later discovers that your organization tried to mislead the surveyors, it is quite likely that your facility will be put on probation or lose its accreditation. Your boss may never know that you were the one who contacted the Joint Commission.	0
Refuse the request.	I will not participate in an action that I feel is unethical.	Taking this action could cause your boss to take disciplinary action or fire you from your job. It could also cause your facility to receive improvement recommendations from the Joint Commission.	17 (50%)

Write-In Actions

No "write-in" actions.

The ethical decision-making matrix is a tool to help you organize complex, ethical problems; however, there is no simple fill-in-the-box approach to ethical decision making. The objective is to follow each step of the process and not move from the question directly to what should be done or how to prevent it next time. If you skip steps, you will not fully understand all of the values and options for action. Also, the matrix provided for each scenario in this book is not the only way to examine the problem. You can make an equally compelling ethical argument for a different decision—just be sure to follow all the steps of the matrix.

SCENARIO 6-D: HIDING INCOMPLETE MEDICAL RECORDS

Steps	Information	
1. What is the ethical question?	Should you hide the incomplete records?	
2. What are the facts?	**KNOWN**	**TO BE GATHERED**
	• The JCAHO survey will take place in 15 days. • Your immediate boss has asked you to hide any incomplete records that are more than 30 days old.	• Are there any incomplete records that are more than 30 days old? • Would hiding these records be illegal? • What are the customary practices in such cases? • What does your boss expect you to do? • What is the likely impact on self and family of changing jobs?
3. What are the values? Examine the shared and competing values, obligations, and interests of the stakeholders (i.e., patient, HIM professional, healthcare practitioner(s), administrators, society, and other advocates) involved in order to fully understand the complexity of the ethical problem(s).	**Patient:** Values accuracy of medical records; values integrity of healthcare institutions. **HIM professional:** Truth, integrity, accuracy, reliability; disclose all relevant information to the JCAHO; fairness; follow the rules and obey the law; loyalty to employer; avoid harm (inaccurate documentation could jeopardize welfare of patients and facility); personal values (promote welfare of self and family by avoiding loss of job). **Healthcare professionals:** Promote patient welfare; obligation to complete medical records; refuse to participate or conceal unethical practices; report violations of practice standards to the proper authorities. **Administrators:** Benefit patients and keep from harm; promote welfare of facility; fairness in disclosing all appropriate information. **Society:** Preserve integrity of JCAHO surveys.	

4. What are my options?	• Hide incomplete records. • Do not hide incomplete records.	
5. What should I do?	Do not hide incomplete records.	
6. What justifies my choice?	**JUSTIFIED**	**NOT JUSTIFIED**
	• Obligation to tell the truth. • Support accuracy of JCAHO survey. • Preserve professional integrity. • Follow rules and respect the law. • Demonstrate loyalty to employer, unless asked to push legal boundaries.	• Hide incomplete records. • Make special exception to the rules to protect hospital. • Not fair to the other institutions that follow rules. • Not fair to patients who value completion of medical records. • Not fair to physicians who complete records to protect those who don't. • Jeopardize professional integrity.
7. How can I prevent this ethical problem?	• Determine if system changes are needed. • Learn more about disclosure and JCAHO surveys. • Discuss standards and the values that support them with colleagues. • Evaluate institutional integrity at job interview and subsequently as ethical problems arise.	

SCENARIO 6-E: AUDIT RESULTS INDICATE INAPPROPRIATE HEALTH CARE

Table 6–5 Survey Results

Alternative Actions	Rationale for This Action	Probable Consequence(s) of This Action	Survey Results $N = 34$
Do nothing more.	It's the leaders' job to take action. I've done my job by supplying them with accurate information.	Taking this action could mean that the new physician will continue to practice and patients may be harmed by his incompetent behavior.	2 (6%)
Continue providing data to leaders in hopes that they will finally see that a problem exists.	It's the leaders' job to take action. I'll continue to supply them with accurate data in hopes that they'll eventually acknowledge the problem.	Taking this action will increase the amount of information the leaders have about the physician and hopefully cause them to take appropriate action at some future date. It could also mean that the new physician will continue to practice, and patients may be harmed by his incompetent behavior while you gather and report the data and the leaders are deciding what to do.	13 (38%)
Notify the hospital compliance officer of your concerns.	One of the guiding principles of this organization is the provision of quality patient care. I feel that this principle is being compromised, and the compliance officer needs to know this.	Taking this action would mean that a person in a position of power was made aware of the situation and hopefully would deal with it in accordance with the organization's rules of ethical conduct. Taking this action could result in some ill will from the leaders, your colleagues, and other physicians. However, taking this action could hasten an investigation of the physician's behavior and prevent future patients from being harmed.	17 (50%)

Alternative Actions	Rationale for This Action	Probable Consequence(s) of This Action	Survey Results *N* = 34
Notify the governing board chair of your concerns.	The hospital governing board is ultimately responsible for the quality of care, and I feel that they should be made aware of the situation.	Taking this action would mean that the governing board chair was made aware of the situation. Taking this action could result in loss of your job or disciplinary action and/or could invoke the ill will of other physicians. However, taking this action could hasten an investigation of the physician's behavior and prevent future patients from being harmed.	1 (3%)
Anonymously notify the State Board of Medical Examiners concerning this physician's inappropriate medical practices.	I feel the board of medical examiners needs to be made aware of the physician's repeated instances of alleged negligent patient care.	Taking this action could bring negative publicity to your hospital if the board determined that the physician was impaired and the community discovered that the hospital failed to act on information that was available to the leadership. However, taking this action could bring about a formal investigation of the physician's behavior and prevent future patients from being harmed.	0

Write-In Action

One respondent (3%) indicated a decision to notify the head of the medical staff department to which this physician belonged.

The ethical decision-making matrix is a tool to help you organize complex, ethical problems; however, there is no simple fill-in-the-box approach to ethical decision making. The objective is to follow each step of the process and not move from the question directly to what should be done or how to prevent it next time. If you skip steps, you will not fully understand all of the values and options for action. Also, the matrix provided for each scenario in this book is not the only way to examine the problem. You can make an equally compelling ethical argument for a different decision—just be sure to follow all the steps of the matrix.

SCENARIO 6-E: AUDIT RESULTS INDICATE INAPPROPRIATE HEALTH CARE

Steps	Information	
1. What is the ethical question?	Should you report the physician's conduct to a higher authority?	
2. What are the facts?	**KNOWN**	**TO BE GATHERED**
	• A staff physician routinely undertakes questionable behavior. • The QM problems have been twice reported to superiors and both times no action has been taken.	• Is the physician engaging in practices that could be detrimental to patients? • What are the customary practices in such cases? • What does your boss expect you to do? • What is the likely impact on self and family of changing jobs? • What is the likely impact on the physician if the audit results are reported?
3. What are the values? Examine the shared and competing values, obligations, and interests of the stakeholders (i.e., patient, HIM professional, healthcare practitioner(s), administrators, society, and other advocates) involved in order to fully understand the complexity of the ethical problem(s).	**Patient:** Values good health and quality care. **HIM professional:** Truth and integrity; report problems that may endanger patients; loyalty to employer; avoid harm (inappropriate treatment may harm the patient, reporting the physician may harm him and his family, as well as the supervisors and their families). **Healthcare professionals:** Promote welfare of patients through provision of appropriate care. **Administrators:** Benefit patients and keep from harm; promote welfare of facility; truth and integrity. **Society:** Enforce QM standards equally for all.	

4. What are my options?	• Ignore physician's conduct. • Report physician and superiors' conduct to board of ethics, compliance officer, or chair of the governing board.	
5. What should I do?	Report physician's and superiors' conduct to board of ethics, compliance officer, or chair of governing board if facts indicate that the physician is putting patients in danger.	
6. What justifies my choice?	**JUSTIFIED**	**NOT JUSTIFIED**
	• Obligation to tell the truth. • Obligation to maintain QM standards. • Preserve professional integrity.	• Ignore physician's conduct. • Loss of professional integrity. • Violate QM standards. • Endanger patient health.
7. How can I prevent this ethical problem?	• Learn more about QM responsibilities. • Discuss standards and the values that support them with colleagues. • Evaluate institutional integrity at job interview and subsequently when ethical problems arise.	

7

RESEARCH AND DECISION SUPPORT

Merida L. Johns, PhD, RHIA
J. Michael Hardin, PhD

Abstract

The roles of research specialists (RSs) and decision support specialists (DSSs) are intimately related to the use of various information technologies that gather and store data and perform sophisticated analyses. The incorporation of new technologies to support the work of these specialists, particularly the Internet and computerized networks, makes it easy to track individuals, identify their characteristics, and pinpoint their preferences and inclinations. Furthermore, the massive increase of information collection, storage, and retrieval associated with new technologies and industry demands for more information introduces a greater likelihood of data integrity concerns. RSs and DSSs have always been challenged in their work by ethical considerations with regard to informational privacy and data integrity. The purpose of this chapter is to discuss how these ethical considerations have expanded and what new challenges face these professionals given the current advances in the use of information technologies.

Learning Objectives

After completing this chapter, the reader should be able to:

- Discuss the ethical responsibilities of research specialists (RSs) and decision support specialists (DSSs).
- Describe how the advances in information technologies have intensified the ethical challenges in research and decision support.
- Identify how RSs and DSSs can meet their ethical responsibilities with regard to ensuring data integrity and confidentiality, with a focus on the impact of HIPAA.
- Describe the role of institutional review boards (IRBs).
- Discuss the ethical responsibility of the professional to maintain and enhance professional competence.

Scenario 7-A: Designing a Survey to Bias the Results

A research specialist (RS) has been asked to construct a survey instrument to obtain data about how patients feel after receiving a certain treatment modality. The RS designs a three-point ordinal with the rating categories of good, fair, and poor. The principal investigator of the study asks the research analyst to change the scale from a three-point to a five-point scale, with the categories of excellent, very good, good, fair, and poor.

The RS can see that adding excellent and very good does not just break up the good category into three categories. Rather, it changes the whole sense of the scale, because people respond not only to the words in the scale, but also to their placement on the scale. The word fair is now on the negative side of the scale. Thus, one would expect considerably more people to give a rating of good or better with the five-point scale than with the three-point one (Fowler, 1988).

Questions

1. What are the possible ethical implications of such a change?

2. What should the RS do?

A completed ethical decision-making matrix for the scenario is provided at the end of the chapter.

The information age brings with it new and more profound ethical issues related to the management of information. Uncovering ethical issues that grow out of information technology and providing ethical guidelines are the major challenges for business and business ethics at the start of the new millennium (DeGeorge, 1999). With the rise of the Internet and more sophisticated ways of storing data and performing data analysis, it is now much easier to track individuals, identify their characteristics, and pinpoint their preferences and inclinations than it was just a few years ago. Certainly, these new technological capacities raise many ethical questions. What data ought to be collected? How should these data be collected? How should they be reported? Who should be able to see and use information that has been collected, synthesized, and processed? Frequently, the people who have oversight in determining the answers to these questions are research

specialists (RSs) and decision support specialists (DSSs). RSs and DSSs face many ethical issues in the course of their work that can affect employees, patients, research subjects, and other members of the public. Examples of such issues are presented throughout this chapter as we discuss these professionals' roles and special responsibilities. For example, the RS in Scenario 7-A constructed the scale according to her or his best scientific ability following standard practices for scale development and seeking to avoid response bias. In this case, the RS could ask the principal investigator for his or her reasons for wanting to change the scale. Perhaps the principal investigator is aware of other scales using such a five-point scale that have been accepted by other researchers in the area and are known to provide a more useful representation of patient responses. If such reasoning is true, then other scientific evidence would alleviate the RS's concern. A possible compromise for the RS might be to suggest that only the extremes of "excellent" and "poor" be placed on the scale, leaving the adjectives off the other three points. The guiding principle, however, should be to avoid response bias and to anticipate and to eliminate as many sources of response and measurement bias as possible. In essence, the RS should draw upon her or his scientific knowledge and training and seek to develop the best instrument possible to measure the particular patient effect under study (Streiner & Norman, 1989).

ROLES OF THE RS AND THE DSS

In 1996, the American Health Information Management Association (AHIMA) launched Vision 2006 (AHIMA, 1999), an initiative to move health information management (HIM) professionals forward into new roles that have emerged with the information age. Two of the emerging roles identified are those of the RS and the DSS. In 2004, the Center for Health Workforce Studies confirmed that HIM professionals are "increasingly being asked to help with tasks related to the distillation, organization, analysis, and interpretation of patient information for both clinical and business decisions" (AHIMA, 2004a, p. 7). Important roles that will emerge well into the future include professionals who investigate and compile data for different purposes including clinical research, data auditing, quality assessment, cost estimation, risk assessment, and management of resources, among others (AHIMA, 2004a, p. 34). Information technologies for sharing health information will proliferate, and "the information explosion will focus attention on the need to maintain individual privacy" (AHIMA, 2004a, p. 16).

RS and DSS professionals play important roles in contributing to the quality of patient care by ensuring data integrity and by applying information technology for data analysis. Recent studies show that the use of data throughout the healthcare organization is growing at a rapid rate, and the need for decision support and business intelligence analysts, likewise, continues to grow (Krohn,

2004a,b). At the same time RSs and DSSs must uphold ethical principles in the handling of personal health information.

RSs create new knowledge by gathering and analyzing data. They work, for example, on clinical trials and outcomes research with scientific and medical investigators. They are involved in research studies that are usually highly structured and follow a strict research methodology. The sample position description in Table 7–1 (retrieved from a Web page) for a "Research Analyst" and the sample position description in Table 7–2 (developed by AHIMA's Delphi Group) for a "Research Specialist" illustrate possible responsibilities and skills of the RS role.

DSSs analyze data to support strategic planning and operational improvements at the organizational level (Lawrence, 1997). Unlike RSs, DSSs are not necessarily concerned with gaining new clinical and scientific knowledge. Rather, they are concerned with how data may be used to assist management activities. The sample position descriptions in Table 7–1 for a "Decision Support Analyst" and a "Decision Support Specialist" and AHIMA's sample position description in Table 7–3 for a "Decision Support Specialist" illustrate the responsibilities and skills involved. The description in Table 7–3 shows that the DSS has a managerial as well as an analytic role. For example, the DSS will participate and assist in the design of a comprehensive program for the enterprise for decision support. This means that the DSS must be able to see the big picture of the organization's strategic objectives and then be able to match information requirements to the strategic direction of the company. The analytic portion of the job is to analyze selected data and provide decision support overviews and demonstrations to a wide variety of audiences within the organization.

Although their application areas may differ, RSs and DSSs must have essentially the same skills in manipulating and analyzing data. They both use computer software, such as **SPSS** and **SAS,** that includes database

Table 7–1 Sample Position Descriptions

Decision Support Analyst: Provides analysis of quality and performance measurement initiatives, such as patient satisfaction survey programs, data analysis and reporting for operational/clinical departments, external benchmarking efforts, 'quality of care' and clinical outcome performance tracking, and measurement support for patient safety improvement efforts.

Analyzes and organizes qualitative and quantitative clinical, financial and administrative data from multiple sources, and synthesizes results into meaningful reports and presentations on a regular basis.

Provides analytic and QA support for the development and implementation of the Balanced Scorecard throughout BWH and Faulkner Hospitals.

Provides development, implementation, support, and evaluation of a variety of departmental and institutional databases to support Center for Clinical Excellence activities at Brigham and Women's and Faulkner Hospitals.

Bachelor's degree required, master's degree or healthcare experience preferred, preferably in public/health management or the sciences.

Exceptional judgment and discretion in interacting with physicians and senior management on sensitive political and confidential issues.

Knowledge of current issues in the healthcare environment preferred, particularly regarding quality measurement, outcomes studies, healthcare finance, and patient safety.

Knowledge and application of statistical analyses including financial variance analysis and statistical significance preferred.

Proficiency in IBM PC systems and applications including Access, Excel, Lotus, PowerPoint, Paradox, WordPerfect, publishing, and other database management software.

Source: Retrieved September 2005 from http://jobsearch.monster.com/getjob.asp?JobID=33711493& AVSDM=2005%2D09%2D07+15%3A01%3A40&Logo=1&q=finance+decision+support+systems

---

Decision Support Analyst: This position will generate and prepare Decision Support information for clinical and administrative staff. The analyst will work with clinical and financial personnel to determine their information needs. They will also install software and train personnel in the use of the software. This position develops, interprets, and presents cost accounting information within the hospital environment using EPSi cost accounting system

Education: Bachelors degree in business, finance, accounting or the equivalent. CPA and MBA/MHA preferred. Minimum of 3 years of cost accounting experience, preferably within health care.

Source: Retrieved September 2005 from http://jobsearch.monster.com/jobsearch.asp?q=finance+ decision+support+systems

---

Research Analyst: The successful candidate will have work experience in describing and presenting health research results. Experience with statistical techniques and research methodologies necessary. Must have excellent writing skills and ability to access research resources. Qualifications include a bachelor's degree in social sciences or health related discipline with emphasis on research plus two years experience in summarizing statistical analyses. An advanced degree is a plus. Excellent oral and written skills and experience with MS Office is required.

Source: Retrieved September 2005 from http://www.nahdo.org/projects/projects.asp?homepage= true&page=news&option=display&id=355

Table 7–2 AHIMA Sample Position Description: Research Specialist

Position Title: Research Data Analyst

Immediate Supervisor: Department Director

General Purpose: The Research Data Analyst ensures the quality of data collection, coordination, and analysis for clinical research projects.

Responsibilities:

- Verifies, examines, and collects data
- Ensures that clinical data are quality assured, consistent, and relevant to project's and the organization's goals
- Ensures the integrity of the data and safe and proper management of study parameters
- Maintains expert knowledge of relevant FDA guidelines and other regulatory procedures
- Monitors protocol at study sites
- Retrieves data from numerous clinical databases within the organization as well as from proprietary and nonproprietary databases available through outside sources
- Uses structured query language and downloads data into the organization's custom databases for review and analysis
- Manipulates and analyzes data by using statistical software, such as SPSS and SAS, and identifies and determines significant variances and trends for quality control
- Reviews proposed research design to ensure that the data collected are adequate to meet the project's goals
- Prepares periodic progress and monitoring reports on study recruitment, data collection, and data quality
- Participates in team meetings
- Prepares and provides overviews, demonstrations, and presentations to wide variety of audiences

Qualifications:

- Master's degree in health science or related field
- Baccalaureate degree in health information management, business, or closely related area
- Experience in health science and administration
- Certification as RHIA preferable

Source: Reprinted with permission from American Health Information Management Association's Delphi Group, *Evolving HIM Careers: Seven Roles for the Future, Vision 2006,* © 1999, American Health Information Management Association.

development, data analysis, graphic, and presentation tools specifically for assisting in conducting research, decision support, and business and marketing intelligence. They both are involved in development and maintenance of computer databases. Therefore, they must understand basic concepts about databases, including structure models, data

Table 7–3 AHIMA Sample Position Description: Decision Support Specialist

---

Position Title: Decision Support Specialist

Immediate Supervisor: Director, Decision Support

General Purpose: The Decision Support Specialist coordinates data and research for senior managers at the corporate level of the integrated system.

Responsibilities:

- Participating and assisting in the design of a comprehensive program to lend support and analysis to management

- Performing scientific and technical planning, direction, and analysis of selected surveillance systems used by management

- Investigating existing national data and performing descriptive and analytic studies using statistical techniques

- Providing ongoing data analysis to entity decision makers that is relevant to the healthcare market and assisting in problem solving, solution development, decision making, and strategic planning

- Recommending focus and direction of resources toward management goals

- Preparing and providing decision support overviews, demonstrations, and presentations to a wide variety of audiences

- Serving as technical expert advisor and consultant to collaborating organizations in the area of management goals

Qualifications:

- Bachelor's degree in health information management, business, health care, or information systems technology

- Certification as RHIA or RHIT

- Understanding of healthcare delivery systems and health science administration

---

Source: Reprinted with permission from American Health Information Management Association's Delphi Group, *Evolving HIM Careers: Seven Roles for the Future, Vision 2006,* © 1999, American Health Information Management Association.

---

modeling, and database normalization. They must also be familiar with data dictionary development and maintenance and how to perform storage, retrieval, and updating functions in a computer database. They must be familiar with statistical techniques to analyze and manipulate data and be proficient in computer languages such as SQL Server, a Microsoft relational database management system, designed to query databases. Expertise includes report and presentation abilities and project management skills, including managing teams of people, identifying project tasks and priorities, developing timelines and milestones, and balancing resources. In addition, they must have a broad knowledge of the theory and practice in data administration, research design, statistical methods, decision making, and the visual display of quantitative information.

Because each of these positions has a complex relationship with health information management, both RSs and DSSs must have a strong foundation in computer and information ethics and regulatory issues affecting the handling and management of personal health information. This includes not only knowledge of ethical responsibilities in the critical areas of data acquisition, reporting, and access, but also the ability to apply a general framework for ethical analysis to HIM.

ETHICAL RESPONSIBILITIES OF THE RS AND DSS

RSs and DSSs, as HIM professionals, have the responsibilities outlined in the HIM profession's code of conduct set forth by the AHIMA Code of Ethics (2004b; see Chapter 1 of this book, Appendix 1-E) to ensure the integrity and the confidentiality of health information. Further, RSs in particular have responsibilities regarding the protection of human subjects that include special issues related to the confidentiality of research data. Because they are often directly collaborating with clinical investigators, they are, like those investigators, answerable to **institutional review boards (IRBs),** which are advisory boards composed of physicians, scientific colleagues, and concerned nonscientists (frequently administrators and private citizens) that have been set up by federal legislation to oversee research on human subjects and ensure protection of those subjects from research abuses. Both RSs and DSSs must comply with regulatory requirements for handling personal health information. Many of the privacy and security standards resulting from the Health Insurance Portability and Accountability Act (HIPAA) affect how information is used and managed for research and analytical purposes. For example, in most cases an individual's written authorization is required before personal data can be used for research purposes. We will first outline general responsibilities of RSs and DSSs regarding the management and control of information for integrity and confidentiality and then discuss the special issues facing the RS.

Ensuring Data Integrity and Confidentiality

Data integrity usually refers to the entire set of characteristics associated with data quality; that is, how "good" the data are. Data integrity has been described in terms of six dimensions (Cash, 1994):

1. Content, including currency (whether data are up-to-date or current), relevance to the decision-making purpose, and accuracy (whether data are correct)
2. Scope (comprehensiveness)
3. Level of detail
4. Composition (issues involved in database structure and the definition of entities and attributes)
5. Consistency, including both semantic consistency (consistency in the definitions of data elements, such as "patient number," across entity types, such as "patient" and "encounter") and structural consistency (consistency in the business rules that define the relationships among data elements)
6. Reaction to change, which concerns how data elements are updated, deleted, or added to a database

Data stewardship is the obligation to protect data integrity and security. RSs and DSSs have responsibilities of data stewardship with regard to all six dimensions of data integrity. As custodians of health information, they must verify and maintain the accuracy and consistency of their data and exercise control over how those data are matched or recombined with other data (Cash, 1994, pp. 248–250). They must guard against the contamination of data by user errors, program errors, and intentional manipulation that could harm patients. Methods should be in place to review data collection procedures and the data themselves for likely sources of errors and to apprehend and correct defects in composition that might affect the ability to identify and retrieve data appropriately. Methods should also be implemented to identify and rectify any potential security breaches. Security procedures should allow for authorized additions and deletions to the data, and edit checks should be conducted to ensure that correct domain values are entered into the database.

As Johns (1997), Redman (1992), and Brandel (2004) have described, data stewardship must involve collaborative and multidisciplinary efforts to oversee processes from the point of data collection through the data's various transformations and usages. Data policies should be established for all the various levels of job tasks involved with data collection, aggregation, synthesis, and use. Table 7–4, from Spinello (1997, p. 9), provides a guideline for policy development.

Because decisions about patient care, employee and provider performance, organizational performance, competitive analysis, and strategic issues are made on the basis of the collection and analysis of data by RSs and DSSs, these specialists must be held to a high level of accountability. Lack of data integrity can profoundly affect large numbers of individuals in many ways. For example, if data are not accurate or up-to-date, then decisions made based on these data may be faulty. As such, they may affect the quality of patient care and the reputation and viability of healthcare organizations. For instance, let's say that an insurance company is benchmarking the mortality rates of hospitals by clinical services. The insurance company discovers that the respiratory service at City Hospital has a 25% higher-than-average mortality rate than the same service at other similar hospitals. The insurance company concludes that City Hospital is providing less than optimal care in its respiratory service and sanctions the hospital on the basis of this analysis. Further examination of the data shows, however, that not all of the final diagnosis codes of these mortality cases coincide with those normally associated with a respiratory clinical service. The DSS discovers that many of the service codes were inaccurately assigned at the time of patient admission and that many of the mortality cases actually belong to another service.

In a real example, faulty data contributed to the reporting of extraordinarily high rates of breast cancer in Marin County, California. Marin County, one of the wealthiest counties in the United States, was reported in 2003 to have one of the highest breast cancer rates in the country. Activists seized upon this data, and pollution was cited to explain the high cancer rate. But as it turned out, pollution was not the reason for the reportedly high rate. Instead if was found that the estimate used faulty data from the U.S. Census Bureau that dramatically undercounted the total population of women in Marin County by almost 20%. This undercount was the cause of the inflated breast cancer statistic (Pritchard, 2003).

Data confidentiality, as discussed in Chapter 3, has become a major concern for many patients. As the amount, diversity, and intimacy of health-related data recorded have increased, and as computerization has made it increasingly possible to interlink and transfer information from one database to another, opportunities to gain access to this information have multiplied. Meanwhile, more and more parties are seeking access to health data, including employers, schools, insurers, courts, and news media, with potentially drastic consequences for the individuals on whom these data are released. Because DSSs and RSs frequently have oversight for determining who should get what information, they play a crucial role in protecting patient health information from unauthorized access and use.

Concerns regarding data integrity and confidentiality must be addressed in practices regarding data acquisition, reporting, and access. We will discuss each of these areas in more detail as follows.

Data Acquisition

Acquisition of data, a principal task of both the RS and the DSS, seems as if it would be fairly straightforward. What possible ethical

Table 7–4 Sample Data Policy

Individuals who are responsible for the following activities have an obligation to treat data as a valuable corporate asset and to respect the rights of any stakeholders affected by use of that data.

Collectors and Processors of Data

- Implement data quality and security procedures to ensure data integrity.

- Review systems and methods of data collection for likely sources of errors.

- Review systems for possible security breaches.

- Establish and maintain a technology infrastructure that facilitates the sharing of data across functions and departmental units.

- Monitor and update data on a timely and regular basis.

- Make sure that databases reflect the current state of the business and that the proper information is available for strategic decision making.

- Understand how and by whom the data will be used.

Database Custodians and Those Controlling Access

- Protect data from undesired or unauthorized access.

- Make data available to users within the organization who can demonstrate a legitimate business need for the data.

- Restrict the information available to those outside the company unless they have a legitimate business need for that information.

Data Users

- Users are fully responsible for the data that they request.

- Ensure that data are correctly used and interpreted.

- Use data only for valid business purposes.

- Protect the privacy rights of fellow employees, customers, and all other organization stakeholders. This means that users must prudently weigh the implications for those stakeholders if certain information is made public, redistributed, or recombined in some fashion.

Source: R. A. Spinello, *Case Studies in Information and Computer Ethics*, © 1997, page 9. Reprinted by permission of Prentice-Hall, Inc., Upper Saddle River, NJ.

*Reprinted with permission of W. W. Lawrence, PhD Report to the United States Secretary of Health and Human Services, Privacy and Health Research, Office of Assistant Secretary, Division of Data Policy, Office of Program Systems, Washington, DC.

concerns could there be with capturing information required for the care and treatment of the patient or for the operation of the organization?

One of the primary concerns dealing with data acquisition is the quality of the data being collected. The degree of quality that data have begins at the source of their collection (Johns, 1997). How well data are collected determines to a large part the degree to which project results will have integrity. If data are collected from a poor sampling distribution, are poorly defined, or are inaccurately entered in a database, then the outcomes of analysis will not be valid and reliable. That is, such results will not be truthful to the extent that they do not measure what they claim to measure. Therefore, the amount of care taken in the initial collection of data is a paramount consideration. Any errors at the initial point of collection will continue to infiltrate and possibly escalate problems of data integrity throughout the project.

RSs and DSSs must carefully consider the previously listed dimensions of data integrity in any data collection effort. For example, with regard to content, are the data relevant (i.e., meaningful) to the decision-making purpose at hand? With regard to scope, are the data being collected comprehensive enough for the decision-making purposes for which they will be used? This is an important question in outcomes and evidence-based medicine, where the lack of comprehensive data may have grave consequences for decision making. The detail level at which the data are gathered is important, because collection of imprecise data may have significant ramifications and may lead to false conclusions.

Scenario 7-A at the opening of this chapter raises an ethical issue related to data acquisition. A significant portion of research relies on surveys that use rating scales. It is therefore important that any rating scale that is used be both reliable and valid. However, there are many ways in which a rating scale can be biased, and researchers can intentionally bias the results of a study by choosing a particular type of rating scale (Friedman & Amoo, 1999).

Here, the principal investigator may want the RS to change the rating scale because a much more favorable response to the treatment is likely to be given by patients if the five-point scale is used. The principal investigator is attempting to bias the response of the patients so that the treatment modality will have a higher chance of receiving a more favorable or positive rating. Although such an alteration, even if intentional, would not be outright fraud, it could unethically distort the pattern of patient responses, ultimately biasing decisions about the treatment's adoption and use.

If the principal investigator is trying to manipulate the scale to achieve a desired outcome, then he or she is behaving unscientifically and unethically. The RS should calmly and logically demonstrate to the principal investigator how the suggested changes are unscientific and, if solely changed for purposes of skewing the data, unethical. The RS may consider writing a memo to the principal investigator, thereby documenting his or her concerns for the record. After discussions with the principal investigator, if he or she remains committed to such behavior, the RS must decide whether to report the principal investigator to the appropriate organizational authorities or to resign from the project. The RS should realize that by doing nothing or going along with the principal investigator, the RS can be held liable for misconduct or perhaps be placed in the position of being assigned the entire blame for the misconduct of the principal investigator.

Patient-related data collection is not the only type of data collection engaged in by healthcare organizations. Provider information is also collected and used to make determinations about the quality of care that a physician or other healthcare professional supplies. RSs and DSSs must take the same care in determining data acquisition quality in these cases as when collecting patient-related data.

Other ethical questions in the area of data acquisition concern privacy and confidentiality. Today's advanced technologies allow acquisition of data on healthcare consumers by "passive" means such as monitoring systems. For example, monitoring systems can track an individual's use of a healthcare organization's Web page. For what purposes is this information being collected? Is the information individually identifiable? Will personal information and/or the identification of individual preferences collected from such monitoring systems be subsequently used in ways that may annoy or inconvenience the individual? For example, will these data be used in marketing campaigns? Will they be used to individually identify persons who may use specific products or services that the company provides? What are the ethical responsibilities to inform the public that individually identifiable information is being collected about them?

RSs and DSSs must adhere to regulatory standards. Several HIPAA privacy standards address data collection and use. For example, most uses and disclosures of patient-specific information for research purposes require a written patient authorization, unless an alteration or waiver of authorization has been granted by an IRB or privacy board. Such an authorization, as defined by HIPAA, has several core elements and must include specific notifications to the patient authorizing release of information for research purposes. When gathering or using data for research purposes, RSs should be sure that appropriate authorizations have been obtained. Table 7–5 provides an outline of HIPAA privacy rules that affect data used for research purposes.

A closely related issue is the use of monitoring systems to collect information on employees. For example, companies can monitor and archive electronic messages for future in-

spections. Sophisticated systems can measure the duration of telephone calls and the time it takes for an employee to perform a work task. Electronic identification badges that serve as door keys provide physical security for a business, but they also allow monitoring of the movements of employees. Before deciding on a course of action, the enterprise must weigh carefully the philosophical and practical questions. Does the employee's right to privacy take precedence over the employer's right to monitor its employees? The ethical situation here consists of defining a reasonable balance between, on the one hand, the employer's property rights, protection of company assets, the need for access to business information, and the need to monitor for possible legal and liability problems and, on the other hand, the employee's right to personal privacy (Baase, 1997). Certainly, the company should state in writing and during orientation sessions to employees that their performance may be monitored using any one of these methods.

Today's healthcare environment is extremely competitive. In addition to issues involving the collection of internal data, many

Table 7–5 HIPAA Privacy Standards Affecting Research

Covered entities must obtain an individual's authorization for the creation, use, and disclosure of personal health information (PHI) for research purposes, except when

- An alteration or waiver of the authorization has been approved by an IRB or privacy board.

- Covered entities must obtain an individual's authorization for the creation, use, and disclosure of PHI for research purposes, except when the researcher, either in writing or orally represents that:

  - the use or disclosure is solely to prepare a research protocol, and

  - no PHI will be removed from the covered entity, and

  - PHI requested is necessary to conduct the research

- Covered entities must obtain an individual's authorization for the creation, use, and disclosure of PHI for research purposes, except when the researcher, either in writing or orally, represents that the use or disclosure being sought is solely for research of decedents and provides, if requested, documentation of the death of the individuals, and represents that the PHI requested is necessary to conduct the research

Source: M. Johns, *Computer-Based HIPAA Privacy Training Series* © 2001. Reprinted with permission.

companies are interested in the acquisition of competitive data. Moral norms, however, are sometimes ambiguous, so there is a gray area where it is difficult to differentiate industrial espionage from competitive analysis (Spinello, 1997). Certainly, healthcare enterprises must engage in competitive analysis and devote resources to business intelligence. These activities, however, should not be at the expense of ethical practice. DSSs, who may play an important role in gathering such data, must be concerned with the methods and techniques used for data acquisition.

Another ethical concern relates to the collection of data from outside sources or external data banks. Organizations must ensure that data collected from external sources meet the same stringent ethical requirements as those imposed internally. For example, external data sources should be able to provide assurances that their data collection techniques have not been illegal or unethical.

Data Reporting

As we saw previously, there are many ways to introduce bias into data during data collection. The same is true for data reporting. There is a saying that says that it is easy to "lie with statistics." In other words, by using statistical or reporting techniques incorrectly, you can make your results look better (or worse), depending on the bias desired. Let's take a simple example. Suppose that a research analyst is presenting data on central tendency (i.e., mean, median, and mode) regarding compliance of a specific clinical unit with documentation standards. The analyst has a close relationship with the chief of the service, so he or she might be motivated to look at how the results differ depending on which measure is used and might decide to use the measure (say, in this case, the median) that was most favorable to the service because of his or her friendship with the chief of the service. However, this course of action would not be ethical. Data should always be presented in a way that will provide for the most accurate interpretation of the

findings. If several measures are needed to present the data accurately, then all of them should be used.

Data Access

RSs and DSSs, as professionals who may have security clearance to access a broad spectrum of data, must confront several ethical issues regarding data access. It is their responsibility to contribute to the development of policies and procedures with regard to these issues and to ensure that they are implemented properly.

First, they have the responsibility to ensure that data in reports and analyses are released only to authorized individuals. For example, an analyst may be requested by a medical provider to do a trend analysis on a specific condition. The information requested may include not only clinical findings, but also information about other providers. If the requesting individual does not have clearance for this type of data, then it is the responsibility of the analyst to turn the request down. This would also be the case if an employer requested personally identifiable information about employees' health records.

Second, they have a responsibility to ensure that patient data, particularly personally identifiable patient data, are released only for authorized purposes. The primary purpose of sharing patient data is to serve the needs of the patient in the current care encounter. But additional authorized purposes are, typically, to document and support the diagnosis and treatment the patient received, to substantiate charges for professional fees and ancillary tests, and to provide evidence in cases of legal dispute. Then, beyond purposes directly related to the patient's care, is a series of secondary, larger purposes: education (both continuing education for the current providers and academic programs for the providers of the future), maintenance of quality of care, compliance with regulatory and accrediting agencies (including credentialing), planning for new services or new healthcare delivery systems, public health uses (reporting of communicable diseases), and medical and social research. For these larger purposes, typically information may be released, but not in a form that allows individual patients to be identified unless special circumstances require it. For example, consider the request of a facility administrator who wants information from the facility's DSS on the demographics, including patient names, of all patients treated in the facility for the diagnosis of clinical depression in order to compile a report for management purposes. The DSS should not give the administrator access to that information. Normally, personally identifiable information coupled with specific diagnoses should not be used for decision support purposes. Policies and procedures should be in place that provide guidance on how such circumstances should be handled.

A situation that raises a similar ethical issue is one in which administrators attempt to access data originally collected for one purpose in order to use them for an unrelated purpose. For example, let's say that a DSS at a hospital helps to conduct a satisfaction survey of patients who have been hospitalized. On the survey instrument is the question "If you had to have another inpatient hospitalization, how likely would you be to choose this hospital again?" This type of data helps the hospital determine how good its services have been and provides opportunities to improve them.

Now suppose that the foundation arm of the hospital is mounting a fund-raising campaign. The foundation knows that the hospital has gathered satisfaction information from patients and asks the DSS for a list of those patients who provided high satisfaction ratings, on the assumption that patients who reported high satisfaction are more likely to give a charitable contribution to the hospital than those patients who reported low satisfaction. The ethical issue in this case is that the information collected is not being used for its original intended purpose, but is being used as a way to identify potential contributors to the hospital.

Still another ethical issue concerns the secondary use of data by external parties. As Ware (1993) observed, "Traditional record-keeping privacy has taken a new face, namely, data about people are used not for the internal business purposes of the organization that collected them, but for the business purposes of whoever is willing to buy the data" (p. 195). Because of the intensely competitive nature of the environment and the value of information, policies and procedures should be in place that protect organizational and patient-related data from brokers who specialize in the buying, recombining, and selling of information.

HIPAA privacy standards specifically address the de-identification of data for research purposes (Amatayakul, 2003; Burrington-Brown & Wagg, 2003). De-identified health information is information that does not identify an individual and for which there is no easy way to link the information back to a specific individual. Information that has been de-identified can be used and disclosed without an individual's authorization. HIPAA explicitly states that de-identification of information can be performed in one of two ways. First, de-identification can be performed by a person with appropriate knowledge who oversees the process of de-identification and can verify that information has been de-identified. This person must use appropriate principles and methods to ensure that the information, either used alone or in combination with other information, cannot be linked back to an individual. The methods for de-identification of data in this manner must be documented along with the rationale that supports the determination. The second way that HIPAA allows de-identification of data is through removal of specific identifiers. Table 7–6 provides a list of all the identifiers that must be removed in order for data to be considered de-identified.

Human Subject Research

Because of the strict requirements for clinical and scientific research, RSs must be especially attentive to issues of data integrity in data acquisition and reporting. Errors in

Table 7–6 Identifier Removal Required for De-identification of Data

Identifiers of the individual or of relatives, employers, or household members including:

- Names
- All geographic subdivisions smaller than a state, including street address, city, county, precinct, ZIP code, & their equivalent geocodes, except for the initial three digits of a ZIP code if
  - The geographic unit formed by combining all ZIP codes with the same three initial digits contains more than 20,000 people
  - The initial three digits of a ZIP code for all such geographic units containing 20,000 people or less is changed to 000
- All elements of dates (except year) directly related to an individual
  - Birth date, admission date, discharge date, date of death
  - All ages over 89 and all elements of dates, including year, indicative of such age
  - Ages may be aggregated into a single category of age 90 or older

Identifiers of the individual or of relatives, employers, or household members:

- Telephone numbers
- Fax numbers
- E-mail addresses
- Social Security numbers
- Medical record numbers
- Health plan beneficiary numbers
- Account numbers
- Certificate/license numbers
- Vehicle identifiers
- Device identifiers and serial numbers
- Web URLs
- Internet Protocol (IP) addresses
- Biometric identifiers
- Full-face photographic images
- Any other unique characteristic or code

Source: M. Johns, *Computer-Based HIPAA Privacy Training Series* © 2001. Reprinted with permission.

methods or reporting are often unintentional. However, numerous cases of intentional misconduct have been reported (Lynoe, Jacobsson, & Lundgren, 1999). Intentional misconduct ranges from improperly changing observation data to taking discarded research data, laundering it, and then including it in another research project. Thus, RSs must be concerned with avoiding both intentional and unintentional scientific misconduct.

As stated earlier, RSs, as collaborators in human subjects research, are answerable to IRBs, which were founded as a response to publicized abuses in research. The Tuskegee Syphilis Experiment provided a dramatic illustration of the need for controls over the use of human subjects in research projects. The study, conducted from 1932 to 1972, involved 399 black men in the later stages of syphilis and was expected to discover how syphilis affected blacks as opposed to whites. It purported to test the theory that whites had more neurological complications than blacks, who were said to have more cardiovascular complications. How this knowledge would have changed the treatment is uncertain. The study was later described as an experiment that was an inefficient study using human beings as laboratory animals (Jones, 1993). In 1997, President Clinton delivered an apology to the eight remaining survivors of the experiment, stating, "The United States government did something that was wrong— deeply, profoundly, morally wrong. It was an outrage to our commitment to integrity and equality for all our citizens" (Clinton, 1997).

The atrocities of Nazi Germany were another grim example of cruel behavior toward human subjects. Physicians and scientists performed medical experiments in concentration camps against the subjects' will. When this information became public, it stunned the research community. Those who prosecuted the war criminals at Nuremberg asked practical questions about experiments on humans, including whether they should be conducted at all. In the final analysis, the answer was that using human subjects could be justified "if a wall of protection" could be built around them.

That wall of protection is provided by IRBs. Their determinations of adequate protection for potential research subjects are made with reference to three basic principles of ethical research: (1) beneficence (avoid harm, promote good); (2) justice (fairness); and (3) respect for persons (personal autonomy). Application of the standards involves a determination that a study is morally justified by

(1) adequate design, (2) a favorable risk/benefit ratio, (3) equitable selection of subjects, and (4) **informed consent** by study subjects (i.e., assurance that when individuals give consent to participate in research or to release information, they have explained to them, and clearly understand, their rights as research subjects and the consequences, benefits, and risks that participation or release of information will involve) (DHEW, 1978).

The role of the IRB is to ensure that the institution has a set of policies and procedures that guide the conduct of research according to the following principles:

- Conduct health research in an atmosphere with respect for the privacy of people whose health experience is being studied.
- Collect personally identifiable data only if the research is worthwhile and identifiability is required for scientific reasons.
- Publicize the existence of data collection and give subjects the opportunity to review data about themselves.
- Obtain informed consent.
- Safeguard personal identifiers as close to the point of original data collection as possible.
- Enforce the policy of no access to person-identifiable information as a default rather than as a general rule.
- Maintain and monitor access "audit trails."
- Remove the data subject's personal identifiability as thoroughly as is compatible with research needs.
- Maintain proper physical safeguards and cybersecurity measures.
- Develop policies on seeking or allowing secondary use of personally identifiable data.
- Sensitize, educate, answer for, and certify all personnel who handle personally identifiable data or who supervise those who do (Lawrence, 1997).

As stated previously, a written authorization must be obtained from the patient before personally identifiable information is used for research purposes. Table 7–7 provides a listing of all required authorization elements and notifications. An exception to this rule is when an IRB or Privacy Board has granted an alteration or waiver of the authorization. An alteration or waiver of an authorization means that the authorization for uses and disclosure of information has been waived or required elements altered for a specific situation. Specific conditions must be met before an IRB or Privacy Board grants an alteration or waiver of authorization. To be valid, an alteration or waiver must include the following:

- Identification of the IRB or Privacy Board granting the alteration or waiver
- The date of the alteration or waiver
- A description of protected health information to be used or accessed
- A statement that alteration or waiver has been reviewed and approved under normal or expedited review procedures as stipulated by HIPAA
- Signature of chair or other designee of the IRB or Privacy Board

Eight criteria must be satisfied for an alteration or waiver of authorization to be issued. These include documentation that:

- Use and disclosure involve minimal risk.
- Use and disclosure do not adversely affect privacy rights or the welfare of the individuals.
- The research could not practicably be conducted without the waiver or alteration.
- The research could not be practicably conducted without access to and use of the protected health information.
- The privacy risks to individuals are reasonable to the anticipated benefits.

Table 7–7 Required Authorization Elements and Notifications for Use and Disclosure of Information

Authorizations must be written in plain language so that individuals can understand the conditions of the authorization and must include:

- A description of the information that is to be used or disclosed
- The identification of persons or classes of persons who are authorized to make the request
- The identification of the persons or classes of persons to whom the requested information is to be used or disclosed
- The description of the purpose of the use or disclosure
- Identification of the expiration date or event of the authorization
    - A specific expiration date is not required for research. The authorization may simply state "at the end of the research study." In cases where the authorization is for inclusion of information in a research database or repository, the statement "none" or similar language is sufficient.
- Signature of the individual
- Date of the signature

Individuals must be notified that they can revoke the authorization in writing and be provided with instructions on how to revoke the authorization. The authorization must also notify individuals that treatment, payment, enrollment, or eligibility for benefits is not dependent upon providing the authorization and that privacy requirements only apply to covered entities.

Source: U.S. Department of Health and Human Services, Office for Civil Rights. (2002). Standards for Privacy of Individually Identifiable Health Information.

- An adequate plan to protect the identifiers from improper use and disclosure is in place.
- An adequate plan to destroy identifiers at the earliest opportunity is in place.
- There are adequate written reassurances that the protected health information will not be reused or disclosed to any person or entity, except as required by law, for authorized oversight of the research project or for other research for which the use or disclosure of protected health information would be permitted.

Researchers conducting any publicly funded study must submit a protocol to the IRB (including the study's aims, significance, relation to prior research, design and methods, budget, and consent forms) and get the IRB's approval before the study begins. Any expansion or modification of approved protocols requires a new review, at least at the executive committee level. Then, once the study is begun, the research protocol is subject to annual review based on evaluation of findings and consent form use. All serious adverse events, whether expected or unexpected, must be submitted to the IRB for review. Serious but non-life-threatening events are to be reported and documented. Reports of life-threatening events are required within 24 hours of the occurrence for committee review; reports of non-life-threatening events, within five working days. Committee review can result in modification of the study, modification of the consent form, or suspension of enrollment in the study, up to and including suspension of the study itself (Mayo Clinic, 2000).

Though the IRB creates, endorses, and enforces its policies, the RS puts them into practical application. As a member of the study team, the RS ensures that the information being collected matches the approval from the IRB review, that all of the IRB strictures regarding protection of privacy and confidentiality are met, and that patients are included in the study only if they have given informed consent and that all regulatory standards regarding information privacy are met. Ensuring appropriate informed consent involves ensuring not only that the signature of the patient on the informed consent form is obtained, but also that the form itself includes the elements required by law. For non-English-speaking subjects, the requirements must be in a form that will be understood (Public Welfare and Human Services, Title 45, Code of Federal Regulations, Part 46, secs. 46.116-7).

Special privacy and confidentiality issues arise regarding the relation of the research record to the clinical record. One such concern is the disposition of information gathered as part of a research protocol. Is this information part of the research database, or is it part of the clinical record? The simple answer is that it can be either or both.

In academic healthcare centers (teaching hospitals), subjects are frequently solicited to participate in research, either for minimal-risk protocols or non-minimal-risk protocols. Data about the research subject are documented outside the usual clinical record as part of the research protocol. Although it is appropriate that this information be retained separately, its existence needs to be documented. A summary of subjects participating in a nonclinical event is useful for both clinical investigator and the clinician if the subject is admitted to the hospital or when a complication occurs. The information collected as part of the research protocol must be immediately available, and a note documenting the event and the extent of the complication must be included as part of the documentation in the patient's medical record.

Of equal concern is the access of researchers to the medical record. Although secondary uses of the medical record to heal the sick through advancing science are important, RSs must ensure that the central principle of the Hippocratic Oath, "First, do no harm," is respected. Thus, they will need to employ safeguards to indicate when clinical information is not authorized for use beyond direct clinical care. These must be maintained as part of the data architecture in system design.

Meeting requirements for the ethical use of medical record information implies being able to block access to selected information for research while allowing that same information to be visible for patient care. The prospect of designing a system with such capabilities is daunting at best. Yet as long as we do not have such a system, we may be hampered in our ability to use information for research without specific authorization for each research encounter. Putting such a system in place will add a cost burden to both the design and implementation of the research project and may result in delays of outcome information as well. But, as suggested by Gary Ellis, director of the National Institutes of Health Office for Protection from Research Risks, we owe our best effort to citizens who contribute to the common good by participating in research studies (Ellis, 1999).

The use of medical record data in retrospective studies, often initiated years after the medical event, poses special research opportunities and ethical problems. For formal clinical trials and some other types of research, informed consent is routinely sought, the IRB supervises the research, and other protections are enforced. But for some other kinds of research—retrospective epidemiological studies, for example—neither notice nor explicit consent has always been required. Should the patients be contacted for release authorization in these longitudinal studies?

Still another concern is the use of secondary data sources, such as indexes, registries, and reports that typically contain patient-identifiable data. Although these secondary sources are designed to locate relevant health information, they in and of themselves may contain sufficiently sensitive data that can identify an individual patient. A process must be in place to protect patient privacy with regard to secondary data sources as well as the source document, which is the medical record. It is in these areas that the greatest opportunity for ethical compromise may occur. The cost to the facility of creating a system to meet these require-

ments when little research is done may either seem prohibitive or receive such a low priority in terms of information technology support that the anxious researcher may simply circumvent the requirements and include patients in a study who have not given their approval. When this occurs, the IRB or institutional policies of IRB notification and review must be followed. If the facility does not have an IRB, then its ethics committee will be the appropriate review body to consider the issue. In the state of Minnesota, for example, the penalty for unauthorized disclosure of medical information is loss of license to the practitioner via sanctions by the Board of Medical Practice. The consequences are high and reflect the importance ascribed to the patient's right to privacy.

Federal legislation provides RSs some protection against the compelled disclosure of research information on socially sensitive topics such as mental health, alcohol use, drug use, and sexually transmitted diseases to "any federal, state, or local civil, criminal, administrative, legislative, or other proceedings" (Ellis, 1999, p. 282). Such information is often urgently sought by such parties as law enforcement, but it is potentially stigmatizing, and its disclosure may have such consequences as job loss or criminal prosecution. The federal Public Health Service Act allows the Assistant Secretary of Health to grant certificates of confidentiality to biomedical, behavioral, clinical, and other researchers who are investigating these topics. The certificates, by providing researchers with a legal defense for nondisclosure, aims to protect the privacy rights of people who participate in these important areas of research so that the research can continue.

MAINTAINING AND ENHANCING PROFESSIONAL COMPETENCE

We have provided a general discussion of the ethical considerations involved in the roles of the RS and DSS. These were related primarily to activities involved with the management of information and the protection of human subjects. There is, however, another dimension to ethical practice by RSs and DSSs. These professionals have a responsibility to maintain an expected level of competence and to be current on professional standards and techniques (Baase, 1997). The consumer of their work product, whether an employer, patient, or colleague, should be able to expect a certain minimum level of expertise based on current knowledge, industry best practices, and standards of the profession. As professionals, RSs and DSSs have an ethical responsibility to do a thorough and careful job, to minimize harm to the organi-zation and individuals, and to not increase risk to the organization or individuals.

Specifically, then, what are the knowledge and skill areas in which RSs and DSSs should be competent? An adaptation of a skill and knowledge inventory created by AHIMA is presented in Table 7–8. RSs and DSSs should assess their competency in these areas, enhance their knowledge and skills as needed, seek out knowledge of best practices among their colleagues, and participate in national professional organizations to advance their learning and abilities.

Table 7–8 Skill and Knowledge Inventory

Data Analysis		
Skill Area	**Tasks**	**My Knowledge** 1 = No knowledge 2 = Awareness 3 = Understand concepts 4 = Good understanding and can perform 5 = Skilled use
Computer fundamentals	Proficiency in SPSS and/or SAS Proficiency in SQL Proficiency in Excel or similar spreadsheet application Knowledge of principles of decision support system development and design	
Data quality management	Ability to understand and apply techniques and develop policies and procedures to ensure data quality, including: ▪ data content ▪ data scope ▪ data detail ▪ data composition ▪ data consistency ▪ reaction to change	
Statistical and research skills	Knowledge of research design Knowledge of sampling techniques Ability to apply descriptive and inferential statistical techniques Knowledge of theory and rules of probability Knowledge of basic principles of epidemiology	
Visioning	Knowledge of principles of decision making Problem-solving ability	

continues

Table 7–8 continued

Report Preparation and Presentation	
Report presentation	Ability to present and display data clearly: ■ Understanding of frequency distributions, cumulative distributions, histograms, frequency polygons, bar graphs, line graphs, pie charts ■ Ability to use computer software such as SPSS, SAS, Excel for production of reports and analyses ■ Strong written communication skills ■ Ability to synthesize data
Project Design and Management	
Data collection	Ability to develop a data dictionary Knowledge of and ability to develop surveys, questionnaires, and collection instruments Ability to conduct quality assurance and control reviews Ability to design validation procedures for surveys, questionnaires, and other collection instruments
Design	Ability to develop relational databases and model data Ability to use DBMS software Knowledge of research design parameters
Research design	Knowledge of survey research design Knowledge of scientific design Knowledge of qualitative design
Leadership	
Communication skills	Ability to design and facilitate meetings Ability to communicate orally and written
Initiative	Ability to learn new things Commitment to lifelong learning Willingness to take risks Self-motivator
Personal effectiveness	Ability to maintain good working relationships Ability to interact effectively with others Political savvy and tact

Source: Reprinted with permission from American Health Information Management Association's Delphi Group, *Evolving HIM Careers: Seven Roles for the Future, Vision 2006,* © 1999, American Health Information Management Association.

CONCLUSION

Advances in information technology coupled with the emergence of the information age bring new and more profound issues related to the ethics of information management. Centralization of data, large storage capacities, sophisticated analysis and data-mining tools, implementation of enterprise-wide intranets, and use of the Internet all contribute to this phenomenon. These are all tools and capacities on which RSs and DSSs rely in their daily work. Although the ethical responsibilities of these professionals may not have changed with the information age, the context in which these professionals practice is more complex and requires execution of good management practices and constant vigilance to support ethical responsibilities.

As HIM professionals, RSs and DSSs need to embrace within their ethical responsibility an organizational leadership imperative to further best practices. This includes creating opportunities for members of the organization to know and understand the dimensions of ethical responsibility with regard to information management; articulating and supporting policies that protect the dignity of users and others affected by computing systems; and acknowledging and supporting proper and authorized uses of an organization's information resource.

Key Terms

- **Data integrity**
- **Data stewardship**
- **Informed consent**
- **Institutional review boards (IRBs)**
- **SAS**
- **SPSS (Statistical Package for the Social Sciences)**

Chapter Summary

- Research specialists (RSs) create new knowledge by acquiring and analyzing data. They work, for example, on clinical trials and outcomes research with scientific and medical investigators. Decision support specialists (DSSs) analyze data to support strategic planning and operational improvements on the organizational level. Unlike RSs, DSSs are not necessarily concerned with gaining new clinical and scientific knowledge. Rather, they are concerned with how data may be used to assist management activities.

- As HIM professionals, RSs and DSSs are custodians of data with specific responsibilities regarding data integrity and data confidentiality that they must consider in the areas of data acquisition, data access, and data reporting. Good management practice requires data policy development that encompasses all of these areas.

- For data collection and processing, policies, standards, and procedures should be in place to ensure data quality and security. A total data quality and monitoring program should be implemented that covers all of the dimensions of data quality (Johns, 1997). It is important to consider the relevance, comprehensiveness, and precision of the data collected and the ways in which selection of measures may bias results.

- For access control, data must be protected from undesired or unauthorized access. Data should be made available only to users within the organization who can demonstrate a legitimate business need for them. The issue of legitimate business need must be defined through policy and procedure.

- With data reporting, as with data acquisition, there are many ways that bias can be introduced into data. Data should always be presented in a way that will provide for the most accurate and complete interpretation of the findings.

- RSs in particular have responsibilities regarding the protection of human subjects that include special issues related to the confidentiality of research data. Like the principal investigators with whom they collaborate, they are answerable to IRBs, institutions established by federal law to ensure that human subjects research is beneficent and just and shows respect for persons. RSs ensure that the information being collected matches the approval from the IRB review, that all of the IRB strictures regarding protection of privacy and confidentiality are met, and that patients are included in the study only if they have given informed consent.

- Both RSs and DSSs have an ethical obligation to maintain their competence and to perform their work in a thorough and responsible manner. Because their analyses may have a profound impact, these professionals must ensure that good practices of research design and data management are implemented. They must also ensure that the interpretation of data is relevant, correct, and as thorough as possible.

References

Amatayakul, M. (2003). Another layer of regulations: Research under HIPAA. *Journal of AHIMA, 74*(1), 16A–D.

American Health Information Management Association [AHIMA]. (1999). *Vision 2006. Evolving HIM careers: Seven roles for the future.* Chicago: Author.

American Health Information Management Association [AHIMA]. (2004a). *Data for decisions: The HIM Workforce and Workplace. Recommendations to the AHIMA Board of Directors from the Center of Health Workforce Studies based on the HIM Workforce Research Study.* Chicago: Author.

American Health Information Management Association [AHIMA]. (2004b). *AHIMA code of ethics.* Chicago: Author.

Baase, S. (1997). *A gift of fire: Social, legal, and ethical issues in computing.* Upper Saddle River, NJ: Prentice Hall.

Brandel, M. (2004, March 15). Data stewards seek data conformity. *ComputerWorld.* Retrieved October 2004 from http://www.computerworld.com/databasetopics/businessintelligence/datawarehouse/story/0,10801,91146,00.html?SKC = datawarehouse-91146.

Burrington-Brown, J., & Wagg, D. G. (2003). Regulations governing research (AHIMA Practice Brief). *Journal of AHIMA, 74*(3), 56A–D.

Cash, J. I. (1994). *Building the information age organization.* Homewood, IL: Richard D. Irwin.

Clinton, W. J. (1997). *Remarks by the president in apology for study done in Tuskegee.* Retrieved September 13, 2005, from http://clinton4.nara.gov/textonly/New/Remarks/Fri/19970516-898.html.

DeGeorge, R. T. (1999). Business ethics and the information age. *Business and Society Review, 104,* 261–278.

Department of Health, Education, and Welfare (DHEW). (1978). *The Belmont Report: Ethical Principles for the Protection of Human Subjects.* U.S. National Commission for the Protection of Human Subjects of Biomedical and Behavioral Research. DHEW Publication no. (OS) 78-0013 and (OS) 78-0014. Washington, DC: U.S. Printing Office.

Ellis, G. B. (1999). Keeping research subjects out of harm's way. *Journal of the American Medical Association, 282*(20), 1963–1965.

Fowler, F. J. (1988). *Survey research methods.* Newbury Park, CA: Sage.

Friedman, H., & Amoo, T. (1999). Multiple biases in rating scale construction. *Journal of International Marketing and Marketing Research, 24*(3), 115–126.

Johns, M. L. (1997). *Information management for health professionals.* Albany, NY: Delmar.

Jones, J. H. (1993). *Bad blood: The Tuskegee syphilis experiment.* New York: Free Press.

Krohn, R. (2004a). Data analytics throughout the healthcare enterprise. *Journal of Healthcare Information Management, 18*(2), 15–18.

Krohn, R. (2004b). JHIM Quick Study: Healthcare Business Intelligence and real-time decision support systems. *Journal of Healthcare Information Management, 18*(3), 14–16.

Lawrence, W. W. (1997). Report to the United States Secretary of Health and Human Services, Privacy and Health Research, Office of Assistant Secretary, Division of Data Policy, Office of Program Systems. Washington, DC.

Lynoe, N., Jacobsson, L., & Lundgren, E. (1999). Fraud, misconduct or normal science in medical research: An empirical study of demarcation. *Journal of Medical Ethics, 25,* 501–506.

Mayo Clinic. (2000). *Manual for investigators conducting research involving humans.* Rochester, MN: Author.

Pritchard, J. (2003, April 4). Marin County breast cancer rates not as high as once thought. Associated Press. Retrieved October 2004 from http://www.skepticism.net/discussion/fullthread$msgnum = 623.

Public Health Services Act sec. 301(d), U.S. Code, vol. 42, sec. 241.

Public Welfare and Human Services, Title 45, Code of Federal Regulations, Part 46, secs. 46. 116–117.

Redman, T. C. (1992). *Data quality management and technology.* New York: Bantam.

Spinello, R. A. (1997). *Case studies in information and computer ethics.* Upper Saddle River, NJ: Prentice Hall.

Streiner, L., and Norman, G. R. (1989). *Health measurement scales: A practical guide to their development and use.* Oxford: Oxford University Press.

Ware, W. H. (1993). The new faces of privacy. *Information Society, 9,* 195.

The ethical decision-making matrix is a tool to help you organize complex, ethical problems; however, there is no simple fill-in-the-box approach to ethical decision making. The objective is to follow each step of the process and not move from the question directly to what should be done or how to prevent it next time. If you skip steps, you will not fully understand all of the values and options for action. Also, the matrix provided for each scenario in this book is not the only way to examine the problem. You can make an equally compelling ethical argument for a different decision—just be sure to follow all the steps of the matrix.

SCENARIO 7-A: DESIGNING A SURVEY TO BIAS THE RESULTS

Steps	Information	
1. What is the ethical question?	Should the RS insist on the original three-point ordinal?	
2. What are the facts?	**KNOWN**	**TO BE GATHERED**
	• Visual bias will negatively affect the integrity of the data.	• Would changing to a five-point scale constitute fraud? What are the customary practices in such cases? • What is the RS's supervisor expecting? • What is the likely impact on the RS and family of changing jobs?
3. What are the values? Examine the shared and competing values, obligations, and interests of the stakeholders (i.e., patient, HIM professional, healthcare practitioner(s), administrators, society, and other advocates) involved in order to fully understand the complexity of the ethical problem(s).	**Patient:** Benefit from improvements in service. **HIM professional:** Integrity, accuracy, and reliability (RS has an ethical obligation to generate the most accurate data possible); personal values (promote welfare of self and family by avoiding loss of job); promote and participate in research. **Healthcare professionals:** Promote welfare of patients through provision of best possible care. **Administrators:** Benefit patients.	
4. What are my options?	• Use five-point scale. • Insist on three-point scale.	
5. What should I do?	Insist on three-point scale.	
6. What justifies my choice?	**JUSTIFIED**	**NOT JUSTIFIED**
	• Obligation to preserve integrity of data. • Preserve professional integrity.	• Use five-point scale. • Compromise data integrity. • Compromise professional integrity.
7. How can I prevent this ethical problem?	• Review standards for preserving integrity of data and creating surveys. • Discuss standards and the values that support them with colleagues. • Evaluate institutional (or departmental) integrity at job interview and subsequently when ethical problems arise.	

8

PUBLIC HEALTH

Babette J. Neuberger, JD, MPH

Learning Objectives

After completing this chapter, the reader should be able to:

- Describe how the government uses private medical information in protecting the public's health.
- Conduct an ethical analysis of a proposed policy concerning government access to private medical information.
- Participate more meaningfully in public debate about government uses of private health data.
- Advocate more persuasively for policy measures using well-reasoned arguments.

Abstract

Government access to, and use of, patient information is critical for protecting the public's health. At the same time, it raises ethical challenges to doctor–patient confidentiality and respect for the individual's privacy. This chapter explores the use of patient data to assess and protect the health of the population. It raises the difficult question of when the government's need to know should prevail over the interests of the individual and his or her desire to keep personal information solely within the provider–patient relationship. A theoretical framework is provided for addressing difficult policy choices about when patient information ought to be reported to health authorities.

Scenario 8-A: Reporting HIV Status

In 1998, Dr. Moe, the medical director of a state health department, was faced with the difficult challenge of determining whether to require healthcare providers to report to state health authorities the names of people who tested positive for the human immunodeficiency virus (HIV). Word that he was considering this proposal spread to the gay community. The Alliance to End Discrimination, a patient advocacy group for persons afflicted with AIDS, staged a protest in front of the medical director's office. The group argued that the proposed regulation would substantially interfere with the privacy and autonomy of HIV-positive persons. Moreover, the group argued that because of the often severe stigma associated with the disease, anything other than anonymous testing would likely discourage persons from getting tested. This would diminish their ability to seek much-needed medical treatment. In the end, patient advocates argued, mandatory reporting would result in a further spread of the virus.

The Coalition for Responsible Reporting, a coalition of concerned parents, emergency response paramedics, and other healthcare workers, argued equally vociferously (if not as publicly) in support of Dr. Moe's proposal. The coalition predicted that the proposed law would have exactly the opposite effect. According to this group, the notification law would enable the state to find and warn partners of infected individuals of the risk of infection. It would further enable health authorities to counsel partners on effective preventive measures. The coalition also contended that mandated reporting would allow the state to provide infected persons with the help they need more quickly.

Faced with these emotionally charged and competing perspectives, Dr. Moe was counseled by his chief of staff to delay a decision indefinitely, or at least until after the next gubernatorial election. The chief of staff recommended that Dr. Moe announce a decision to "convene a study panel to examine the conflicting facts before making a final decision." That recommendation was immediately and strongly opposed by the bureau chief for the state's Infectious Disease Control Unit. The bureau chief maintained that, as the state's leading health official, Dr. Moe had a responsibility to take a public stand on the issue.

You are the chief information officer for the state health department, and Dr. Moe has turned to you for advice.

Questions

1. What would you advise Dr. Moe to do?

2. Does Dr. Moe have a duty to take immediate action on this issue?

3. Does the proposed rule create an ethical conflict between the patient and his or her healthcare provider? Between the patient and society? Examine the proposed rule from the competing perspectives of the patient, physician, the state health director, and the public as you think about what action you would advise the health director to take.

4. What are the ethical issues involved in this scenario? What ethical principles might guide you as you advise the health director in making this extraordinarily difficult decision? How would you decide this conflict?

A completed ethical decision-making matrix for the scenario is provided at the end of the chapter.

This chapter explores government access to and use of patient information to protect the public's health. Although health information management (HIM) professionals think primarily of the clinical uses of patient information, such data also are essential to protecting the health of the public. For example, medical records of a tuberculosis (TB) patient are used by the medical team to establish an appropriate treatment regime for the patient. The hospital administration may use such data to ensure compliance with infection control guidelines for the facility. Public health researchers may map the aggregated data of all TB cases within a city, looking for a correlation between TB and high-risk groups, such as the city's homeless population and/or HIV-infected population. The research results may be used by public health authorities to design intervention measures to prevent TB from spreading further. All of these uses depend initially on the proper diagnosis and coding of the patient's medical condition.

As the ability to capture large data sets in an electronic format improves, data are becoming more centralized. The field of public health has responded to this data explosion by relying increasingly upon the collection and analysis of data to carry out its mission. HIM professionals play an emerging role in this exciting field. As you read through this chapter, you will see that HIM professionals possess many of the skills that are needed in public health. Readers are likely to identify a broad range of positions that could best be filled by those who are educated in the management of health information. But even if you work in a more traditional HIM setting, such as a hospital or outpatient health clinic, you will discover that the work you do is integrally related to, and will significantly affect, the ability of public health officials to guard the public's health. By learning how local, state, and federal governments use patient data, you will gain a new appreciation of the importance of ensuring data quality and accuracy. This chapter also challenges you to think about the HIM professional's role as a patient advocate. It provides you with tools to help you decide whether to support or oppose public policies requiring the sharing of private medical information.

This chapter's opening scenario exemplifies an ethical challenge to an HIM professional in public health. It is followed by an introduction to the field of public health and government uses of patient data. Relevant ethical principles are then explained and discussed and are related back to the opening scenario. A second scenario is presented giving students further opportunity to practice skills of ethical reasoning. The chapter continues with a discussion of the HIM professional's role as a patient advocate within the policy arena. The chapter concludes with a brief discussion and case scenario relating to the emerging issues of bioterrorism and global infections.

PUBLIC HEALTH: AN OVERVIEW

Generally speaking, public health encompasses all those activities that we as a society undertake to ensure conditions in which people can be healthy. Such conditions include clean air, clean water, and proper sanitation; a safe work environment that is free from physical and chemical stressors; a healthy food supply; access to medical care and preventive diagnostic screenings; a good diet; and participation in physical exercise. To completely understand public health, one must think broadly about all those who are involved with accomplishing its mission. The systems for public health delivery include not only an extensive array of public actors, encompassing local, county, state, and federal health departments and environmental agencies, public health clinics and hospital systems, clinical laboratories, and school nursing programs, but also the efforts of a multitude of private actors, persons and institutions delivering the services and care that are essential to ensuring the health and well-being of our populace. A large component of this latter group is, of course, private medical care providers.

Though public health and medicine are integrally related, there are essential differences between them. Historically, medical care was focused on the care, treatment, and/or cure of diseased individuals. More recently, we have witnessed a shift in focus, with great interest and attention paid to prevention in addition to cure, due in some measure to a restructuring of the medical care delivery system. Nevertheless, it is still safe to say that the medical profession's primary focus is on the individual; its concern is the one-on-one, provider-to-patient relationship. In contrast, the field of public health has prevention as its primary focus, with particular attention paid to populations rather than to individuals. Table 8–1 illustrates these differences.

The Evolution of Public Health and Government Access to Private Medical Information

The first large-scale advances in public health were made in the 1800s, during what was known as the "Great Sanitary Movement." During this period, enormous advances occurred in the eradication of the conditions that gave rise to such diseases as malaria, typhoid fever, cholera, yellow fever, dysenteries, and summer diarrheas. Prior to the 1800s, diseases and contagions were largely accepted as the norm, and ill health was generally seen as evidence of a person's poor moral character. Public health measures

were primarily directed at separating diseased individuals from the rest of the population through isolation and quarantine laws (Institute of Medicine, 1988).

The Great Sanitary Movement coincided with an unprecedented influx of rural Americans and immigrants into cities and industrial towns seeking work. The numbers overwhelmed the capacity of urban areas to absorb and serve the needs of the newly arrived. The first wave of migration to urban areas occurred in the 1830s. Between 1860 and 1910, the number of Americans living in urban areas rose from 19 to 45 percent (Rosen, 1971).

Overcrowded urban areas were an ideal breeding ground for infectious diseases of all kinds, as reports by investigators of the time vividly show (Rosen, 1972). The contagions that thrived there affected the rich and poor alike, causing an outcry for a public response and undermining the assumption that the ill were morally deficient. Two early crusaders, Edwin Chadwick in London and Lemuel Shattuck in Massachusetts, published reports that called attention to the need for improved sanitation and other social measures that could reduce the spread of disease (Chave, 1984; Rosenkrantz, 1974). The response was overwhelming. Inadequate public health measures such as quarantine and isolation were supplemented with rigorous attention to improved systems of sanitation; provision and supervision of sanitary water supplies; sewage disposal facilities; better control of sanitary

Table 8–1 Distinctions between Medical Care and Public Health Interventions

	Medicine: A Biomedical Paradigm	**Public Health: A Population-Based Paradigm**
Focus	Individual patient	Population or community
Goals	Care, treatment, and cure—and more recently prevention	Health promotion, disease prevention
Diagnosis	Physical examination, medical tests	Epidemiologic studies, toxicologic studies
Treatment	Drugs, therapeutic procedures, patient education and counseling	Laws and policies, government-funded programs, community-based interventions

conditions affecting the food supply; and better housing codes that eliminated crowded tenement structures in the industrial cities (Rabe, 1990). New government programs were created to provide services for infants and children, and public boards, agencies, and institutions were created to assume the greater social responsibility for the health of citizens. Overall, there was a dramatic shift from reaction to planned prevention. By the end of the 1800s, 40 states and several cities had established health departments.

Simultaneous with the new commitment to social improvements in the late 1800s came the discovery of bacterium and its role in spreading infectious diseases. This discovery led to the establishment of laboratories in local and state health departments. It also created the impetus for many health departments to require or mandate the reporting of infectious disease cases to health authorities (Institute of Medicine, 1988).

With the introduction of mandated reporting came the ability of government to institute more aggressive infection control strategies. Health authorities were able to investigate reported cases to gather information on the patient, inspect the premises, and give instruction on isolation and disinfection. Patients who were convalescing in isolation in their own homes were visited regularly by health authorities during the course of their illness. At the end of the illness, the authorities required elaborate and quite expensive disinfection of the patient's sick room and personal belongings. Those who could not successfully be isolated at home were moved to isolation hospitals, where, unfortunately, deaths occurred frequently because of cross-infection by other diseases (Eyler, 1986).

Mandatory reporting laws were not accepted without controversy. The laws offended notions of individual rights and liberties, threatening both the "right" of individuals to convalesce privately and the "right" of physicians to practice their profession without state interference. Physicians protested that the laws forced them to violate the ancient Hippocratic Oath, which obliges physicians not to use acquired information for any purpose other than the patient's care. Doctors objected to being used as a tool to further the public's interest at potentially grave expense to their patients, because, for many patients, quarantine or removal to a hospital resulted in grave financial difficulties or devastating social stigma. Those opposing the laws further argued that due to the fear of public exposure, notification laws would deter patients from calling in a physician, thereby adding to the disease burden.[1]

Although compliance initially was quite low, notification laws slowly gained acceptance (Lerner, 1993). Today, mandatory reporting of infectious diseases is standard public health practice in all 50 states. This change was due in some measure to the growing credibility and influence of public health as a profession. The laws also gained acceptance as health authorities successfully demonstrated their ability to take control of an epidemic when equipped with timely notification and the ability to adopt early preventive measures.

During the early part of the twentieth century, the role of state and local health departments expanded greatly. Several states established disease registries in an effort to centralize information about the occurrence of specified diseases. Registry data revealed that high rates of morbidity continued to predominate among children and the poor. In response, within the larger metropolitan areas, home nursing programs were created and school-based clinics were established. Also during this period, the science of **epidemiology** became an integral discipline of state and local health departments. Discoveries of disease agents and the systematic collection of data opened the way for developing programs targeted at both community improvements

---

1. For an interesting historic account of the development and controversies surrounding disease notification laws, see Mooney (1999).

and individual behavior-based interventions (Institute of Medicine, 1988).

Since the early twentieth century, the range of activities and health agency concerns has continued to expand at a rapid pace. Health authorities now engage in an extremely broad array of activities that are designed to ensure healthy conditions for the populace. Activities include the delivery of personal health services, environmental regulation and sanitation measures, **surveillance** (the systematic monitoring of the occurrences of diseases, deaths, events, procedures, and/or risk factors), clinical laboratory investigation and services, immunization programs, maternal and child health interventions, and health education and health promotion campaigns that are designed to promote healthier lifestyles and nutritional habits. Exhibit 8–1 offers a more inclusive list of governmental public health activities.

These modern public health efforts are facilitated by government access to a full range of individual medical and health-related data. Agencies at the local, state, and federal levels collect such data as vital statistics records of births, deaths, marriages, divorces, adoptions, and abortions. These are used to calculate birth rates, identify conditions during pregnancy and congenital malformation, tabulate causes of death, and provide other indices of public health. State and federal governments maintain registries that capture and compile statistical data in a centralized database, enabling population-based research and analysis. Most common are disease registries, specifically cancer

---

Exhibit 8–1 Local Health Department Activities

Local public health agencies provide numerous services to the residents of their jurisdictions. According to a 2000 survey conducted by the National Association of County and City Health Officials (NACCHO), among the most common services provided by agencies were the "core" public health programs associated with traditional local public health:

- Adult and childhood immunizations
- Communicable disease control
- Community assessment
- Community outreach and education
- Environmental health services
- Epidemiology and surveillance programs
- Food safety
- Health education
- Restaurant inspections
- Tuberculosis testing

Less common were those programs related to primary care services and chronic disease:

- Cardiovascular disease, diabetes, and glaucoma treatment
- Behavioral and mental health services
- Programs for the homeless
- Substance abuse services
- Veterinary public health

Source: Reprinted from the NACCHO (2001), *Local Public Health Agency Infrastructure: A Chartbook,* p. 18, Washington, DC.: Author.

and tumor registries, and more infrequently exposure registries. Other, less common registries capture events as diverse as mental retardation, strokes, accidents, and enteric diseases. The data come from public agencies, medical care providers, and medical institutions that are required by law to submit patient information about the event. Disease registries serve as a rich resource for patient tracking, detection of trends in the rate of diseases, and epidemiologic studies to detect causal relationships between exposure and disease.

Another significant data source is the information reported to government by medical providers in compliance with state "**reportable diseases and conditions**" statutes. A *reportable disease* (sometimes referred to as a *notifiable disease*) is one for which regular, frequent, and timely information on individual cases is considered necessary for the prevention and control of that disease (Friis & Sellers, 1999). A common example is the outbreak of an apparent food-borne illness among children and adults attending a company picnic. Healthcare providers who treat the stricken individuals are legally required to report the illness to health authorities. The data are shared among local and state health officials as needed to investigate and contain the outbreak. The list of notifiable diseases varies by state; it also varies over time. Exhibit 8–2 illustrates a typical state mandatory reporting law for diseases and health conditions.

Data collection, including registry data and reports of notifiable diseases, raises ethical concerns because the data include patient identifiers, such as the patient's name, age, sex, race, ethnicity, and address; the name and address of the responsible physician;

Exhibit 8–2 Mandatory Reporting Laws for Diseases and Health Conditions in the State of Colorado

Colorado regulations require healthcare providers, including attending physicians, laboratories, coroners, hospital administrators, and persons in charge of other institutions licensed by the Colorado Department of Public Health and Environment (such as nursing homes and day care centers), and persons in charge of schools (including school nursing staff), and any "other persons either treating or having knowledge of a reportable disease," to report an array of diseases and conditions to the health department. Most reports must be filed within 24 hours of learning about a confirmed or suspected case.

The occurrence of a single case of any unusual disease or manifestation of illness that the healthcare provider determines or suspects may be caused by or related to a chemical, radioactive, or bioterrorist agent or incident must be reported immediately by telephone to the state or local health department by the healthcare provider and the hospital, emergency department, clinic, healthcare center, and laboratory in which the person is examined, tested, and/or treated. The same immediate reporting is required for any unusual cluster of illnesses that may be caused by or related to a chemical, radioactive, or bioterrorist agent or incident. Chemical terrorist agents include, but are not limited to, Sarin (GB), VX (V agent), and HD (distilled mustard). Bioterrorist agents include, but are not limited to, anthrax, plague, smallpox, tularemia, botulism, viral hemorrhagic fever, and brucellosis.

The following diseases and conditions (confirmed or suspected) must be reported within 24 hours:

- Acquired immunodeficiency syndrome
- Animal bites by dogs, cats, bats, skunks, or other wild carnivores

Exhibit 8–2 continued

- Anthrax
- Botulism
- Cholera
- Diphtheria
- Group outbreaks, including food poisoning
- Hepatitis A
- Human immunodeficiency virus (HIV)
- Measles (rubeola)
- Meningitis or other invasive disease caused by *Haemophilus influenzae*
- Meningitis or other invasive disease caused by *Neisseria meningitidis*
- Plague
- Poliomyelitis
- Rabies in human (suspected)
- Rubella
- Severe Acute Respiratory Syndrome (SARS)
- Smallpox
- Syphilis (first-degree, second-degree, or early latent)
- Active tuberculosis disease
- Typhoid fever

Other diseases and conditions must be reported within seven days. For certain diseases (those designated with an asterisk), reports are based on the physician's diagnosis, whether or not laboratory tests have confirmed the doctor's findings.

The following diseases and conditions must be reported within seven days:

- Amebiasis
- Bites by animals not included in the previous list
- Brucellosis*
- Campylobacteriosis
- Chancroid
- Cryptosporidiosis
- Cyclospora
- Encephalitis*
- *Escherichia coli* O157:H7* and shiga-toxin-producing *Escherichia coli*
- Giardiasis*
- Gonorrhea, any site
- Hantavirus
- Hepatitis B*
- Hepatitis C, acute
- Hepatitis, other viral
- Hemolytic uremic syndrome if < 18 yrs
- Influenza-associated hospitalization
- Influenza-associated death if < 18 yrs
- Kawasaki syndrome
- Legionellosis*
- Leprosy

Exhibit 8–2 continued

- Lymphogranuloma venereum
- Listeriosis
- Lyme disease
- Malaria*
- Meningitis, aseptic*
- Mumps*
- Pertussis syndrome*
- Psittacosis
- Q fever*
- Relapsing fever*
- Rocky Mountain spotted fever
- Rubella, congenital*
- Salmonellosis
- Shigellosis
- Tetanus*
- Toxic shock syndrome
- Transmissible spongiform encephalopathy if >50 years*
- Trichinosis*
- Tularmeia*
- Varicella*

Other Colorado regulations require healthcare providers to report a host of environmental and chronic conditions (State of Colorado Rules and Regulations Pertaining to the Detection, Monitoring and Investigation of Environmental and Chronic Diseases, 6 CCR-1009-7).

With very few exceptions, a report must include the patient's name, age, sex, race, ethnicity, and address; the name and address of the responsible physician; and other information needed by the health department to locate the patient for follow-up. In addition, for animal bite cases, the healthcare provider must also report the name and locating information of the owner of the biting animal, if known.

*Reports are to be based on the physician's diagnosis, whether or not laboratory tests have confirmed the doctor's findings.

Source: Data from State of Colorado Rules and Regulations Pertaining to Epidemic and Communicable Disease Control 6 CCR-1009-1 (last amended July 21, 2004, effective September 30, 2004). See also State of Colorado Rules and Regulations Pertaining to the Detection, Monitoring and Investigation of Environmental and Chronic Diseases, 6 CCR-1009-7 (last amended July 21, 2004, effective September 30, 2004).

and other information needed by the health department to permit record linkages and/or to locate the patient for follow-up investigation. Further, the information is reported to the government without the patient's permission, raising some concerns that will be discussed later in this chapter.

Diseases and conditions reported at the state level are funneled into a national database system called the National Electronic Telecommunications System for Surveillance (NETSS). NETSS is maintained by the CDC. The 50 state health departments and the health departments of New York City, the

District of Columbia, and five U.S. territories submit reported information on a weekly basis. Data are submitted in aggregate form; that is, without personal identifiers. Aggregated data allow the federal government to track national trends, to monitor the incidence and prevalence of diseases and conditions, and to assess the progress of the nation's prevention efforts. (The **incidence** of a disease or condition refers to the number of occurrences of the event during a defined unit of time, such as a week, month, or year. It is often expressed as a rate: the number of new cases occurring within a specified period/ the population at risk for the event. In contrast, **prevalence** refers to the total number of cases (new and old) ascertained at one point in time and again may be expressed as a rate: total number of cases / the population at risk for the event). For example, data are used to track drug-resistant communicable diseases, such as drug-resistant tuberculosis, so that the government can develop and evaluate control strategies. NETSS data also enable the government to identify areas in the United States with high proportions of

particular diseases, such as later-stage breast cancers or invasive cervical cancer among women. The information informs the CDC's decisions on allocation of program resources and enables the government to target communities for prevention messages and education campaigns (CDC, 1999). Exhibit 8–3 describes government uses of surveillance data.

Sexually Transmitted Disease Contact Tracing and Partner Notification

Utah's experience with its sexually transmitted diseases (STD) program dramatizes the value of disease-reporting laws. Utah's program for contact tracing and partner notification, a program typical of those nationwide, uses reported cases of STDs to contact, interview, and counsel infected individuals. Reports are received from health clinics, private physicians, hospitals, blood banks, the state prison system, and local health departments. During an interview, patients receive counseling and referral for medical follow-up and community-based services. Patients also are asked to

---

Exhibit 8–3 Government Uses of Surveillance Data

The government uses surveillance data for, among other purposes,

- Quantitative estimates of the magnitude of a health problem
- Portrayal of the natural history of disease
- Detection of epidemics
- Documentation of the distribution and spread of a health event
- Facilitating epidemiologic and laboratory research
- Testing of hypothesis
- Evaluation of control and prevention measures
- Monitoring of changes in infectious agents
- Monitoring of isolation activities
- Detection of changes in health practices
- Planning

Source: Reprinted from S. M. Teutsch (2000), "Considerations in planning a surveillance system," in S. M. Teutsch and R. E. Churchill (Eds.), *Principles and practice of public health surveillance,* 2d ed., Table 1-1 p. 8. New York: Oxford University Press.

name all sexual and needle-sharing partners for the past five years or back to the date of their infection, if known.

Although health authorities encourage infected patients to voluntarily notify their partners, they will use the reported names to contact named individuals if voluntary notification does not occur. The state aggressively searches for all partners for whom reasonable identifying information is available. This is accomplished by interviewing neighbors and apartment managers, obtaining records from the Department of Motor Vehicles and utility companies, and/or examining telephone and cross directories. When a partner has relocated to another state, an interstate referral notice is sent to the other state's health department. Partners that are located are interviewed and counseled face to face in sessions that last from 30 to 90 minutes. The identity of the infected patient is never revealed to the partner. If the partner tests positive, the process is repeated for his or her contacts (Pavia, Benyo, Niler, & Risk, 1993).

The yield from contact tracing and notification can be quite dramatic. In April 1993, a man incarcerated in a Pennsylvania prison voluntarily requested an HIV-antibody test and was diagnosed with HIV infection. Following an interview and counseling by the Pennsylvania Department of Health authorities, the person provided contact information about four persons with whom he had shared syringes to inject drugs before his incarceration. The resulting investigation uncovered an HIV-positive diagnosis in two of the four named individuals. One of them provided contact information about 47 partners, including 41 partners with whom he had shared syringes only and 6 with whom he had had sex and shared syringes. By May 1994, activities of the health authorities had produced a social network of 124 persons linked by syringe sharing and/or sex (CDC, 1995).

This program illustrates the difficulties that public health officers face in trying to "walk the line" between using confidential medical information to slow the spread of STDs while at the same time protecting an infected person's privacy. Imagine yourself as a public health officer faced with the difficult job of notifying someone that he or she has been exposed to an STD while not being able to identify the person who gave you the partner's name and contact information.

State Use of Health Data for Planning Purposes

Efforts are under way nationally to engage in more systematic statewide planning to protect the public's health. The following example illustrates how data are used in one state, Illinois, to assess and provide for the health needs of its residents. Illinois law requires every local health department to conduct a series of planning activities, resulting in the development of an organizational capacity assessment, a community health needs assessment, and a community health plan. This effort is called the State of Illinois Project for Local Assessment of Needs (IPLAN Data System, 2000).

The community health needs assessment phase calls for local health departments to bring together community stakeholders to identify, describe, and/or predict the health status of community residents. Stakeholders are people who are interested in and who contribute to the health of community residents. Information is collected about disease agents and hazards, risk factors, exposures to unhealthy substances such as hazardous chemicals, and exposures to unhealthy conditions such as high-fat diets and sedentary lifestyles. A computerized data resource, called the IPLAN data system, serves as a primary source of information to counties that are conducting community health needs assessments. The IPLAN data system is a dynamic database that can provide statewide, county, or community-level profiles of the health status of Illinois residents. The database derives information from such sources as the Adverse Pregnancy Outcomes Reporting System (APORS), to which all certified Illinois hospitals are required to report; the Behavioral Risk Factor Surveillance System (BRFSS), a monthly telephone survey of self-reported data on health behaviors conducted by the Illinois Department of Public Health and the CDC; the U.S. Bureau of the Census; vital statistics on births and deaths for Illinois residents; the Illinois Health Care Cost Containment Council (data tabulating hospital discharge forms for inpatients discharged from Illinois hospitals); and the Illinois State Cancer Registry.

The collected data are used by the stakeholders to prioritize the community's diseases, conditions, and public health needs. A plan is then established to address the highest ranked of the community's needs. Following the assessment phase, local health departments are expected to advocate for programs and policies that will address the identified needs (Illinois Administrative Code, title 77, chap. 1, subchap. H, pt. 600).

As this overview of public health illustrates, the professional backgrounds of those working in the field are as broad and multidisciplinary as the previously described activities. Professions represented within the public health workforce include physicians, dentists, public health nurses, and other healthcare providers; social workers; health educators; laboratory technicians; environmental sanitarians; toxicologists; program planners; analysts and statisticians; epidemiologists; and administrators (Turnock, 1997). HIM professionals are well positioned to enter this exciting, multidisciplinary, data-rich field.

ETHICAL CHALLENGES IN PUBLIC HEALTH

Improvements in the government's technologic capacity, combined with an increase in governmental data gathering and reporting requirements, lead inevitably to ethical dilemmas in the treatment and management of private medial information. The next section will explore some of these challenges and provide a road map for ethical reasoning.

When the Public's Right to Know Conflicts with the Individual's Right to Privacy

Let's return to the scenario that appears at the beginning of the chapter. To answer the questions on Dr. Moe's predicament, and on your predicament as his advisor, you should think about the public health mission described earlier in this chapter and how that mission applies to the scenario. The following pages describe the ethical principles that one should apply in trying to resolve the questions raised previously. After you have made an initial attempt to answer the questions, read the next few pages to see how one might apply the ethical principles of autonomy, nonmaleficence, beneficence, and reciprocity to address the questions. But before you begin, an initial issue must be addressed—the question of when there is a duty to make a decision.

▪ An Antecedent Issue: The Duty to Decide

As with most cases involving conflicting ethical principles, there is no right answer for this scenario, yet the situation calls for a decision to be made. In challenging situations of this nature, it may be tempting for a policymaker simply to avoid the conflict and look the other way. Yet if the health director were to ignore the question entirely, then the present state of affairs would continue: HIV-positive persons would remain anonymous, and the government—and the public—would be left without the possible benefits of early intervention. As is often the case with issues of public policy, a failure to act or to make a decision has as many ramifications as a decision to act. In short, the health director has an ethical duty as the state's chief public health officer to address the question and to reach a well-reasoned conclusion. Policymakers may be faulted for failing to make a decision or for making a hasty, ill-informed, or poorly reasoned choice, but they cannot be faulted, regardless of their decision, as long as they make the most reasoned decision possible given the circumstances. A reasoned decision requires us to justify why we give priority to one set of ethical principles over another.

▪ Making a Reasoned Decision

How should the state health director weigh the competing ethical values? What principles would you use in developing a recommendation for the director? To address these questions, you could revisit Beauchamp and Childress's (2001) four ethical principles of autonomy, nonmaleficence, beneficence, and justice, which were discussed in Chapter 2. How might these concepts help guide you? How would the information you learned about public health in the first part of this chapter color your answer?

Autonomy. As Beauchamp and Childress (2001) suggested, respect for the person and the autonomy of the individual runs deep in common morality. This notion subsumes the right of autonomous individuals to make their own choices about matters affecting the most intimate aspects of their lives. The right to privacy, including a right to the confidential treatment of private medical information, flows directly from the concept of respect for the individual. The basis for this ethical principle can be found in the works of both Immanuel Kant and John Stuart Mill. Although starting from drastically different philosophic beliefs, their worldviews about the primacy of individual autonomy converge in the world of practice. To Kant, a deontological philosopher, it is morally right to respect the autonomy of individuals. Respect for the individual necessarily means "respecting" or "honoring" the individual's values and choices (Beauchamp & Steinbock, 1999).

As a utilitarian, or consequentialist, Mill's view of "right behavior" differs significantly from that of Kant's. To Mill, the world is most correctly ordered when every individual is free to "self-maximize": that is, to act in his or her own best interest free from government interference. According to Mill, the only exception to this rule, and an exception that turns out to be of significance to us, is that government may interfere with an individual's liberty "as necessary to prevent harm to others" (quoted in Dworkin, 1999, p. 115).

Applying these concepts to Scenario 8-A, we see that implicit in the arguments of the Alliance to End Discrimination is a strongly felt respect for the autonomy of infected individuals. This group is arguing that individual patients are in the best position to know whether, and to what extent, they may suffer as a consequence of disclosing their medical condition. Those individuals who believe that the benefits of reporting their status outweigh the risks to themselves can authorize their physicians to report the information to the state health department. And those who fear the release of such information, whether such fear is realistic or not, should be respected—first, because if their fears are correct, damage may be inflicted upon them if their HIV status is made known, and second, because even if their fears are unwarranted, the unintended and unfortunate consequence of mandated reporting could cause such individuals to forsake testing and avoid seeking needed medical attention altogether.

Although these arguments have potency, they are not decisive. As Beauchamp and Childress (2001) pointed out, the ethical principle of autonomy has only prima facie standing and thus may be overruled by more compelling arguments to the contrary, as the following discussion illustrates.

Nonmaleficence. One such argument is the "do no harm" principle. This principle suggests that an individual's autonomy and freedom may be properly constrained to prevent harm to others. Although often thought of within the medical setting as the physician's dictum "first, do no harm," it is also used as a justification within the political arena to take action that interferes with individual rights and liberties when necessary to prevent harm to others or to the community at large. To this, both Kant and Mill would agree.

In our case study, the Coalition for Responsible Reporting argues the need for community protection. They feel that because government intervention might stem the spread of this deadly virus, the public's interest substantially and significantly outweighs the prima facie rights of infected individuals.

Asserting that the "do no harm" principle should take precedence over all other ethical principles is very persuasive; nevertheless, the proponents' arguments should not be accepted blindly. A cautious decision maker must scrutinize the facts upon which the assertions were based before agreeing with either the policy's supporters or its opponents. Among the questions you might ask: Is it true that governmental intervention could stop or slow the virus' spread? What has the experience been in other states where reporting of HIV-positive status is mandated? Has the HIV incidence rate declined? Have potentially infected individuals shied away from medical testing and treatment? You might also question the state legislature's intentions. Would a mandatory reporting rule be supported by budgetary allocations to fund intervention measures? If not, should the rule be promulgated? Based on what logic? What other facts might you want to know?

To address some of these questions, it is helpful to place the case study within a historical context. In 1988, the arguments of the Coalition for Responsible Reporting would have been much weaker, because the "care" to be provided to infected patients was at best palliative in nature. This had to be weighed against the dangers of reporting. To a greater extent than has occurred with most other reportable diseases, persons infected with the HIV virus have suffered discrimination in housing, jobs, health and life insurance; loss of support from family and friends; and occasionally violence. By 1998, the balance had shifted. Due to the development of a new cocktail of drugs, the ability to prolong the lives of HIV-infected individuals has been greatly enhanced. However, the drugs are expensive, and many infected individuals lack health insurance and the ability to pay for the drugs themselves.

Beneficence. The third ethical principle that must be considered is that of beneficence. Beneficence is closely related to concepts of morality generally and refers to the moral obligation, generously inspired by religious doctrine, that it is morally correct to take actions that promote the health and welfare of others. Beneficence and the closely allied principle of nonmaleficence are among the primary justifications supporting public policies that interfere with the autonomy of individuals. However, unlike nonmaleficence, which suggests a duty to refrain from acting, beneficence implies an obligation to affirmatively act to promote "good for others."

One argument used to justify the principle of beneficence is that of reciprocity. According to Hume, one basis for the formation of society is the idea that each of us as a member of society benefits from the collective good of the whole, and therefore each of us owes a duty in turn to promote the good of others in society (Beauchamp & Childress, 2001). This raises a challenging question: How much does each of us owe to society? One suggested answer is that we ought to give as much as possible until we reach a level at which, by giving more, we would cause as much suffering to ourselves as we would relieve through our giving. Stated another way, we should give up to the point where our giving would diminish our own life plan (Beauchamp & Childress, 2001). This maxim seems to be overly demanding as a moral obligation and probably would not be followed by any but the most altruistic. Other, more forgiving standards have been suggested, including that we expect others to give as much (or as little) as we ourselves are willing to sacrifice. How would you answer the question?

The principle of beneficence is often used to support paternalistic public policies. Beauchamp and Childress (2001) defined *paternalism* as involving "some form of interference with or refusal to conform to another person's preferences regarding their own good" (p. 274). The justification for this interference with autonomy is that the policy will benefit the person whose preference is overridden; that is, the policy is "for his (her) own good." Laws against assisted suicide are examples of this. In Scenario 8-A, strains of paternalism may be found in the arguments of the Coalition for Responsible Reporting. The coalition argued that the proposed rule will enable the government to render care more quickly to those afflicted with the virus.

Under what circumstances the beneficence principle should take primacy over the autonomy principle has been the subject of lengthy philosophical discussion. The debate often centers on the question of whether the person has the capacity to make a knowing, voluntary, and informed choice or whether the person is of such diminished capacity (due to, for example, outside influences, cognitive impairment, age, emotion, or coercion) that his or her ability to decide the best course of action for him- or herself is impaired (Dworkin, 1999). In the scenario, one could argue that patients who are HIV positive might be under such severe emotional distress—due not only to their compromised health status, but also to the social stigma attached to the virus—that they might not be able to make an informed choice concerning disclosure of their condition. But it could also be argued that these patients can make a more informed choice about disclosure than others could make for them because they know more about the discriminatory environment in which they must live.

The obligation to promote "good" for society requires us to think about the concept of utility. In an era of scarce public resources, a decision by the government to affirmatively act for the social welfare generally means that limited public resources cannot be ex-pended elsewhere. Thus, beneficence requires that we ensure that government expenditures to promote the "social good" are being put to their best possible use. This is known as the *utility principle*. The concept of utility has three main components: cost, benefit, and risk.

Cost refers to the resources required to bring about a benefit, as well as any unintended consequences resulting from pursuing that benefit. In Scenario 8-A, one cost of imposing a mandatory reporting law is the resources required to enforce the provision. A potential unintended consequence of the law, but one that must also be considered, is the possibility that the law will discourage infected individuals from getting tested.

Risk, in turn, refers to a possible future harm, or, as Beauchamp and Childress (2001) explained, "a possible future setback to interests in life, health and welfare" (p. 292). Risk is expressed in terms of both the probability, or chance, of a future event occurring and the magnitude, or severity, of the potential harm. Using the scenario as an example, one must consider the likelihood or probability that infected persons will feel forced to forgo medical attention, and one must estimate the extent of harm that could result from that possibility.

The term *benefit* has several meanings. It refers to cost avoidance or risk reduction and also to the positive value that would result from implementing a policy. One benefit of the proposed mandatory reporting law is the positive value that could result from enabling the state to provide infected persons with the help they need more quickly. The benefit may also be expressed as avoiding the costs associated with failing to warn the partners of infected persons about the dangers of unprotected sexual activity and/or syringe sharing.

The costs and benefits of a public policy are usually expressed in monetary terms. Thus, before opting for a particular policy, a decision maker may demand proof that the cost of implementing a program (in dollars) is outweighed by the resulting benefits (again, expressed in dollars). The difficulties this presents should be obvious. In the scenario, both the costs and the benefits involve, to some degree, promoting health and preventing morbidity and early death. But how does one determine the monetary value of a life? This is much more than a metaphysical question. Government (and the judicial system) routinely assign dollar values to lives saved or to the preservation (or loss) of a "quality life." The dollar value of a life is not, of course, an objectively determined scientific fact. Nevertheless, economists, health outcomes specialists, and other "experts" are often called upon to make cost-benefit determinations. This lends an unwarranted aura of "science" or dignity to the cost-benefit decision and engenders greater deference to the outcome than is due. The great potential to manipulate the weight assigned to costs and benefits has been used by critics to oppose the utility principle. Critics maintain that cost-benefit analysis is often used as a means of justifying, after the fact, an already decided-upon course of action.

Notwithstanding these criticisms, the rigor of the utility technique has its value as long as its limitations are well understood. A danger occurs when policymakers accept the technique as dogma. Utilitarians rely on cost-benefit analysis as the deciding basis for public policies. To a rigid utilitarian, no policy should be adopted unless it can be demonstrated that the benefits of the policy outweigh its costs and that it achieves the greatest good for the greatest number. This is referred to as the *efficiency principle*. Unfortunately, the principle is often accepted as the basis for public decision making without critical analysis. The approach has been criticized for focusing on a single, unidimensional measure of value, usually expressed in dollars, rather than inviting a full exploration of other ethical concerns.

Like the other ethical concerns that have been discussed, the principle of beneficence is only a **prima facie argument;** that is, although at first glance beneficence seems to be the controlling principle, deeper analysis is re-

quired. Actions based on the beneficent principle of efficiency have been criticized as placing misguided primacy on a single ethical litmus test. Other values, it is argued, may be as compelling or more compelling than that of efficiency and may compel an alternative action even when the solution may "cost more" in dollars. To demonstrate this argument, one might imagine a rule that would permit health authorities to quarantine HIV-infected individuals in state-run institutions "until such time as they are cured." This rule would absolutely prevent contact between infected and non-infected individuals, and economists could probably demonstrate significant cost savings resulting from the quarantine. Under the efficiency principle, this would be a justifiable action. Nevertheless, the law would probably not withstand public criticism in this country, as it would amount to a life sentence based on disease status. This example highlights a significant criticism of the utilitarian approach. **Utilitarianism** is concerned only with the "aggregate good"; that is, with whether the good to society outweighs the aggregated costs or risks to individuals. It does not consider whether a rule is administered fairly; in particular, it fails to consider whether the benefits of a policy fall on one group while the costs are borne by others. This latter concept is called *distributive justice,* and it is explained in the next section.

Justice. Distributive justice seeks to ensure that the benefits and burdens of a policy are distributed evenly, or at least fairly, throughout the community. As applied to Scenario 8-A, this principle would lead us to ask whether a mandatory reporting law would be fair or just if it was enacted to protect the community but offered little benefit to infected individuals. Would the law be more ethically justifiable if, in addition to containing the spread of infection, the reported medical information was used to ensure that infected individuals received appropriate medical care and social service interventions?

How does society determine the fair and equitable allocation of benefits and burdens?

This section explores two leading theories for doing just that: social justice theory and communitarianism.

Prominent philosophers have wrestled with the notion of distributive justice, trying to describe an ideal set of norms or rules to govern society. Among these is the political philosopher John Rawls (1971), who, in his elegantly constructed argument in *A Theory of Justice,* propounded a theoretical basis upon which to determine the fair and equitable distribution of rights and privileges among all individuals in society. Rawls's argument rests on two fundamental principles. His first principle of justice is that "each person has an equal right to a fully adequate scheme of basic rights and liberties, which scheme is compatible with a similar scheme for all" (p. 227). His second principle states that "social and economic inequalities are to satisfy two conditions: first, they must be attached to offices and positions open to all under conditions of fair equality of opportunity; and second, they must be to the greatest benefit of the least advantaged members of society" (p. 227).

Though written in fairly dense language, Rawls's theory is really quite simple and elegant. At issue is the challenge of navigating the political terrain between the twin goals of individual liberty and social equality. Rawls's first principle suggests that society should first determine the basic set of rights and liberties to which every member of the society is entitled. Using a clever metaphor, Rawls proposes that we determine the content of the basic collection of rights and liberties by imagining ourselves "behind a veil of ignorance" (p. 235) concerning what our own station or lot in life will be; whether, for example, we will be born rich or poor, sick or healthy, and of majority or minority ethnicity. From behind this "veil of ignorance," we determine what are the basic necessities for leading a good life, such as food, clothing, shelter, education, work, medical care, freedom of thought and expression, and a right to association. It is these basic rights and liberties that Rawls argues should be equally distributed among all.

Rawls's second principle recognizes that some degree of social inequality is necessary for society to progress. This idea flows from a belief that without reward, persons will lack the incentive to engage in creative and productive activity. Rawls suggests, however, that there be limits to the extent of the inequality. The first limitation is that each person should have the same fair opportunity to get ahead as any other person. The second limitation is that the equality gap should only be as great as is needed to benefit the least advantaged among us. This idea suggests that the reward to those at the top should not be any greater than is needed to stimulate creativity and progress and, further, that the gap in equality is too great if those at the bottom do not benefit from social progress.

Although Rawls's theory of justice does not lend itself very readily to direct application, in thinking more generally about how his principles might apply to Scenario 8-A one might argue that a basic need of life is the right to medical care. Thus, although society might decide, irrespective of individual rights, that it is essential to track and control the spread of deadly infectious viruses, a fair distribution of benefits and burdens would also mean a societal responsibility to ensure treatment and care for the afflicted.

An approach that is somewhat at variance with the social justice theory is that of **communitarianism**. Rather than determining what each individual in society is due, a communitarian ethic focuses on those goods that are enjoyed collectively by society. For example, we as a society benefit collectively from an educated populace, a low infant mortality rate, safe roads and highways, clean air, and a healthy citizenry. Enjoyment of these social goods is meaningless when expressed as individual preferences. To promote the collective social good, a communitarian ethic envisions an affirmative role for government. Beauchamp (1999a) argued that

> . . . our country is founded upon a "republican legacy" that permits limits to individual rights of property

and liberty in order to protect the common good. The government's duty is to protect both the private good and the public good, as we are both private individuals pursuing our own individual interests as well as members of a political community. Within this public realm, is a legitimate area for the government to intervene for purposes of promoting the common social good. (p. 58)

Communitarians would argue that policy decisions must rest upon the core values of a community and that these decisions represent choices that benefit and are enjoyed by the community as a whole. In contrast, utilitarians would approach policy decisions by summing the aggregated preferences of individuals. According to communitarian theory, alternative policies should be evaluated not in monetary terms, but on the basis of the best, most well-reasoned, or persuasive ethical argument. Proponents of a policy must be prepared to address such moral questions as: Which action is best for our community? What is the most fair, most right, most equitable thing to do given the circumstances? How will the policy affect the long-term goals or vision for our community?

From a communitarian perspective, HIV is a common problem affecting the community at large, as well as presenting a threat to individuals; collective measures are the appropriate response to something that threatens the community; and preference ought to be given to solutions that strengthen and affirm attachments of all members to the community, thus forging a more cohesive whole (Beauchamp, 1999b). To quote Beauchamp (1999b), "When we face problems as a group and use group methods to solve our problems, we achieve both security for individuals and a stronger sense of community" (p. 55). If we apply this analysis to our scenario, the mandatory reporting law offers a community-level solution to a community problem, so it should be enacted. At the same time, to advance the concept of community, and especially the ideal of protecting all members of the society, the solution must also provide for assistance to infected individuals who are brought into the system as a result of the law.

As an ideal, communitarianism seems to be unassailable. Critics suggest, however, that group norms are not, in reality, always fair, just, or beneficent. Unfortunately, history bears this out. One need only think of Nazi Germany or the historical treatment of African Americans within the United States to recognize the need to proceed cautiously.

We have looked at four ethical principles that may be used to design, analyze, and justify government regulations affecting private medical information. None of these principles is absolute, but each offers an essential perspective that must be considered and addressed to reach a well-reasoned decision.

Scenario 8-B: When Duty to One's Employer Conflicts with a Duty Owed to the Public

Mary Ruiz is the HIM manager for an HMO in Autotown, Indiana. In 1999, she noticed an unusually large number of recorded cases of neurologic damage to the bladders of patients who were seen by several of the group's physicians. Mary alerted her supervisor, Mr. King, about the apparent increase in cases and proposed that she create a special database to track the occurrence of this condition. Mr. King told her not to waste her time.

Against her supervisor's directives, Mary developed the database. Upon analyzing the data, Mary realized that all the affected patients worked in the same plant—a facility that manufactured automobile and truck seats. Alarmed by this discovery, Mary again approached her supervisor, this time with the suggestion that health authorities be notified of the increased incidence of this rare form of bladder disease. Again Mr. King rejected her suggestion. He reminded Mary that her primary responsibility was to provide data management services to the HMO healthcare team and to protect the confidentiality of patient records. He also reminded Mary that the manufacturing facility had the largest employee enrollment of any of the HMO's clients and that the company was one of Autotown's largest employers.

Questions

1. Should Mary take it upon herself to notify the health authorities? Assume that Mary lives in a state with a law similar to that of Colorado, which requires "persons or employees having knowledge of exposure of large numbers or specific groups of persons to a known or suspected public health hazard [to] report such disease, outbreak or epidemic" (State of Colorado Rules and Regulations Pertaining to the Detection, Monitoring, and Investigation of Environmental and Chronic Diseases, 6 CCR-1009-7).

2. What if Mary's state does not have that kind of law on the books? Should Mary still take it upon herself to notify the health authorities? Are there any actions that Mary can take to fulfill her conflicting obligations to the HMO's patients, to her employer, to the automotive company, and to the public?

3. Does the HMO have an ethical duty to report the situation to governmental authorities?

4. Does Mary have an ethical obligation to come forward with the evidence, even though she was told not to by her supervisor? What are the consequences if Mary does so? If she fails to do so?

5. How would you resolve Mary's ethical dilemma?

A completed ethical decision-making matrix for the scenario is provided at the end of the chapter.

Making a Reasoned Decision

Mary's dilemma in Scenario 8-B might be framed as follows: Does Mary have an ethical duty to report her findings of an increased number of rare bladder cases to public health authorities? Clearly, if Mary lives in a state with a law similar to that of Colorado's, she has a legal duty to report the increased cases of bladder disease to public health authorities.[2] The more difficult question arises when the law is silent about this duty. As noted in

Chapter 2, compliance with laws and regulations is the minimum guideline for ethical

---

2. Colorado rules state, "In addition to physicians, health facilities, and laboratories, any person having knowledge of a reportable disease, outbreak, or epidemic, such as coroners, persons in charge of schools (including school nursing staff), *or persons or employees having knowledge of exposure of large numbers or specific groups of persons to a known or suspected public health hazard shall report such disease, outbreak, or epidemic*" (emphasis added) State of Colorado Rules and Regulations Pertaining to the Detection, Monitoring and Investigation of Environmental and Chronic Diseases, 6 CCR-1009-7. (Last amended July 21, 2004, effective September 30, 2004.)

behavior. Ethical considerations may compel the HIM professional to act even when the law does not address an issue or situation or does so unsatisfactorily.

The AHIMA Code of Ethics for HIM professionals (AHIMA, 2004; see Appendix 1-D in Chapter 1 of this book) promotes the core values of integrity, objectivity, and trust. Among other things, the AHIMA Code exhorts HIM professionals to adhere to truth and accuracy in the reporting of medical information. Is there anything in the Code that says—or implies—that Mary has an affirmative obligation to notify authorities about a possible disease cluster occurring in one of the plants served by her HMO?

Analyzing the Ethical Conflict. This case highlights a situation in which a duty to one's employer conflicts with a duty to promote the best interests of patients. The ethical principles of nonmaleficence, beneficence, and justice apply. On its face, the "do no harm" principle, or the principle of nonmaleficence, seems to suggest a course of inaction; that is, by simply remaining quiet, Mary would do no harm to her employer. This is, however, a weak application of the principle. A more careful examination could lead one to argue persuasively that by remaining silent Mary would be doing great harm—particularly if she were in a unique position to identify and disclose the disease's pattern.

The principles of beneficence and justice arguably outweigh any duty to remain silent to protect one's employer. Beneficence, the moral duty to take actions that promote the health and welfare of others, would clearly suggest that Mary has an obligation to notify those who have the authority to investigate the workplace and to determine whether exposures in the plant are causing neurologic bladder damage to the plant employees. If the authorities detect a causal relationship between chemical exposures in the plant and the workers' bladder disease, the health officials could require the company to take actions to prevent further harm to the plant's employees.

Similarly, the principle of justice supports the argument that Mary ought to notify authorities about this potential health threat. Recall that we spoke about justice as the fair and equitable distribution of benefits and burdens within society. Thus, Mary's dilemma may be framed as follows: Is it fair to protect the HMO's business relations at the potential expense of the HMO's patients? When the question is framed this way, we may easily see that it would be unjust for Mary to remain silent. Her silence would protect the business relationship between her employer and its client, the automobile seat manufacturer. However, Mary's failure to warn officials about a potentially preventable disease would unjustly burden the HMO's patients. The added pain and suffering of the plant workers and their families could not be justified.

This is not to say that Mary's dilemma is easily resolved. Her situation is extremely difficult because her professional obligations directly conflict with her personal interests. If she tells the government officials about the increased cases of bladder disease, she may seriously jeopardize her employment. In deciding what course of action to take, she needs to weigh the possibility that if she disobeys her supervisor, she could lose her job. What would that mean to her and to her family? However, Mary also must consider the importance of working for an organization that has virtue and integrity.

Even if Mary decides that she cannot go to the public health authorities, she may decide to work for change within her organization. Some other actions that Mary might take include seeking the advice of the HMO's ethics committee, if one exists, or the advice of peer professionals. Mary might also consider alerting the group's physicians concerning the increased number of bladder disease cases and seeking their help in alerting the public health authorities. She might also implore those in higher positions within the HMO to take action. Can you think of anything else Mary might do?

Scenario 8-B highlights a situation where an HIM professional must act courageously when faced with a conflicting set of values. Because

HIM professionals are responsible for maintaining medical records from a variety of providers over a period of time, they may be the first to notice the outbreak of a previously undetected disease or epidemic. The astute HIM professional is thus able to alert public health authorities to situations and conditions that require a government response. As Scenario 8-B shows, however, this opportunity to serve the public may challenge the HIM professional's other allegiances and give rise to an extremely difficult situation in which professional duty conflicts with personal interests and loyalty to an employer. In the end, when faced with this kind of dilemma, each of us must make our own decision about what to do. Hopefully, by applying the ethical principles discussed in this chapter and throughout the book, you will gain the necessary tools for making a well-reasoned decision.

THE HIM PROFESSIONAL'S ROLE AND RESPONSIBILITY AS AN ADVOCATE

The 2004 Code of Ethics adopted by AHIMA states that HIM professionals should "advocate, uphold and defend the individual's right to privacy and the doctrine of confidentiality in the use and disclosure of information." The association interprets this duty to include a responsibility to

> Engage in social and political action that supports the protection of privacy and confidentiality, and be aware of the impact of the political arena on the health information system. Advocate for changes in policy and legislation to ensure protection of privacy and confidentiality, coding compliance, and other issues that surface as advocacy issues as well as facilitating informed participation by the public on these issues.

In this section, we explore the ethical basis for this obligation.

To begin, we must introduce two new concepts: **obligatory action** and **supererogatory action**. According to Beauchamp and Childress

(1994), the former serves as guidance to the minimum moral conduct required of everyone within the profession, whereas the latter serves as the ideal; that is, action that is neither required nor expected but that, if done, is exemplary or praiseworthy. As the authors suggested, it is helpful to identify supererogatory actions because they illuminate the pathway toward more beneficent performance in the service of patients and the public.

Is the HIM professional's duty to advocate for quality laws obligatory or supererogatory? One can argue that the duty is obligatory based on principles of reciprocity, superior knowledge, and the unambiguous responsibility of HIM professionals to protect patient privacy.

A Reciprocal Duty Owed to Society

One basis for claiming that the duty of advocacy is obligatory is the ethical argument of reciprocity. According to Hume, each of us has received the benefits of society, and therefore we have a responsibility to further promote it. Our success as professionals is due not just to our own hard work and labor, but also to the long list of persons in our lives who have supported us and enabled us to reach this far in our professions. The list includes not only family members who may have provided financial and emotional support, but also our teachers and other professionals who went before us and paved the way for our professional development. This concept of reciprocity pervades our entire social life and lends strength to the notion that we should not only act for our individual best interests but also contribute to furthering "good" in society. As members of the community, we must repay our debt and pave the way for others as others have done for us. Indeed, the nature of both giving and receiving is part of the very special benefit one gains from belonging to a "community" (Beauchamp & Childress, 1994).

Superior Knowledge

One may argue that the expert knowledge possessed by HIM professionals also confers an obligation to act on behalf of the public. In an era when information systems are increasingly maintained and shared electronically, there is growing concern about the potential erosion of health information privacy. As noted in a 1999 report of the President's Advisory Commission on Consumer Protection and Quality in the Health Care Industry,

> The changing structure of the health-care system and rapid advances in information technology and medical and health care research have increased the demand for and supply of health information among traditional users, such as the treating physician, and new users, such as large networks of providers, information management companies, quality and utilization review committees, and independently contracted service providers. Concerns have been raised that, under the current system of information exchange, various entities can access individually identifiable information without sufficient security safeguards and consent requirements. Other activities undertaken to improve quality and efficiency may present new risks to the confidentiality of health information. For example, quality oversight activities by plans, providers, accreditation bodies, and regulatory agencies require detailed information about the treatment and benefit status of individual consumers. The growing role of employers in workforce health issues has also contributed to the confidentiality debate. (Appendix A, Chapter 6)

Because HIM professionals have superior knowledge about the uses and potential abuses of confidential medical information and the threats to confidentiality posed by technology, they have a special duty to inform the public and policymakers about the potentials for abuse and the precautions to be taken.

An Unambiguous Duty to Protect Patient Privacy

Given their superior knowledge and unequivocal obligation to safeguard the accuracy and privacy of medical information, HIM professionals are uniquely qualified to provide germane and influential testimony relating to laws and policies protecting the confidentiality of patient data. As the various levels of government seek to pass comprehensive laws protecting healthcare consumers, opportunities for patient advocacy abound. HIM professionals are encouraged to maintain contact with their professional association so that they can remain current on pending laws and policies, assist in drafting position papers on behalf of the association, and provide testimony on pending bills. Knowledge of the ethical bases for making policy choices will enable HIM professionals to offer well-reasoned arguments in support of policy positions.

Resources for Advocacy

The Internet has greatly increased the ability of professionals to remain current on pending federal and state legislative matters. One excellent resource is AHIMA's Web site at http://www.ahima.org. This site includes access to AHIMA's "Policy and Government Relations" pages where one can find analyses of pending legislation pertinent to HIM professionals and membership alerts that warn members about important votes and issues under consideration by Congress. One may also research the status of pending bills, look up the contact information of Congressional representatives, and link to the Library of Congress's Legislative Information Service, the Federal Register, and the Centers for Medicare and Medicaid Management Services (CMS). AHIMA has also made it easy to send a member of Congress a message in support of, or in opposition to, pending policies. Draft letters reflecting AHIMA's position are provided, along with ready access to congressional e-mail accounts, permitting advocacy literally with the push of a button. The Web site also presents tips for communicating effectively with Congressional representatives and their staff and provides a brief description of the legislative process, from the drafting of a bill to the president's signature or veto. The ease with which professionals can access relevant information over the Internet and become involved with policy development activities strengthens the argument that the advocacy role is a fundamental component of the HIM professional's responsibilities.

Emerging Issues: Bioterrorism and Global Infections

The September 11, 2001, attacks on the World Trade Center towers in New York City and the Pentagon in Washington, D.C., and the crash of a hijacked plane in Pennsylvania have mobilized our nation's political leaders to take actions to combat terrorist threats on U.S. soil in unprecedented ways. National policies have spawned vigorous debate over how best to protect the public's security while safeguarding civil liberties. For example, the USA PATRIOT Act of 2001,[3] which passed Congress with very little scrutiny in the immediate aftermath of 9/11, greatly expands the government's authority to obtain private records (including medical records), documents, books, and other personal items. The government now has the ability to obtain these items simply by certifying to the court through written statement that they are sought "for an investigation to protect against international terrorism or clandestine intelligence activities." The government need not suspect the person who owns or controls the records of any wrongdoing. In short, the Act expands the government's right to conduct essentially warrantless records searches on U.S. citizens and permanent residents who are not themselves terror suspects, with little or no judicial oversight.

A draft bill prepared by the Department of Justice as a sequel to the USA PATRIOT Act,

known as the Domestic Security Enhancement Act of 2003,[4] would have authorized the government to collect and maintain a database of private genetic information of persons "for terrorism investigation purposes," without a court order or the person's consent, even if such persons have not been convicted of a crime. Due in part to public outcry, this particular bill was not passed into law. However, it is likely that a new version of the bill will be introduced into a future session of Congress.

Although some argue that these types of laws are necessary given the post–9/11 climate, others believe that such provisions undermine our democratic ideals. Wherever you stand on this issue, HIM professionals must follow the legal trends and reach reasoned decisions about whether the laws are necessary or whether they violate the carefully constructed balance of privacy with respect to health information (Working Group on "Governance Dilemmas," 2004).

This scenario depicts the classic conflict between the privacy rights of individuals and the needs of the community to access health information to protect the public interest. Among the ethical duties included in the 2004 AHIMA Code of Ethics is the obligation to "advocate, uphold and defend the individual's right to privacy and the doctrine of confidentiality in the use and disclosure of information." This is interpreted as a duty to "advocate for changes in policy and legislation to ensure protection of privacy and confidentiality, coding compliance, and other issues that surface as advocacy issues as well as facilitating informed participation by the public on these issues."

All the scenarios in this book reflect ethical dilemmas that have actually occurred. However, the following scenario differs because it is offered as a potential future issue rather than a formal scenario; therefore, it has not been analyzed in a decision-making matrix. It is offered as a source for discussion.

3. See section 215 Uniting and Strengthening America by Providing Appropriate Tools Required to Intercept and Obstruct Terrorism (USA PATRIOT) Act of 2001, Pub. L. No. 107-56, 115 Stat. 272.

4. A draft bill, the Domestic Security Enhancement Act of 2003. Retrieved September 24, 2004, from http://www.dailyrotten.com/source-docs/patriot2draft.html.

Scenario 8-C: The Terrorism Preparedness Act

A bill pending in your state legislature entitled the "State Terrorism Preparedness Act" gives the governor or his designee the authority to seek a court order compelling the production of any tangible items that are relevant to an investigation into international or domestic terrorism. The term *tangible items* includes medical records, books, papers, recordings, and documents.

The bill further provides that the court shall grant the order whenever the state "has knowledge of any individual attempting, threatening, or conspiring to engage in an act of terrorism." The bill defines *terrorism* as:

> The use of any biological agent, chemical or radioactive substance or device to cause death, disease or biological malfunction in humans, plants, animals, or other living organisms in an effort to influence the conduct of government or to intimidate or coerce a civilian population.

The State Mental Health Society contacted the State Health Information Management Association (SHIMA) to ask its support in opposing this section of the bill. The Society fears the law could be used to coerce psychiatrists and other mental health providers to divulge patient mental health records based on nothing more than an individual's threat to engage in an act of terrorism.

SHIMA has not yet taken a stand on the bill. The association's director for policy, legislation, and advocacy has asked for your advice.

Questions

1. What would you recommend the director do?

2. Does the 2004 AHIMA Code of Ethics address the inherent conflict between individual and community rights?

3. Can you suggest alternate language that would improve the balance of protections between individuals and the community?

The Code implies an ethical obligation on the part of SHIMA and individual HIM practitioners in the state to take a stand against legislation authorizing unacceptably broad access to private mental health records. SHIMA ought to consider the legislation and take political action if indeed it agrees with the State Mental Health Society's assessment that the proposed Act is unduly harmful to individual privacy.

The principles of autonomy, nonmaleficence, beneficence, and justice apply in determining whether SHIMA should oppose the pending legislation. When taken together, these concepts suggest that a balance must be reached between absolute individual protections and the public's interest. The balance must also consider the public's multifaceted interests. Not only is the community concerned with protection against terrorist acts, but also protection against unreasonable government intrusion into individuals' private affairs.

One way to assess the bill is to ask whether, as worded, it gives the state an unacceptable reach into the private lives of individuals.

Could state officials use the bill to subpoena a person's mental health records based on mere allegations that someone has "threatened to blow up a building"? If so, than the bill's language is overly broad. For example, we would not want the government to use unsubstantiated knowledge from an informant (who may have a grudge against someone) that he overheard a person threatening to bomb a government office building.

Similarly, we would not want to give the government authority to compel mental health providers to turn over the records of any individual who ever threatened during the course of treatment to engage in a terrorist act.

However, if mental health records could corroborate or help substantiate the intent or motive of a person caught with a lethal quantity of bioterrorist agents, then arguably the balance might shift in favor of allowing the government access to the person's mental health records.

Language could be proposed to assure that the government is acting on more than mere suspicion that someone may be about to commit a terrorist act. For example, the bill could be reworded to require the government to demonstrate by "clear and convincing evidence" that it has reason to believe the person is about to engage in a terrorist act. Alternatively, the bill could require a hearing to afford the court an opportunity to assess the reliability of the state's information. The state would have to show why the information they have is reliable. Finally, the bill could provide for an in-camera inspection of the person's mental health records by the judge or a special master to determine if there is anything in the records that might help the state. (An in-camera inspection means that a judge or a special master appointed by the judge takes the first look at the records to see whether they should be given to the state.)

Hopefully, this scenario will stay in the potential future context.

CONCLUSION

Maintaining the privacy of patient data is of paramount importance, but it is not absolute. At times and for various reasons, including legitimate research needs and protection of the public's health, data must be shared with parties outside the provider–patient relationship. Finding the proper balance between the individual rights of patients and the competing needs and demands of the community and the government is often difficult. Legitimate but conflicting claims to the data may be made by several stakeholders, without there being a single correct answer. In these situations, the best one can demand is that a reasoned decision be made; that is, a decision based on a thorough analysis of the competing facts and ethical principles.

An extensive and growing array of persons and offices, both inside and outside the healthcare industry, has access to patient health information. The large number of individuals and organizations with such access strongly supports the argument that HIM professionals have an obligatory duty to advocate for responsible confidentiality legislation; that is, legislation that both protects the privacy of patient information and recognizes the legitimate need for government access to such data to protect the public's health.

Key Terms

- Communitarianism
- Epidemiology
- Incidence
- Obligatory actions
- Prevalence
- Prima facie argument
- Reportable diseases and conditions
- Supererogatory actions
- Surveillance
- Utilitarianism

Chapter Summary

- Public health encompasses all those activities that we as a society undertake to ensure conditions in which people can be healthy. Such conditions include a clean, healthy, and safe natural and work environment; a healthy food supply; a good diet; access to medical care and diagnostic screenings; and opportunities for physical exercise.
- Government access to and use of patient information are critical for protecting the public's health.
- Although government agencies use patient data to prevent or slow major epidemics and to otherwise bring harmful conditions under control, such advances may come at a cost to individual liberty and privacy.
- Decisions about the use of or access to patient information often involve dilemmas that involve conflicting ethical principles and for which there are no right answers. Difficult choices can be made by applying ethical reasoning to reach a principled decision.
- HIM professionals play an expanding role in protecting the public's health. They are often in a position to first detect the outbreak of a previously undetected disease or epidemic.
- HIM professionals have a duty to advocate for ethical HIM policies that best serve the interests of patients and the public.

References

American Health Information Management Association [AHIMA]. (2004). *AHIMA code of ethics.* Chicago: Author.

Beauchamp, D. (1999a). Community: The neglected tradition of public health. In D. Beauchamp and B. Steinbock (Eds.), *New ethics for the public's health*, pp. 57–67. New York: Oxford University Press.

Beauchamp, D. (1999b). Introduction to Part II: Public health as community perspective. In D. Beauchamp and B. Steinbock (Eds.), *New ethics for the public's health*, pp. 53–57. New York: Oxford University Press.

Beauchamp, T., and Childress, J. F. (2001). *Principles of biomedical ethics*, 5th ed. New York: Oxford University Press.

Beauchamp, D., and Steinbock, B. (1999). Introduction: Ethical theory and practice. In D. Beauchamp and B. Steinbock (Eds.), *New ethics for the public's health*, pp. 3–23. New York: Oxford University Press.

Centers for Disease Control and Prevention [CDC]. (1995, March 24). Notification of syringe-sharing and sex partners of HIV infected persons—Pennsylvania 1993–1994. *Morbidity and Mortality Weekly Report, 44*(11), 202–204.

Centers for Disease Control and Prevention [CDC], National Center for Chronic Disease Prevention and Health Promotion. (1999). National program of cancer registries. Retrieved August 30, 2004, from http://www.cdc.gov/cancer/npcr/register.htm.

Chave, S. P. W. (1984). The origins and development of public health. In W. W. Holland, R. Detels, G. Knox, with assistance of E. Breeze (Eds.), *Oxford textbook of public health. Vol. 1: History, determinants, scope, and strategies,* pp. 3–19. New York: Oxford University Press.

Dworkin, G. (1999). Paternalism. In D. Beauchamp and B. Steinbock (Eds.), *New ethics for the public's health,* pp. 115–128. New York: Oxford University Press.

Eyler, J. M. (1986). Public health then and now: The epidemiology of milk-borne scarlet fever: The case of Edwardian Brighton. *American Journal of Public Health, 76,* 573–583.

Friis, R. H., and Sellers, T. A. (1999). *Epidemiology for public health practice.* Gaithersburg, MD: Aspen.

Institute of Medicine. (1988). *The future of public health.* Washington, DC: National Academy Press.

IPLAN Data System. (2000). 1990 IPLAN Data System Homepage. Retrieved August 30, 2004, from http://app.idph.state.il.us/IPLANDataSystem.asp?menu=1

Lerner, B. H. (1993). Public health then and now: New York City's tuberculosis control efforts: The historical limitations of the "War on Consumption." *American Journal of Public Health, 83,* 758–766.

Mooney, G. (1999). Public health versus private practice: The contested development of compulsory infectious disease notification in late nineteenth-century Britain. *Bulletin of the History of Medicine, 73,* 238–267.

National Association of County and City Health Officials (NACCHO). (2001). *Local Public Health Agency Infrastructure: A Chartbook,* p. 18. Washington, DC: Author. Retrieved December 5, 2005, from http://www.archive.naccho.org/documents/chartbook.html.

Pavia, A., Benyo, M., Niler, L., & Risk, I. (1993). Partner notification for control of HIV: Results after 2 years of a statewide program in Utah. *American Journal of Public Health, 83,* 1418–1424.

President's Advisory Commission on Consumer Protection and Quality in the Health Care Industry. (1999). 1999 Report [online]. Retrieved September 19, 2005, from http://www.hcqualitycommission.gov/final/append_a.html#exec.

Rabe, B. (1990). Environmental health policy. In G. Pickett and J. J. Hanlon (Eds.), *Public health administration and practice,* 9th ed., pp. 317–330. St. Louis: Times Mirror Mosby.

Rawls, J. (1971). *A theory of justice.* Cambridge, MA: Harvard University Press.

Rosen, G. (1971). Public health then and now: The first neighborhood health center movement—its rise and fall. *American Journal of Public Health, 61,* 1620–1637.

Rosen, G. (1972). Public health then and now: Tenements and typhus in New York City, 1840–1875. *American Journal of Public Health, 62,* 590–593.

Rosenkrantz, B. G. (1974). Cart before the horse: Theory, practice and professional image in American public health. *Journal of History of Medicine and Allied Sciences, 29,* 55–73.

Turnock, B. (2004). *Public health: What it is and how it works,* 3d ed. Sudbury, MA: Jones and Bartlett.

Working Group on "Governance Dilemmas" in Bioterrorism Response. (2004). Leading during bioattacks and epidemics with the public's trust and help. *Biosecurity and Bioterrorism, 2*(1), 25–40.

The ethical decision-making matrix is a tool to help you organize complex, ethical problems; however, there is no simple fill-in-the-box approach to ethical decision making. The objective is to follow each step of the process and not move from the question directly to what should be done or how to prevent it next time. If you skip steps, you will not fully understand all of the values and options for action. Also, the matrix provided for each scenario in this book is not the only way to examine the problem. You can make an equally compelling ethical argument for a different decision—just be sure to follow all the steps of the matrix.

SCENARIO 8-A: REPORTING HIV STATUS

Steps	Information	
1. What is the ethical question?	Should you advise Dr. Moe to require healthcare providers to report the names of people who test positive for HIV?	
2. What are the facts?	**KNOWN**	**TO BE GATHERED**
	A blood-borne disease, HIV can be transmitted to sexual partners, to people with whom the infected person shares a needle, and from mother to unborn child.	• Would requiring healthcare providers to report the names of HIV-infected persons promote nonmaleficence and beneficence to the extent that it is worth compromising the patients' autonomy? • Is there a way in which such a mandate could achieve distributive justice? • What are the customary practices in such cases? • What does your boss expect you to do?
3. What are the values? Examine the shared and competing values, obligations, and interests of the stakeholders (i.e., patient, HIM professional, healthcare practitioner(s), administrators, society, and other advocates) involved in order to fully understand the complexity of the ethical problem(s).	**Patient:** Interest in maintaining privacy and autonomy; interest in receiving quality health care. **HIM professional:** Integrity (protect public health, preserve patients' privacy and autonomy); avoid harm (not requiring the release of names could endanger individuals who are unaware of their exposure to HIV); fairness (promote distributive justice). **Healthcare professionals:** Maintain doctor–patient confidentiality; avoid harm (protect individuals who are unaware of their exposure to HIV); offer treatment to HIV-positive patients. **Administrators:** Duty to decide; obligation to protect public health. **Society:** Promote public health through disclosure of names of infected persons.	

4. What are my options?	• Advise Dr. Moe to not require healthcare providers to report names. • Advise Dr. Moe to wait to make a decision. • Advise Dr. Moe to require healthcare providers to report names.
5. What should I do?	Advise Dr. Moe to require healthcare providers to report names, but also to use the information to ensure that infected individuals receive medical care and support services.

6. What justifies my choice?	**JUSTIFIED**	**NOT JUSTIFIED**
	• Obligation to promote public health. • Obligation to promote distributive justice.	• Advise Dr. Moe to not require healthcare providers to report the names of infected individuals. • Protect privacy and autonomy at the expense of public health, which is not fair to parties who may have been exposed to HIV. • Lack of a means of ensuring that HIV-positive individuals receive needed medical care and social support services.

7. How can I prevent this ethical problem?	• Learn more about the principles of autonomy, nonmaleficence, beneficence, and justice. • Determine if system changes are needed. • Discuss standards and the values that support them with colleagues.

The ethical decision-making matrix is a tool to help you organize complex, ethical problems; however, there is no simple fill-in-the-box approach to ethical decision making. The objective is to follow each step of the process and not move from the question directly to what should be done or how to prevent it next time. If you skip steps, you will not fully understand all of the values and options for action. Also, the matrix provided for each scenario in this book is not the only way to examine the problem. You can make an equally compelling ethical argument for a different decision—just be sure to follow all the steps of the matrix.

SCENARIO 8-B: WHEN DUTY TO ONE'S EMPLOYER CONFLICTS WITH A DUTY OWED TO THE PUBLIC

Steps	Information	
1. What is the ethical question?	Should Mary notify the health authorities about her findings?	
2. What are the facts?	**KNOWN**	**TO BE GATHERED**
	• There is an increased incidence of a rare disease among workers at a single facility. • The facility has the largest employee enrollment of all of the HMO's clients.	• What are the customary practices in such cases? • Would failing to report the cases jeopardize public health? • What is the likely impact on self and family of changing jobs?
3. What are the values? Examine the shared and competing values, obligations, and interests of the stakeholders (i.e., patient, HIM professional, healthcare practitioner(s), administrators, society, and other advocates) involved in order to fully understand the complexity of the ethical problem(s).	**Patient:** Values quality health care; values confidentiality and autonomy; interest in knowing if workplace is putting patient in physical jeopardy. **HIM professional:** Truth and integrity; obligation to protect public health; loyalty to employer; avoid harm (reporting incidence of disease may put patients' privacy and autonomy in jeopardy; not reporting incidence could put others at risk); personal values (promote welfare of self and family by avoiding loss of job). **Healthcare professionals:** Promote welfare of patients through appropriate treatment. **Administrators:** Benefit patients and keep from harm; maximize financial income without compromising public health. **Society:** Promote public health through the disclosure of incidence rate.	

4. What are my options?	• Do not disclose incidence rate. • Disclose incidence rate.	
5. What should I do?	Disclose incidence rate to public health authority.	
6. What justifies my choice?	**JUSTIFIED**	**NOT JUSTIFIED**
	• Obligation to tell the truth. • Obligation to protect public health. • Preserve professional integrity.	• Do not disclose incidence rate (not fair to the public, especially those who work in the plant). • Lack of disclosure undermines the public health system.
7. How can I prevent this ethical problem?	• Determine if system changes are needed. • Learn more about the principles of autonomy, nonmaleficence, beneficence, and justice. • Discuss standards and the values that support them with colleagues. • Evaluate institutional integrity at job interview and subsequently as ethical problems arise.	

MANAGED CARE

Ida Critelli Schick, PhD, MS, FACHE

Learning Objectives

After completing this chapter, the reader should be able to:

- Understand the key elements that describe managed care.
- Understand the role of the health information management (HIM) professional in the managed care environment.
- Identify key ethical issues regarding privacy of personally identifiable patient information in a managed care environment.
- Discuss possible policies to address ethical problems related to managed care.

Abstract

In the maturing managed care environment, the control of healthcare costs is increasingly dependent on information regarding individual patients/consumers, clinicians, and healthcare organizations. Health information management (HIM) professionals have a crucial role to play in obtaining and analyzing this information. Further, HIM professionals deal constantly with questions of access to information—both access to patient or provider information by other parties and patients' access to information that they require in order to give informed consent to their care and to their insurance plans. Consequently, HIM professionals are at the center of ethical dilemmas regarding these questions in the managed care environment. This chapter explains how managed care works and explores ethical issues raised by managed care that are of particular relevance to HIM professionals.

Scenario 9-A: Complexity of Choosing a Managed Care Plan

The Airtite Packaging Company in Middleburg is a small, privately owned company with 150 employees. Over the past several years, the cost of employee health insurance has increased precipitously. This year the owners will be offering managed care products to their employees in an effort to rein in expenses. Airtite has contracted with one insurer, ABC Insurance Co., to provide four products: indemnity insurance, a health maintenance organization (HMO), a preferred provider organization (PPO), and a point-of-service (POS) plan.

Alice, Betty, and Charlie are employees who each chose different insurance products after hearing the insurance representative's talk. Alice is aged 62 and will retire in 3 years. She had a mild heart attack last year, so she doesn't want to change doctors or hospitals and wants the greatest guarantee from her insurance that her care will be covered. Alice has had indemnity, or fee-for-service, insurance all of her 25 years at Airtite, and she would like to continue with it. However, it will now cost her an additional $175 a month, and she cannot afford it. Her primary care doctor is not on either the HMO or the PPO list, but her cardiologist is on the HMO specialty list. So she joins the HMO, thinking she can use his services. She does know that she must choose a new primary care physician who is a member of the HMO panel.

Betty is a 25-year-old, recently married woman who has just moved to Middleburg. She doesn't know when, but she knows she will need an obstetrician soon, because she and her husband plan to start a family. Having a baby can be expensive. The HMO package will cover everything with a small copay ($5.00) at the doctor's office. This looks like a good product to her. Betty is also considering the POS product, because it offers her the possibility of going outside the HMO if she should so desire, but it could be expensive, especially if the newborn has any problems. She'll talk to her husband before she makes her selection.

Charlie is a 45-year-old, married father of three teens ranging in age from 14 to 18. He and his wife, Cindy, are natives of Middleburg. They have utilized the services of a Middleburg internist for 20 years. They have a pediatrician for their youngest teen; however, she, too, will soon want to move from the "baby doctor" to the internist. Cindy has looked at the list of physicians and found that the pediatrician and the internist are not on the HMO list of physicians; however, they are on the PPO list. Charlie and Cindy don't really want to change physicians, because they have a good rapport with their current physicians. Their young teen daughter plays soccer and has had some knee injuries. She has developed an amicable, working relationship with an orthopedic surgeon whom she likes. In order not to change physicians and to eliminate inconveniences for the whole family, Charlie has signed up for the PPO package.

All these employees signed up for a plan on the basis of the information made available to them. They know nothing about the strategies that their managed care organization (MCO) uses to hold down healthcare costs, such as its financial arrangements with their healthcare providers, even though these may present their physicians with conflicts of interest and affect what kind of care and how much care they receive. Alice, for example, is mistaken in believing that she can see her cardiologist just because he is on the HMO provider list. After enrolling in the HMO, she visits her primary care physician, Dr. Smith, an internist, several times because she is experiencing some light-headedness and a little tightness in her chest and because she has difficulty at times catching her breath. Initially, Dr. Smith is able to control these symptoms with medication. However, eventually the symptoms recur, and it becomes clear that the medication is not working. Alice asks to be referred to her cardiologist, who is on the HMO panel, but Dr. Smith refuses. Why does the doctor refuse to make the referral?

According to the contract between the HMO and Dr. Smith's group practice, the group is paid a capitated amount per member per month for each enrollee who chooses this group. The group is then to provide all primary and medically necessary specialty care for each enrollee for that month. Any fees for specialists outside the group must be paid by the group. Any payment amount remaining at the end of the month belongs to the group; any deficit is the physician group's liability.

One condition of the group's policy is that referrals are to be kept internal to the group. Although the cardiologist that Alice wants to see is on the HMO provider panel, he is not in Dr. Smith's group practice. Specialists outside the group are paid on a fee-for-service basis, which puts the group at financial risk. Referral to specialists outside the group will most likely require fee-for-service payments, which are much higher than the capitated amounts allotted to the group.

Question

1. **You are an HIM professional who has just been hired by the ABC Insurance Co. to develop policies regarding the information that consumers will receive about the insurance plans in which they have the option to enroll. What kinds of information do you think the MCO should be obliged to provide its enrollees and why?**

A completed ethical decision-making matrix for the scenario is provided at the end of the chapter.

WHAT IS MANAGED CARE?

Managed care is a term that is much used and abused in our society. To its supporters, managed care is a response to an expensive, fragmented, and unaccountable medical care system that devotes its attention to sickness, disease, and injury, with little attention to health promotion and disease prevention. To its critics, it is an ill-conceived payment system for medical care services that has turned physicians into technicians by obstructing their professional autonomy and that has limited patient choice to the designated physicians, hospitals, and other healthcare entities that it will pay for approved services to enrollees. According to critics, managed care disrupts the physician–patient relationship, which develops over long periods of time, because those who enroll in these managed care products often find that the lists do not include their physicians and that they must find new physicians on the managed care product's list.

Managed care is not simple; it has many forms. Its primary forms are **health maintenance organizations (HMOs), preferred provider organizations (PPOs), point-of-service (POS) plans,** and managed **indemnity (fee-for-service) plans.** Managed care plans are owned by Blue Cross/Blue Shield, physician groups, hospitals, commercial insurance companies, and community cooperatives, among others. They can be for profit or not for profit.

HMOs are prepaid medical plans that provide and manage healthcare services to their members for a fixed premium price. There are several different models of HMOs: staff, group,

independent practice association (IPA), and network. In a staff-model HMO, the physicians and others are salaried employees, and they provide care only to the members enrolled in the HMO. In a group model, the HMO contracts with a large group of multispecialty physicians to provide care to its members. The group-model and staff-model HMOs are transparent to the HMO members. In an IPA model, the HMO contracts with individual physicians and small-group practices to provide care to the HMO enrollees in the individual physician offices. The physicians see their own patients as well as the HMO patients. In a network-model HMO, the HMO contracts with several large-group practices, not individual or small-group practices, and the contracted physicians see their private patients as well as HMO patients. HMOs are risk-bearing organizations; that is, if the cost of rendering services outpaces the income, then the HMO must bear that cost itself. The HMO itself provides utilization management and quality assurance services.

PPOs are networks of physicians, hospitals, and other healthcare providers and services that provide for services under a negotiated fee. PPOs do not bear risk for those to whom they render service. The risk is borne by the insurance company that sponsors the product, by the self-insured employer, or by the third-party administrator. PPOs usually contract for services, such as quality assurance and utilization management.

Point of service (POS) is usually an addition to an HMO product. It allows the member to go outside the HMO for services, but at a copay that varies in size with the level of benefit sought. The copay can be substantial.

Although managed care has no simple definition and has many forms, its essence is captured in the following characteristics (Knight, 1998, p. 22):

- Integration of healthcare delivery and health insurance
- Network-based arrangements with physicians, hospitals, and other healthcare professionals

- Provision of a defined set of healthcare services to enrollees
- Criteria and a process for selecting and monitoring healthcare providers
- Systems to gather, monitor, and measure data on health service utilization, physician referral patterns, and other quality and performance measures
- Incentives or requirements for members to use providers and procedures associated with the plan
- Incentives for providers to encourage the appropriate use of resources
- Activities aimed at improving the health status of members

These descriptors are in themselves ethically neutral to positive; however, the implementation of plans with these characteristics presents ethical issues.

GROWTH OF MANAGED CARE

Despite negative opinions, managed care, in its many forms, has grown significantly in the last 10 years. HMOs, which are considered the strongest form of managed care, increased nationally among those who were enrolled in health plans from 18% in 1988 to 30% in 1998. PPOs increased from 11% in 1988 to 33% in 1998. Finally, POS products increased from 0% in 1988 to 23% in 1998. Fee-for-service plans, however, decreased from 71% of those enrolled in health plans in 1988 to 14% in 1998 (VHA & Deloitte and Touche, 1999, p. 25).

Managed care has not increased uniformly across the United States. Geographically, managed care in the form of HMOs has penetrated 15 states with more than 31% of their population; 10 states with 21% to 30%; 14 states with 11% to 20%; and 11 states with less than 10% (VHA & Deloitte and Touche, 1999, p. 27).

The variability in healthcare market penetration is due to the economic factors of supply and demand. Low managed care penetration can be traced to low hospital market concentration, a low number of physician solo practices, and low hospital occupancy. This kind of situation is not appealing to managed care: There is no competition and little opportunity to increase market share. On the demand side, managed care penetration is inversely related to the proportion of the population that is minority and not highly educated. Again, this is not an appealing environment, because of the generally small numbers of privately insured. Managed care penetration is positively related to the large, urbanized markets that have significant segments of the population who are college educated (Dranove, Simon, & White, 1998). Again, this is an attractive environment due to the large number of privately insured individuals. Further, the high ratio of providers to population allows for competition and market share growth.

MANAGED CARE STRATEGIES

The growth of managed care is due to its strategies regarding (1) pricing, (2) access to providers, and (3) quality of care.

Pricing

Until recently, managed care has been able to decrease the increasing price of health care through pricing strategies. Managed care's emphasis on price was originally due to the influence of (1) government, which had already instituted diagnostic-related groups (DRGs) in Medicare hospital payments and had begun to research resource-based relative value systems (RBRVSs) for physician payments, and (2) large employers who were (and remain) very concerned about the increasingly high prices of American products in the competitive global market. Health insurance has been singled out as a significant factor in the cost of American-made products.

Under traditional indemnity (fee-for-service) insurance, physicians, hospitals, and other providers of care are paid for each procedure,

medication, piece of equipment, and supply item used in delivering patient care. Thus, the healthcare provider has incentives to use more services than may be appropriate or necessary for the care of a patient, a situation that both increases healthcare costs and potentially harms patients—for example, through the overuse of x-rays, the overuse of medications, or iatrogenic disease contracted in hospitals. In contrast, in a managed care environment, there may be a financial incentive to underutilize services, which may also cause harm to a patient.

Managed care aims to hold down the cost of health care (1) by ensuring that the services used for the patient's care are appropriate and necessary, (2) by eliminating services that are not necessary, and (3) by eliminating services of marginal value to patient care. Managed care uses pricing to control utilization. Although it uses a variety of pricing methods, the basis for each is to have a fixed price for necessary and appropriate services within a determined time frame.

In its attempts to control price, managed care focused first on hospitals, then on physicians, and finally on enrollees (consumers). Although managed care is not the originator of prospective pricing, it uses a variety of prospective pricing methods. The most common forms of price discounts are those based on usual and customary charges of individual providers. Hospitals and physicians alike may agree to a percentage discount of their usual and customary charges for a DRG or an office visit. UCR ("usual, customary, and reasonable") price discounts are established for a given service area. This requires a database for charges for each item or services from virtually all providers in a designated area. The charges are then arrayed, and a reasonable amount may be set at a certain level, such as the 75th percentile. Managed care also uses bundling of services. That is, managed care may pay a determined amount for a day in the hospital, which includes the pharmacy, laboratory, and other ancillary services. This is called a **per diem**.

Bundling is more complete when it is defined as an admission or discharge rather than a patient day (e.g., payment by DRG).

Physician payment systems under managed care include discounted fees; salaries, as in some HMO plans; and capitation. *Capitation,* simply put, is a defined payment amount **per member per month (PM/PM).** Payment to physicians under this method is independent of volume of services. The fewer services required by members, the greater the physician income. The inverse is also true: the greater the use of services, the smaller the income. Often, there is also a "withhold" if the physician does not meet utilization goals set by the plan. Finally, there may be bonus arrangements whereby physicians are awarded a bonus for not exceeding a referral threshold (Curtiss, 1989). These payment methods put physicians at financial risk, which means they lose money if they provide too many services to patients. Managed care hopes that by putting physicians at risk, they will determine what services are necessary and valuable and eliminate those services that are unnecessary and of marginal value (Ezekiel, 1995).

However, incentives such as capitation, "withholds," and bonus arrangements create a conflict of interest for physicians. Their economic interest, which is tied to clinical decision making, is pitted against maximizing benefit to patients. The greater the intensity of the incentives, the greater the impact on the physicians' clinical decision making. Further, the need for clinical and diagnostic interventions for a current patient may be pitted against the potential needs of the enrolled population. Pellegrino (1997) characterized this conflict as a conflict between the "responsibilities of the physician as a primary advocate of the patient and as a guardian of society's resources" (p. 324).

Managing price occurs not only through managing payment methods, but also through channeling (limiting care to a specified network of providers), benefit design (designating in advance which services will or will not be covered under particular plans), retrospective and concurrent utilization review, and case management, which reviews the current and future methods of care for patients, particularly those requiring intensive or extensive care. For example, in the early years of managed care, because inpatient hospitalization is typically the most expensive portion of healthcare services, managed care focused on limiting its use not only by obtaining discounted fees and charges from providers, but also by requiring preadmission review and authorization for hospitalization, by conducting utilization reviews, and by substituting, whenever possible, ambulatory for inpatient services.

Physicians have objected to many of these cost-lowering MCO strategies as challenging their role and capability to advocate for their patients. For example, utilization review involves the adoption of practice guidelines, or treatment protocols for certain diagnoses, that MCOs then expect physicians to use. Practice guidelines represent a standard of quality treatment for the average patient. One of their purposes is to limit utilization of costly procedures when they are not medically necessary. But sometimes the physician who is required by the MCO to adhere to a guideline may conclude that it is actually in the best interest of the patient to deviate from the guideline. In this situation, the physician may be unable to provide the care that he or she feels is in the patient's best interest (Eastman, Eastman, & Tolson, 1997).

Physicians are also extremely concerned when it appears that a treatment will be denied and they cannot reach a peer, such as the MCO medical director or physician designee, to confer with. When a treatment is denied, the physician can initiate the steps in the appeals process. However, the process is lengthy, consuming considerable time and effort. Physicians have not been trained to operate in this process and view it negatively, because it takes time away from the treatment of the patient in question as well as from their other patients (Mechanic & Schlesinger, 1996).

Access

In forming their panels of providers, MCOs have generally included primary care physicians who are conveniently located in the community so that geographic access has not been negatively affected. Members, however, balk at the limitation of their choice of providers. The same is generally true regarding hospitals and other providers.

The concern that many enrollees have is that their physicians may not be included on the panel of physicians. Then enrollees will need to find another physician and begin a new relationship with him or her. If the employer who sponsors the insurance benefits contracts with different insurance companies or different insurance products to decrease the company's cost whenever a contract period ends, the employee may once again need to find a new physician.

Such disruptions raise issues about how to ensure the continuity of patient information in a managed care system. Enrollees' frequent physician changes under such a system can make it very difficult to coordinate the documentation of a patient's medical history in one location. In fact, if patients move often between employers or managed care organizations, the task can be impossible. As a result, the documentation is fragmented, and those currently treating the patient do not have access to the historical health information.

Another concern regarding access is hidden from the consumer. It is tied to the financial incentive. Contracts may prevent physicians from referring to specialists who are outside the panel or within the panel but who are external to the primary care physician's group. These contracts may stipulate that all services, both primary and specialty care, must be paid within the capitation amount monthly provided to the physician group. These may become ethical issues, particularly if the quality of the provider is questionable or if the price of the premium for the family coverage is so high that the employee cannot pay for the insurance coverage.

Quality

Competence and diligence are integrally related to quality of healthcare services. A healthcare professional who is competent has skills to undertake the cure or care of the patient. That same professional exercises diligence when he or she takes the time needed to deliver the cure or care. Managed care may present professionals with conflicts between exercising competence and diligence and their own financial interests. For instance, under capitation or through deep discounts, the primary care physician (PCP) may feel pressure to see greater numbers of patients; as a result, the PCP devotes less time than required or may fail to order a test to rule out a more serious but less likely disease. Further, in a capitated system, a PCP may be pressured to keep a patient rather than refer the patient to a specialist. Competence may also become an issue for hospitals. In downsizing, for instance, hospitals may substitute other caregivers for nurses. These substitute workers may not be qualified to deliver the care previously provided by the registered nurse. The insurer's ethical obligation is to credential competent physicians and to be circumspect in payment systems so that competent professionals and providers are not bankrupted or do not leave the plan.

Quality, in any healthcare delivery system, is difficult to define and measure. One of the methods used by managed care to determine physician quality is *credentialing*. This is a process of checking physician qualifications, such as education, continuing education, licensure, board certification, fellowship, privileges, and reputation. The forms that the MCOs use are as varied as the number of managed care organizations and their insurance products. This is not an ethical problem as much as it is administratively inefficient for the physicians and hospitals. It can become an ethical issue, however, if the number of resources devoted to administrative work negatively affects the ability of the provider organization to employ caregivers needed for patient care services or if the very existence of providers (particularly those who traditionally serve the poor) is threatened.

A negative feature surrounding credentialing is the inclusion of *economic credentialing.* That is, if physicians consistently use too many resources, they undergo *deselection,* which means they are terminated as providers for this managed care product. There is controversy over whether use of resources is really an acceptable indicator for quality and thus for credentialing.

A method for regulating the quality of practice (and for controlling its costs, as mentioned earlier) is the use of practice guidelines. HMO critics often cite practice guidelines as instances of "cookbook" medicine.

One study showed that the chance of having a major surgical procedure varied significantly according to where the person lived (Wennberg, 1984). The variations seemed to be related to physician practice styles. The conclusion from this and other similar studies was that the scientific evidence to support medical practices may be lacking, ambiguous, or unheeded. Practice guidelines attempt to find the scientific basis for medical practice. However, medicine is as much an art as a science. The scientific findings need to be tempered with the input of practicing physicians.

The National Committee on Quality Assurance (NCQA) has developed a set of performance measures to help employers and plans to evaluate and trend health plan performance. The performance measures are included in a data set, the Health Plan Employer Data and Information Set (HEDIS). The five major areas of performance included in HEDIS are (1) quality of care, (2) access and patient satisfaction, (3) membership and utilization, (4) finance, and (5) descriptive information on health plan management. Steps such as the creation of HEDIS are important to define a core set of measures and then to systematize the measurement process. NCQA has recently developed an Internet-based Health Plan Report Card. It allows consumers to create a customized report that shows how well a specific MCO meets NCQA standards available at http://hprc.ncqa.org/index.asp. The process of developing quality measures is essential to enhancing the knowledge, measurement, and trending of quality in health plans.

Like fee-for-service plans, managed care is but a tool, method, or process; however, it differs from fee-for-service plans, because managed care integrates the financing and delivery of healthcare services. The opposing perspectives on managed care cited earlier in this chapter do not exhaust the reality of managed care. Many of the features of managed care have been absorbed into and have penetrated the healthcare provider and payer environment. This is particularly clear in those areas where managed care has had a significant market penetration for several years.

Managed care has provided the impetus for the development of integrated delivery systems (IDS). Although the number of integrated delivery systems as a total has declined over the last nine years, the number of highly integrated systems has nearly doubled. Highly integrated means vertically integrated systems with three or more delivery components plus a systemwide contract (Aventis Pharmaceuticals Inc., 2005). In 1995, there were 531 integrated systems and only 159 highly integrated systems. In 2003, there were 490 integrated systems and 311 highly integrated systems.

Integration consists of the following:

- Horizontal integration, which is the linking together of similar organizations, such as hospitals, to form a multiple-hospital system, or linking nursing homes to form a multiple–nursing home system. The goal is to enhance economies of scale and to develop greater purchasing power.
- Vertical integration, which is the linking together of organizations along the continuum of care, for instance, primary

care physicians, hospitals, long-term care organizations, outpatient organizations, home care, and hospice. The goal is to keep the patient population in one system for as many health-related needs as possible and to develop systemwide contracts with insurers.

- Integrated health systems (IHS) that include providers *and* payers who may compete with other systems for enrollees. In this situation, the IHS becomes both provider and payer.

The IHS has characteristics remarkably similar to those of an HMO. Both include the following: (1) a panel of primary care and specialty care physicians, (2) ownership of or contracts with hospitals for allocated beds, (3) enrollees and members who pay a fixed fee for predetermined services. In both arrangements, physicians may be salaried or capitated and, in some instances, paid on a discounted fee basis. HMOs undertake risk because they deliver services as providers at a fixed fee and not a la carte. An IHS also presents risks for both providers and payers.

Further, managed care has had a great influence on the healthcare field with its emphases on the following:

- Reduction of cost
- Cost-effectiveness of primary care
- Quality measures
- Practice guidelines
- Preventive care

Reduction of cost. The goal of cost reduction has not been reached, even though, until recently, there has been a reduction in the increase of the cost of healthcare services. The awareness of the high cost of healthcare services has increased as the population of the uninsured and underinsured has increased. Healthcare organizations have used a variety of strategies and tactics to reduce the cost of the delivery of services, including such methodologies as the familiar cutbacks as well as more novel approaches, such as activity-based cost accounting.

Primary Care. Managed care has emphasized the importance of a single primary care physician to direct and coordinate health services. This has led to medical schools placing more emphasis on primary care by developing family practice specialties and emphasizing general internal medicine and pediatrics.

Quality Measures. Managed care has emphasized that the quality of health services can be measured. The new information systems are an essential ingredient in the quest for quality measures. Reports can be generated using standardized data sets, such as the HEDIS format. Through the use of the electronic health record (EHR) and computerized physician order entry (CPOE), more accurate and measurable quality and utilization data can be developed and used both by insurers and providers.

Practice Guidelines. In *Evidence-Based Medicine, How to Practice and Teach E.B.M.*, D. L. Sackett and his co-authors define clinical practice guidelines as "A systemically developed statement designed to assist clinician and patient decisions about appropriate health care for special clinical circumstances" (Sackett, Straus, Richardson, Rosenberg, & Haynes, 2000, p. 245). Practice guidelines are not necessarily cookbook medicine. They should be based on (1) practice questions, (2) best evidence from systematic reviews of all relevant worldwide literature about diagnosis, prognosis, therapy, and harm, and (3) decision points where this evidence can be added to the physician's individual clinical judgment (Sackett et al., 2000). Practice guidelines, within these parameters, should assist physicians to provide care based on the best knowledge in the medical community, which is, at the same time, combined with the best overall interests of the patient.

Preventive Care. Managed care has emphasized that preventive care in the long term can reduce the utilization of subsequent costly acute care. However, currently, it is difficult to measure the cost-effectiveness of preventive care with the turnover of insurance products and/or insurance through employer contracting.

These five elements will continue to influence the delivery and financing of healthcare services. The medium for these elements is the electronic information system.

THE ROLE OF INFORMATION AND HIM PROFESSIONALS IN A MANAGED CARE ENVIRONMENT

Early managed care focused on cost reduction through utilization review, second opinions, and discounted fee for service (as it still does). As the market matures, it has become clear that the gains from these strategies will plateau and that managing healthcare costs will increasingly depend on the collection and analysis of information—on individual patients/consumers, clinicians, and healthcare organizations. Both the payer (employer and insurer) and the provider have a stake in obtaining this information. For instance, from a payer (employer and insurer) perspective, it is essential to have access to information about the practice patterns of physicians and the cost-effectiveness of hospitals and other facilities so that unnecessary and inappropriate services are not utilized. From this information base, the employer/insurer selects or deselects providers. It is equally important for physicians and institutions to have access to this information (1) to develop strategies and actions to become more efficient and to continue to deliver quality care and (2) to negotiate contracts with MCOs.

Further, from a provider and a payer perspective, information about the health status of current and prospective members is also essential. Managing cost depends on managing utilization, which in turn depends on (1) selecting a healthy population that will not use so many healthcare services and (2) obtaining information about the health status of the prospective and current enrollees so that projections about future costs of care can be made and appropriate projections for premium payments can be calculated.

Still another category of information is that required for the purposes of benchmarking, developing practice guidelines, measuring outcomes measures, and tracking patient health status. All of these are very important for the delivery of efficient, quality care.

Finally, all this information must be integrated across episodes of care, sites of care, and a variety of professionals. For this reason, it is clear that the electronic information network and information systems and technology will become more and more central to managed care efforts both to reduce costs and to enhance quality.

HIM professionals will play a crucial role in these developments. They provide accurate data so that administrators can make effective choices. They understand that the data that are made available can make or break an organization. They know the full data system, from clinical care to coding to flows of information. Often, information technology experts act as if they understand what is in the computerized databases when in fact they do not. HIM professionals must constantly teach others what the data really mean through data-mining activities and interpretation of reports.

The increased sophistication of EHR and the continued standardization of reporting will increase the ability of healthcare providers to produce quality care at cost-effective and cost-efficient prices. The complexity of these changes increases the critical importance of the HIM professional. HIM professionals deal constantly with questions of access to information—both access to patient or provider information by other parties and patient access to information that they require in order to give informed consent to their care or their choice of insurance plan. Consequently, HIM professionals are also at the center of ethical dilemmas regarding these questions in a managed care environment. These dilemmas will be discussed next.

ETHICAL DILEMMAS FOR HIM PROFESSIONALS

Limiting Access to Information by Managed Care Organizations

As healthcare has increasingly come to emphasize the participation of patients in their own care, it has become clear that the more information patients have, the more easily they can plan and make decisions. In Scenario 9-A, Alice did not know the financial limitations on her and on the group practice by looking at the panel of physicians. If she had had that information, she might have made a different decision not only about her choice of plan, but also about which physician to choose within the plan.

As discussed earlier, many aspects of provider–MCO contracts can have a bearing on the care that a patient receives, particularly when they tie physicians' financial interest to their clinical decision making, but enrollees to MCO plans seldom know anything about these arrangements. Nor do they know about other strategies that their MCO is using to hold down costs, such as requirements limiting treatment, requirements to replace one therapy with another that is less expensive, economic credentialing of their physicians, quality assurance measures, and utilization review procedures. In fact, some MCOs include confidentiality clauses in their contracts with providers that prohibit physicians from discussing such MCO-related business matters or from making statements to patients that would undermine the patient's confidence in the MCO. They may also prohibit physicians from making any suggestions to patients about the MCO or MCO plan that might be best for them. Confidentiality clauses are just one set of clauses in a larger group of what are called "gag rules" that restrict what information physicians can tell their patients. Some of these gag rules prohibit physicians from discussing treatment options with patients until the plan approves payment for an option; others prohibit physi-

cians from referring patients to physicians either inside or outside the plan for services that the plan does not offer and from charging a patient for a service that the plan does not cover, even if the physician deems it necessary and the patient wants it. Physicians who ignore gag rules requirements risk being deselected by the plan.

Gag rules have attracted a great deal of controversy in recent years. Critics have pointed out that these rules interfere with physicians' carrying out their responsibilities to patients; violate the physician–patient trust relationship, because patients expect physicians to give them the kind of information prohibited by the rules; and force physicians to withhold from patients the information that they need to make an informed decision. For all these reasons, in 1995–1996 legislation prohibiting gag rules with or without sanctions was proposed in 33 states; 18 states adopted legislation. The state laws vary, with some prohibiting gag rules and providing sanctions and others simply prohibiting them (Miller, 1997).

Just what obligation do MCOs have to provide information regarding their resource policies to consumers? It has been persuasively argued that insurers in a managed care environment assume special professional obligations toward the patients whose care they pay for and oversee. A professional–client relationship, such as a physician–patient relationship, is a fiduciary relationship. That is, it is one in which the professional's superior knowledge is recognized but the client retains significant authority and responsibility in decision making (Bayles, 1989). Such a relationship is based on the mutual respect that each party has for the other. The ultimate principle upon which this relationship relies is the principle of respect for persons. The more proximate principle is the principle of respect for persons' autonomy.

In this relationship, the client (patient) trusts the professional (physician) to analyze a situation correctly, present feasible alternatives and their likely consequences, present this information to the client, make a recommendation, and then work with the client to effect the chosen alternative. In this relationship, the client assumes that the professional is competent and that the information provided is correct and sufficient within reason. Generally, the client does not determine what the options are, but consents to or rejects an option provided. The client relies on the superior knowledge of the professional and on the professional's ability to communicate needed information intelligibly. In a physician–patient relationship, the patient's self-determination is protected, although the patient does not make the decisions regarding what the feasible options are. Self-determination is protected through the adequacy and intelligibility of information presented and through the patient's free (uncoerced) and voluntary consent or dissent; that is, through informed consent. Informed consent is a mechanism, a protection, for self-determination.

This model has worked well in one-to-one relationships in medicine, law, engineering, and accounting between the professional and the individual client. However, health care has become more complicated. In the past, the delivery of services and the payment for services were entirely separate: Physicians determined what medical and hospital services were to be used and the insurer or the individual paid for the services. Under managed care, the delivery and financing of services are intertwined. The insurers/payers are determining the services covered, the services appropriate to specific conditions, the location of services provided, and the providers of services. The covered and appropriate services provided by designated physicians, hospitals, and so forth will be paid by the insurer, either totally or after deductibles and copayments, and other services provided outside the limits of the plan will not. Given the role assumed by insurers in developing the plans, it appears that insurers have assumed the role of the professional in the professional–patient relationship.

What are the implications of this conclusion? Upon assuming the role of the professional in a professional–client relationship, the insurer becomes bound by the same responsibilities (as well as having the same rights) as the individual professional in a fiduciary relationship. As far as the provision of information is concerned, these obligations include candor and loyalty to the client.

The value of candor requires full disclosure of information, particularly when the information relates to the client's values. In a fee-for-service environment, the patient relies on the physician to provide the needed information for decision making. But in a managed care environment, candor can be fulfilled only by eliminating all kinds of gag clauses and by providing the necessary information to the potential client (enrollee) at the time that the potential enrollee decides to contract with a designated insurer. This information includes a clear and complete explanation of benefits, of the advocacy process, and of reimbursement systems.

Conflicts of interest are the most common problem related to loyalty. A significant conflict of interest occurs in any profession between the professional's interest in accruing income and the client's interest in services. It is impossible to remove all conflicts of interest in a professional relationship. However, it is essential to minimize them to retain trust. If MCOs are to be loyal to their enrollees, then they must first give them the information concerning potential conflicts of interest—for example, in their payment systems; for-profit MCOs should publish their dividend goals and disbursement of income so that their enrollees are aware of the proportionality between administrative and healthcare costs. This is particularly important in a for-profit situation, because corporate interests in profitability can lead to lack of concern for client services.

Where MCOs do not give out critical information for patients concerning their care, the responsibility for doing this falls on the provider. Consequently, if the MCO does not reveal its method of physician payment, then the physician should inform patients. This can be done with a simple explanation in a one-page document that emphasizes the physicians' loyalty to patients. The document can state that the practice is required to live within the MCO's guidelines, but it can also promise that if the rules conflict with needed patient care, the physician will become a patient advocate with the MCO.

Scenario 9-B: Provision of Information by Physician Practices

When Alice (see Scenario 9-A) asks Dr. Smith to refer her to her cardiologist, he is placed in a very awkward situation. Should he tell Alice that he will refer her only to a specialist in his own group because his group's contract with the MCO makes it difficult for him to refer outside his group for specialty care? Should he insist that Alice see his group's cardiologist? He ends up strongly recommending that Alice see his group's cardiologist, Dr. Sanford, for reasons having to do with professional experience and quality of care. In fact, he has no reason to believe that Dr. Sanford is better equipped to deal with Alice's case than Alice's own cardiologist. He makes the referral for financial reasons. Alice agrees to the in-group referral, but Dr. Smith feels ethically compromised as a result and uneasy enough to bring up the matter the next day with Dr. Osgood, the head of the group practice.

Dr. Smith's story leads Dr. Osgood to propose a plan that he has been thinking about for quite some time. He feels that it would be a novel idea to hire an HIM professional to provide information about the patient population to the physicians, such as data that indicate major diagnostic groups or common procedures performed. This is something Dr. Osgood did not have during his lifetime as a physician, when HIM professionals were mostly employed by hospitals, but he knows that those days are over and that the members of his practice will need the expertise of the HIM professional in the ambulatory setting.

Questions

1. You are an HIM professional considering the position that Dr. Osgood is offering. What kinds of information might you include about the practice's patient population?

2. What impact do you think the information will have on patient care?

A completed ethical decision-making matrix for the scenario is provided at the end of the chapter.

Access to Information about Patients

In 1982, Mark Siegler, a physician and ethicist, responded to a patient's privacy concern by counting those health professionals and hospital personnel who had authorized access to the patient's medical record. He came up with the number of 75—and this was in a predominantly paper environment. Now, with the transition to an electronic environment, much more information on patients is gathered, stored, replicated, transmitted, and analyzed, and the number of health professionals, support personnel, and administrative personnel who have gained access to patients' records has increased exponentially.

Now this information is used not only for patient care, but also for claims, billing, marketing, cost reports, quality assurance and improvement, utilization review, and a multitude of administrative reports.

Despite the anticipated benefits of the electronic information system infrastructure, there is significant public concern regarding the privacy and confidentiality of personally identifiable patient information. These concerns have been amply identified both anecdotally in popular newspapers and magazines as well as in well-documented studies (Harris & Westin, 1993; Donaldson & Lohr, 1994). Simply stated, there are concerns that personally identifiable patient information may be (1) inaccurate, (2) accessed by unauthorized persons, and (3) used by authorized or unauthorized persons for negative or undesired reasons, such as marketing (Schick, 1996). HIM professionals, whether working for MCOs or for providers, must address these concerns.

HIM Professionals in MCOs

In a managed care context, the insurer becomes bound by the same responsibilities to the patient as the individual professional in a fiduciary relationship. As far as the access to the patient's information is concerned, insurers, and the HIM professionals who work for them, have the obligation to exercise discretion. Like physicians, they have the responsibility not to reveal the information that they obtain from the patient unless it is in the patient's best interest.

From the claims presented to them over many years, insurers have collected an immense amount of information about the insured. Patient claims data can be used with other data to build profiles of enrollee populations. Because insurance covers risk and risk is dependent on the health characteristics of the population covered, the more information about this population, the more closely the insurer can estimate the use of services and the cost of services. These estimates can be achieved without identifying the individuals in the enrolled population.

But what about personally identifiable patient data? Clearly, insurers require information related to payment of claims. But, like other professionals, they should use it only for the purpose for which it was acquired. Positive uses would be to develop programs to educate consumers about their preconditions or diseases and to educate physicians about services for these patients.

But then there are the more problematic uses. One is the use of personally identifiable patient information to deny coverage to certain individuals or to charge them higher rates. Another is the sharing or sale of this information to other businesses. Still another is the release of personally identifiable medical information, without the patient's knowledge or consent, to employers who are self-insured or, for MCOs acting as third-party administrators, the release of this information to employers who may or may not be self-insured. This last is a common practice, but it would be unwise to place the responsibility for it on the insurance industry alone. Insurers often react positively to employer demands, because employers are key customers for them. Because large employers are self-insured and exempt from ERISA, insurance companies that act as third-party administrators answer information requests from these employers without question.

Employers demand that health care be delivered at a low cost. One way that employers can keep costs under control is to gain access to individually identifiable patient information. With this information, they can (1) identify who might be an expensive enrollee in the long run, (2) target the expensive enrollee for job loss or not to promote him or her so that the employee might leave, or (3) develop limits on benefits or redesign the benefits package. Harris and Westin's (1993) survey and the Institute of Medicine study by Donaldson and Lohr (1994) show that consumers are very much concerned about these possibilities.

Scenario 9-C: HIM Professionals in Provider Organizations

Beth Blank is the medical records director for Community Hospital. The employees of the department are constantly busy processing medical records, collecting information sent by other providers by fax, and handling walk-in and telephone requests. Beth has just received a request from an MCO to fax a patient's entire medical record (it is two volumes in size). Beth refuses the request because she does not have a signed authorization from the patient. She also tells the MCO representative that she is not authorized to copy the entire medical record. The MCO clerk becomes upset and shouts into the telephone, "The previous clerk always sent the information without question."

If Beth does not comply with the demands of the MCO, payments to the hospital will be slowed, withheld, and eventually denied. The hospital administrator has been very supportive, but Beth knows that if she persists, the hospital may lose the contract. The CEO seems to be wavering in his support and is now telling Beth to "just send the records."

Questions

1. What are the ethical issues? What arguments could be made for Beth's decision to refuse the MCO's request?

2. How can Beth both protect patient privacy and help sustain the hospital's financial stability?

3. With whom should Beth discuss this problem?

A completed ethical decision-making matrix for the scenario is provided at the end of the chapter.

Healthcare providers, and consequently the HIM professionals who work for them, encounter conflicts of interest when MCOs demand personally identifiable patient information beyond claims information. For instance, it is not unusual for an MCO to require parts of or entire individual patient records without patient consent. Forms requesting information or entire medical records are sent without patient signatures or requests are made by clerks via telephone or e-mail. Of course, MCOs may claim that enrollees have agreed to the transmission of their information to the MCO at the time of enrollment. But many consumers and ethicists maintain that this is not free, informed

consent, but rather coerced consent. It is coerced because there is no other avenue for insurance for most employees and their dependents.

The HIM professional in this kind of situation is in an awkward position of trying to adhere to ethical guidelines regarding patient privacy while at the same time trying to balance the good of the institution. Without the patient information, the MCO will refuse to make payments to the provider.

HIM professionals who work for hospitals may encounter another confidentiality issue related to MCOs as well. Case managers who are employees of the MCO regularly visit hospital units to audit medical records. Often, they do not check in with the appropriate hospital officer to do so. The MCO assumption is that the patient has provided prior consent when enrolling in the plan. The HIM professional may be additionally concerned because the case manager, as an employee of the MCO, is biased toward the MCO, and is therefore not primarily concerned with the well-being of the patient.

POLICIES FOR WHICH THE HIM PROFESSIONAL CAN ADVOCATE

Clearly, some of the ethical dilemmas faced by HIM professionals in a managed care environment cannot be resolved at the individual level; they will require systemic change. How can we evolve an ethically acceptable healthcare system from this patchwork, evolving health system? What are some policies for which the HIM professional can advocate?

Managed Care Plans

First, MCOs and providers of all kinds should collaboratively examine the payment systems currently used and devise a system that separates payment and clinical treatment insofar as possible. This, in itself, will help eliminate some of the conflicts of interest related to income versus patient interest that providers experience. Although these conflicts cannot be totally eliminated, they can be mitigated. From an ethical perspective, capitation (when calculated based on a community's health) can be a better payment system than most of the current systems based on discounting and utilization or clinical management. In a capitated system, there is no need for the payer to have personally identifiable health information. Consequently, the pressure on medical records departments is relieved.

Bonus arrangements can also be designed that minimize clinical decision making by lengthening the payment periods and by spreading the payment over larger groups of enrolled populations in larger physician group practices. This is a contractual issue.

Second, incentives are usually aimed at the provider of service, such as the physician.

In a true partnership, the enrollee/patient should be an equal partner. In a managed care contract, usually physicians alone have incentives; enrollees do not. Morreim (1995) has suggested that enrollees have incentives such as points or dollars for following treatments or recommendations, such as stopping smoking or losing weight. This information can be stored in the patient record. The payer does not need to know this information in a capitated system. The provider remains at risk in this situation, but clinical autonomy is not challenged.

Third, in a managed care environment, the familiar term *alignment,* which usually refers to aligning the interests of managed care plans and providers, should be extended to include subscribers to the plan. Currently, subscribers are removed from the important resource allocation decisions that affect them. And physicians on the panel of physician providers are placed in conflict situations that threaten their fiduciary obligations of loyalty and honesty. Both problems can be resolved in the short term and in the longer term. In the short term, MCOs must fully inform subscribers about their resource policies, including incentive systems, and other controls, such as therapeutic substitution requirements and limitations of treatment. In the long term, MCOs must bring subscribers into decision making at the policy level by representing the enrolled population on boards of directors and boards of trustees. This is not an unusual requirement. In the past, federally qualified HMOs were required to have consumers on their boards.

Provider Organizations

Provider organizations must install electronic information systems that have security measures that protect patient privacy and confidentiality. Beyond the appropriate technology, they must (1) develop policies and procedures related to privacy, (2) empower HIM professionals and all managers to implement them, (3) provide orientation and continuing education regarding privacy and confidentiality for their staffs, and (4) ensure that executives and managers model the behavior that they expect their organizations to exhibit.

CONCLUSION

Developing an ethically acceptable framework for financing and delivering quality health care while at the same time protecting privacy and confidentiality of personally identifiable information is no easy task; however, it is possible. The ethical principle of respect for persons, and specifically of respect for autonomy, supports both candor in revealing managed care financial arrangements and care restrictions and discretion in guarding the privacy and confidentiality of

patients' health information. Efforts to deliver quality health care at an affordable price must be balanced by policies that address the numerous ethical concerns that managed care has raised. Our society has only begun this process.

Key Terms

- Health maintenance organization (HMO)
- Indemnity (or fee-for-service) insurance
- Independent practice association (IPA)
- Managed care
- Per diem
- Per member per month (PM/PM)
- Point-of-service (POS) plan
- Preferred provider organization (PPO)

Chapter Summary

- Managed care attempts to deliver accessible quality health care at an affordable price, primarily by controlling utilization through fixed prospective payment systems, financial incentives to providers, benefit design, channeling of care to a specified network of providers, utilization review, and case management.
- In the managed care system, keeping health care costs down, for both payers and providers, is increasingly depending on the collection, analysis, and integration of information—on individual patients/consumers, clinicians, and healthcare organizations. HIM professionals are increasingly playing a major role in fulfilling these information needs.
- HIM professionals deal constantly with questions of access to information—both access to patient or provider information by other parties and patients' access to information that they require in order to give informed consent to their care and to their insurance plans. Consequently, HIM professionals are at the center of ethical dilemmas regarding these questions in a managed care environment.
- Many aspects of provider–MCO contracts can have a bearing on the care that a patient receives, particularly when they tie physicians' financial interest to their clinical decision making. Enrollees to MCO plans seldom know anything about these arrangements or treatment limitations, required therapeutic substitutions, economic credentialing of their physicians, quality assurance measures, and utilization review procedures. In fact, in some states, MCOs are allowed to prohibit physicians from discussing these matters with their patients or from discussing treatments and referrals that the insurance plan will not cover. HIM professionals working for providers or insurers may be involved in developing informative materials for patients regarding insurance plan business arrangements and business procedures.

- Ethical issues involving access to information about patients include the use of personally identifiable patient information to deny coverage to certain individuals or to charge them higher rates; the sharing or sale of this information to other businesses; and the release of personally identifiable medical information, without the patient's knowledge or consent, to employers who are self-insured or, for MCOs acting as third-party administrators, the release of this information to employers who may or may not be self-insured. In provider organizations, HIM professionals may encounter MCO demands for excessive and unauthorized patient information.
- Systemic changes are necessary to support ethical practice in a managed care environment. Some of the changes for which an HIM professional might advocate are a capitated payment system rather than one based on discounting and utilization or clinical management so that there is no need for the payer to have personally identifiable health information; bonus arrangements that minimize clinical decision making by lengthening the payment periods and by spreading the payment over larger groups of enrolled populations in larger physician group practices; the legal prohibition of "gag rules"; insurer and provider policies of fully informing patients/consumers about insurer resource policies and business arrangements; and the representation of consumers on MCOs' boards of directors and boards of trustees.

References

Aventis Pharmaceuticals Inc. (2005). *Managed Care Digest Series*. Retrieved September 15, 2005, from http://www.managedcaredigest.com/index.jsp.

Bayles, M. D. (1989). *Professional ethics*, 2d ed. Belmont, CA: Wadsworth.

Curtiss, F. (1989). Managed health care: Managed costs. *Personnel Journal, 68*(6), 72–85.

Donaldson, M., & Lohr, K. (Eds.). (1994). *Health data in the information age*. Washington, DC: National Academy Press.

Dranove, D., Simon, C. J., & White, W. D. (1998). Determinants of managed care penetration. *Journal of Health Economics, 17,* 729–745.

Eastman, J. K., Eastman, K. L., & Tolson, M. A. (1997). The ethics of managed care. *Marketing Health Services, 17*(3), 26–39.

Ezekiel, E. (1995). Medical ethics in the era of managed care: The need for institutional structures instead of principles for individual case. *Journal of Clinical Ethics, 6*(4), 335–338.

Harris, L., & Westin, A. (1993). *Health information privacy survey 1993*. New York: Louis Harris & Associates.

Knight, W. (1998). *Managed care: What it is and how it works*. Gaithersburg, MD: Aspen.

Mechanic, D., & Schlesinger, M. (1996). The impact of managed care on patients' trust in medical care and their physicians. *Journal of the American Medical Association, 275,* 1693–1695.

Miller, T. E. (1997). Managed care regulations: The laboratory of the states. *Journal of the American Medical Association, 278,* 1102–1108.

Morreim, E. H. (1995). *Balancing act: The new medical ethics of medicine's new economics*. Washington, DC: Georgetown University Press.

Pellegrino, E. (1997). Managed care at the bedside: How do we look in the moral mirror? *Kennedy Institute of Ethics Journal, 74,* 321–330.

Sackett, D. L., Straus, S. E., Richardson, W. S., Rosenberg, W., & Haynes, R. B. (2000). *Evidence-based medicine. How to practice and teach E.B.M.* Edinburgh: Churchill Livingstone.

Schick, I. C. (1996). Personal privacy and confidentiality in an electronic environment. *Bioethics Forum, 12*(1), 25–30.

Siegler, M. (1982) Confidentiality in medicine—a decrepit concept. *New England Journal of Medicine, 307*(24), 518–521.

VHA and Deloitte and Touche. (1999). *Environmental assessment 1999: Rising to the challenge of a new century*. Irvine, TX.

Wennberg, J. (1984). Dealing with medical practice variations: A proposal for action. *Health Affairs, 3*(15), 6–32.

The ethical decision-making matrix is a tool to help you organize complex, ethical problems; however, there is no simple fill-in-the-box approach to ethical decision making. The objective is to follow each step of the process and not move from the question directly to what should be done or how to prevent it next time. If you skip steps, you will not fully understand all of the values and options for action. Also, the matrix provided for each scenario in this book is not the only way to examine the problem. You can make an equally compelling ethical argument for a different decision—just be sure to follow all the steps of the matrix.

SCENARIO 9-A: COMPLEXITY OF CHOOSING A MANAGED CARE PLAN

Steps	Information	
1. What is the ethical question?	Should the HIM professional ensure that the MCO provides full disclosure to its enrollees?	
2. What are the facts?	**KNOWN**	**TO BE GATHERED**
	• The MCO offers a variety of plans and the employer has selected several from which employees may choose. • MCOs can be somewhat selective about the information they provide enrollees.	• Could the MCO be affected adversely by full disclosure to enrollees? • Could enrollees be affected adversely by a lack of full disclosure from the MCO? • Would withholding some plan information from enrollees constitute fraud? • What are the customary practices in such cases? • What does your supervisor expect you to do? • What is the likely impact on self and family of changing jobs?
3. What are the values? Examine the shared and competing values, obligations, and interests of the stakeholders (i.e., patient, HIM professional, healthcare practitioner(s), administrators, society, and other advocates) involved in order to fully understand the complexity of the ethical problem(s).	**Patient:** Interest in receiving high-quality health care; interest in controlling healthcare costs. **HIM professional:** Truth, integrity, accuracy (provide enrollees with appropriate and adequate information regarding coverage plans); avoid harm (inappropriate coverage plan selection could result in patient frustration or harm); full disclosure could encourage enrollees to select more expensive plans, resulting in a financial loss for the MCO; personal values (promote welfare of self and family by avoiding loss of job). **Healthcare professionals:** Promote welfare of patients by being allowed to discuss all appropriate treatment options; interest in protecting institution from financial loss. **Administrators:** Benefit patients and provide with adequate health care; control healthcare costs. **Society:** Control costs.	

4. What are my options?	• Provide enrollees with limited information on plans. • Allow for full disclosure of plan information to enrollees.	
5. What should I do?	Allow for full disclosure of plan information to enrollees.	
6. What justifies my choice?	**JUSTIFIED**	**NOT JUSTIFIED**
	• Obligation to ensure that enrollees have access to appropriate care. • Preserve professional integrity. • Demonstrate loyalty to employer, as well as fairness to enrollees.	• Provide enrollees with limited information on plans. • Jeopardize professional integrity. • Enrollees do not select appropriate plans and cannot receive appropriate treatment.
7. How can I prevent this ethical problem?	• Determine if system changes are needed. • Learn more about disclosure in the managed care environment. • Discuss standards and the values that support them with colleagues. • Evaluate institutional integrity at job interview and subsequently when ethical problems arise.	

The ethical decision-making matrix is a tool to help you organize complex, ethical problems; however, there is no simple fill-in-the-box approach to ethical decision making. The objective is to follow each step of the process and not move from the question directly to what should be done or how to prevent it next time. If you skip steps, you will not fully understand all of the values and options for action. Also, the matrix provided for each scenario in this book is not the only way to examine the problem. You can make an equally compelling ethical argument for a different decision—just be sure to follow all the steps of the matrix.

SCENARIO 9-B: PROVISION OF INFORMATION BY PHYSICIAN PRACTICES

Steps	Information	
1. What is the ethical? questions?	Should you discuss potential conflicts between obeying MCO policies and providing good patient care?	
2. What are the facts?	**KNOWN**	**TO BE GATHERED**
	• In some cases, decisions doctors make for the sake of patient care compromise the practice financially. • MCO policies are designed to maximize cost effectiveness without jeopardizing patient care.	• What are the customary practices when discussing conflicts between MCO policies and patient care? • What does your supervisor expect you to do? • What is the likely impact on self and family of changing jobs?
3. What are the values? Examine the shared and competing values, obligations, and interests of the stakeholders (i.e., patient, HIM professional, healthcare practitioner(s), administrators, society, and other advocates) involved in order to fully understand the complexity of the ethical problem(s).	**Patient:** Values appropriate care; interest in controlling healthcare costs. **HIM professional:** Truth, integrity, and accuracy (obligation to provide complete and accurate information on plan benefits); loyalty to employer; avoid harm (opting for MCO-recommended services may negatively affect patient care); disobeying MCO recommendations may have a negative financial impact on practice. **Healthcare professionals:** Promote welfare of patients through provision of appropriate care; interest in financial success of practice. **Administrators:** Benefit patients and keep from harm; interest in financial viability of MCO and control of healthcare costs. **Society:** Control costs.	

4. What are my options?	• Encourage physicians to opt for MCO-recommended treatments in all instances. • Encourage physicians to opt for MCO-recommended treatments when appropriate, but to put patient care above MCO policies.
5. What should I do?	Encourage physicians to opt for MCO-recommended treatments when appropriate, but to put patient care above MCO policies.

6. What justifies my choice?	JUSTIFIED	NOT JUSTIFIED
	• Obligation to support full disclosure. • Preserve professional integrity. • Demonstrate loyalty to employer and patients.	• Encourage physicians to opt for MCO-recommended treatments in all instances. • Jeopardize professional integrity. • Jeopardize quality and appropriateness of patient care.

7. How can I prevent this ethical problem?	• Determine if system changes are needed. • Learn more about disclosure in the managed care environment. • Discuss standards and the values that support them with colleagues. • Evaluate institutional integrity at job interview and subsequently when ethical problems arise.

The ethical decision-making matrix is a tool to help you organize complex, ethical problems; however, there is no simple fill-in-the-box approach to ethical decision making. The objective is to follow each step of the process and not move from the question directly to what should be done or how to prevent it next time. If you skip steps, you will not fully understand all of the values and options for action. Also, the matrix provided for each scenario in this book is not the only way to examine the problem. You can make an equally compelling ethical argument for a different decision—just be sure to follow all the steps of the matrix.

SCENARIO 9-C: HIM PROFESSIONALS IN PROVIDER ORGANIZATIONS

Steps	Information	
1. What is the ethical question?	Should Beth send the records to the MCO?	
2. What are the facts?	**KNOWN**	**TO BE GATHERED**
	• The MCO has requested the entire medical record. • Beth does not have a signed authorization from the patient.	• Can a signed authorization be obtained? • Would sending the records violate confidentiality? • What are the customary practices in such cases? • What is the likely impact on self and family of changing jobs?
3. What are the values? Examine the shared and competing values, obligations, and interests of the stakeholders (i.e., patient, HIM professional, healthcare practitioner(s), administrators, society, and other advocates) involved in order to fully understand the complexity of the ethical problem(s).	**Patient:** Values confidentiality and privacy; interest in efficient processing of insurance claims. **HIM professional:** Integrity and reliability (expedite claims processing without violating patient's confidentiality); fairness (follow the rules and obey the law); avoid harm (denial of claims could cause financial harm to the hospital and its workers and their families); personal integrity (promote welfare of self and family by avoiding loss of job). **Healthcare professionals:** Interest in preservation of confidentiality of medical records; interest in welfare of hospital. **Administrators:** Benefit patients and protect rights; promote welfare of facility; ensure expeditious processing of healthcare claims. **Society:** Promote preservation of confidentiality and privacy.	

4. What are my options?	• Release the records. • Do not release the records.	
5. What should I do?	If patient authorization cannot be obtained, do not release the records.	
6. What justifies my choice?	**JUSTIFIED**	**NOT JUSTIFIED**
	• Support confidentiality of the medical record. • Preserve professional integrity. • Respect the law. • Demonstrate loyalty to employer, unless asked to push legal boundaries.	• Release the records without patient authorization. • Violate confidentiality. • Break the law. • Jeopardize professional integrity.
7. How can I prevent this ethical problem?	• Determine if system changes are needed. • Learn more about laws regarding confidentiality and right to privacy. • Discuss standards and the values that support them with colleagues. • Evaluate institutional integrity at job interview and subsequently when ethical problems arise.	

CLINICAL CARE: END OF LIFE

James F. Tischler, MD

Abstract

Advances in medical care have added years to the life expectancy of individuals with serious chronic and terminal illnesses. These years may be associated with significant frailty, which often requires patients and their healthcare providers to make difficult treatment decisions. This chapter presents the role of information exchange in scenarios commonly encountered in today's healthcare systems. These scenarios portray the impact of information exchange on patient autonomy and the manner in which information exchange reflects a healthcare provider's sense of beneficence. They also reveal the challenges healthcare providers face as they address sensitive topics in an effort to support their patients across a tenuous healthcare continuum.

Scenario 10-A: Bad News

Mr. Smith is 62-year-old man who has just retired from a very successful grocery business. He started the business as a young man and invested many long hours, rarely taking vacations and often sacrificing time with his wife and children. Over the last month, he has experienced nausea and abdominal pain and has lost 10 pounds. He makes an appointment with his primary care physician, whose physical examination detects a large mass in the upper abdomen. The physician recommends that a CAT scan be performed the next day. It indicates that the mass arises from the stomach and is probably a gastric carcinoma.

The physician schedules Mr. Smith for an appointment for the following day, but receives a telephone call from Mrs. Smith urging the physician not to tell her husband the diagnosis, if it is one with a poor prognosis. The physician documents his conversation with Mrs. Smith in the medical record, indicating, "the standard of practice is to fully inform a patient, and that informed consent for subsequent testing and treatment will require Mr. Smith's understanding of the diagnosis. However, Mrs. Smith has told me that she and her husband have 'waited all their lives for the opportunity to enjoy his retirement, and that hearing bad news will kill him.' "

Questions

1. Should the physician inform Mr. Smith of his diagnosis and potentially poor prognosis?

2. Should he respect Mrs. Smith's request?

3. What is the standard of practice? What are the prevailing laws?

4. What ethical principles guide the physician's choice?

A completed ethical decision-making matrix for the scenario is provided at the end of the chapter.

AGING, FRAILTY, AND INFORMATION ETHICS

When people face illnesses that place their independence and their lives at risk, the importance of information sharing becomes critical. Patients' understanding of the diseases they are facing, their confidence and trust in healthcare professionals, their choice of treatments, their movement through the healthcare continuum, and the support they receive from personal and organizational communities all depend on timely, accurate, and comprehensive information exchange.

As is true in any important interpersonal process, it is probable that difficult decision points will be reached in such information exchange. Healthcare professionals, their patients, and their patients' families are likely to find that they must make difficult choices, including difficult choices about the sharing of information. Ethical principles such as autonomy, justice, beneficence, and equity can guide us through these decision points, but, as is true with many difficult decisions, there may not always be an unequivocally correct choice or one agreed upon by all, which is why ethical decision making, taking into account the competing interests of all of the stake-holders, is necessary.

EVOLUTION OF AUTONOMY

Over the past century, the average life span in the United States has increased from fewer than 60 years to just below 80 years. This has occurred in concert with the development of technologies that have allowed physicians to more accurately diagnose diseases and offer their patients a broad array of treatment choices. At the same time, the provision of care for **serious, chronic,** and **terminal illnesses** has moved out of the home and into institutional settings, distancing the community from the everyday impact of these illnesses. However, the end of the twentieth century saw a reversal of this trend (HCFA, 2001).

Physician practice has evolved as well. To meet the expectations of an American public that anticipates accurate diagnoses, effective treatment, and long survival, physicians have shifted the standard of practice to one of open information exchange. That openness has also evolved into more explicit and precise information. A vague phrase such as "you have a *growth*" has been supplanted by "you have a *tumor*," which has been supplanted by "you have *cancer*." At a time when patients can get very detailed information over the Internet, physicians are often challenged to provide even more detailed diagnostic information, such as the cell type and stage of the cancer.

This standard of practice has also been expressed in regulations that not only require physicians to be open in their communications, but also to ensure that their patients understand what they are being told. The guiding ethical principle behind this expectation is *autonomy,* which holds that an individual should be given the opportunity for self-determination. As Mr. Smith's physician indicated in the opening scenario, Mr. Smith should be sufficiently informed (should have the autonomy) to understand his diagnosis and his treatment choices.

CULTURAL INFLUENCES ON AUTONOMY

Studies have shown that physicians often have difficulty giving bad news and that they find doing so to be very stressful (Baile, Lenzi, Parker, Buckman, & Cohen, 2002). The degree of difficulty varies with the physician's national background, age, location of practice, and academic affiliation. As many ethicists have asserted, such physician variables should not influence the information a patient receives. But, are there patient variables that should affect that determination?

Several cultures (including some American Indian and some Asian cultures) regard the receipt of information about a poor prognosis as a curse or as an irretrievable loss of dignity (Betancourt, Green, & Carillo, 2000).

Also, some patients, for a variety of reasons, may not want to be the recipients of bad news or may have very specific informational needs (Curtis, Wenrich, Carline, Shannon, Abrozy, & Ramsey, 2002). For this reason, some ethicists have advised that physicians discuss information exchange with their patients before a serious illness occurs. This would give a patient the "autonomy to choose how much autonomy" he or she desires.

PHYSICIAN BIAS AND EQUITY: A SYSTEMS ISSUE

Because Mr. Smith and his physician have not previously discussed information exchange in the event of a serious illness, the physician does not know what Mr. Smith expects. It also makes it impossible for the physician to individualize an informational approach for Mr. Smith. Although such discussions are not the standard of practice at this time, they represent an opportunity for improvement, because their absence prevents a systematic approach to the individualization of information sharing. Without such a systematic approach, it is unlikely that physicians can exclude personal bias from their information exchanges. This, in turn, prevents the establishment of an equitable approach to information exchange in practices that include seriously, chronically, and terminally ill patients.

Although the relationship of bias to equity is of great ethical importance, it may be more practical to approach it as a systems problem, rather than as a moral one. In the context of physician–patient relationships (as in all interpersonal relationships), the familial, cultural, and religious background of the physician (person) will always result in a unique perspective that contributes to the decisions she or he will make. Although it is noble to have an expectation that all professionals consistently exclude personal bias from their decision making, it may be best to develop processes that systematically reduce the role of bias. Systematically asking patients when they are well if they would want to receive bad news, instead of assuming that they do or do not, is an example of such a process and is one way of reducing bias.

Scenario 10-B: Treatment Choices

Mrs. Jones is a 75-year-old woman who experienced a myocardial infarction when she was 71. Until that time, she had led an active life, including many years of teaching elementary school, raising three children, enjoying the birth of her grandchildren, and sharing 50 years of marriage with her husband. Since the myocardial infarction, she has experienced recurring bouts of angina pectoris and has developed congestive heart failure. Her cardiologist has determined that the extensive damage from the initial infarction and the nature of her coronary blockage precludes any benefit from cardiac bypass surgery. The cardiologist has regularly adjusted her medication in response to bouts of heart failure, with good, but time-limited, improvements.

Mrs. Jones had been admitted to the hospital three times in the past six months. The last admission included an ICU stay and 48 hours of mechanical ventilation. Since returning home, she has been unable to walk more than a few feet without becoming short of breath. She depends on her husband to prepare her meals and feed her, to dress her, to wash her, and to help her with toileting. Her primary care physician has ordered the services of a visiting nurse, who provides Mrs. Jones with education and assesses her environment for potential adaptive equipment. The nurse recommends a hospital bed and a bedside commode, as well as a home health aide to assist Mr. Jones in her care. The nurse also asks Mrs. Jones if she has considered hospice care. When asked about hospice care, Mrs. Jones becomes visibly upset, saying that she has "much to live for" and that she will complain to her physician and to the nurse's agency about such a "troubling remark."

Questions

1. Was it inappropriate for the nurse to provide information about hospice care?

2. What is the physician's responsibility to inform Mrs. Jones about her prognosis and to facilitate discussion about hospice care?

3. Did information move appropriately across the healthcare continuum?

A completed ethical decision-making matrix for the scenario is provided at the end of the chapter.

INFORMATION ACROSS A HEALTHCARE CONTINUUM

Although Mrs. Jones survived a serious illness (myocardial infarction), she developed a chronic illness (heart failure) that is known to be life limiting and that has created significant functional impairment. Her physicians have provided her with optimal medical treatment, prolonging her life and providing the support that makes it possible for her to remain in her home. The visiting nurse completed an excellent assessment and, as part of the service, made Mrs. Jones aware of another treatment option, hospice. Mrs. Jones was offended by this information.

It is not unusual for individuals with chronic illnesses to receive care in more than one setting. Care may start in an outpatient clinic, then expand to include home care or admission to the hospital, and pass through or end in a nursing home. Along this continuum, many healthcare professionals participate in the care. The opportunity for effective, collaborative care is always great, with the patient benefiting from a seamless provision of services free of duplication and conflict. Unfortunately, however, care may be fragmented and ineffective if there is not good communication and collaboration between settings.

In this scenario, it is apparent that effective communication has occurred, resulting in excellent care in several settings. One opportunity that appears to have been missed is that of eliciting (and documenting) Mrs. Jones's understanding of her illness, of its prognosis, and of her goals in light of that prognosis. Her physician could have engaged Mrs. Jones in a compassionate discussion about her experience of this illness and asked her about her expectations.

TREATMENT GOALS AND BENEFICENCE

This becomes particularly important for individuals with chronic illnesses when the burden imposed by the illness (and its treatment) grows and the benefits of treatment diminish. Although medical technology has given us the opportunity to survive serious illnesses, it has not been accompanied by an ability to reduce the disability associated with ensuing chronic illness. Individuals with chronic, progressively debilitating illnesses experience a dwindling number of treatment options. It is appropriate for physicians to ensure that their patients with chronic disease have a realistic understanding of what can be achieved with treatment, especially when those treatments impose significant burdens.

Individuals like Mrs. Jones, with advanced congestive heart failure, typically experience episodic exacerbations from which they often recover, but with further loss of function and with growing frailty. Admissions to the hospital, especially to the ICU, can be particularly burdensome and traumatic. They are invariably associated with poorly relieved physical pain and emotional stress, and devastating comorbidities, such as delirium, thrombotic events, or falls with fracture, often complicate them. When any individual *chooses* to receive such burdensome treatment, their autonomy is preserved only if they understand the potential benefits of the treatment. It would not be unusual to find medical record documentation in which Mrs. Jones's physician documents a clear sense of beneficence in describing the benefits of admitting her during an exacerbation of heart failure. The documentation might include goals such as reduction in edema, improved oxygen saturation, and return to normal sinus rhythm. But what do these goals mean to Mrs. Jones? Do they translate into improvements in function and quality of life? Perhaps they do, but without a frank discussion regarding their relationship to Mrs. Jones's goals in life, it is difficult to say that she is sufficiently informed.

Ideally, Mrs. Jones's physician would elicit and document her real-life goals. These may include, for instance, being well enough to travel to a grandchild's graduation or to go on a vacation with her husband. If her physician informs her that these are not realistic goals and that it is unlikely that she will be able to live independently outside her home, then Mrs. Jones may decide that the burdens of recurring admission to the hospital would outweigh any foreseeable benefits. The documentation of that discussion and decision process would guide a visiting nurse to comfortably introduce the option of **hospice care.**

However, Mrs. Jones may inform her physician that her only goal is to survive as long as possible and that the burdens of hospitalization are acceptable to her. Her physician's documentation of this choice would guide the visiting nurse to be less direct in introducing the hospice option.

This scenario is common and shows how a physician's sense of beneficence may not be in alignment with the patient's goals. This nonalignment occurs because a failure to translate medical goals into real-life goals results in a failure to sufficiently preserve autonomy.

Scenario 10-C: Advance Care Planning

Mr. Lee is a 68-year-old veteran who has been admitted from the hospital to a VA nursing home. He contracted hepatitis C several years ago and has developed cirrhosis. In the hospital, his physicians treated him for the complications of cirrhosis, attempting to reduce his ascites and encephalopathy and correct his coagulopathy. Although Mr. Lee never married and did not maintain contact with any other family members, he has had an enduring friendship with a neighbor in his apartment house. A year ago his friend brought him to a routine appointment in the VA clinic, where Mr. Lee's physician advised him that his prognosis was poor. The physician recommended that Mr. Lee complete an advance directive, which he did with the assistance of a social worker in the clinic. On the advance directive he indicated that, if he became terminally ill and unable to speak for himself, that he would not want such life-prolonging treatments as CPR, mechanical ventilation, or tube feeding. He also named his friend to be his power of attorney for healthcare decisions.

On his arrival to the nursing home, Mr. Lee was awake and alert, but disoriented. He did not understand where he was or why he was there. He did not know the day or date, and although he seemed to recognize his friend, he could not recall his friend's name. He was jaundiced and weak. The nurse who admitted him correctly assessed that, although he appeared stable, he was at risk for serious and potentially fatal complications of cirrhosis at any time. She noted his advance directive and immediately contacted his attending physician in the nursing home to consider a Do Not Resuscitate (DNR) order. That evening the physician evaluated Mr. Lee and placed a DNR order on his record. He described this order to Mr. Lee's friend, who did not understand why the order was written. Specifically, he questioned whether Mr. Lee was terminally ill.

Questions

1. Was it appropriate for Mr. Lee's physician to write a DNR order?

2. What (and who) determines whether Mr. Lee is terminally ill?

3. Is there any information that could have obviated the conflict and the need to ask these questions?

4. What laws pertain to this situation?

A completed ethical decision-making matrix for the scenario is provided at the end of the chapter.

ADVANCE CARE PLANNING: AN OPPORTUNITY

More than 50% of adults over the age of 65 lose their decision-making capacity when they become seriously ill. Healthcare professionals are known to be uninformed about the healthcare choices of their patients, especially during serious illnesses. Family members do not know their loved ones' preferences for treatment, because they rarely discuss them. These are the findings from a series of studies that began with a hallmark report in the *Journal of the American Medical Association* in 1995 (SUPPORT Principal Investigators, 1995). The findings underscore the importance of effective advance care planning.

Advance care planning gives us the opportunity to state in writing (or verbally) the kind of treatment we would want if we were to lose the ability to speak for ourselves. The most important parts of an advance care plan are a statement of preferences ("Living Will") and a designation of an individual who will speak for us if we cannot speak for ourselves ("Power of Attorney for Health Care"). Many states have developed forms that reflect state laws governing advance care planning. These and other forms can be obtained from healthcare agencies, attorneys, and various Internet sites. In most states, the forms may be completed and the advance care plan established without the assistance of a healthcare professional or a lawyer. However, most individuals will not fully understand the implications of their choices if they do not discuss them with a healthcare professional.

The effectiveness of advance care planning depends on the usefulness of the information provided in the advance directive and on the quality of the communication between the patient and his or her family and healthcare providers. In this scenario, Mr. Lee's autonomy has been greatly supported by giving the opportunity to initiate advance care planning. Still, his friend, who earnestly cares about Mr. Lee's best interests (beneficence), doubts that the physician's order truly represents Mr. Lee's wishes.

THE MEANING OF *TERMINAL*

The use of the word *terminal* has carried different meanings in different settings. In the setting of hospice regulation and reimbursement, a life expectancy of six months or less is equated with terminal illness. This has put physicians in the position of having to articulate prognoses with far greater accuracy than they are capable of doing, and it has also excluded large numbers of individuals from hospice whose chronic illnesses have disabled them, but whose physicians cannot honestly say that they will die within six months.

Regulations have relaxed somewhat, allowing physicians to "recertify" that patients who do not die within six months are still terminally ill. This gives this group of chronically and terminally ill patients greater access to hospice care. Also, the National Hospice and Palliative Care Organization (Stuart, Alexander, & Arenella, 1996) has established criteria for terminal illness in noncancer diagnoses (such as cirrhosis, chronic obstructive pulmonary disease, congestive heart failure, Alzheimer's disease, end stage renal disease, and AIDS).

Although these criteria allow physicians and patients to procure needed services, they do not address the specific decision-making needs of patients who are no longer able to speak for themselves and who have not defined what *terminal* means to them. For Mr. Lee, *terminal* may mean any condition from which he is unlikely to recover independently and with full cognitive functioning. If that is the case, then the physician's order would be consistent with the advance directive and would be appropriate. However, Mr. Lee might regard *terminal* as a stage in his illness when he becomes permanently unconscious.

In that case, the physician's order would not be consistent with his advance directive. Similar issues arise for individuals with Alzheimer's disease who have completed advance directives, but who have not specified at what point in the illness they would want to be considered terminally ill.

One approach to preventing this dilemma is to include "scenario planning" (Pearlman, Starks, Cain, Cole, Rosengren, & Patrick, 2001) in the advance directive documentation. This involves describing specific scenarios to patients and giving them an opportunity to describe their choices and express the values they would want considered when any decisions are made for them. This becomes especially effective when the power of attorney is included in the discussion and when the discussion is well documented in the medical record. Most healthcare systems have not raised the standard of advance care planning to this level.

ADVANCE CARE PLANNING AND THE LAW

Laws governing advance care planning, including the institution of DNR status, vary from one jurisdiction to the next. In the United States, jurisdiction belongs to the states, but federal entities, such as the Department of Veterans Affairs, may have their own regulations that are not deferent to state regulations. For instance, at the VA nursing home in which Mr. Lee resides, his preference to designate a friend as his power of attorney for health care is supported by established VA directives. Those same directives establish an order of decision-making priority in which Mr. Lee's stated wishes are preeminent over all other parties, including his power of attorney. The ability to designate a friend as power of attorney and the preeminence given to wishes stated in an advance directive vary by jurisdiction.

Scenario 10-D: Palliative Care

Mrs. Harris is a 57-year-old woman who developed breast cancer 3 years ago. Despite a mastectomy and aggressive hormonal and chemotherapeutic therapy, she developed extensive metastases to her brain and bones. Although she went through a period of confusion due to hypercalcemia and brain metastases, she responded well to IV fluids and radiation therapy and regained decision-making capacity. Her physician approached her about the completion of an advance directive, to which she agreed and in which she documented that she wanted to continue to receive treatment that could potentially prolong her life.

Her advance directive contained specific information about her desire to receive antibiotics for intercurrent infections and IV fluids for dehydration and hypercalcemia. Mrs. Harris's advance directive also contained information that directed the healthcare team not to introduce tube feeding and not to attempt CPR. These latter requests were based on her physician's opinion that neither of these would be life-prolonging and that both would impose significant burdens and risks. Finally, Mrs. Harris's advance directive urged that her healthcare providers aggressively manage all of her symptoms to assure that her pain and discomfort are minimal at all times. Her physician responded to her advance directive with a note in which he said, "Although the patient has requested a degree of life-prolonging treatment, her request for palliative symptom control is inconsistent with life-prolongation. An ethics consult will be requested."

Questions

1. Are there any situations in which palliative care is not appropriate?

2. Are palliative care and life-prolonging treatments incompatible?

3. How should physicians document their intentions to provide palliative care?

A completed ethical decision-making matrix for the scenario is provided at the end of the chapter.

MANAGING PAIN

Many studies have documented the absence of adequate symptom control for patients with serious, chronic, and/or terminal illnesses. The reasons for this are many, but have consistently included reluctance by physicians to prescribe opioid analgesics. This reluctance is often based on fears regarding the potential for drug abuse and the potential for liability against licensure. In the treatment of chronic pain, these fears are unfounded when prescribing is appropriate.

Many organizations, including the Joint Commission on the Accreditation of Hospital Organizations (JCAHO, 1999), the Veterans Health Administration (2003), the American Medical Association (2001), and the World Health Organization (1990), have issued position statements and guidelines directing the appropriate use of analgesics, including opioid analgesics. Recently, the Drug Enforcement Agency (DEA) published a consensus statement and a list of "Frequently Asked Questions" (2004) to encourage the appropriate use of opioid analgesics in the management of pain. These guidelines include specific recommendations for physician documentation, which should clearly identify the diagnosis being treated, the goals for pain relief (e.g., a pain scale), and a discussion in which the patient is informed about the risks and benefits of opioid use.

ETHICS COMMITTEES

A patient's goals for the prolongation of life should not be seen as conflicting with aggressive **palliative care.** Although her physician may be more comfortable providing Mrs. Harris with aggressive pain relief in a hospice setting, such relief should not be withheld from her simply because she still desires life-prolonging treatment.

Most hospitals and many other healthcare organizations have established ethics committees to advise physicians and other healthcare professionals when difficult decision points are reached. The ethics committee is usually an interdisciplinary team composed of physicians, nurses, ethicists, social workers, chaplains, dietitians, and others with experience in ethical deliberation in healthcare. Their role is often that of facilitating communication, clarifying expectations, and reducing misunderstandings over treatment options and goals. Ethics committee members face the challenge of remaining objective and unbiased in deliberations over emotionally charged cases.

PALLIATIVE CARE

In Mrs. Harris's case, the committee might advise her physician that there is no evidence that individuals in the terminal stages of life-limiting illnesses experience shorter lives by virtue of receiving palliative care. In fact, they may point out that there is preliminary evidence that individuals receiving palliative care may enjoy better nutrition, decreased heart failure, and fewer procedure-related complications (palliative care includes increased use of advance directive documentation) than individuals not receiving such care. Their longevity may, on average, be better.

The committee may also remind the physician and other healthcare professionals that it is important for them to attend to the needs of dying patients. Studies have shown significantly diminished visitation rates to dying patients by physicians and nurses in nonhospice settings. Yet, it is at this time that a patient's needs may be the greatest. Physicians should document their attention to troubling symptoms and patient needs on a regular basis. This becomes especially important in the case of patients who are near death and who receive sedatives and opioid analgesics. There is often great concern (often unspoken) that when a patient dies, there will be a claim that the medications shortened the patient's life, and that a physician ordered or a nurse gave the fatal dose. Documentation should show regular attendance by staff, discussions in which the patient or family were given an understanding of the disease course and the effects of these medications, and clear statements indicating that the entire treatment team and the patient (or family) understand that these medications are given with the intent of reducing symptoms, not shortening life. Because there is no evidence that palliative treatment at the end of life does shorten life, this intent should be confidently expressed.

EMERGING ISSUES

The following are some emerging issues in end-of-life care:

- **Palliative care specialization.** An increasing number of physicians are acquiring experience and certification in pain management and hospice care. Many organizations are creating palliative care consultation teams to respond to the palliative care needs of individuals in such venues as intensive care units, where palliative care has not historically been practiced. Palliative care will increasingly be recognized as not being in conflict with other, curative treatments.

- **Home health care.** Although federal and state funding for home health care (and the corresponding benefits) has varied, the demand for this service has not. As the U.S. population ages, older individuals will see increasing value in receiving care at home, from the time of onset of chronic illness until the time of death (home hospice). Notwithstanding unusual political and economic forces, communities will see continued growth of home and community-based services and linkages between these and traditional institutional services.

- **Dementia.** The number of individuals with dementia will grow in proportion with the aging of society. Specifically, as many as 45% of individuals over the age of 85 will develop dementia. The care of these individuals will exact a significant burden on families, communities, and the healthcare system. The role of effective advance care planning and the integrity of information exchange across the care continuum will become even more important.

Key Terms

- Chronic illness
- Hospice care
- Palliative care
- Serious illness
- Terminal illness

Chapter Summary

- As people age, their vulnerability to illness grows. Many people will face serious illnesses that will become chronic and disabling or terminal in nature. The timely, accurate, and comprehensive exchange of healthcare information plays a pivotal role in ensuring that patients experience optimal healthcare outcomes.

- This exchange of information evolves over time, from the patient's initial receipt of "bad news" through difficult decisions and advance care plans to the provision of palliative and hospice care. The exchange also bridges healthcare venues, from hospital and clinic care to home care and nursing home care.
- The way in which information is exchanged can support patient autonomy, but the kind of autonomy that patients desire will vary. The ability of physicians and other healthcare providers to remain free of bias depends on the development of systems that reduce bias and that support effective information exchange. These include systems that establish each patient's preference for information and the articulation of treatment goals in terms that are meaningful to each patient's life.
- Good care of seriously, chronically, and terminally ill patients includes advocacy at difficult decision points and the provision of treatment that effectively treats symptoms, especially pain. This care should be meticulously documented to reflect the intent and continuing effectiveness of the decisions and the treatment selected.

References

American Medical Association. (2001). Promoting pain relief and preventing drug abuse: A critical balance act. *AMA*. Retrieved August 20, 2004, from http://www.ama-assn.org/ama1/pub/upload/mm/455/jointstatement.pdf.

Baile, W. F., Lenzi, R., Parker, P., Buckman, R., & Cohen, L. (2002). Oncologists' attitudes toward and practices in giving bad news: An exploratory study. *Journal of Clinical Oncology, 20*(8), 2189–2196.

Betancourt, J. R., Green, A. R., & Carillo, J. E. (2000). The challenges of cross-cultural healthcare—diversity, ethics, and the medical encounter. *Bioethics Forum, 16*(3), 27–32.

Curtis, J. R., Wenrich, M. D., Carline, J. D., Shannon, S. E., Ambrozy, D. M., & Ramsey, P. G. (2002). Patients' perspectives on physician skill in end-of-life care. *Chest, 122,* 356–362.

Drug Enforcement Agency. (1994). *Prescription pain medications: Frequently asked questions and answers for health care professionals, and law enforcement personnel.* Retrieved May 12, 2004, from http://www.medsch.wisc.edu/painpolicy/domestic/DEA_faq.htm.

HCFA, Center for Information Systems, Health Standards and Quality Bureau. (2001, February). *Basic statistics about home care.* Retrieved August 29, 2005, from http://www.nahc.org/consumer/hcstats.html.

Joint Commission on Accreditation of Hospital Organizations [JCAHO]. (1999). *Pain management standards.* Retrieved August 20, 2004, from http://www.jcaho.org/news+room/health+care+issues/jcaho+focuses+on+pain+management.htm.

Pearlman, R., Starks, H., Cain, K., Cole, W., Rosengren, D., & Patrick, D. (2001). *Your life, your choices.* Seattle, WA: Office of Research and Development, Department of Veterans Affairs. Retrieved August 20, 2004, from http://www.hsrd.research.va.gov/publications/internal/ylyc.htm.

Stuart, B., Alexander, C., & Arenella, C. (1996). *Medical guidelines for determining prognosis in selected noncancer diseases,* 2d ed. Arlington, VA: National Hospice and Palliative Care Organization.

SUPPORT Principal Investigators. (1995). A controlled trial to improve care for seriously ill hospitalized patients: The Study to Understand Prognoses and Preferences for Outcomes and Risks of Treatments (SUPPORT). The SUPPORT Principal Investigators. *JAMA, 274,* 1591–1598.

Veterans Administration. (2003). *Pain management.* Retrieved August 20, 2004, from http://www1.va.gov/vhapublications/ViewPublication.asp?pub_ID=246.

World Health Organization. (1990). *Cancer pain relief and palliative care.* Retrieved August 20, 2004, from http://www.who.int/medicines/library/qsm/who-edm-qsm-2000-4/Balance%20in%20Nat%20Opioids%20Control%20Policy%20final.pdf.

The ethical decision-making matrix is a tool to help you organize complex, ethical problems; however, there is no simple fill-in-the-box approach to ethical decision making. The objective is to follow each step of the process and not move from the question directly to what should be done or how to prevent it next time. If you skip steps, you will not fully understand all of the values and options for action. Also, the matrix provided for each scenario in this book is not the only way to examine the problem. You can make an equally compelling ethical argument for a different decision—just be sure to follow all the steps of the matrix.

SCENARIO 10-A: BAD NEWS

Steps	Information	
1. What is the ethical question?	What is the role of autonomy in information exchange?	
2. What are the facts?	**KNOWN**	**TO BE GATHERED**
	• Mr. Smith, a recently retired 62-year-old, has abdominal mass, probable cancer. • Mrs. Smith requests that the physician not tell Mr. Smith because it will "kill him."	• What is the relationship between the physician and Mr. Smith? • What is the relationship between Mr. and Mrs. Smith? • Is there documentation about Mr. Smith's values about receiving healthcare information? • What is the standard of practice? • What legislation affects communication with patients? • Does HIPAA influence the information exchange? • Has potential cancer been discussed with the patient prior to this? What are boundaries of autonomy?
3. What are the values? Examine the shared and competing values, obligations, and interests of the stakeholders (i.e., patient, HIM professional, healthcare practitioner(s), administrators, society, and other advocates) involved in order to fully understand the complexity of the ethical problem(s).	**Patient:** Expects accurate diagnosis, effective treatment, and long survival; can access Internet for information about diseases and treatment options. **HIM professional:** Accurate and timely information documented in the medical record; compliance with advance directives and informed consent. **Physician:** Some physicians support a standard of practice for open information exchange with patients; some physicians do not want to share bad news with patients; reduce or eliminate bias to equity for information sharing. **Administrators:** Open, honest, ethical conversations between patients and physicians. **Society:** Patient autonomy when making decisions; family participation in decision making, as appropriate.	

4. What are my options?	• Honor Mrs. Smith's request not to tell Mr. Smith. • Communicate directly with Mr. Smith.	
5. What should I do?	Communicate directly with Mr. Smith.	
6. What justifies my choice?	**JUSTIFIED**	**NOT JUSTIFIED**
	Mr. Smith sought health care and has an expectation of truth-telling, unless he specifically indicated that he did not want to know the results.	• Placing autonomy for decision making with Mrs. Smith, unless that is the expressed desire of Mr. Smith. • Keeping the truth from the patient.
7. How can I prevent this ethical problem?	Establish desires for communication with patients in advance, while they are in the healthy state, so that the physician and the patient are prepared for difficult decisions.	

The ethical decision-making matrix is a tool to help you organize complex, ethical problems; however, there is no simple fill-in-the-box approach to ethical decision making. The objective is to follow each step of the process and not move from the question directly to what should be done or how to prevent it next time. If you skip steps, you will not fully understand all of the values and options for action. Also, the matrix provided for each scenario in this book is not the only way to examine the problem. You can make an equally compelling ethical argument for a different decision—just be sure to follow all the steps of the matrix.

SCENARIO 10-B: TREATMENT CHOICES

Steps	Information	
1. What is the ethical question?	Should the visiting nurse ask the patient about hospice care?	
2. What are the facts?	**KNOWN**	**TO BE GATHERED**
	• Mrs. Jones, a 75-year-old woman, had a myocardial infarction at 71, which has limited her activity. • Mrs. Jones is not eligible for by-pass surgery. • She is dependent on her husband for daily activities. • A visiting nurse asks her whether she wants hospice care, which upsets Mrs. Jones.	• What is the relationship between the physician and Mrs. Jones? • What is the physician's responsibility to discuss hospice care? • What is the relationship between the nurse and Mrs. Jones? • What is the practice standard about nurses discussing hospice care with patients? • What is Mr. Jones's perspective, as the caretaker? • What are boundaries of patient autonomy? • Have conversations about future care episodes been discussed and documented? • Does Mrs. Jones understand the treatment options?
3. What are the values? Examine the shared and competing values, obligations, and interests of the stakeholders (i.e., patient, HIM professional, healthcare practitioner(s), administrators, society, and other advocates) involved in order to fully understand the complexity of the ethical problem(s).	**Patient:** Expects accurate diagnosis, effective treatment, and long survival. **HIM professional:** Accurate and timely information documented in the medical record; compliance with advance directives. **Healthcare professionals:** Many participate in the care of chronic illness and seek effective, collaborative care based on the availability of information. **Administrators:** Open, honest, ethical conversations between patients and physicians. **Society:** Patient autonomy when making decisions; family participation in decision making, as appropriate.	

4. What are my options?	• The visiting nurse should ask the patient about hospice care. • The visiting nurse should not discuss hospice care with the patient, unless requested by the physician or documented patient values indicate the acceptance of this model of care.	
5. What should I do?	The nurse should contact the physician to identify whether this has been discussed or verify the discussion and values in the patient's medical record, prior to the discussion with the patient; if not, the physician should take responsibility to discuss hospice with the patient, so that the nurse could appropriately follow-up or not, depending on the patient's goals.	
6. What justifies my choice?	**JUSTIFIED**	**NOT JUSTIFIED**
	• Build on the existing documentation of patient goals and physician decision making. • Physician–nurse communication regarding patient goals and values about hospice care.	• Physicians failing to discuss and document the treatment goals and outcomes for the various stages of acute and chronic care. • Nurses failing to determine the status of this dialogue. • Making assumptions about what is best for patients.
7. How can I prevent this ethical problem?	• Educational programs for physicians and healthcare providers regarding the importance of documentation of care decisions at the end of life. • Document patients' goals.	

The ethical decision-making matrix is a tool to help you organize complex, ethical problems; however, there is no simple fill-in-the-box approach to ethical decision making. The objective is to follow each step of the process and not move from the question directly to what should be done or how to prevent it next time. If you skip steps, you will not fully understand all of the values and options for action. Also, the matrix provided for each scenario in this book is not the only way to examine the problem. You can make an equally compelling ethical argument for a different decision—just be sure to follow all the steps of the matrix.

SCENARIO 10-C: ADVANCE CARE PLANNING

Steps	Information	
1. What is the ethical question?	Should the Do Not Resuscitate order be written and followed?	
2. What are the facts?	**KNOWN**	**TO BE GATHERED**
	• Mr. Lee, a 68-year-old veteran, was admitted to a VA nursing home with complications of cirrhosis. • Mr. Lee has no family relationships but does have a close friend. • Advance directive indicates that Mr. Lee does not want life-prolonging treatments. • Friend named as power of attorney. • DNR order was questioned by the friend.	• Is Mr. Lee truly terminally ill? • Should the DNR order have been written? • Would other physicians agree with the decision? • What laws pertain to this case? • Did Mr. Lee discuss his wishes in the advance directive with his friend? • Do the principles of autonomy (Mr. Lee) or beneficence (friend) apply? • Was "scenario planning" documented as part of the advance directive?
3. What are the values? Examine the shared and competing values, obligations, and interests of the stakeholders (i.e., patient, HIM professional, healthcare practitioner(s), administrators, society, and other advocates) involved in order to fully understand the complexity of the ethical problem(s).	**Patient:** Expects accurate diagnosis, effective treatment, and long survival; expects that advance directives and power of attorney will be followed. **HIM professional:** Accurate and timely information documented in the medical record; compliance with advance directives. **Healthcare professionals:** Many participate in the care of chronic illness and seek effective, collaborative care based on the availability of information; desire to comply with advance directives. **Administrators:** Open, honest, ethical conversations between patients and physicians. **Society:** Patient autonomy when making decisions, whenever appropriate.	

4. What are my options?	• Implement the DNR order, without further consultation with Mr. Lee or the friend. • Do not implement the DNR order.	
5. What should I do?	Do not implement the DNR order.	
6. What justifies my choice?	**JUSTIFIED**	**NOT JUSTIFIED**
	• Determine Mr. Lee's status and establish presence of autonomy. • Discuss advance directive with friend. • Evaluate existing documentation for guidance by VA physician.	• Assume that both the patient and friend understand the DNR order. • Implement the DNR order without consultation with Mr. Lee or the friend. • Fail to get second opinion about the health and autonomy status of the patient.
7. How can I prevent this ethical problem?	• Educational programs for physicians and healthcare providers regarding the importance of documentation of care decisions at the end of life. • Document the patients' goals.	

The ethical decision-making matrix is a tool to help you organize complex, ethical problems; however, there is no simple fill-in-the-box approach to ethical decision making. The objective is to follow each step of the process and not move from the question directly to what should be done or how to prevent it next time. If you skip steps, you will not fully understand all of the values and options for action. Also, the matrix provided for each scenario in this book is not the only way to examine the problem. You can make an equally compelling ethical argument for a different decision—just be sure to follow all the steps of the matrix.

SCENARIO 10-D: PALLIATIVE CARE

Steps	Information	
1. What is the ethical question?	Should palliative care be given?	
2. What are the facts?	**KNOWN**	**TO BE GATHERED**
	• Mrs. Harris is a 57-year-old woman with metastases of breast cancer to the brain and bones. • Advance directive indicates preferences for prolonging life, including pain management, but no tube feeding or CPR.	• Is palliative care appropriate at this time for Mrs. Harris? • Has a second opinion been sought to collaborate on this question? • Are palliation and life-prolonging treatment compatible? • What is documented in the medical record regarding these choices? The advance directive? • Have guidelines from accrediting agencies been reviewed in relationship to palliative care? • Has an ethics committee consultation been requested? • Are there clinical protocols for end-of-life pain management?
3. What are the values? Examine the shared and competing values, obligations, and interests of the stakeholders (i.e., patient, HIM professional, healthcare practitioner(s), administrators, society, and other advocates) involved in order to fully understand the complexity of the ethical problem(s).	**Patient:** Expects accurate diagnosis, effective treatment, and long survival; expects that advance directives will be followed; wants to avoid pain, whenever possible. **HIM professional:** Accurate and timely information documented in the medical record; compliance with advance directives. **Healthcare professionals:** Many participate in the care of terminal illness and seek effective care based on the availability of information; desire to comply with advance directives. **Administrators:** Open, honest, ethical conversations between patients and physicians. **Society:** Patient autonomy when making decisions, whenever appropriate.	

4. What are my options?	• Give palliative care. • Do not give palliative care.	
5. What should I do?	Give palliative care.	
6. What justifies my choice?	**JUSTIFIED**	**NOT JUSTIFIED**
	• Get an ethics consultation. • Give palliative care, rather than life-prolonging care, if ethics committee determines that this is the wish of the patient.	Prolong life at all costs and regardless of patient wishes.
7. How can I prevent this ethical problem?	• Educational programs for physicians and healthcare providers regarding the importance of documentation of care decisions at the end of life. • Document patients' goals. • Educational programs regarding palliative care versus prolongation of life care; when compatible, when not.	

COMPUTERIZED HEALTH INFORMATION

Part III explores issues related to the computerization of health information, including the electronic health record (EHR), information security, software development and implementation, data resource management, integrated delivery systems, and e-health and e-HIM systems. Chapter 11 explains how demands for greater business efficiency, system performance, and timely access to data have raised new ethical issues regarding privacy, data integrity, and confidentiality in the implementation of electronic health information systems. Chapter 12 discusses security issues that arise from the use of electronic health information systems, including the implications of HIPAA, and presents a model for an information security program. Chapter 13 describes a collaborative decision-making framework for software development and implementation, noting the competing interests of the physician, the chief financial officer, the information technology specialist, and health information management (HIM) professional. Chapter 14 discusses data resource management involving clinical data repositories, data marts, data warehouses, and EHRs. Chapter 15 analyzes the complexities of managing an integrated delivery system, with a focus on balancing competing interests and the importance of confidentiality and data quality. Chapter 16 includes a discussion of e-health technologies and the role of HIM professionals in resolving emerging ethical issues, with a focus on e-health and the changing healthcare system, national health policy, and the ethical issues of choice and interoperability. Chapter 17 concludes this section with a review of e-HIM issues, including the initiatives of the government in support of the EHR.

ELECTRONIC HEALTH RECORDS

Mary Alice Hanken, PhD, CHP, RHIA
Gretchen Murphy, MEd, RHIA, FAHIMA

Abstract

The increasing implementation of electronic health record (EHR) systems and the increasing sophistication of these systems have raised new ethical issues with regard to the potential for compromising data integrity and confidentiality for the sake of greater business efficiency, better system performance, or more convenient and timely access to data. Although EHR systems include security features, technological solutions alone are not adequate to protect the integrity and confidentiality of patient information. This chapter presents ethical dilemmas typically raised during system planning, when working with alliance partners to link organizations' EHRs, and following the implementation of EHR systems. This chapter explores how these dilemmas can be addressed by health information management (HIM) professionals.

Learning Objectives

After completing this chapter, the reader should be able to:

- Recognize the role of ethics in assessing technology and electronic health record (EHR) applications.
- Identify common health information business practice issues that require ethical consideration as health information systems and EHR systems are implemented in healthcare organizations.
- Demonstrate how practice issues can be analyzed on the basis of principles and related values as a framework for identifying ethical questions.
- Apply a model for health information management (HIM) professionals to use in identifying and addressing ethical issues with regard to rapidly developing technologies.

Scenario 11-A: Patient Record Integrity and System Security

Your healthcare organization (Lincoln City Hospital) has selected a vendor for an electronic health record (EHR) system. This vendor has a well-regarded history of solid information systems, and its EHR product has been well received in the user community. The product includes modules for registration (admission/discharge/transfer), order communication, care documentation, basic medical record processing, and discharge and referral. It features financial applications as well as bedside documentation and online transcription displays. A central feature is a clinical data repository to house information captured in the EHR software and selected data sent from departmental systems and ancillary applications.

You are asked to serve on the implementation planning team. Part of the planning for software implementation and education is the institutional readiness process. The system vendor has proposed a patient record definition in its product, and the system features offer new point-and-click options for documenting the care process. Data quality edits and software security features are provided in the new system as well. Because the technology offers new ways to perform current business processes in these areas, existing organizational policies and procedures that govern health information and patient record integrity, clinical documentation, data quality, and confidentiality and security are expected to be reviewed and updated. Your initial review uncovers two problems.

The first problem has to do with the integrity of patient records. The new EHR system does not capture medication data from the existing pharmacy system, which are now included in the organization's patient record, and it does not offer the capability to link to the missing application. The hospital's legacy pharmacy system maintains a list of current medications for Lincoln City Hospital patients that is printed out and included in the paper medical record. In addition, authorized users can access medication data by logging on to the pharmacy system. Pharmacy system medication summaries are defined as part of the Lincoln City Hospital patient record. The vendor product does not accommodate information transfer from the pharmacy system, and the vendor is unwilling to include a link to the system, citing performance concerns about maintaining the EHR system's response time. The vendor's representative points out that medications can be summarized in narrative summaries.

The second problem has to do with security. The new system provides a "temporary user ID" for nursing units. On-call nurses or those assigned to the unit on a temporary basis share a user ID and password to access the EHR. This means that multiple individuals will have the same user ID and password to access the system. Not only will it be difficult to establish accountability policies that hold individuals responsible for their use of information systems, but the audit trail function will be compromised. The hospital will be unable to enforce employee accountability because it will be unable to verify user actions on patient data. The vendor reports that the changes required to implement individual user IDs for temporary staff are not practical due to the time it takes to set up individual user IDs and passwords.

Questions

1. How do you proceed?
2. What is the most ethical course of action?

A completed ethical decision-making matrix for the scenario is provided at the end of the chapter.

In this chapter, we focus on the role of ethics in planning, developing, and implementing electronic health record (EHR) systems. We consider EHRs in their strategic capacity and explain their functions and expected features. Understanding current expectations for EHRs prepares health information management (HIM) professionals to assess their institution's situation more realistically. We present ethical principles of the HIM profession and describe how they are challenged by the capability of EHR systems to combine many sources of patient data and to make more information available to many more users. Finally, we discuss the scenarios, which feature ethical problems in a proposed EHR system, ethical problems involved in linking the information systems of two different organizations that are entering an alliance, and problems encountered following the implementation of an EHR system.

EHR SYSTEMS: FUNCTIONS AND EXPECTED FEATURES

Computer technology has been changing health care and health information business processes for some time. For several decades, computerized **clinical information systems** have been used for collecting data relevant to the health status of an individual and to healthcare processes. For example, such systems are used in physician order entry, laboratory results reporting, and case management. Recently, these systems have become more complex as healthcare organizations have recognized the capabilities of

technology and the need for more sophisticated approaches to managing and using clinical data. Increasingly, these tools have been linked and integrated to form more comprehensive information systems in the clinical environment. Individually, clinical information systems provide the building blocks for a fully operational EHR system. An **electronic health record (EHR)** is any information relating to the past, present, or future physical/mental health or condition of an individual that resides in electronic systems used to capture, transmit, receive, store, retrieve, link, and manipulate multimedia data for the primary purpose of providing health care and health-related services (Murphy, Hanken, & Waters, 1999, p. 5).

This definition specifically includes individual health status and condition to encompass preventive medicine, illness, and patient-contributed information. It intends inclusion of information from birth (or prebirth) to death. It recognizes that genome data could be part of a health record. It lists system functions to denote the broadest capability for using and linking information available through technology and communications. It uses the term *multimedia* to cover the scope of electronic tools currently available. Text, coded data, voice, wave forms, and video may all be delivered through a multimedia workstation or other device. This definition offers a starting point for organizations working to acquire or build EHR systems.

Murphy et al. (1999) described the EHR system as having multiple integral components: the master patient index (MPI), documentation and feeder systems, clinical decision support, and the clinical data repository. The MPI is the application in which the initial patient identification data are captured as a permanent record of the patient's treatment in the facility. One of its core elements is a unique identifying number that links to subsequent patient information captured during care events, resulting in the development of the EHR over time. In complex systems, such as integrated delivery systems that include several institutions, there may be a "super MPI" that links patient identifying information among multiple institutions.

In another case, the clinical data repository represents the gathered patient information maintained in centralized form. The repository is integral to the EHR system because it stores patient data over time within institutions. For example, test result data, encounter data, problem lists, diagnoses, and the like are maintained. Practitioners typically retrieve the necessary clinical information on patients through their workstation or other device. EHR systems also need to be designed to support the functions associated with maintaining a quality HIM system and timely, accurate, accessible patient records.

In 2004 the federal government introduced a national technology initiative with the EHR as the centerpiece. The goal of the EHR system is to improve the quality, safety, and service of health care. This federal initiative is intended to encourage the widespread adoption of electronic health record systems. Four goals were identified: first, inform clinical practice through access to quality clinical information; second, interconnect clinicians so patient information and health records can be accessed as needed; third, personalize care by encouraging individuals to maintain their own records; and fourth, improve population health efforts through more and better data (Thompson & Brailer, 2004).

As today's technology becomes more cohesive and allows for linkages among systems already in place in healthcare organizations, institutional leaders are increasingly planning and implementing EHR systems. In the 2004 Health Care Information and Management Systems Society (HIMSS) Leadership Survey on technology priorities, 33% reported that they had implemented electronic medical records; 44% reported that they planned to replace or upgrade their clinical systems. Perhaps because of the focus on HIPAA security regulations, 48% reported that they planned to upgrade security. In reporting on the status of the EHR system in their facilities, 19% reported fully operational systems, 37% had begun installation, and 23% were developing plans to implement electronic medical record systems. Those reporting on the cost benefits of EHRs recognize that they offer strategic value to the organization (HIMSS, 2004). Table 11–1 portrays the EHR in terms of strategic and operational value (Murphy et al., 1999). Note that EHRs are portrayed as improving satisfaction and fundamental decision-making capabilities over the long term.

The group Connecting for Health has acknowledged the increasing investment and growth in EHRs and has addressed the technical infrastructure required to bring EHR systems together through developing a "national infrastructure through the creation of a network of networks to support the connectivity of patient clinical information and electronic health records" (Versweyveld, 2004).

In 1991, an Institute of Medicine study (Dick & Steen, 1997) published a comprehensive model for computerizing patient records that reflected interdisciplinary participation and the collective experiences of pioneers in automated medical record developments. Exhibit 11–1 depicts the user requirements identified in the study. These serve as a basis for today's expectations of EHR functions.

The section "Record Content" calls for uniform content. Standard coding systems and agreed-upon data dictionaries to define data consistently are recommended. It also specifies that the system have the capacity to track the outcomes of the healthcare process. The expectation that content will be rich enough to track the status of patients over time is based on the computer's potential for storing data over time. ASTM standard E1384

Table 11–1 Strategic and Operational Value of Electronic Health Records

Strategic Value	Operational Value
Improved patient satisfaction	• Optimize registration process • Eliminate data entry • Eliminate duplicate data storage • Reduce identification and billing steps
Improved physician and clinician satisfaction	• Provide greater access to complete and accurate information • Support direct entry of orders by physicians • Provide practitioner reminders • Enable access to new sources of medical information • Enhance development and use of multidisciplinary pathways

Source: Reprinted with permission from G. Murphy et al., *Electronic Health Records: Changing the Vision.* Figure 17–4, © 1999, WB Saunders Company.

addresses the content of an EHR. Periodically, the federal government has specified minimum data sets that serve as uniform ways of describing certain sets of data. Work is continuing in this arena.

The "Intelligence" section specifies that patient data can be used to support decision making. For instance, the EHR system can have **alert and reminder features**. Individual patient data can be used to help providers remember important facts, such as medication allergies; trigger reminders about needed interventions, such as complying with an immunization schedule; avoid unnecessary interventions, for example, reminding the provider about recent tests so that a test will not be conducted twice; and giving alerts so that the provider can respond immediately, for example, to a hospitalized patient's change in status. Multiple examples demonstrate that "by applying automated rules to data gathered in EHRs, providers can be reminded or prompted to take appropriate action for those who need it" (Murphy et al., 1999, p. 235).

Aggregate patient data can be used to provide information on specific populations of patients, such as pediatric patients, so that

care and services can be analyzed to evaluate what has been done and to help provide rationales for new plans. Special registries may collect and manage data in specific chronic disease areas, such as diabetes and cardiac care, to support clinicians in developing individual care plans for their patients. Decision support offers practice profiles for providers so that they can better understand how to assess and plan the use of clinical and management resources. Aggregate data about their own patients may help physicians see which diagnostic tests they order, which medications they prescribe, and much more. These data allow analysis of an individual's practices as well as comparison of a group's practices. Data on patient outcomes enable providers to better understand and act on their practice style. Finally, aggregate data can be used for public health purposes and for such business purposes as quality monitoring and cost analysis.

Navigational features are specified in the "Record Format" and "Reporting Capabilities" sections. Recognizing that users will need to access the information in flexible ways, the requirements indicate how the record should function. The requirements

Exhibit 11–1 CPR User Requirements for Electronic Health Records as Set Forth by the Institute of Medicine

Record Content
Uniform care data elements
Standardized coding systems and formats
Common data dictionary
Information on outcomes of care and functional status

Control and Access
Easy access for patients and their advocates
Safeguards against violation of confidentiality

Intelligence
Decision support
Clinician reminders
"Alarm" system capable of being customized

System Performance
Rapid retrieval
24-hour access
Available at convenient places
Easy data input

Record Format
"Front-page" problem list
Ability to "flip through the record"
Integration among disciplines and sites of care

Training and Implementation
Minimal training required for system use
Graduated implementation possible

Reporting Capabilities
"Derived documents" (e.g., insurance forms)
Easily customized output and other user interfaces
Standard clinical reports (e.g., discharge summary)
Customized and ad hoc reports (e.g., specific evaluation queries)
Trend reports and graphics

Linkages
Linkages with other information systems (e.g., radiology, laboratory)
Transferability of information among specialties and sites
Linkages with relevant scientific literature
Linkages with other institutional databases and registries
Linkages with record of family members
Electronic transfer of information

Source: Reprinted with permission from R.S. Dick and E.B. Steen, eds,. *The Computer-based Patient Record: An Essential Technology for Health Care,* Rev. ed., p. 36, © Copyright 1997 by the National Academy of Sciences.

specified under "Control and Access" reflect a long-standing recognition of the importance of the privacy, confidentiality, and security of patient data. The sections "System Performance" and "Training and Implementation" stress timeliness and convenience of access and "easy to learn" expectations. They call for full understanding of the impact of technology on system users and, in particular, a rec-ognition that change management is needed for achieving success in implementation and user acceptance. Finally, the section "Linkages" exemplifies the potential for comprehensiveness of an EHR system and the dynamic movement of the information in and out of it. Linkages with other information systems allow clinicians to use workstations or other electronic devices to check on diagnostic test results and view transcribed reports. Patient information such as test results can be electronically transmitted from one location to another for expert review or accessed remotely. Telemedicine, which is the exchange of medical information between sites via electronic communications for the care and education of the patient or healthcare provider, allows patient examination and/or treatment to take place with the participation of a consultant at a distant location (Burns, 1999). Linkages to expert systems and clinical resources can also support diagnosis and treatment.

EHR SYSTEMS IN THE TWENTY-FIRST CENTURY

Today's EHR system is likely to include not only the wish list of features set forth in the 1991 Institute of Medicine study, but also several new features. Today, healthcare organizations may purchase a vendor-developed EHR application as a single system or they may design links to existing systems and add an institutional data repository to store data. In the future, healthcare organizations may use intranets with special navigational tools to offer seamless access to their collections of information systems so that EHR features are developed as more of an overall computing environment. Consider the following description of Brigham and Women's Hospital—Partners Healthcare in Boston—ambulatory EHR.

The hospital's system includes treatment notes, problem lists, medications, allergies, vital signs, advance directives, health maintenance information, flowsheets for specific problems, "to do" items, and discharge summaries and offers access to all other online clinical information. Workstations and other electronic devices are located in intake areas and exam rooms or are carried to the point of care. Wireless devices can be used locally or remotely to check on a patient's condition and review updated information. The EHR system features a "patient at a glance" sum-

mary view of problems, medications, allergies, and recent visits. The "day at a glance" feature provides a detailed outline of recent inpatient and outpatient encounters and links to specific notes and lab results (Murphy et al., 1999). The EHR system may also include links to reference databases, reminder systems, and decision-support systems.

In 2004 HL7, a standards development group, proposed a functional model for an EHR system. This interest in what an EHR system should be able to do, that is, the functionality of the system, underscores and expands on the EHR capabilities. The model also proposes a framework for bringing together the required clinical and administrative functions. HL7, in cooperation with a number of other organizations, including the American Health Information Management Association (AHIMA), is working to develop a functional model for the EHR. HIM professionals' expectations have evolved to include use of the Internet and secure Web technology to facilitate electronic mail among providers and between providers and patients; patients' access to their own health information and their ability to schedule appointments, renew prescriptions, and view educational materials via their providers' Web sites; and more advanced applications of telemedicine that encompass not only textual data and text but also sound, still video, and motion video (Murphy et al., 1999; Burns, 1999). Further, information management tools that organize and summarize health record content to suit unique data needs need to be more fully developed, so that, for example, users can view trend data to track blood glucose levels or monitor high blood pressure and input their own data from home to add to the monitoring database. Although these would be major advances in the use of patient record information, such features would make more information potentially available to many more users.

Risks of confidentiality breaches increase exponentially with the expansion of the number of users who may access an individual's information in EHR systems. Technology challenges human behavior and values to apply resources in ways that maintain universal and institutional values. Ethical practices need to be applied to the new questions that present as technology increasingly affects human behavior.

Figure 11–1 illustrates EHR systems in healthcare organizations today. Note the complexity of data interaction and user access.

EHR TECHNOLOGY AND ETHICAL ISSUES

Maintaining the balance between individual and institutional commitments to information management principles and policies and technological expediency requires vigilance. Advances in technology, changes in laws, and changes in expectations raise ethical issues related to the following topics: patient privacy, technology, information integrity, patient care quality review, organizational advocacy, and professional HIM roles.

Patient Privacy

The overriding obligation of HIM professionals is to protect patient privacy by adopting privacy practices that ensure the confidentiality of patient health information and by using secure methods to collect, maintain, and release data for authorized purposes.

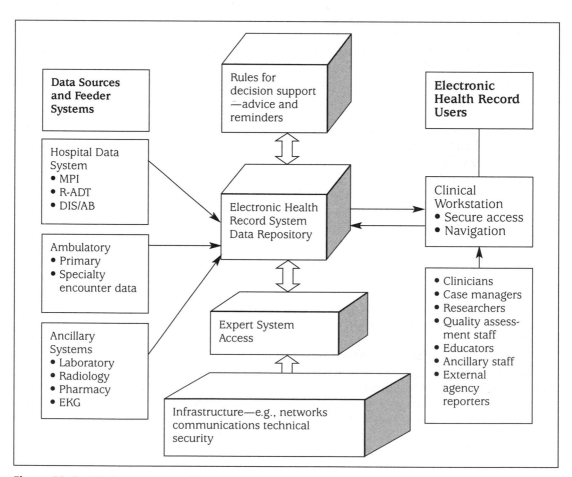

Figure 11–1 EHR Systems in Health Care Organizations

Privacy is the right of an individual to be left alone. It includes freedom from intrusion or observation into one's private affairs and the right to maintain control over certain personal information. Although information is shared with care providers, individuals are entitled to expect that the healthcare system and their care providers will respect their privacy (ASTM, 2004, E1869-04 §7.1.1). In fact, consumer awareness of privacy has grown significantly over the past decade. Patient rights initiatives clearly emphasize more control over healthcare decisions and personal health information; additionally, legislative initiatives that address privacy of health information clearly illustrate the activity in this area (e.g., HIPAA). For example, one of HIPAA's requirements is that consumers be presented with a Notice of Information Practices that describes how an organization will maintain, use, and disclose protected health information.

Confidentiality is the responsibility to limit the disclosure of private matters and includes the responsibility to use, disclose, or release such information with the knowledge and consent of the individual unless permitted or directed by law (ASTM, 2004). HIM professionals are required to practice and promote confidentiality by recommending and developing institutional policies and developing staff education programs. HIM professionals implement privacy practices to oversee health information business processes. This includes secure information-handling procedures, whether the information is hard copy or electronic.

Security is the means to control access to and protect information from accidental or intentional disclosure (Computer-Based Patient Record Institute [CPRI], 1996). Technology can improve collection, storage, and access to information. Adherence to appropriate "need-to-know" rules for granting authorization to access information can be an ethical dilemma in the face of user demands for ease of access. Security measures can be applied, but they are not foolproof. Institu-

tions can implement individual user identification and password protection, but if individuals share user IDs and passwords for convenience, security is compromised. Any comprehensive initiative to create a safe environment to transmit individually identifiable health information will need to ensure that special protections, as well as routine protections, can be addressed through policies, procedures, and technical measures.

The Health Insurance Portability and Accountability Act (HIPAA), passed in 1996, includes specific provisions for the privacy and security of health information. As a follow-up to the law, specific regulations have been developed for privacy and security (45 CFR Parts 160 and 164). The focus of these requirements is on human behavior. Organizations have developed policies and procedures to address privacy and security. Additionally, systems have been reviewed to improve security features. In one commentator's words, "It's absurd for anyone to say they have a 100% technology solution for the security provisions—the rules are 70% about educating people and 30% about possibly using any type of technology" (Gillespie, 2000, p. 48).

Table 11–2 summarizes what computers can and cannot do to protect privacy and maintain confidentiality and security. The information featured in this table illustrates the human-behavior aspects of using technology in health care. Achieving unqualified privacy protection remains an unmet goal. The business-process-efficiency paradigm is the driver. Ethical questions are inherent in making the choice as to how to employ these technologies. This means that the application of ethics to choices made to access and transmit health information using today's available technology is essential to minimize risk, meet consumer concerns, and uphold institutional values for maintaining confidentiality.

HIM professionals will be challenged to strike a balance and make the best possible recommendations, even when full security is not ensured. In one instance, the right choice would be to approve electronic transmission

Table 11–2 Computers and Privacy

Computers Can . . .	Computers Cannot . . .
Maintain more information more legibly than paper systems	Control the quality and integrity of user documentation
Monitor access through individual user identification security procedures	Monitor individuals who share information inappropriately
Provide the capacity for updates in user confidentiality agreements by programming automatic renewal notification through the logon process every 6 months	Establish the institutional policy that all employees be required to sign confidentiality agreements
Use audit trails to monitor data access, updates, and release-of-information systems	Enforce sanctions for unauthorized access or release
Apply encryption procedures for electronic information transfer	Ensure that individuals use authorized methods to transfer information

of critical patient information to meet emergency requirements, because it would still address the best interest of the patient, regardless of the technical security limitations in an organization's procedures for information transfer. Here it might be necessary to accept security limitations to meet the prevailing need. In another situation, the HIM professional might recommend against implementing an institutional policy to allow e-mail communication among providers over the Internet until e-mail encryption is in place and/or institutional policies clearly call for the relevant clinical content of e-mail communications to be included in the patient's record (Burrington-Brown & Hughes, 2003).

Data Quality

HIM professionals are also responsible for promoting data quality. As technology continues to affect information-processing activities, from ancillary systems to data repositories, data integrity issues surface. Ethical commitments to ensure the timeliness and accuracy of health information require resources to be applied to data maintained and interfaced in and among systems. Institutional resources must be invested in ensuring consistent data definitions; for example, organizational computer-stored master files, such as the chargemaster used for accurate billing and ICD and HCPCS codes

used for accurate code assignments, must be updated in a timely manner.

When selecting an information system, it is ethically sound to insist that the selection process include a review and certification of data editing, validation, and interfacing requirements so that data integrity is not compromised. Clearly, identifying data integrity issues for current and proposed systems is the correct action. However, endorsing this action may be difficult when influential leaders in the organization support a system because of personal preference or the preference of an influential group in the organization.

Patient Interest

Placing the patient's interest first is another key value in making ethical decisions. This may require that choices be made among competing principles to select the one that best meets the needs of patients. An institution may decide to implement a results-reporting system for laboratory test results even though the programmers failed to include a module for anatomical pathology results, citing that those results were available in their "own" system. Although the physician who ordered the test would know to access the anatomical pathology application, other clinical users of the new results-reporting application may assume that all test results were included and may base clinical decisions on incomplete information. The information technology (IT) director may insist that the application be implemented to meet institutional goals and that it support the principle of "continually improving information access to support patient care." Consideration of incomplete information compromising the care process should take precedence, and the best interest of the patient should drive a decision to delay implementation until the application is corrected or a notification is included to direct users to another application for additional information.

Institutional Values

Another ethical tenet for HIM professionals is honoring institutional values. Loyalty to institutional values means advocating and representing them in business dealings. It includes upholding principles with customers (patients and other internal and external individuals and groups who use the services of the institution). Data release principles adopted by the organization may state that aggregate data are released for patient populations large enough so that individual identification of patients cannot occur. This protects patient privacy and still provides aggregate information on health services provided. When companies are self-insured and contract to a health plan to provide medical benefits for their employees, they may request aggregate data on their employees from contracting institutions who provide health services in order to evaluate costs and plan for future healthcare benefits for their employees. Upholding this data release principle may be difficult when the company in question has a small number of employees. Because the numbers are small, inference or direct knowledge of some individuals' health problems can identify individual patients. In this case, the ethical action is to deny release and work to explore an alternative way to provide information that does not risk patient privacy. Scenario 11-B will further illustrate how this institutional value can be challenged.

Making Ethical Decisions

The goal is to practice HIM in ways that meet the AHIMA Code of Ethics. Responsible HIM professionals will assemble information from legal, accreditation, policy, and professional practice sources to assist in formulating recommendations and strategies to participate in assessing, planning, and implementing information technology. HIM professionals will draw on a variety of sources to answer the following basic questions:

- What is in the best interest of the patient?
- How does a proposed action support my organization's principles and values?
- Are regulatory and accrediting requirements accounted for?
- Are personal and professional values of honesty and promoting quality health information upheld?

After careful preparation, the HIM professional must make recommendations, specify quality concerns, and exercise voting options to add or delete steps in the organization's technology review process; propose new and revised principles and policies that define the organizational values; and verify that regulatory and accrediting criteria are addressed. Carrying out ethical actions is vested in understanding and accounting for human behavior. People need the leadership and direction provided by clearly expressed and published principles and policies.

Ethical Issues in Implementation Planning

Let's return to Scenario 11-A, which opened this chapter. The vendor's proposed EHR system has two problems, one concerning patient record integrity and another concerning security.

Patient Record Integrity

The new EHR system does not capture medication data that is included in the organization's patient record nor does it offer the capability to link to the missing application. Currently, the hospital's legacy pharmacy system maintains a list of current medications for Lincoln City Hospital patients that is printed out and included in the paper record. In addition, authorized users can access medication data by logging on to the pharmacy system. Institutional policy specifies that pharmacy system medication summaries are defined as part of the Lincoln City Hospital patient record. The vendor product does not accommodate information transfer from the pharmacy system, and the vendor is unwilling to include a link to the system, citing performance concerns for maintaining the EHR application's response time. The vendor representative points out that medications can be summarized in narrative summaries.

The following are some of the organization's options:

- Require the vendor to develop the interface to the pharmacy system at the risk of degrading performance of the application.
- Require the vendor to feature an announcement of the application log on display that instructs users to access the pharmacy system for medication summaries.
- Continue to maintain the medication summary in the paper record and negotiate for the next product update to include the linkage to the pharmacy system, because the paper record is expected to continue to be available during an anticipated transition period.

The right thing to do is based on external legal and accreditation standards and organizational values to ensure that all information required for care purposes is made available to providers. Think through the consequences of each option. If the organization values completeness and integrity of health information based on principles, values, and standards, then the right choice should reflect these values. The second option ac-

knowledges the vendor analysis about performance issues associated with a direct interface between the EHR software and the pharmacy system, but it provides information to the system's users that maintains the institutional values for patient data integrity. The third option will require that clinicians continue to use the paper record along with the computer record for an individual's care.

Security

Security provisions in the new system allow for a "nursing unit on-call ID," whereby on-call nurses or those assigned to the unit on a temporary basis share a user ID and password to access the EHR. This could result in multiple individuals using the same user ID and password to access the system. It will be difficult to establish accountability policies that hold individuals responsible for their use of information systems, because the institution will be unable to enforce such policies because user actions on patient data will not be able to be audited. The vendor reports that the changes required to implement individual user IDs for temporary staff are not practical due to the time it takes to set up individual user IDs and passwords. The security manager in the IT division agrees.

This is in conflict with the current practice at Lincoln City Hospital. Current practice at Lincoln City Hospital prohibits the sharing of user IDs and passwords to access information systems. This policy and technical security practice is based on external standards and security practices recommended by recognized accrediting organizations and standards development organizations. ASTM, an accredited standards development organization, publishes a guide entitled *Confidentiality, Privacy, Access, and Data Security Principles for Health Information, Including Computer-based Patient Records* (2004) that includes guidelines in the areas of privacy, confidentiality, collection, use, and maintenance, ownership, access, disclosure/transfer of data, data security, penalties/sanctions, and education. In addition, HIPAA security regulations require that an organization use reasonable safeguards to secure and protect confidential health information. Identifying individual users and not sharing passwords would be part of a reasonable security system.

A published Lincoln City Hospital institutional principle is: "All employees will be assigned individual user IDs and will be accountable for the actions performed under them." Approved by senior leadership, this principle is an expression of the values held by the organization and defines the individual employee accountability expected, with the associated security capability included.

The following are some of the organization's options:

- Make exceptions to the current principle and policy for temporary employees.
- Hold to the principle and policy and issue individual user IDs for each individual employee, even when he or she is assigned temporarily. The IT manager may require authorization for additional staff to be able to implement this process.

To back away from the ethical practice of individual system user accountability that is currently the organizational standard would violate organizational principles. It might compromise the organization's commitment to patients to ensure, by technical security measures, that their data are protected. Although cost is involved, the second option is the best course of action. What additional justification can be made for this option? Why does this option meet the ethical concerns in the most appropriate way? Finally, could this situation have been prevented? How?

Additional Ethical Issues in Implementation Planning

To prepare your organization to address key issues in implementation planning, consider how EHR systems change basic information collection, validation, processing, updating, and retrieval functions.

Recognize that the EHR provides capabilities that the paper record does not have. The paper record is available to only one user at a time. Multiple users can view the EHR. The paper record is developed in chronological format. The electronic record is a database that can be presented in multiple formats or views. Paper record formats vary according to providers who use different documentation practices. The electronic record offers consistent data collection for encounters, which aids in the acquisition of essential data elements. The paper record maintains diagnostic test results over time on multiple pages. The electronic record can display the same data in a single graph. The paper record does not provide alerts and reminders to the physician without human intervention. The electronic record provides notification to physicians and other clinicians automatically.

Clinical Care Process

The EHR system records each transaction and timestamps the transaction. It is now possible to see how often the practitioner checks the system for new data. The system can track when an entry is made and when an entry is authenticated. It can also track the length of time between the availability of a lab result and a subsequent related order for care. In some instances, it can record exactly when the care or intervention was performed. This level of detail raises potential questions about the use of this data. Are the ethical issues any different from those of the paper record? Should the date/time of "viewing" a result be retained as part of the EHR?

Data Correction and Editing Process

Other capabilities, such as the ability to move data and the ability to "cut and paste," have great potential, but they also present potential problems. Should a practitioner be able to repeatedly "cut and paste" to pull the majority of the previous treatment note into the next treatment note? Are there any controls on "cutting and pasting" the work of another author/clinician? Is there any review to recognize the volume of use of the "cut and paste" function? Are treatment notes audited periodically to see that each note contains timely information? Should data be downloaded by providers to their laptops, PCs, or other personal electronic devices? Who should be able to edit an EHR? What happens if the original author is not available to correct an error? At what point does the EHR document become "official"?

System Problems

When data and/or technical problems arise in the EHR system, how are they addressed? What access should IT staff have to "fix" problems? What facts are needed to address these questions?

Technical staff who are needed to fix system problems and who require access to individual file information to do it fall under the principle of those who "need to know" information for an authorized purpose. In addition, signed confidentiality statements by all employees signal an additional emphasis on confidentiality. This practice recognizes the institutional commitment to confidentiality by giving notice to all employees that confidentiality practices are endorsed and compliance is expected. For contract employees and consultants, agreements should spell out required confidentiality measures. HIPAA refers to these agreements as *business associate agreements*. The IT security provisions for the organization should address standards for accessing, transmitting, updating, and auditing data in a secure fashion.

Health Information Access Capabilities

Typically, HIM professionals use laws, regulations, and the organization's needs to determine who has access to clinical records and to help establish retention policies. In an electronic environment the emphasis is on inputting data and information into the system and making it available to active users. If a provider is seeing a patient over a long period of time, there is an obvious need to maintain at least a core record in an accessible format. However, in acute care settings a large volume of data may be generated over a short period of time and while necessary during the care period the value of keeping all of that information immediately available over a long period of time needs to be evaluated. Given this environment, what is the HIM professional's responsibility to see that system decisions include the capability to access data over time? Is some data more valuable than other data? Will the system used today become outmoded and the data become inaccessible? Will the need to maintain or update access capabilities be a financial rather than a clinical decision? What are the ethical implications when patients trust that the healthcare provider is maintaining important health information on their behalf? How are principles and values used to fully explore this topic?

Expanded Use of Health Information

HIM professionals can use their health information advocacy role to support the appropriate use of health information. For example, EHRs allow a more fine-grained approach to the release of information. It is possible to release only what is needed to answer a specific question or to receive payment for a specific service. It may be possible to remove information about the lives of others that is often found in an individual patient's record or the specifics of a long-ago event that the patient does not want shared at this point in his or her life. This disclosure of information can be made without the record appearing to have been edited or redacted. Mental health, chemical dependency, HIV/AIDS, and other data that have special handling requirements can be monitored for appropriate limited release. It will be possible to screen records to pull only those records and data elements authorized for a particular research project. Instead of releasing a copy of a health history from a clinical record, it will be possible to disclose only the data element that answers an inquiry or meets the needs of a study request.

Infrastructure Strengths and Weaknesses

The EHR has many entry and exit points. The pressure to make the EHR widely available will compete with the need to create the infrastructure needed to manage appropriately in an electronic environment. The HIM professional needs to be able to analyze access and availability with the commitment to protect the individual's expectation of health information privacy.

PC workstation and printer deployment in business and clinical areas requires security analysis for physical placement and system security protections. Simply making the best decision about the physical placement of equipment is not sufficient. All employees and other authorized users must agree to follow the organization's policies. These policies and procedures must be communicated clearly through education and reminders. Deployment of wireless hardware tools is also subject to data integrity and security reviews and requires modification to access and use policies.

New Opportunities for Vendors and Healthcare Organizations

Vendors provide adjunct services that may require access to patient information. For example, drug information sheets can be printed out and given to patients to take with them at an appointment or sent to patients by e-mail. The same system offers to forward prescriptions to the pharmacy. The system also alerts physicians to potential drug interactions. The fee for such services is usually minimal.

The healthcare provider understands that the service is offered to obtain information about prescribing patterns. How can the HIM professional help prevent ethical problems associated with using these adjunct vendor services? Ethical problems arise because the provider cannot control how the vendor uses the patient information.

One way to address such ethical concerns is through formal agreements and contracts. The contract between the vendor and the provider should spell out the precise data that will be maintained in the vendor database. Specific data elements need to be identified. Specific use of the data needs to be clarified. Agreements that prohibit unauthorized use, including redisclosure of patient-identifiable information, should be included. Confidentiality policies from the vendor need to be reviewed as well. If the details about data collected and maintained and information use are satisfactory to the provider, and if appropriate prohibitions for misuse are documented in written agreements, then patients should be informed of the new practices and given the opportunity to decline participation. Without formalizing such agreements for information handling, ethical practices are at risk.

Scenario 11-B: Differences When Linking EHR Systems

You are an HIM professional at Hope Hospital and Physicians' Clinic who is responsible for managing the transition from paper records to EHRs. In your organization, a 300-bed hospital with a large group practice of 300 practicing physicians in 15 clinics, an EHR system has been implemented over the past three years. Not all modules are complete. Currently, your organization has basic health information service functions, including registration, admissions, discharge, transfer, abstracting and encoding, order communication, a clinical data repository, and financial modules. Data from the pharmacy, lab, radiology, cardiology, and nuclear medicine applications are fed into the repository. On the clinic side, appointments and encounters are automated as well. Transcribed reports from both hospital and clinics are maintained online with electronic authentication. The system is widely accessible via workstations, which operate Web-style access tools. These are in place throughout the hospital; they are also located in clinics and physician offices.

Recently, your organization has established a partnership with Southwest Health HMO, which is located in your city. Plans are to collaborate where possible to facilitate shared use of resources for patients and providers. A series of meetings is under way to address the mutual goals of both entities. In your healthcare facility, the stated goals of the EHR system are to

- Improve the health care of the individuals
- Improve patient and practitioner satisfaction
- Contribute to healthcare process efficiencies
- Facilitate compliance with legal and accreditation standards
- Enable research and planning to support healthcare policy decisions

The collaborative process is expected to take several months. The two organizations differ not only in the stages of EHR development, but also in organizational philosophy. Several "boundary" issues have already been identified by you and your HIM colleague:

- Common adherence to professional principles is in question because basic health practitioner user access is determined by user demand in one organization, under the broad principle of providing health information access for all health professionals who directly care for patients. In the other organization, user requests for access are filtered by user role and relationship to the patient before privileges are provided.
- Health information access rights are not specified when patients cross borders and different providers care for them. New access issues are expected.
- Basic security practices that determine time requirements for unattended workstations to automatically log off reflect different philosophies.
- The role and application of audit trails with report generation and follow-up are well specified in one organization but not in the other.
- Infrastructure is not protected. Patient information in the form of e-mail attachments is sent to insurance companies and in referrals. E-mail security is not ensured.
- Data quality issues associated with access and/or transfer of recent lab test results have not been assessed.

Question

1. How do you proceed? Analyze the case and propose the most ethical course of action.

A completed ethical decision-making matrix for the scenario is provided at the end of the chapter.

When individual organizations ally with other organizations to share business processes, patient services, patient data, and information on EHR initiatives, they frequently discover that their partner organization has divergent standards and policies. Practitioners who plan to see patients in the new environment may expect that the familiar standards and practices that have been worked out in their home environment will also apply in the new one, but in fact this is rarely the case. For example, those practicing in a more restricted environment will often want to "loosen" up the practices to reflect what they perceive as more "practical" operations. HIM professionals charged with maintaining ethical practices in handling patient information will confront challenges to their basic organizational principles and policies. They may also face ethical challenges in charting new paths for their organization. Scenario 11-B exemplifies this common situation.

The first step in figuring out how to proceed is to clearly identify how the organizations in this scenario differ in current practice. Table 11-3 illustrates the differences that have been described in this scenario.

The two organizations in Scenario 11-B are exploring how to work together. The initial plan is to keep the two organizations distinct and to focus on how their clinical services complement one another. Southwest Health's strength is primary care and care across a wide spectrum of settings, from outpatient through hospice. Hope

Table 11-3 Practice Comparison Table for Hope Hospital and Clinic and Southwest Health HMO

Hope Hospital and Clinic	Southwest Health HMO	Ethical Strengths	Ethical Issues
Access			
User demand—any user can access data on the system	User must link to data through a role/relationship filter	Southwest practices "need to know" principle	There is no access standard that ensures that each organization's patients' data are treated consistently
Users expect unlimited access to Hope Hospital patient data systems	Users expect to have limited direct access to Southwest Health's patient data systems		
Security Practices			
Unattended/no-use terminals are automatically logged off after 4 hours	Unattended/no-use terminals automatically log off after 30 minutes	Southwest procedures provide more security	Variation to protect patients' data on institutional computers is unacceptable
E-mail			
No specific policies or agreed-upon practices for clinical e-mail	Policies and procedures limit the use of clinical e-mail and specify when to include e-mail in clinical record	Southwest policies and procedures direct the technology options	E-mail practices compromise confidentiality practices for all patients
Audit Trails			
No system in place to review and organize audits of data and flag potential problems	Well-specified system with sanctions for inappropriate access revealed in an audit	Audit trails and sanctions are higher level security features	Auditing for patient access does not meet current recommended standards and legal requirements

continues

Table 11–3 continued

Hope Hospital and Clinic	Southwest Health HMO	Ethical Strengths	Ethical Issues
Confidentiality Agreements			
Employees and medical staff do not sign confidentiality agreements	All employees and medical staff members sign confidentiality agreements; vendors, students, auditors, and researchers are also asked to sign confidentiality agreements	Institutional principles for employee confidentiality practices meet industry recommendations	Southwest patients treated by Hope Hospital have less confidentiality awareness and accountability specified for employees
Information Notice to Patients			
Notice-of-information practices posted in the lobby	Written notice is given to the patient of the organization's information practices	Notice to the patient illustrates organizational commitment to privacy and confidentiality	Notice-of-information practices to patients are out of date and no longer accurate

Hospital and Clinic has some of the same services, but it also has very strong, well-respected specialty services. How does the HIM professional at Southwest Health HMO analyze the professional and ethical issues as this new working relationship between the two organizations is explored and put in place? Can Southwest Health open its patient database to Hope Hospital, knowing that the culture of Hope Hospital is very different? What about the safeguards and practices that have been communicated to patients in the Notification of Information Practices?

Technology drives the decisions at Hope Hospital. If it is technologically possible to do something, then it is implemented. This approach to decision making does not make decisions "correct" in terms of confidentiality of patient information. As the HIM professional, you may seem to be the lone voice of caution at Hope Hospital or you may be labeled as an obstructionist for not immediately supporting a new technology.

Several differences have been highlighted between the two organizations and their approaches to the privacy and security of their EHR systems. This can be viewed as a culture clash, but it also raises ethical issues. If you are the HIM professional at Southwest Health, you will need to examine each security safeguard for its importance to the working relationship between the two organizations and its criticality in terms of the core values that are embedded in the system of patient care.

User Access

At Hope Hospital, all users have equal access to the EHR without regard to their role in the care process or their relationship to an individual patient. All staff members are given an orientation that encourages them to respect the confidentiality of the information. The organization believes that it is not possible to know when any given provider will need access to a particular patient record.

Southwest Health has reviewed the roles of its staff in relationship to the need to access all or part of a patient record. It has been determined that certain staff members need access only to portions of the record and that certain other staff members need access only to patients under their care. Systems have been designed to set up front-end access filters so that staff members are privileged to gain access only to certain information. If a provider or other staff member needs to exceed his or her ordinary privilege level, a screen requests the reason for the access and notifies the user that this access will be reviewed.

The following are some initial options to consider when working through and reconciling practices in each organization in a way that preserves the ethical position of each organization:

- Notify all patients that there will be information sharing between the two organizations. If a patient objects, his or her information will be shared only with a consent or in an emergency.
- Have Southwest Health offer to share its access filter approach and programs with Hope Hospital.
- Establish agreements to govern access. Southwest Health could set up an agreement with Hope Hospital that the only access permitted would be directly related to providing patient care. Additionally, a more complex access process for requests for information by Hope Hospital staff could be agreed upon. The process could include a reason for the access and an audit of all Hope Hospital staff member accesses.

Think through these options. The recommended option should be based on the partner organization's philosophy and values. Each option needs to be evaluated to fully understand the consequences. What will the results be? Among the alternatives presented, it appears that the third option best preserves the current security practices in place at Southwest Health while imposing some limits to access by Hope Hospital staff. A rationale for this option could specify how it meets organizational principles and values and maintains an approach that conforms to national standards, state laws, and regulations and privacy and security provisions in federal legislation (HIPAA).

Security Practices

An ethical issue is one that involves core values of practice. In this case, ethical issues emerge when the core value of professional commitment to patient health information security is challenged because industry customers want technological ease to drive their user responsibilities and/or privileges. The facts are that variance exists in institutional principles to honor self-determination for patients' control over release of their information by placing protections in limiting the display and sharing of patient-identifiable information through workstations or other electronic devices. Options are:

- Southwest Health may maintain all current security practices and negotiate for Hope Hospital to adopt minimal security practices in areas that pose the most risk to confidentiality. The automatic log-off time noted may be reviewed in each facility to negotiate a new mutually acceptable time-out.
- Each organization may elect to employ the security practice it has. When a provider treats a patient, the patient's information is handled in accordance with the policies of the provider's home organization.
- Southwest Health may maintain its log-off standards through application and system software tools so that when Hope Hospital staff access Southwest Health data systems, the system controls the logoff standard at the current level.

What option do you recommend? Why?

Data Quality/Integrity

Another ethical issue emerges when core values of professional commitment to data quality are challenged because the appropriate infrastructure has not been prepared to protect the integrity of patient information. Oversight is necessary to ensure that the most current and reliable results are accessible at the time care is delivered. Established technical protocols to transfer data from ancillary systems can provide assurance that updates are consistently made and that data has not been lost or compromised as it is transferred between systems. In the same way that HIM professionals commit to keeping the paper records current with "up-to-date" maintenance of all data that arrives for interfiling, they need to be involved in ensuring that EHR data are as current as possible by working with technical partners to clearly understand the update details. In addition, policy recommendations may underscore the need for data currency.

Confidentiality Agreements

The ethical issue emerges here when principles established in one institution that call for signed confidentiality statements are not held by the partner organization. Signed confidentiality statements are another well-supported and recommended practice. National forums on privacy and HIPAA regulations encourage heightening privacy awareness for healthcare employees. In ASTM standards, this principle is endorsed in recommended education programs. An example of an institutional principle would be "Documentation of employee (signed) acknowledgment of confidentiality policies will be maintained in permanent files by the human resources department" (ASTM, 2004).

By extending the practice to the partner organization to require all employees requesting user IDs and passwords who demonstrate a "need to know" access to the EHR system, the institutional commitment to confidential information handling practices for all staff is validated. By focusing on the subset of users, this offers a negotiated course of action that ensures that the users of the EHR system will adhere to the same value. This would be a minimal implementation of confidentiality agreements for the institution that has not adopted this practice for all employees.

Notifying Patients About Information Practices

Notifying patients about information practices is a stronger part of the institutional culture in one organization. A Notice of Health Information Practices is required by HIPAA as of 2002. Each organization is charged to develop its own Notice of Information Practices and share it with patients. However, as the two organizations begin to work together and sort out their differences in information practices, they will need to rewrite their notices and inform their patients of any changes. Patient rights documents may also need to be updated to explain interinstitutional access to patient information. How will sharing resources and patient information affect the values held by the organization with regard to patient communication? Should the organizations collaborate and develop a mutual Notice of Information Practices? What are some other options?

Audit Trails and E-Mail

Audit trails and e-mail security practices will need to be examined as well. Audit trails record the access patterns to patient-identifiable data that are used to verify that approved access rules defined by the organization's policy are followed consistently. Because e-mail documents communication among providers and patients, this medium must comply with operational and technical security practices in order to uphold institutional policy. In contrast to Southwest Health HMO, Hope Hospital does not have any system to review and organize audit data and flag potential problems, nor does it meet current recommended standards and legal requirements. Also, Hope Hospital's lack of specific policies regarding clinical e-mail threatens the confidentiality of information on both patients and providers.

CONCLUSION

Information technology (IT), when deployed appropriately, can support organizations in achieving competitive leverage, market position, quality patient care, and efficient operations. These factors will become increasingly important in the future, as the cost of care continues to rise, reimbursement levels decrease, and competition for revenues increases (Mathews, 2000).

As organizations focus on EHRs for strategic value and the EHR becomes a center-piece of the IT initiatives in healthcare organizations, ethical issues will continue to arise. HIM professionals need to be prepared to thoughtfully analyze and share their analysis of the ethical issues related to IT applications with key decision makers. The goal is to help healthcare providers make good ethical choices in the implementation and use of EHRs and the resultant clinical databases.

Key Terms

- Alert and reminder features
- Clinical information system
- Confidentiality
- Electronic health record (EHR)
- Security

Chapter Summary

- EHR systems are being implemented in healthcare organizations, and they encompass increasingly sophisticated approaches to managing and using clinical data.
- The linking features of EHR systems, which are recognized as major advances in the use of patient record information, also make more information potentially available to many more users, and thereby exponentially increase the risk that patient confidentiality will be breached.
- Although EHR systems can include security features, technological solutions alone will not be adequate to protect the integrity and confidentiality of patient information. Any comprehensive solution must also include organizational and perhaps inter-organizational policies and legislation that require, monitor, teach, and sanction various behaviors related to the use of the EHR system and patient data.
- In the process of assessing, planning, and implementing EHR systems, ethical issues often arise that are related to the potential compromising of data integrity and confidentiality for the sake of greater business efficiency, better system performance, or more convenient and timely access to data. Issues include security provisions; application linkages; the data correction and editing process; access to data by technical staff and vendors; the ability to access data over time; and capacities for selectiveness of what data from a patient's record are released for a particular purpose.
- The people involved in developing and implementing systems must choose or develop systems that support the ethical principles of the organization and the healthcare professionals in that setting. Ethics should guide the organization to do the right thing when implementing the systems and using the information contained within them.

- In making ethical decisions, HIM professionals should draw on legal, accreditation, policy, and professional practice sources to consider what is in the best interest of the patient, how a proposed action supports the organization's principles and values, whether regulatory and accrediting requirements are accounted for, and whether personal and professional values of honesty and promoting quality health information are upheld.

References

45 CFR Parts 160 and 164, Standards for Privacy of Individually Identifiable Health Information and Security Standards for the Protection of Electronically Protected Health Information, 2003.

ASTM. (2004). *ASTM Standard E1869-04: Confidentiality, privacy, access, and data security principles for health information including computer-based patient records.* West Conshohocken, PA: Author.

Burns, P. (1999). Telehealth or telehype? Some observations and thoughts on the current status and future of telehealth. *Journal of Healthcare Information Management, 13*(4)(suppl.), 5–15.

Burrington-Brown, J., & Hughes, G. (2003). *AHIMA Practice Brief: Provider-Patient E-mail Security (Update).* Retrieved September 26, 2005, from http://library.ahima.org/groups/public/documents/ahima/pub_bok1_019873.html.

Computer-Based Patient Record Institute, Work Group on CPR Description. (1996). *Computer-based patient record description of content.* Schaumberg, IL: Author.

Connecting for Health. (2004). *Connecting for Health 2004. Connecting Americans to their Health Care.* Retrieved November 5, 2004, from http://connectingforhealth.org/resources/wg_eis_final_report_0704.pdf.

Dick, R. S., & Steen, E. B. (Eds.). (1997). *The computer-based patient record: An essential technology for health care*, Rev. ed. Washington, DC: National Academy Press.

Gillespie, G. (2000). How will CIOs protect data? *Health Data Management, 8*(8), 48.

Health Privacy Project. (2000). Exposed: A health privacy primer for consumers. Retrieved September 21, 2005, from http://www.healthprivacy.org/usr_doc/34775.pdf.

Healthcare Information and Management Systems Society [HIMSS]. (2004). *Annual HIMSS leadership survey, 2004 update.* Retrieved September 21, 2005, from http://www.himss.org/2004survey/ ASP/index.asp.

HealthKey Privacy Advisory Group. (2000, May 15). *A framework and structured process for developing responsible privacy practices.* Retrieved September 21, 2005, from http://www.healthkey.org/tools.htm.

Mathews, P. (2000). Leveraging technology for success. *Journal of Healthcare Information Management, 14*(2), 5–12.

Murphy, G., Hanken, M. A., & Waters, K. A. (1999). *Electronic health records: Changing the vision.* Philadelphia: W.B. Saunders.

Thompson, T. G., & Brailer, D. J. (2004). *The decade of health information technology: Delivering consumer-centric and information-rich health care.* U.S. Department of Health and Human Services. Retrieved September 26, 2005, from http://www.hhs.gov/healthit/documents/hitframework.pdf.

U.S. Department of Health and Human Services. (2004). *HHS health information technology strategic framework, executive summary 2004.* Retrieved September 21, 2005, from, http://www.hhs.gov/healthit/executivesummary.html.

Versweyveld, L. (2004, July 14). Press release: Connecting for Health recommends specific actions for bringing healthcare into the information age. *Virtual Medical Worlds Monthly.* Retrieved September 21, 2005, from, http://www. hoise.com/vmw/04/articles/vmw/LV-VM-08-04-17.html.

The ethical decision-making matrix is a tool to help you organize complex, ethical problems; however, there is no simple fill-in-the-box approach to ethical decision making. The objective is to follow each step of the process and not move from the question directly to what should be done or how to prevent it next time. If you skip steps, you will not fully understand all of the values and options for action. Also, the matrix provided for each scenario in this book is not the only way to examine the problem. You can make an equally compelling ethical argument for a different decision—just be sure to follow all the steps of the matrix.

SCENARIO 11-A: PATIENT RECORD INTEGRITY AND SYSTEM SECURITY

Steps	Information	
1. What is the ethical question?	Should you require the vendor to develop features that would protect record integrity and security?	
2. What are the facts?	**KNOWN**	**TO BE GATHERED**
	• New EHR system does not capture medication data from the existing pharmacy system. • System does not offer capability to link to medication data. • Multiple individuals will have the same user ID and password.	• Would competing vendors' products preserve record integrity and security? • What are the customary practices in such cases? • What does your supervisor expect you to do? • What is the likely impact on self and family of changing jobs?
3. What are the values? Examine the shared and competing values, obligations, and interests of the stakeholders (i.e., patient, HIM professional, healthcare practitioner(s), administrators, society, and other advocates) involved in order to fully understand the complexity of the ethical problem(s).	**Patient:** Values accuracy/integrity of records; values privacy and confidentiality. **HIM professional:** Integrity and accuracy (protect security and integrity of records); loyalty to employer; avoid harm (inaccurate records could harm patient); personal values (promote welfare of self and family by avoiding loss of job). **Healthcare professionals:** Value accuracy/integrity of medical records; promote welfare of patients through accurate documentation for future care. **Administrators:** Benefit patients and keep from harm; promote welfare of facility; maximize efficiency without compromising accuracy and integrity of medical records. **Society:** Promote preservation of privacy and confidentiality.	

4. What are my options?	• Accept the vendor's product as is. • Require the vendor to develop features that will protect record integrity and security.	
5. What should I do?	Require the vendor to develop features that will protect record integrity and security.	
6. What justifies my choice?	**JUSTIFIED**	**NOT JUSTIFIED**
	• Obligation to preserve record integrity. • Obligation to protect security. • Preserve professional integrity. • Demonstrate loyalty to employer unless asked to jeopardize record integrity and/or security.	• Accept the vendor's product as is. Jeopardize record integrity. • Jeopardize security. • Jeopardize professional integrity. • Violate organizational principles.
7. How can I prevent this ethical problem?	• Determine if system changes are needed. • Learn more about ethical issues surrounding EHR systems. • Discuss standards and the values that support them with colleagues. • Evaluate integrity of vendors.	

The ethical decision-making matrix is a tool to help you organize complex, ethical problems; however, there is no simple fill-in-the-box approach to ethical decision making. The objective is to follow each step of the process and not move from the question directly to what should be done or how to prevent it next time. If you skip steps, you will not fully understand all of the values and options for action. Also, the matrix provided for each scenario in this book is not the only way to examine the problem. You can make an equally compelling ethical argument for a different decision—just be sure to follow all the steps of the matrix.

SCENARIO 11-B: DIFFERENCES WHEN LINKING EHR SYSTEMS

Steps	Information	
1. What is the ethical question?	How should the hospital and HMO proceed?	
2. What are the facts?	**KNOWN**	**TO BE GATHERED**
	• The hospital and HMO have agreed to collaborate and share resources. • There is a lack of commonality on several key issues related to access and security.	• What is the nature of each conflict between hospital/HMO standards? • Would creation of joint policies enhance or decrease EHR security? • What are the customary practices in such cases? • What does your supervisor expect you to do? • What is the likely impact on self and family of changing jobs?
3. What are the values? Examine the shared and competing values, obligations, and interests of the stakeholders (i.e., patient, HIM professional, healthcare practitioner(s), administrators, society, and other advocates) involved in order to fully understand the complexity of the ethical problem(s).	**Patient:** Values confidentiality and privacy and security of information; values expeditious processing of medical claims. **HIM professional:** Integrity, accuracy, and reliability (develop a common set of standards that maximize EHR security); loyalty to employer; avoid harm (violation of security could harm the patient, provider, hospital, and HMO); personal values (promote welfare of self and family by avoiding loss of job). **Healthcare professionals:** Promote welfare of patients through accurate documentation and preservation of confidentiality; value confidentiality of medical records; value expeditious processing of medical claims. **Administrators:** Benefit patients and keep from harm; maximize expediency of claims processing without jeopardizing security. **Society:** Promote EHR security.	

4. What are my options?	• Proceed without standardization. • Establish a mutually agreeable set of standards and philosophies that maximize security and record integrity.	
5. What should I do?	Establish a mutually agreeable set of standards and philosophies that maximize security and record integrity.	
6. What justifies my choice?	**JUSTIFIED**	**NOT JUSTIFIED**
	• Obligation to preserve record integrity. • Obligation to protect security. • Loyalty to employer. • Preserve professional integrity.	• Proceed without mutually agreeable standards and philosophies. • Jeopardize record integrity. • Jeopardize security. • Jeopardize professional integrity.
7. How can I prevent this ethical problem?	• Determine if system changes are needed. • Learn more about ethical issues surrounding EHR systems. • Learn more about EHR systems and collaboration with outside organizations. • Discuss standards and the values that support them with colleagues. • Evaluate integrity of organizations with which you might collaborate at initial discussion stage and subsequently as ethical problems arise.	

12

INFORMATION SECURITY

Karen Czirr, MS, RHIA, CHP
Karen A. Rosendale, MBA, RHIA
Emily West, RHIA

Learning Objectives

After completing this chapter, the reader should be able to:

- Recognize how recent advances in information technology are challenging the security of patient health information.
- Define and discuss data integrity, authenticity, and security.
- Understand the implications of the Health Insurance Portability and Accountability Act (HIPAA) for information security.
- Identify potential system vulnerabilities and discuss how these may be addressed in the complex health organization.
- Discuss risk analysis and the role it plays in the security program.
- Adopt a model for a comprehensive information security program.

Abstract

Traditionally, the patient's primary care physician safeguarded the confidentiality of patient information. In the case of the hospital environment, the health information management (HIM) professional was the gatekeeper. Health information was stored and maintained in file cabinets or on file shelves by qualified staff. Today, however, the explosion of available information and the technology utilized to ensure confidentiality and security present challenges. The Internet and e-mail have collapsed the traditional boundaries of the file room. Although security standards are not new to health care, the adoption of the Health Insurance Portability and Accountability Act (HIPAA) of 1996 has introduced a host of security mandates that pertain to the electronic protection of protected health information (PHI). This chapter will focus on security standards and the ethical issues facing HIM professionals as they strive to deal with security as a rule under HIPAA and as good business practice.

Scenario 12-A: A Curious Human Resource Employee

General Hospital Health System's billing director, Robert Johnston, is admitted to the hospital where he is employed and undergoes a major abdominal procedure. He is admitted using an alias, and all computerized patient information is restricted from access except by Barry Miller, the attending physician, Scott Peters, the consulting physician, and the nursing and clinical staff on the unit where the patient is recuperating. The human resources (HR) representative, Marge White, anticipating a short-term disability claim, logs on to the clinical information system, searching for the data to help expedite the disability application for Mr. Johnston.

Questions

1. Did the HR representative violate access privileges or does she have the right to the information as a representative of the employer?

2. Was the proper level of access to clinical information provided to the representative?

3. Did the representative use sound judgment in accessing the patient's information?

4. Should nonclerical staff have access to clinical information systems?

A completed ethical decision-making matrix for the scenario is provided at the end of the chapter.

The key concept behind security is to set standards for protecting electronic personal health information (e-PHI) while it is in use, storage, or transit. The HIPAA Security Rule does not distinguish between e-PHI stored on magnetic or optical disks, hard drives, or servers (Quinsey, 2004). However it is stored, such information must be protected from any real or potential threats to its safety. Although information security is everyone's responsibility, rapid advances in technology have opened the doors to increased vulnerabilities across the enterprise. Consumer concerns regarding privacy and confidentiality have fueled the development of comprehensive information security programs (Exhibit 12–1). Consequently, professional management of information security programs has become a crucial need as well as a mandate for healthcare organizations. The appointment of a security official is required. This official's responsibilities will vary depending on the size and complexity of the organization. The actual title of the designated security official may vary as well. For the purposes of this chapter, the title *information security officer (ISO)* will be used.

THE HEALTHCARE INFORMATION REVOLUTION

We are in the midst of a healthcare information revolution. The explosion of healthcare data to be read, synthesized, applied, and subsequently managed for current care and future reference has resulted in more complex medical practices. Caregivers today must assimilate more procedures, diagnostic tests, medical instrumentation and devices, pharmaceutical products, and medicines. Tools such as the Internet, intranets, extranets, virtual private networks (VPNs), and video, voice, and wireless networks are changing the way we access information.

Exhibit 12–1 A Model Outline for an Information Security Program: Your Approach to Security

1. **Understand the security rule.** The security rule sections are in part 164 of the Federal Register.
2. **Assign responsibility.** Assign an ISO. Coordinate with the privacy officer, chief medical officer, physicians, and the board of directors.
3. **Develop a plan.** Complete a time line, identify a budget, and allocate adequate resources.
4. **Conduct a risk analysis.** A risk analysis is your road map to implementation.
5. **Develop security policies.** These are your overall directives that the security plan will accomplish.
6. **Implement administrative, physical, and technical controls**. Involves selecting, testing, and developing procedures to implement your plan.
7. **Develop and deliver a security training and awareness program.**
8. **Develop an ongoing security monitoring process.** You will need to develop a process to make sure your security plan works.

Source: M. Amatayakul, S. Lazsarus, T. Walsh, C. P. Hartley. (2004). *Handbook for HIPAA security implementation.* Chicago: AMA Press.

Electronic health records (EHRs), picture archive communication (PAC) systems, e-prescribing, document imaging, and clinical decision support are changing the way health care is being conducted. Securing such systems requires comprehensive administrative policies and procedures and documented formal practices designed to manage the selection and implementation of security measures. The escalating costs of health care and the likelihood of both continuing expensive technological advances and consumer demand give a special sense of urgency to the issues of managing information security.

To illustrate, say that a patient is taken to the local hospital emergency department for acute pain. Upon arrival, demographic information is entered into the hospital's computerized registration system and interfaced with the hospital's EHR system. While examining the patient, the physician, x-ray technician, and nurse enter findings into the EHR system as well. The physician requests recent lab values and current history and physical from the hospital lab and primary care physician (PCP). The information is electronically transferred from their respective EHR systems. At discharge, the physician enters and transfers an e-prescription to the patient's preferred pharmacy and sends an e-message with discharge instructions to the patient's personal e-mail address. A summary of the findings is sent electronically to the PCP. The ability to electronically combine and cross-match health information from divergent sources saves the patient from unnecessary testing and the providers from redundant documentation. The volume and complexity of data available virtually at our fingertips are increasing as technology becomes more powerful and readily available. Demand for information systems that are robust (i.e., that prove trustworthy even under varying circumstances) and that also allow instantaneous access by a multitude of users continues to increase. Coupled with a belief that anything is possible with computers, it is easy to understand the risks of using e-PHI without security controls. Consequently, implementing reliable systems to communicate and transmit patient and institutional information in a secure format is paramount. The complex nature of protecting the information is a primary responsibility of the ISO.

THE ROLE OF THE ISO

The security program requires an organization-wide commitment that is championed by the CEO, the CIO, and the board of directors. The ISO's responsibilities range from coordinating the security policies and procedures of the organization to making staffing decisions to producing routine reports for administration. The specific duties will depend, as mentioned earlier, on the size and complexity of the organization. To be effective, the ISO should have authority and responsibility to do the following (CPRI, 1996):

- Implement and maintain the goals of the information security program and the methodology to accomplish those goals.
- Propose and implement policies to senior management.
- Determine which security incidents and findings will be communicated to senior management.
- Determine the adequacy of the risk assessment.
- Make personnel and administrative decisions in the supervision of information security and computer access.
- Control the use and expenditure of budgeted funds.
- Prepare reports per administrative directives.

CONCEPTS IN INFORMATION SECURITY

Privacy, Confidentiality, Disclosure, and Need to Know

To begin discussing information security, we should examine more closely several terms surrounding this concept. When we use the word **privacy,** we mean the right of the patient to be autonomous—that is, to retain control over the individually identifiable in-

formation held by healthcare workers and their institutions. The American Society for Testing and Materials (ASTM, 1997) standard E1869 defines *informational privacy* as:

1. A state or condition of controlled access to personal information.
2. The ability of an individual to control the use and dissemination of information that relates to himself or herself.
3. The individual's ability to control what information is available to various users and to limit re-disclosure of information.

Confidentiality is the responsibility to limit the disclosure of private matters. In health care, it includes the responsibility to use, disclose, or release information only with the patient's knowledge and consent. Two more words whose definitions are important to keep in mind are *disclosure* and *external disclosure.* *Disclosure* is the access, release, transfer, or divulging of health information to any internal or external user or entity other than the individual who is the subject of such information. *External disclosure* is the access, release, transfer, or other divulging of confidential information beyond the boundaries of the provider, healthcare organization, or other entity that collected the data or holds the data for a specific health-related purpose. Other helpful terms can be found in Exhibit 12–2.

PRIVACY-RELATED SECURITY

The implementation of the HIPAA Privacy Rule set in motion a number of security-related initiatives. Sometimes referred to as the "mini security rule," the goal of the security rule is to preserve the confidentiality, integrity, and availability of protected information stored electronically. The security rule does not mandate any particular technology, in fact it is "technology neutral" to allow for flexibility in implementation. Although the requirements of the rule apply to all healthcare organizations, the exact method and technology adopted to meet the requirements will vary from organization to organization.

Exhibit 12–2 Definitions for Security

Knowledge of the following terms will make it easier to understand the HIPAA security regulations.

- *Protected health information (PHI)*—medical information that contains any of a number of patient identifiers including name, social security number, medical record number, and ZIP code, to name a few. Privacy regulations protect all individually identifiable health information in any form (electronic, paper based, oral).
- *Security*—efforts to protect the confidentiality, integrity and availability of individually identifiable information in electronic form. Security measures can be administrative (policies and procedures addressing access to information and disciplinary actions for violations), physical (locking rooms, storage facilities), or technical (encryption of electronic data and use of IDs and passwords to gain access to information).
- *Security incident*—attempted or successful unauthorized access, use, disclosure, modification, or destruction of information stored in an information system (45 CFR 164.304).
- *Information systems*—an interconnected set of information resources under the same management control that shares common functionality. It normally includes hardware, software, information, data, applications, communications, and people (45 CFR 164.304).
- *Workstation*—electronic computing device such as a laptop, desktop, or similar device, and electronic media storage device in its immediate environment (45 CFR 164.304).

Source: Adapted from D. Kibbe. (2001). A problem-oriented approach to the HIPPA security standards. *Family Practice Management, 8*(7), 37–43.

Deciding factors as to how to meet the rule include the organization's size, complexity, infrastructure, and hardware and software capabilities. Additionally, the cost of implementing security measures is a consideration, but cannot be the only deciding factor: "The cost should be proportionate to the value and degree of reliance on the computer system and the severity, probability and extent of potential harm—the requirements for security will vary depending on the particular organization and computer system" (NIST, 1995).

Confidentiality, Integrity, Availability

Confidentiality, in the context of security, is the responsibility to protect personal health data stored electronically from unauthorized use, sharing, and disclosure. **Integrity** is the dependability or trustworthiness of information. It refers to those qualities that give data internal consistency and ensure that data cannot be accidentally or intentionally modified, destroyed, or disclosed. It also involves ensuring the *authenticity;* that is, ensuring that whoever is entering information into the system has the right to do so. Standards must be developed to guarantee that information remains consistent with its sources. *Availability* is the assurance that the e-PHI that is collected, maintained, created, or transmitted is available for the proper use and to the proper user as necessary. Referring back to the patient's visit to the emergency department, imagine the consequences if the critical information needed by the treating physician had not been available due to loss, alteration, or inaccessibility, either because the system was down or failed in some way.

Sanctions

Applying and documenting sanctions for failure to comply with HIPAA standards is yet another requirement that spans both privacy and security. The organization is required to employ safeguards to ensure that information is not breached. These safeguards are security solutions such as passwords, encryption, biometrics, and automatic log-off mechanisms used to authenticate individuals and control access to confidential information. Sanctions, generally part of the organization's disciplinary policy, include actions such as retraining, oral and written warnings, suspensions, or terminations.

ESTABLISHING A SECURITY BASELINE

Policies and Procedures

First and foremost, an organization must develop a formal security management program for creating, administering, and overseeing organization-wide policies. Policies are guides to human behavior. More than 50% of the requirements under the HIPAA Security Rule address the development and implementation of policies and procedures. For instance, a policy for access to the master patient index (MPI) may state that only the MPI coordinator and patient registrars have access to editing functions and all other personnel have view-only access. Similarly, the policy may also state that only the MPI coordinator has deletion rights. Defining the current policy and the degree to which it adhered to is reinforced throughout the HIPAA rule. Proof of compliance is the documentation of adherence to established policies and procedures.

In the past, the paper record provided single user access; therefore, the risk of inadvertent or deliberate misuse, improper disclosure, or destruction was minimal. The healthcare provider controlled the record either by a manual or an electronic chart-tracking mechanism. Access to the EHR, however, is controlled primarily by policy, and multiple user access is the norm. An HIM department policy may stipulate that all employees have full access to the EHR, and release-of-information staff plus risk managers have full access to the EHR, including all correspondence.

The EHR promises enhanced efficiency, but without proper protection the door is open for unauthorized and remote access to virtually unlimited amounts of health and financial data. A strong security framework shows that policies are the foundation. The following example demonstrates the importance of policy. General Hospital Health System (GHHS) has established a protocol to provide an electronic notice to community-based physicians when their patients register at the hospital. A physician's office receptionist, a previous chart analyst at GHHS, notices that her neighbor was recently seen at the hospital. Logging on to the hospital lab system, she accesses her neighbor's records, which reveal a positive pregnancy test. The receptionist phones her neighbor to offer congratulations on the good news.

- Are adequate security policies and procedures in place at GHHS? At the physician's office?
- Has access control to hospital systems been properly implemented? Is it enforced?
- What ethical standards have been compromised?

Need to Know and Data Sharing

In the previous example, is there a "need to know"? There must be adequate balance between a patients' need for confidentiality with the physician's "need to know." Best practices dictate that only those with the need to know should have access to PHI. It would seem reasonable, then, to expect that only individuals such as physicians, nurses, therapists, and healthcare professionals who provide direct patient care would be granted that privilege. However, others, including the following, may also have a genuine need to know:

- Billing clerks charged with claims processing
- Social workers who arrange visiting nurse services following discharge
- Educators who supervise the clinical experience of students
- Student practitioners who must demonstrate core competencies in their area of learning
- Researchers evaluating drug therapies or the effectiveness of new product services
- Insurers who pay for services provided
- State and federal public health user groups, such as registries, communicable disease reporting agencies, and child and elder abuse agencies
- Regulatory and accreditation surveyors

At the administrative level, access to and reporting of patient-specific and aggregate data can help meet the short- and long-term healthcare needs of the individual patients, the healthcare enterprise, and society at large. Such information can help establish healthcare guidelines; aid in the development of treatment protocols and best practice standards; increase the quality and convenience of care at the point of service; provide decision support; speed up reimbursement; reduce operating costs; create better products and services, including more effective pharmaceuticals and medical devices; improve public health; make medical benefits more affordable; and facilitate more timely research outcomes. Considered in this light, the definition of *need to know* can easily become very broad. Policies and procedures that establish the appropriate level of access based on the employee's role in the organization or job functions help to guide the organization faced with such decisions.

One could argue that if the ultimate good of the "universal patient" is being served, then data sharing on individual patients is justifiable. However, tension may exist between the benefit of privacy for the individual patient and the benefits of disclosure for society as a whole. Other forms of data sharing could be seen as exploitative of patients and patient information; for example, the sharing or sale of data for marketing purposes. Demographic information regarding the patient population enables hospitals to plan activities that promise profits, such as fund-raising events and solicitation of donations for worthy causes, research, or the building of a new wing. Similar patient information could be used to develop an outreach program targeted to a specific neighborhood or area of the county where medical services are limited and access to adequate health care is a hardship. Does the intent of the party acquiring the data then become the deciding factor as to who should have access to the information?

In the case of data sharing with immunization registries, the American Academy of Pediatrics (1999) has suggested that patients, immunization providers, and parents should receive copies of written policies that describe the privacy and security standards of the registry and explain the purposes for which the data are to be used, the parties that will be allowed to input and receive data, and the requirements for written authorization before data are released for purposes other than those intended by the registry.

Still another issue with data sharing is the authorized release of confidential information to an unsecured system. For example, the director of marketing and development contacts the information systems (IS) department and requests an ad hoc report that lists the patient name, complete address, diagnoses, discharge status, and insurance information on all inpatients admitted during the last 15 days. The patient data will be entered into a database that is loaded onto a laptop computer. The enterprise is planning a fundraiser and wants to solicit donations from all patients who had a positive experience while in the hospital. Because the goal is success, they are narrowing their target to patients from affluent neighborhoods who are more likely able to make sizable donations. If the report proves worthwhile, the marketing and development department will be requesting that the report be generated automatically on a monthly basis. Is this appropriate use of patient information? What additional issues should be of concern to the ISO?

In Scenario 12-C, the research project was initially approved by the IRB, which is responsible for explaining the policy and procedures associated with research and publication of findings; therefore, the IRB is ultimately responsible for the breach of patient confidentiality. But what is the responsibility of the HIM director? Further, the researcher bears responsibility because he has been provided with the policies, procedures, and reminders associated with research and the IRB approval process under HIPAA.

Access Control

In the HIPAA security matrix (Federal Register 164.312), access control falls under technical safeguards and is one of the required regulations. What kind of access do employees have to confidential information in electronic form? Does the organization use passwords and user IDs for access to its networks and servers? Is access available from off-site locations? Can the organization track which users are accessing what information? Consider the following example: A coder reviewing an online medical record leaves her desk at noon for lunch without logging off her workstation. Besides the inconvenience of logging off and logging in, she feels that since everyone in HIM has access to the EHR anyway, it is hardly a serious issue. The hospital does prescribe to automatic logoff after 2 minutes of inactivity; however, coder workstations are set to log off after 15 minutes to

allow for the intense review of complex medical records.

- What are the ramifications of this type of behavior?
- Is there a true threat to confidentiality?
- Could an unauthorized individual gain access to the electronic files?

Scenario 12-A, which opened the chapter, raises the issue of unauthorized use by an authorized user. In many ways the greatest risk to e-PHI lies with the people who already have access. The HR representative was an authorized user. It was also an authorized user that accessed former President Bill Clinton's medical records following bypass surgery in September 2004. Events such as employee carelessness or thoughtlessness by those who have little regard for organizational policy are more common than one might expect and collectively expose the organization to civil and criminal liability.

Unique User IDs

Sometimes preventive security measures conflict with operational efficiency and clinicians' desire for convenient and timely access to data, and consequently security measures are ignored or circumvented. HIPAA requires that all electronic systems that store PHI be password protected. Therefore, to gain access to computer-stored data, each employee must have his or her own unique logon identifier and password. Typically, employees have access to more than one system and are educated not to share or post their passwords in plain view. Creating and protecting passwords are critical, but often there is little enforcement because the number of passwords a person is expected to remember becomes a problem of efficiency. When tools designed to make data more secure become a larger burden in their own right, they cease to be effective. In these instances, the organization may need to explore new technological options that can reduce the conflict. One option is to create one single but easy-to-remember password for each user that will link to all accessible systems for that employee. The security issue is that if the password is stolen or shared with another person, PHI is compromised.

Another solution is **biometrics**. Biometric authentication is the marriage of access control and a human attribute—something that cannot be stolen, faked, or lost (Tabar, 2003). Implementation of such a system at South Jersey Healthcare provides an excellent example. They have implemented fingerprint login for physicians who need access to the hospital's system from their office and home. This mechanism helps prevent security breaches and provides ease of access at the same time. Once physicians log into the site, a touch of their finger gets them directly into the system. The system is further protected by automatic logoff after 60 seconds of inactivity. Some other human attributes that can be used to identify individuals include voice patterns, handwritten signatures, retinal blood vessel patterns, hand geometry measurements, and facial characteristics.

As sophisticated as such systems seem to be, they are not without error. Problems exist when such systems do not work reliably, denying access to legitimate users and/or permitting access to unauthorized individuals. Also, there is nothing to prevent the user from logging into the system and then letting staff use the system to access information on the physician's behalf. With proper security education for the workforce, and with frequent reminders, the organization can expect the appropriate behavioral changes necessary that would ensure that those viewing the e-PHI do so in a secure location and log off immediately at the conclusion of the session.

Audit Trails

Security audits are the systematic review of an organization's information systems activity. They are used to evaluate compliance with policies and procedures. With the exception of some legacy systems, the auditing capabilities of various information systems are able to track those who have accessed patient information and when. However, **audit trails** (also called **audit logs**) will not necessarily reveal unauthorized use and disclosure by authorized employees, as was the case in

---

Scenario 12–B: Failure to Log Off of the System

At General Hospital Health System, patient care is expedited by real-time reports generated by the laboratory, pathology, or radiology departments that are then sent to the electronic record system. Barry Miller, a staff physician, can retrieve these results on his office PC or at the bedside of his patient Robert Johnston. This type of access permits him to make informed treatment decisions for optimal patient care. The risk is he may forget to log off of the system. If this occurs, others working in the vicinity of those PCs may deliberately or accidentally view patient information.

Questions

1. Is the failure to log off placing patient confidentiality in jeopardy?
2. Is the failure to log off a system vulnerability?
3. What are the risks of this system?
4. Are there safeguards that could help reduce the risk?

Scenario 12-A, nor unauthorized access using a stolen or shared password. Auditing functions should be set to target specific categories of data or patients. Security events commonly audited are access to restricted information such as HIV or other communicable disease results, data on VIPs (such as diagnosis, procedures, and perhaps demographic information), and sensitive information such as substance abuse and psychiatric data. Also audited are simultaneous logons to more than one workstation. This could be an indication that a password has been stolen or shared with someone who might not have access to the system. As mentioned previously, oftentimes such internal vulnerabilities are overlooked. Completing a security-driven risk analysis can effectively highlight these pitfalls. A completed ethical decision-making matrix for the scenario is provided at the end of the chapter.

Workstation Use and Security

The organization must have documented policies and procedures for workstation use and security. The procedures should explain proper functions such as logging in and logging out and policies on the use of unauthorized software. Procedures regarding the most appropriate placement of workstations that are used to access PHI should address limited viewing, password access, and automatic logoff. With automatic logoff, the ISO must ensure that the procedure does not corrupt data on the system. Particularly vulnerable are PCs at the nursing stations and in the patient care areas.

Particular attention should be paid to the use and maintenance of laptops, personal digital assistants (PDAs), and other handheld and wireless computers. Such devices are targets for theft and vandalism (Barmettler & Bauer, 2004). Power-on passwords and file encryption should be implemented, at a minimum. Locking cables and alarms for laptops provide additional physical security if such equipment is left in unattended areas or in

areas with only partial security. Other security mechanisms available are Secure Sockets Layer, VPNs, tracking devices that can be concealed from the untrained eye, and erasing software that automatically destroys files when improperly accessed (Young, 2004).

The Internet, E-Mail, and E-Health

The use of the Internet, intranets, and extranets, and particularly e-mail, by both providers and patients has escalated exponentially over the last few years. Electronic transmission of information is rapidly becoming widely accepted as a means to communicate and deliver e-PHI, and e-mail has taken increased significance as a mode of communication that is readily available to both patients and healthcare professionals. Patients want to be able to communicate with their physicians by e-mail to schedule appointments and access information. More and more healthcare organizations are adopting Internet technologies and implementing Web interfaces to their EHRs. Although there is no mandate that strictly forbids the use of such technologies, stringent policies, and corresponding safeguards are required. Likewise, the HIPAA Security Rule does not expressly prohibit the use of e-mail for sending e-PHI as long as the data are adequately protected.

For physician–patient communication, e-mail is especially useful for follow-up care, clarification of instructions, and to provide such information as addresses, telephone numbers, and directions on how to take or apply a medication. Although such communication technologies should never take the place of the crucial interpersonal contacts, issues of privacy and security should be taken seriously. The American Medical Association (AMA, 2004) recommends encryption of messages at all times. The AMA also recommends that security mechanisms, such as encryption, that are in place be described to the patient in advance of an e-mail relationship.

The use of the Internet to access health information and manage personal health data is on the increase as well: "Maintaining a personal health record is one of the best ways to have constant access to your health information over the course of your lifetime" (AHIMA, 2003). Online consumer-oriented services are now available that allow individuals to store and regularly update basic medical information about themselves so that information is available when changing providers, traveling outside the country, or in the event of an emergency. The major issue at this time is that patients will not update their information or that they may incorrectly enter information required for safe patient care.

Conducting a Risk Analysis

A comprehensive risk analysis is the foundation of any information security program (Gross, 2004). Basically, a **risk analysis** identifies the risks, vulnerabilities, and threats to the organization's assets (information systems, applications, physical plant, equipment). The outcomes assist the organization in determining potential loses or exposure should the vulnerabilities be realized or the threats be carried out. Risk analysis also involves estimating how much applied safeguards could reduce the risks. Consider the MPI access policy mentioned earlier. Limiting access to editing functions reduces the risk of inappropriate changes; limiting deletion rights reduces integrity risks.

▪ Identifying Vulnerabilities

A **vulnerability** is any gap in policies and procedures or in technical and physical safeguards. A **threat** takes advantage of a vulnerability. Threats can be material (e.g., power failure, broken pipes), environmental (e.g., water, snow), or human (e.g., input errors, fraud, snooping). Consider the example of a staff member (threat) whose access privileges were not terminated (vulnerability) at

the time she resigned. Ways to identify organizational vulnerabilities are to:

- Review audit trails.
- Review Joint Commission on Accreditation of Healthcare Organizations (JCAHO) or state licensure reviews.
- Make sure patches for hardware and/or software have been implemented.
- Walk through your organization or department and observe how staff utilizes systems, workstations, etc.
- Review help desk logs, patient complaints, and privacy issue reports.

Protecting data, whether from theft and vandalism, alterations, deletions, additions, and other tampering or unauthorized copying, transfer, or disclosure, requires that the ISO (1) address system vulnerabilities and (2) minimize the risk of threats to the integrity of e-PHI. Both of these tasks must be accomplished in ways that recognize not only the needs of patients and their families and the requirements of regulatory and accrediting agencies, but also the sometimes-conflicting needs of clinicians, administrators, researchers, vendors, insurers, and public health agencies. Suppose, for example, that a famous professional athlete from another city is brought to the emergency department via ambulance following a car accident after playing a winning game. Returning to his metropolitan city, the player visits his PCP, who requests and receives an e-mail copy of the emergency department record for follow-up care. The attached lab results showed alcohol levels in excess of the legal limit. During transmission, a hacker for the local newspaper sports section intercepts the message, and the star athlete is front-page news. The player is suspended due to the alcohol-related accident. Where are the vulnerabilities in this example? What security practices could have helped to reduce the risk?

Scenario 12–C: Storing Data on a Laptop Computer

With IRB approval, Marvin Jenkins, MD, a researcher, is completing a postdischarge record review. He is looking for cases where children under the age of three were treated for complications resulting from motor vehicle accidents. In particular, the researcher is looking for data to support the use or nonuse of child safety restraints, such as a car seat or seat belt. Dr. Jenkins asks the HIM director for permission to bring his laptop computer to the HIM department for purposes of entering the data captured from the medical record. Abstracted information includes patient name, diagnoses, procedures, length of stay, and any complications that existed as a result of the accident. Overwhelmed by the findings, Dr. Jenkins publishes his findings and is subsequently invited to present his paper to physician colleagues at an upcoming convention. In preparation, the researcher creates a PowerPoint presentation using data stored in his laptop computer and patient-specific data to support an interesting course of treatment or outcome. At the end of his presentation, he volunteers to provide copies of his presentation to anyone who leaves his or her business card.

Questions

1. What are some of the potential consequences and ethical complications of this proliferation of the data?

2. What could have the HIM director done differently?

3. Does the HIM director bear any share of the responsibility for the proliferation of data?

A completed ethical decision-making matrix for the scenario is provided at the end of the chapter.

Managing the Partnerships

As discussed earlier, data sharing for legitimate uses raises questions regarding the costs in terms of loss of privacy to the individuals on whom the data are shared. Prime examples are health registries that are organized systems implemented for purposes of collecting, storing, analyzing, and disseminating information on individuals with a particular disease, risk factor, or exposures to a substance or circumstance known to cause adverse health effects. The development of health registries indicates that certain elements of an individual's medical record may need to be accessible by the public. More than 20 states have begun to establish immunization registries, and many others are considering legislative proposals to authorize them. Such public health measures are intended to protect the community from outbreaks of vaccine-preventable diseases, to assess the cost-effectiveness of care, and to simplify the reporting of data to state health agencies or local schools. California has enacted legislation granting health professionals access to immunization databases without the patient's consent. Yet without appropriate security protections and prospective patient authorization to release immunization data, immunization registries may contribute to the erosion of privacy of patient health information.

When the benefits to the public outweigh the need for patient privacy, the ISO may choose to support certain data-sharing programs, but the ISO should ensure that e-PHI is protected to the fullest extent possible and that potential liability risks associated with releasing patient data are minimized. Policies to be considered involve (1) how patients should be notified about handling and release of e-PHI and what would constitute their informed consent and (2) whether data can be released in a de-identified format. Of equal concern is (3) whether the receiver of the data has a secure system and (4) might the receiver, in turn, share the data with still other users.

Patient Notification and Informed Consent

As discussed earlier, HIPAA states that for certain national priority purposes, such as research, oversight, and public health, PHI can be disclosed without patient authorization. Patient authorization should be sought when the information being requested was collected for other purposes or was not a type of information whose disclosure is mandated by law (e.g., gunshot wounds). Suppose, for example, that the U.S. Department of Health and Human Services (DHHS) is conducting an asthma study in the Northeast corridor of the country. The request is for basic information about the patient population requiring emergency treatment due to acute asthma. DHHS is asking for an upload of patient data from all urban hospitals within a given region to determine the extent of the problem.

- What are the patients' rights in this scenario?
- Would there still be value if the data were de-identified?
- What constitutes informed consent to data sharing?

Key Terms

- Audit trail (audit log)
- Biometrics
- Confidentiality
- Integrity
- Privacy
- Risk Analysis
- Security Audits
- Threat
- Vulnerability

Chapter Summary

- The ISO is responsible for determining appropriate practices regarding data security; that is, the physical and technical protection of the confidentiality, integrity, and availability of computer-based information and the resources used to enter, store, process, and communicate it.
- The rapid expansion of information technology and the increase in groups seeking patient health information for a variety of uses have greatly increased security risks and dilemmas involving the management of this information.
- In addressing system vulnerabilities that threaten data confidentiality and integrity, the ISO must find solutions that do not compromise clinical and operational efficiency.
- The ISO faces ethical questions in balancing patients' need for confidentiality with other parties' "need to know." In data-sharing arrangements, they must address ethi-

320 CHAPTER 12: INFORMATION SECURITY

cal and legal issues regarding patient authorization and informed consent and the use and protection of the data without sacrificing the benefits of data sharing for legitimate uses.

- A comprehensive security program should include policies and procedures based on need to know, identification and authentication mechanisms, detailed audit trails, and enforceable policies and procedures.

References

Amatayakul, M., Lazsarus, S., Walsh, T., Hartley, C. P. (2004). *Handbook for HIPAA security implementation*. Chicago: AMA Press.

American Academy of Pediatrics, Committee on Practice and Ambulatory Medicine. (1998). *Policy on the development of immunization tracking*. Retrieved May 23, 1999, from http://www.aap.org/policy/01398.html.

American Health Information Management Association [AHIMA]. (2003). *myPHR, a guide to understanding and managing your personal health information* [Brochure]. Chicago: Author.

American Medical Association [AMA]. (2004). *Guidelines for physician–patient electronic communication*. Retrieved March 31, 2004, from http://www.ama-assn.org/ama/pub/category/2386.html.

American Society for Testing and Materials [ASTM]. (1997). *Confidentiality, privacy, access, and data security principles for health information including computer-based patient records*. Standard E1869-97. West Chester, PA: Author.

Barmettler, J., & Bauer, J. C. (2004). Protecting the wave of the future: Establishing security for the electronic health record. *Journal of the American Health Information Management Association, 75*(8), 25–28.

CPRI. (1996). *CPRI toolkit: Managing information security in health care*. Retrieved February 24, 2003, from http://www.cpri-host.org/resource/toolkit/toolkit.html.

Federal Register. (2003). *Security standards final rule. 45 CFR Parts 160, 162, and 164*. Retrieved August 18, 2004, from http://www.hhs.gov/ocr/hipaa.

Gross, L. (2004). HIPAA security alert: A race to the finish. *Advance for Health Information Management Professionals, 14,* 26.

Kibbe, D. (2001). A problem-oriented approach to the HIPPA security standards. *Family Practice Management, 8*(7), 37–43.

National Institute of Standards and Technology [NIST]. (1995). *An introduction to computer security: The NIST handbook*. Washington, DC: National Institute of Standards and Technology, Technology Administration.

Quinsey, C. A. (2004). A HIPAA security overview. *Journal of the American Health Information Management Association, 75*(4), 56A-C.

Tabar, P. (2003). *Nine tech trends. Healthcare informatics online*. Retrieved April 2, 2004, from http://www.healthcare-informatics.com/issues/2003/02_03/cover.htm.

Young, C. (2004). Maximizing the return on investment in information technology by incorporating best practices. *Journal of Healthcare Information Management, 18*(2), 51.

The ethical decision-making matrix is a tool to help you organize complex, ethical problems; however, there is no simple fill-in-the-box approach to ethical decision making. The objective is to follow each step of the process and not move from the question directly to what should be done or how to prevent it next time. If you skip steps, you will not fully understand all of the values and options for action. Also, the matrix provided for each scenario in this book is not the only way to examine the problem. You can make an equally compelling ethical argument for a different decision—just be sure to follow all the steps of the matrix.

SCENARIO 12-A: A CURIOUS HUMAN RESOURCE EMPLOYEE

Steps	Information	
1. What is the ethical question?	Should you continue to allow HR employees to access medical records?	
2. What are the facts?	**KNOWN**	**TO BE GATHERED**
	• The HR liaison accessed the patient's record. • The HR liaison was not authorized to access the record.	• Did the HR liaison violate the patient's confidentiality? • What are the customary practices in such cases? • What does your boss or supervisor expect of you? • What is the likely impact on self and family of changing jobs?
3. What are the values? Examine the shared and competing values, obligations, and interests of the stakeholders (i.e., patient, HIM professional, healthcare practitioner(s), administrators, society, and other advocates) involved in order to fully understand the complexity of the ethical problem(s).	**Patient:** Values confidentiality of medical record; values expeditious processing of claims. **HIM professional:** Truth, integrity, reliability (protect record integrity and confidentiality); fairness (follow rules for all); loyalty to employer; avoid harm (inaccurate documentation in disability record could harm patient); personal values (promote welfare of self and family by avoiding loss of job). **Healthcare professionals:** Promote welfare of patients through accurate documentation. **Administrators:** Benefit patients and keep from harm; promote welfare of the facility; value expeditious processing of claims. **Society:** Promote preservation of confidentiality.	

4. What are my options?	• Allow HR liaison to handle claims in this manner. • Do not allow HR liaison to handle claims in this manner.	
5. What should I do?	Do not allow HR liaison to handle claims in this manner.	
6. What justifies my choice?	**JUSTIFIED**	**NOT JUSTIFIED**
	• Obligation to protect confidentiality. • Obligation to protect record integrity. • Preserve professional integrity.	• Allow HR liaison to handle claims in this manner. • Make exceptions to the rules to allow expeditious claims processing. • Jeopardize confidentiality. • Jeopardize record integrity. • Jeopardize professional integrity.
7. How can I prevent this ethical problem?	• Determine if system changes are needed. • Learn more about security issues surrounding EHR systems. • Discuss standards and the values that support them with colleagues.	

The ethical decision-making matrix is a tool to help you organize complex, ethical problems; however, there is no simple fill-in-the-box approach to ethical decision making. The objective is to follow each step of the process and not move from the question directly to what should be done or how to prevent it next time. If you skip steps, you will not fully understand all of the values and options for action. Also, the matrix provided for each scenario in this book is not the only way to examine the problem. You can make an equally compelling ethical argument for a different decision—just be sure to follow all the steps of the matrix.

SCENARIO 12-B: FAILURE TO LOG OFF OF THE SYSTEM

Steps	Information	
1. What is the ethical question?	Should you require the implementation of a timed logout system?	
2. What are the facts?	**KNOWN**	**TO BE GATHERED**
	• The current system expedites patient care. • Physicians must log off of the system to close access to patient records.	• What information is accessible via the system? • Could the use of such a system increase the probability of confidentiality violations? • Is it possible to implement a timed logout if physicians forget to log out? • What are the customary practices in such cases? • What does your boss or supervisor expect you to do? • What is the likely impact on self and family of changing jobs?
3. What are the values? Examine the shared and competing values, obligations, and interests of the stakeholders (i.e., patient, HIM professional, healthcare practitioner(s), administrators, society, and other advocates) involved in order to fully understand the complexity of the ethical problem(s).	**Patient:** Values privacy and confidentiality; values protection of record integrity; has an interest in prompt, accurate care. **HIM professional:** Integrity and accuracy (preserve accuracy and confidentiality of records); avoid harm (patients could be harmed if their records are accidentally altered); personal values (protect welfare of self and family by avoiding loss of job). **Healthcare professionals:** Value prompt, accurate patient care; promote the welfare of patients through accurate documentation. **Administrators:** Promote welfare of the facility; benefit patients and keep from harm. **Society:** Preservation of record integrity; preservation of confidentiality.	

4. What are my options?	• Allow the system to operate as is. • Require the implementation of a timed automatic logout system.	
5. What should I do?	Require the implementation of a timed logout system.	
6. What justifies my choice?	**JUSTIFIED**	**NOT JUSTIFIED**
	• Obligation to preserve record integrity. • Preserve professional integrity.	• Allow the system to operate as is. • Jeopardize confidentiality. • Jeopardize record integrity. • Jeopardize professional integrity.
7. How can I prevent this ethical problem?	• Determine if system changes are needed. • Learn more about the issues surrounding the security of EHR systems. • Discuss standards and the values that support them with colleagues.	

The ethical decision-making matrix is a tool to help you organize complex, ethical problems; however, there is no simple fill-in-the-box approach to ethical decision making. The objective is to follow each step of the process and not move from the question directly to what should be done or how to prevent it next time. If you skip steps, you will not fully understand all of the values and options for action. Also, the matrix provided for each scenario in this book is not the only way to examine the problem. You can make an equally compelling ethical argument for a different decision—just be sure to follow all the steps of the matrix.

SCENARIO 12-C: STORING DATA ON A LAPTOP COMPUTER

Steps	Information	
1. What is the ethical question?	Should you allow the researcher access to the database?	
2. What are the facts?	**KNOWN**	**TO BE GATHERED**
	• The researcher downloaded information into the laptop with the HIM director's permission. • The IRB approved the researcher's project. • The research disseminated the information widely. • The abstracted information includes patient-identifiable information.	• What information did the patient's signed release authorization cover? • What are the customary practices in such cases? • What does your boss or supervisor expect you to do? • What is the likely impact on self and family of changing jobs?
3. What are the values? Examine the shared and competing values, obligations, and interests of the stakeholders (i.e., patient, HIM professional, healthcare practitioner(s), administrators, society, and other advocates) involved in order to fully understand the complexity of the ethical problem(s).	**Patient:** Values the confidentiality of medical record; could benefit from study results. **HIM professional:** Integrity (protect confidentiality); personal values (promote welfare of self and family by avoiding loss of job). **Healthcare professionals:** Value confidentiality. **IRB:** Protect confidentiality; protect institutional integrity; protect the welfare of the facility. **Society:** Preservation of confidentiality; could benefit from study results.	

4. What are my options?	• Allow access to the database. • Do not allow this type of access to the database.	
5. What should I do?	Do not allow this type of access to the database.	
6. What justifies my choice?	**JUSTIFIED**	**NOT JUSTIFIED**
	• Obligation to protect confidentiality. • Preserve professional integrity. • Demonstrate loyalty to employer, unless asked to push legal boundaries.	• Allow this type of access to the database. • Jeopardize confidentiality. • Jeopardize professional integrity.
7. How can I prevent this ethical problem?	• Determine if system changes are needed. • Learn more about security issues surrounding EHR systems. • Discuss standards and the values that support them with colleagues.	

13

SOFTWARE DEVELOPMENT AND IMPLEMENTATION

Susan H. Fenton, MBA, RHIA

Learning Objectives

After completing this chapter, the reader should be able to:

- Appreciate the differing perspectives of individuals who give input into the development and implementation process of the electronic health record (EHR).
- Articulate the ethical responsibilities of the health information management (HIM) professional.
- Identify potential development and implementation conflicts and propose solutions to those conflicts.

Abstract

Development and implementation of an **electronic health record (EHR)** is a multidisciplinary undertaking. The various professionals involved will have differing opinions and needs. Because health information management (HIM) professionals have a major role in this development and implementation, they must decide how to resolve conflicting requests from stakeholders in ways that conform to the AHIMA Code of Ethics, are compatible with established standards, and meet the needs of their organization. This chapter explores typical conflicts among stakeholders, offers possible solutions to such conflicts, and presents a collaborative model for making decisions by integrating input and reconciling conflicting interests.

Scenario 13–A: Planning the EHR: Competing Interests

Mercy Hospital has decided to begin implementing an electronic health record (EHR) system. Senior management has tasked the chief information officer to hire a consultant to suggest a structure for the management of the EHR implementation project and to recommend a chairperson for the committee. The hospital has hired a consultant who must answer the following questions.

Questions

1. Who are the opinion leaders in the organization?
2. Who should be the leader of the implementation project?
3. What is best for the organization? What will meet the needs of the clinicians, patients, and the members of the committee?

A completed ethical decision-making matrix for the scenario is provided at the end of the chapter.

As the healthcare industry has become increasingly computerized, software applications have become pervasive. HIM professionals are increasingly faced with the need to participate in the development and/or the implementation of software applications. Because health care is multidisciplinary, so, too, are the software development and implementation processes, especially those concerning the EHR.

Both **software development** and implementation involve the perspectives of many different professionals and require many decisions about everything from the programming language in which the application will be written to how the screen looks and the actual functions or tasks performed by the software. Very often the task to be completed, or functionality, will determine the best programming language. Data entry, clinical information processing, report writing, and communications are all very different tasks, which may be written in Perl, JavaScript, Visual Basic, and C++, among others.

Who will make these decisions? Sometimes this in and of itself is an important decision. Possible choices are senior man-

agement, clinicians, information services, HIM professionals, or any combination. How will they make the decisions? Autocratically or democratically? What are the implications of a wrong decision? If a wrong decision is made, who will be affected? Who will be held accountable?

Depending on the software being developed or implemented, a wrong decision could mean something as inconsequential as the failure to complete a patient record within the regulation time frame or as serious as a breach of patient confidentiality or even endangerment of a patient's life. Of course, the consequences should be proportional to the results of the wrong decision. An incomplete patient record could have financial implications, such as an inability to bill, or it could result in survey recommendations from the Joint Commission on Accreditation of Healthcare Organizations (JCAHO). A breach of patient confidentiality could be more serious, resulting in the patient's being refused life insurance or even losing his or her job.

CONSULTANT'S APPROACH

The consultant is treating this assignment as a pre-EHR implementation project. She begins by outlining the steps she needs to take to help Mercy Hospital. She falls back on her project management training. Although every project has an identified sponsor, at this time she feels she does not have enough information about the organization to recognize the best leader for this project. She can, though, identify many of the stakeholders, most of whom are already on the project team. From these stakeholders, she will be able to establish the project parameters. These parameters include the scope or magnitude of the work to be done; the required resources, such as personnel, equipment, or even vendors; and the project schedule. She knows that the project manager will need to have strong managerial, communication, analytical, facilitation, and leadership skills (Seidl, 2002). After interviewing key stakeholders, the consultant will write a report with recommendations—the final outcome of this project. Of course, as with all projects, Mercy Hospital has imposed a deadline for the report.

INFORMATION GATHERING

The consultant meets with a number of the stakeholders and ultimate end users of the system to gather information.

Physician, Chief of the Medical Staff

The first person the consultant meets with is the physician who represents the medical staff. Here is what he has to say:

> I'm Dr. Smith in Internal Medicine. I'm here to tell you that all of the documentation requirements that exist today frustrate me enormously. I didn't go into medicine to write in a patient record or to interact with a computer terminal for extended periods of time. My goal is to take care of patients! Keeping that in mind, I need an EHR that takes no more time than my current system. Knowing what computers can do, I also need help managing my patients. I need to

> know the latest clinical guidelines. I need to be able to check drug interactions and look up answers to the questions of patients.

The following are Dr. Smith's criteria for the EHR:

- It must make it easier for him to care for patients efficiently and effectively.
- It must offer easy access to decision-support information on recommended preventive care, drug interactions, clinical guidelines, and other reference materials.
- Patient information must be available when and where he needs it.
- It must enable him to easily find the information he needs about his patients.
- It must allow speech-recognition data entry.
- It must be accessible over a wireless network on lightweight screens.
- It must be accessible from home.

In reviewing the interview with Dr. Smith, the consultant can see that he faces many ethical dilemmas. Upon graduation from medical school, he swore to care for patients to the best of his abilities. Because of increased financial pressures in the healthcare industry, he is being pressured to care for more and more patients within the same time frame. Of course, this means he has more documentation to complete, but no time during his busy workday to do it. If he does not do quality documentation, it could affect patient care. In addition, poor record keeping could mean the organization could not bill insurance companies and it would run the risk of being charged with fraud and abuse. Of course, Dr. Smith always has the option of not caring for the number of patients required by his organization, but that could result in the loss of needed income or his job.

Furthermore, the information-intensive nature of medicine has only increased. He can spend many hours trying to keep up with the medical literature; however, that has proven to be impossible. He needs help. He is often faced with making the decision of having something left undone or having someone unhappy with him.

Chief Financial Officer

Next, the consultant interviews the hospital's chief financial officer (CFO). The CFO says:

> My name is Jeff Jones, and I am the chief financial officer for this organization. Money, money, money—that's the mantra if we are going to keep our doors open! These doctors just don't understand. If we close, where will they send their patients? Getting them to document completely so that we can send the patient bills to the insurance companies in a timely fashion and keep our accounts receivable low is difficult at best. We need an EHR that sets the rules for documentation and enforces them. Functionality, such as computerized physician order entry (CPOE), is also becoming important as large employers and the government begin to require it of their healthcare providers (Leapfrog Group for Patient Safety, 2004).

The CFO would like the EHR to meet the following criteria:

- Enforce the requirement that all discharge summaries be dictated and typed within 24 hours of discharge. If they are not done within that time frame, the doctor's pay should be reduced. All physicians sign agreements to abide by the medical staff bylaws. The organization should enforce the bylaws.
- Codes should be entered automatically from the record into the billing system, thus allowing the organization to file the claim that much earlier.
- Physicians and staff should have the capability to print, fax, or e-mail patient record documents. The business office needs to be able to respond quickly to requests for information in order to maintain the organization's cash flow.
- Physician partners should be allowed to sign for each other if it is determined that this is necessary to keep the accounts receivable down.

The CFO wants an EHR that supports bill collection in order to help the organization to save money. The CFO is extremely worried about the impact of the Medicare Reform Act. It is going to be very complicated, not to mention expensive, to determine a patient's eligibility and whether the patient or Medicare is responsible for the bill (Centers for Medicare and Medicaid Services, 2003).

In reviewing the interview with Jeff Jones, the consultant concludes that Jones' main goal is to keep the organization financially solvent by all legal means.

Information Technology Specialist

The consultant's next interview is with the organization's information technology (IT) specialist. She had the following to say:

> I'm Sandra Jameson, and I have no background in health care other than what I have learned since I was hired at Mercy Hospital last year. However, I am an excellent project leader and have a lot of knowledge about different software development languages (C++, VisualBasic, Perl, etc.) and their capabilities.

Sandra has the following questions and requirements regarding the EHR:

- What kind of user interface will the system use? Will it be a Web-type interface or a more traditional screen interface?
- Who, outside of IT, will be her main point of contact? She does not want five people giving her directions. Someone must be responsible for making the day-to-day decisions for the project.

- The project must have a deadline for functionality specifications. Sandra has had a lot of experience with "functionality creep." Every time something new is added, it delays the implementation of the application (Seidl, 2002).
- The security of the application must meet the organization's legal and privacy requirements, especially given the requirements of HIPAA (Centers for Medicare and Medicaid Services, 1996; Federal Register, 2003; Quinsey, 2004).
- Users, especially the physicians, must be satisfied or at least neutral, because the IT department will have to educate them, and IT will be blamed for what the physicians do not like about the application.
- Senior management must support the project.
- A physician champion or sponsor must sell the change to the medical staff.
- How standards-based will the implementation be? Which standards will be used? (AHIMA Workgroup on Core Data Sets as Standards for the EHR, 2004).

The IT specialist wants direction and support. She can help manage the project, but she does not want to be the project leader. She needs someone to help secure senior management support and buy-in, which are vital to any successful project. She can help to define the necessary tasks, identify responsible parties, and estimate a time line for the project. Many of the decisions required for the project are outside of her area of responsibility, and she needs someone higher up in the organization to provide leadership (Seidl, 2002).

The consultant can certainly empathize with Sandra. Invariably the failure of any technology implementation is thought to be due to the technology, not the human users. Also, Sandra will have some difficult decisions to make if the project takes a path that she does not believe is legal or correct for the organization. She is not placed highly enough in the organization to put pressure on persons who make many of the decisions.

HIM Director

The HIM director, Susan Hancock, is interviewed next.

> I want to be actively involved in the project. I have so many ideas about what is possible with the EHR. I want to provide the right information to the right providers at the right time. I am very concerned about adverse events and patient safety (medication errors, etc.), and I want to ensure that these are addressed by the EHR. I also know that, although implementing the EHR in this organization is important, interoperability with the rest of the healthcare industry in the future must be considered.
>
> I will play an integral role in the development and management of the EHR, and Mercy Hospital cannot implement an EHR without complying with the information and documentation requirements of JCAHO, Medicare, HIPAA, and the many stakeholders involved in the clinical information system. I am so excited that we are finally going to begin working on our EHR. I have spent a lot of time considering the current processes and determining how I believe an EHR will help our organization.

Susan would like the EHR to meet the following criteria:

- The EHR should conform to standards promulgated by the Department of Health and Human Services, Health Level-7, and the American Society for Testing and Materials (ASTM). The developers should look at the standards the federal government is using for the Consolidated Health Initiative (CHI) project (AHIMA Workgroup on Core Data Sets as Standards for the EHR, 2004; Health Level-7, 2004).

- It should be compatible with HIPAA privacy and security rules (Centers for Medicare and Medicaid Services, 1996; Federal Register, 2003; Quinsey, 2004).
- The printing, faxing, and e-mailing of discharge summaries should be restricted to the HIM department so that patient confidentiality can be protected.
- It should generate automatic audit trails for any access to the discharge summaries and have any fax or e-mail tracked as a part of the patient record. Audit trails can be used to ensure patient confidentiality.
- The system should receive the necessary ICD-9-CM and/or CPT codes and transfer them to the billing office. This will allow the HIM department to effectively and efficiently process discharge summaries.
- It must be easy for the HIM department to use.

The Consultant's Recommendations

The consultant has to decide on recommendations for Mercy Hospital. Among the questions to be answered are:

- How much should the interested parties (head physician, CFO, CIO, IT director, HIM director) be expected to participate in the process of developing and implementing the EHR?
- What role should each have in the process?
- How much weight should be given to the concerns of different parties?
- How should decisions be made?
- What are some of the conflicts of interest of the different parties?
- What are some ways that specific conflicts of interest might be resolved?

A Collaborative Approach to Decision Making

After much thought and deliberation, the consultant decides to recommend a multidis-

ciplinary task force to manage this project. Senior management agrees with this approach, but they decline to designate a task force chair, asking that the consultant do this.

Sandra (IT) and Jeff (CFO) have both stated that they are not interested in chairing the task force, although both agree that they have a vital role to play in implementing the EHR. After considering the competencies and skills required of a project manager (Seidl, 2002), as well as the skills and knowledge base of all the different task force members, and discussing the issue of who should be made chair, either Dr. Smith (physician) or Susan Hancock (HIM director) must be selected to lead the task force.

The consultant convenes the first task force meeting. The selection of the task force chair is the first item on the agenda. When the topic of task force chair comes up for discussion, the task force members make the following statements:

- Physician, Dr. Smith: "I would like to be the task force chair to ensure that physician needs are met. While this will be yet one more demand on my time now, the potential for making my life and the lives of my colleagues easier in the long run is enormous. This project cannot possibly be successful without a physician advocate and champion."
- CFO, Jeff Jones: "I do not want to be the task force chair, but I want to ensure that our needs are met."
- IT, Sandra Jameson: "While I can certainly operate as task force chair, I would rather not. My role in this process is to ensure that the EHR is consistent with our long-term technical plan and that it meets user needs and legal requirements."
- HIM director, Susan Hancock: "I feel that I am the best choice for task force chair. I know what the legal and regulatory requirements are for the EHR and the confidentiality of patient records. I consider it part of my job to work with everyone on this task force to ensure that all of

their needs are included in the software if at all possible."

The question remains: *Who should be selected to chair the task force?*

The task force must begin the process of developing and/or selecting the software. The team needs to define the project such that everyone agrees with the project's scope, deliverables, and deadlines (Seidl, 2002). With regards to the actual software, the task force will be responsible for guiding the EHR application through the first three steps of planning, selection, and implementation. The fourth step of **project management** (maintenance) is outside the scope of this task force, but this will need to occur as the software is implemented (Homan, 1999).

As the task force begins the planning process, they do not want to reinvent the wheel, so they begin with the Health Level-7 EHR Functional Model (HL-7, 2004). This model separates the functional specifications into three main areas:

1. Direct care functions—those with a direct impact upon patient care
2. Supportive functions—items such as registries, scheduling, bed assignments, and financial operations
3. Information infrastructure functions—these include security, record management, unique identifier management, interoperability standards, business rules, and workflow management

In the end, all of the parties generally agreed on functionality and the use of the record; however, when all of the bids were in and it was time to make a purchase, the CFO began insisting that Mercy choose the cheapest product. The other members of the group have used their strongest arguments with him to no avail. They must now decide whether to live with that product, which they happen to believe will not be best for patient care, or go around and over the CFO to the CEO, and possibly the board of trustees.

What should the task force do in response to the CFO?

CONCLUSION

The EHR implementation scenario that opened this chapter illustrated the often-competing perspectives of the multiple parties who will be using the software and the system features that each party wants. How do healthcare organizations decide what to do in such instances? They must not only meet the needs of this task and the needs of the organization, but also act ethically (AHIMA Code of Ethics, 2004).

As is true for most tasks performed by HIM professionals, there are few easy ethical answers. According to Harman (2000), the AHIMA Code of Ethics, from the founding of AHIMA to the present, has espoused values that include, but are not limited to,

- Providing service
- Protecting, preserving, and securing personal information
- Promoting collaboration and cooperation
- Complying with laws, regulations, and policies
- Refusing to participate in or conceal unethical practices
- Being truthful

Within this abbreviated list, you can begin to see that these values are not always congruent with one another. HIM professionals will encounter many ethical dilemmas during their careers. They should call upon all of their resources: knowledgeable colleagues, coworkers, their association, their organizational ethics committee, and possibly legal counsel to help determine their best course of action.

Key Terms

- Collaborative decision making
- Software development
- Project management
- Electronic Health Record (EHR)

Chapter Summary

- HIM professionals often have a major role in developing and/or implementing new software. This is a multidisciplinary process, which requires input from many different stakeholders who have differing, and often conflicting, requirements.
- Clinicians may well request features that speed up time-consuming review procedures and allow them to access and share information more quickly and easily. Administrators may also request such features for efficiency reasons. The legal and regulatory requirements with which the HIM professional must comply may rule out these features or require compromises to modify them. Even in the absence of legal restrictions, ethical concerns to ensure accuracy and protect security of information require the HIM professional to suggest special safeguards for these features.
- A collaborative process of decision making that involves a multidisciplinary task force to oversee the software project can ensure that the opinions, rationales, and suggested solutions of all stakeholders are heard and considered.

References

AHIMA Code of Ethics. (2004). AHIMA Website. Retrieved November 7, 2004, from http://library.ahima.org/xpedio/groups/public/documents/ahima/pub_bok1_024277.html.

AHIMA Workgroup on Core Data Sets as Standards for the EHR. (2004). E-HIM strategic initiative: Core data sets (AHIMA Practice Brief). *Journal of AHIMA*, 75(8), 68A–D.

AHIMA Workgroup on Electronic Health Records Management. (2004). The strategic importance of electronic health records management. *Journal of AHIMA*, 75(9), 80A–B.

Centers for Medicare and Medicaid Services. (1996). *The Health Insurance Portability and Accountability Act of 1996*. Washington, DC: Department of Health and Human Services.

Centers for Medicare and Medicaid Services. (2003). Medicare Modernization Update. Washington, DC: Department of Health and Human Services.

Federal Register. (2003). *Security Standards Final Rule*. 45 CFR Parts 160, 162, and 164. Retrieved August 18, 2004, from http://www.hhs.gov/ocr/hipaa.

Harman, L. B. (2000). Confronting ethical dilemmas on the job: An HIM professional's guide. *Journal of AHIMA*, 71(5), 45–49.

Health Level-7. (2004). Index Page. Retrieved November 7, 2004, from http://www.hl7.org/.

Homan, C. (1999). *Beyond the basics: Systems development life cycle*. Online Course, AHIMA.

Leapfrog Group for Patient Safety. (2004). *Rewarding higher standards*. Retrieved November 7, 2004, from http://www.leapfroggroup.org/.

Quinsey, C. A. (2004). A HIPAA security overview [AHIMA Practice Brief]. *Journal of AHIMA*, 75(4), 56A–C.

Seidl, P. B. (2002). Project management. In K. LaTour & S. Eichenwald (Eds.), *Health information management: Concepts, principles, and practice* (pp. 631–660). Chicago: AHIMA.

The ethical decision-making matrix is a tool to help you organize complex, ethical problems; however, there is no simple fill-in-the-box approach to ethical decision making. The objective is to follow each step of the process and not move from the question directly to what should be done or how to prevent it next time. If you skip steps, you will not fully understand all of the values and options for action. Also, the matrix provided for each scenario in this book is not the only way to examine the problem. You can make an equally compelling ethical argument for a different decision—just be sure to follow all the steps of the matrix.

SCENARIO 13-A: PLANNING THE EHR: COMPETING INTERESTS

Steps	Information	
1. What is the ethical question?	How should Mercy Hospital approach the project?	
2. What are the facts?	**KNOWN**	**TO BE GATHERED**
	• A new electronic health record (EHR) will be implemented. • Each group of participants has different requirements. • Some of the suggested capabilities could increase the risk of security violations.	• Who has the authority among the participants? • Which capabilities could threaten security or confidentiality, or violate the law? • Who is responsible for the final product? • What are the customary practices in such cases? • What are the convenience, timeliness, accuracy, legal, and regulatory requirements?
3. What are the values? Examine the shared and competing values, obligations, and interests of the stakeholders (i.e., patient, HIM professional, healthcare practitioner(s), administrators, society, and other advocates) involved in order to fully understand the complexity of the ethical problem(s).	**Patient:** Values accuracy; values expeditious claims processing. **HIM professional:** Truth, integrity, accuracy, and reliability: ensure development of a system that is effective, but that does not violate ethics; loyalty to employer; avoid harm (protect patients by ensuring the creation of an ethical system). **Healthcare professionals:** Protect welfare of patients without compromising confidentiality or data integrity; value a time-saving system. **IT:** Values an efficient, accurate system that does not compromise legal or regulatory requirements. **Financial administration:** Values expeditious claims processing; values maximum product for a minimum price.	

4. What are my options?	• Proceed alone relying on information garnered from interviews. • Form a multidisciplinary task force to develop the system.	
5. What should I do?	Form a multidisciplinary task force to plan for the system.	
6. What justifies my choice?	**JUSTIFIED**	**NOT JUSTIFIED**
	• Obligation to ensure the accuracy and legality of the system. • Obligation to meet regulatory requirements. • Obligation to protect confidentiality. • Demonstrate loyalty to employer. • Preserve professional integrity. • Support interdisciplinary collaboration and decision making.	• Proceed alone. • Take responsibility for the entire project. • Jeopardize confidentiality. • Potential violation of regulatory and legal requirements. • Jeopardize professional integrity. • Jeopardize accuracy of records.
7. How can I prevent this ethical problem?	• Determine if system changes are needed. • Learn more about the ethical issues surrounding the implementation of EHR systems. • Discuss standards and the values that support them with colleagues. • Evaluate institutional integrity at job interview and subsequently as ethical problems occur.	

14

DATA RESOURCE MANAGEMENT

Frances Wickham Lee, DBA
Andrea W. White, PhD
Karen A. Wager, DBA, RHIA

Abstract

Information age technologies are profoundly affecting health care. Clinical data repositories, data marts, data warehouses, and electronic health records (EHRs) are enhancing or replacing paper medical records. In this new environment, health information management (HIM) professionals face new challenges of combining the best practices of medical record management with the best practices of database management. The chapter explores these challenges and the ethical questions that may raise.

DATA RESOURCE MANAGEMENT IN HEALTH CARE

Information age technologies are profoundly affecting health care. Clinical data repositories, data marts, data warehouses, and electronic health records (EHRs) are enhancing or replacing paper medical records. Patient-specific information has been an essential component of patient care for decades. Today, however, health information administrators face new challenges of combining the best practices of medical record management with

Learning Objectives

After completing this chapter, the reader should be able to:

- Describe the role of a data resource manager in health care.
- Discuss the ethical questions facing data resource managers.
- Understand the impact of Health Insurance Portability and Accountability Act (HIPAA) regulations on data resource management.
- Explain the differences among the following: databases, clinical data repositories, data warehouses, data marts, data mining, and visual integration of data.
- Describe the features associated with an electronic health record.

the best practices of database management. These practices are merging in the role of data resource manager.

A **data resource manager** is a person who uses technical tools, such as computer-based health record systems, data repositories, and data warehouses "[to] ensure that the organization's information systems meet the needs of those who provide and manage patient services along the continuum of care and that the organization's data resources are secure, accessible, accurate, and reliable" (American Health Information Management Association [AHIMA], 1999, p. 111). The data resource management role is defined as having two primary goals: (1) providing leadership for the data resource management functions and (2) ensuring that the data are secure, accessible, accurate, and reliable.

The skills required to perform the data resource management function include a thorough understanding of health information administration, as well as a working knowledge of the technical aspects of health information systems. The data resource manager should be comfortable as a participant in healthcare database and computer network management and design. Knowledge of the Internet and its use as a "front end" to access patient information is essential in today's electronic healthcare environment. Health information management issues such as confidentiality, access, release of information, and security are equally important in the electronic environment and must be thoroughly understood by the data resource manager. The underlying principles governing these issues remain the same, but the implementation of safeguards is quite different (AHIMA, 1999).

IMPACT OF HIPAA REGULATIONS ON DATA RESOURCE MANAGEMENT

Most health information administrators are very familiar with the **Health Insurance Portability and Accountability Act (HIPAA),** Public Law 104-191. Passed in 1996 by Congress, HIPAA was designed not only to improve the portability and continuity of health insurance coverage, but also to address administrative simplification, data privacy, and security. HIPAA requires that healthcare plans, providers, and clearinghouses adopt standards or safeguards to ensure the integrity and confidentiality of health information and protect against threats to the security or integrity of the information and against unauthorized uses of the information. HIPAA does not mandate the use of EHRs; rather, it sets forth rules for those who use electronic records.

HIPAA (and other laws and standards) require that data resource managers assume an active role in formalizing healthcare privacy, confidentiality, and security practices within their organizations. They need to demonstrate that the organization has in place reasonable and appropriate administrative, technical, and physical safeguards for transmitting health information electronically. Such practices are essential to ensuring the integrity and confidentiality of patient information.

DATA RESOURCE MANAGEMENT TOOLS

Data resource managers may use a variety of data storage and data analysis tools. Data stores take the form of small and large databases, clinical data repositories, EHRs, data warehouses, and data marts. Data analysis tools may range from standard query tools to sophisticated data mining applications. We will briefly describe each of these tools and how they compare or interact with one another.

Database and Data Decision Tools

A **database** is a collection of related data designed to meet the information needs of its users. Although there are other models for database design, many data stores today were developed as relational databases. The relational database model represents data in the form of tables. The relational database has many advantages over older "flat" file computer systems, including improved data integrity and decreased data redundancy (Rob & Coronel, 2002).

The term *data repository* is used in a variety of ways. However, it generally implies a large database structure that stores data that were originally captured within a smaller, application-specific database. The **clinical data repository (CDR)** is a database designed to aggregate and store patient-specific clinical data that have been captured via other information systems within the healthcare facility (Fox & Jesse, 1999). Relevant patient-specific data from disparate information systems throughout the healthcare facility, such as the laboratory, radiology, or medical record systems, are electronically screened and translated into a standard format that can be stored permanently in the CDR (see Figure 14–1).

Data warehouses and data marts differ from databases and clinical data repositories. Whereas the CDR is more or less a large relational database, the data warehouses are more sophisticated decision support systems. A **data warehouse** is defined as an integrated, subject-oriented, time-variant, nonvolatile database. Data warehouses are designed for decision support; usually they are read-only databases optimized for data analysis and query processing. Typically, data are captured from various sources and passed through an extraction process that will filter, transform, integrate, classify, aggregate, and/or summarize the data. This extraction process creates "data cubes" that allow for multidimensional presentation of the data with "drill-down" capabilities (Rob & Coronel, 2002). Database and data repository use is basically transactional in nature, whereas data warehouse use is historical. Databases and data repositories generally rely on transactional processing tools to generate reports, but data warehouses employ online analytical processing tools (AHIMA, 1999) (see Figure 14–2).

A **data mart** is a small single-subject data warehouse. The difference between a data warehouse and a data mart is the scope of the problem being addressed. The data mart is generally confined to a department or other business unit within the organization (Rob & Coronel, 2002).

Data mining tools are used in conjunction with data warehouses or large databases. They are used to analyze data for anomalies and possible relationships. They differ from standard query languages in that they uncover

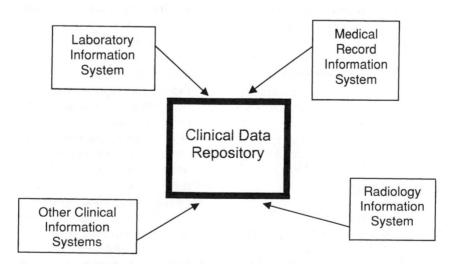

Figure 14–1 Clinical Data Repository. Disparate information systems feed information into a central CDR.

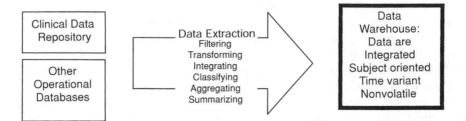

Figure 14–2 Data Warehouse. Advanced data extraction processes create "data cubes" that allow multidimensional presentation tools with drill-down capabilities.

possible problems or opportunities that are "hidden" in the data relationships. Querying a database using a standard query language requires the user to know what question to ask. Data mining requires very little end-user intervention (Rob & Coronel, 2002).

Another model of integrating patient information is emerging within the healthcare community. With the rise in the use of the Internet and World Wide Web, new tools are being developed for accessing and extracting data from disparate clinical information systems. These new tools use a "visual integration" approach to present patient-specific information at the workstation. Rather than physically moving data from the department-level clinical information systems into a new data store, **visual integration tools** grab data from the original databases and visually present data to the user so that it looks like it comes from one record. However, the sources have not been physically integrated as belonging to one patient (Seliger, 2001). Arguments for visual integration are its flexibility and elimination of the extraction processes required for data repositories. Arguments against it generally involve a loss of control over the data source and security fears (see Figure 14–3).

Electronic Health Records

A host of different terms has been used over the years to describe the concept of an electronic health record system. The two most common terms include the *computer-based patient record (CPR)* and the *electronic health*

record *(EHR)*. Depending on the source, the terms may be used interchangeably or viewed quite differently. The term *CPR* was officially defined by the Institute of Medicine (IOM) in 1991 in its report entitled *The Computer Based Patient Record—An Essential Technology for Health Care.* The IOM (1991) defined the CPR as "an electronic patient record that resides in a system specifically designed to support users by providing accessibility to complete and accurate data, alerts, reminders, clinical decision support systems, links to medical knowledge and other aids" (p. 11).

Nearly 12 years later, the IOM (2003) adopted the term **electronic health record (EHR)** to include the attributes of the CPR as well as the following core components:

- **Health information and data**—includes defined data set such as medical and nursing diagnoses, a medication list, allergies, demographics, clinical narratives, and laboratory test results
- **Results management**—manages all types of results (e.g., laboratory test results, radiology procedure results) electronically
- **Order entry/management**—incorporates use of computerized provider order entry, particularly in ordering medications
- **Decision support**—employs computerized clinical decision support capabilities such as reminders, alerts, and computer-assisted diagnosing
- **Electronic communication and connectivity**—enables those involved in pa-

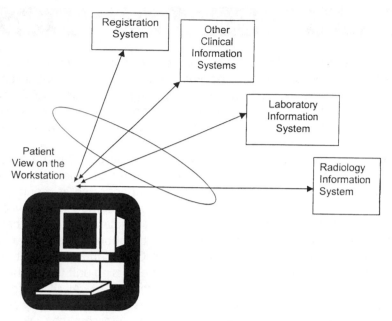

Figure 14–3 Visual Integration. Rather than physically extracting data into a new data store, visual integration tools use data from the data source.

tient care to communicate effectively with each other and with the patient; possible technologies to facilitate communication and connectivity include e-mail, Web messaging, and telemedicine

- **Patient support**—includes everything from patient education materials to home monitoring to telehealth
- **Administrative processes**—facilitates and simplifies administrative processes such as scheduling, prior authorizations, insurance verification; may also employ decision support tools to identify eligible patients for clinical trials or chronic disease management programs
- **Reporting and population health management**—establishes standardized terminology and data format for collecting public and private sector reporting requirements

The initial IOM report, along with numerous other studies published over the years, concluded that the EHR is, in fact, an essential technology for health care. In fact,

President George W. Bush recently called for the adoption of the EHR within the next decade and appointed a National Health Information Technology Coordinator to help lead and orchestrate the effort. This renewed interest in the widespread adoption of EHR systems stems from increased pressure to decrease medical costs, ensure quality, decrease medical errors, and promote patient safety and public health. A recent HIM workforce report published by the American Health Information Management Association (AHIMA) states that "the conversion of the EHR will be a pivotal event for HIM professionals" (Russell & Patena, 2004, p. 24).

Widespread EHR adoption also has direct implications for the data resource manager. Healthcare organizations will need to store large amounts of clinical data. The actual data store may be a relational database, a clinical data repository, or even a data warehouse. Some EHR-type systems may employ multiple data storage, data analysis, and visual integration tools.

Scenario 14-A: The Physicians Resist a New Password Policy

General Health Care Center (GHCC) is a large tertiary care facility in the southeastern United States. Several years ago, the organization began to develop an enterprise-wide EHR system. The GHCC EHR is to be built upon an existing CDR that was created for GHCC five years earlier. Implementation of the full EHR, however, has been problematic. The original time line for achieving an EHR for all inpatients was three years. This has now been expanded to six years.

The current legal medical record for inpatients seen at GHCC is the paper record that is housed in the medical record department. The CDR does not include electronic signatures, so information within it is not authenticated as required by state law and JCAHO regulations. The CDR receives information electronically from throughout the institution. At present, it includes all dictated notes, discharge summaries, histories and physicals, and operative reports; laboratory data; and radiological reports (but not images) for inpatients seen at GHCC during the past five years. Currently, there is no direct entry into the CDR. One nursing unit within the facility is testing an order entry module that can be used with the CDR. All CDR information is accessed through workstations located on each nursing unit and in key administrative areas throughout the medical center. Physicians can access the CDR from home via a secure Web interface. Because of numerous organizational issues associated with the development of the EHR at GHCC, the EHR steering committee recommended the creation of a data resource management position. The data resource manager would be responsible for coordinating the clinical, administrative, and technology aspects of the current CDR and, eventually, the EHR.

After much deliberation, Sarah Jones, RHIA, was hired into the data resource manager position. Sarah has a bachelor's degree in health information management and a master's degree in information systems. Her primary job responsibilities include the following:

- Developing and maintaining CDR/EHR management policies and procedures
- Monitoring compliance with the CDR/EHR policies and procedures
- Developing and implementing a plan for ensuring the quality (accuracy, reliability, and security) of the data within the CDR/EHR
- Assessing and providing for the education needs of clinical and administrative staff related to the use of the CDR/EHR
- Monitoring laws, regulations, and accreditation standards as they apply to management of the CDR/EHR
- Participating in the strategic planning for the EHR implementation

One of the first policies to be drafted by Sarah was one governing the assignment and use of passwords to access the CDR. As a first step, Sarah attempted to survey the current users of the CDR. She found, however, that identifying current users was a difficult task. Five hundred passwords had been assigned for accessing the CDR. Of those 500, approximately half appeared to be inactive accounts that could not be traced to any individual currently employed at GHCC. Other employees appeared to have duplicate passwords. Sarah also found that it was common for clinicians, particularly residents, to share passwords.

In Sarah's view, the problems associated with duplicate passwords, shared passwords, and unaccounted-for passwords were numerous. The most serious problem, from Sarah's perspective, was the potential for violating patient confidentiality and HIPAA regulations. Without a better system to control passwords, she feared that almost any employee (or former employee) could access patient records. Because Sarah had been charged with oversight of the quality of the data within the CDR, she was also concerned about her ability to monitor exactly who would have access to the CDR and the impact this could have on data integrity. According to the current CDR policies, attending physicians had limited privileges to request corrections and amendments to the CDR for their assigned patients, but residents did not. When an attending physician shared a password with a resident, the attending physician was essentially granting those privileges to the resident. Sarah's final concern was managerial in nature. She believed that the number of passwords that were not accounted for reflected a lack of administrative oversight.

Sarah researched and drafted a complete policy to protect the integrity of passwords, including rather stiff penalties for sharing passwords among providers. When Sarah presented her draft proposal to the EHR committee, however, it was not adopted. In fact, it was met with some resistance. A few of the influential physicians on the committee felt that patient care would be negatively affected if residents could never share passwords among themselves and with the attending physician. They argued that any physician at GHCC had a right to access patient information as long as the access was related to patient care. They further argued that the medical staff was capable of policing itself and did not need rigid rules that could inhibit their workflow. They felt that the new policy would inhibit rapid access to patient care information. They cited examples of it taking up to three days for a new resident to be assigned a CDR password and pointed out that residents' passwords had to be changed for each rotation to reflect new access privileges.

The physicians on the committee asked Sarah to concentrate on procedures that would make it easier for them to gain access to the patient information. They were particularly concerned about the "timing out" of the computers after three minutes. Most of the physicians admitted that it had been common practice to post the attending physician's password at the computer workstations. They felt that this was necessary to prevent delays in obtaining vital clinical information from the CDR.

Question

1. What should Sarah do about the resistance by the physicians to adopt the new password policy?

A completed ethical decision-making matrix for the scenario is provided at the end of the chapter.

ETHICAL DILEMMAS FOR DATA RESOURCE MANAGERS

Scenario 14-A and the two scenarios that follow explore problems that Sarah Jones encoun-tered in her new job and represent situations that could create ethical dilemmas for HIM professionals who serve as data resource managers. New technologies and new roles for HIM professionals lead to new ethical situations.

Is the sharing of passwords in this scenario an ethical issue? Although the paper record in GHCC is still the legal record, the

CDR provides healthcare practitioners in the facility quick and ready access to needed patient information. Physicians appreciate the availability of patient information and have begun using shortcuts, such as sharing or posting passwords, to permit even faster access to patient information. They also would prefer the system to remain up and not to "time out" when there is evidence of its not being currently in use. They view ready access to patient information as helping them provide quality care in a timely fashion, and they want nothing to interfere with that access.

Sarah Jones, however, is alarmed at removing the safeguards. An important aspect of her job is to protect and ensure the security of the data residing in the CDR. She wants to protect patients' privacy by ensuring that their potentially sensitive health information is not needlessly exposed to unauthorized access. She knows that sharing and posting passwords can clearly compromise the patient's protection, as can the practice of allowing screens to remain open, exposing confidential patient information to anyone happening by. Sarah knows that sharing passwords prevents electronic audit trails from offering useful, reliable information about who accesses the record. She also knows that posting physician passwords can permit anyone to enter the system and obtain or perhaps amend information. Excessive password availability prevents management from knowing whether access information has been limited to only those with a true need to know.

In this situation, Sarah finds herself caught between conflicting duties. As the data resource manager, she is charged with doing all that she can to create systems that permit clinicians to provide care with accurate, reliable, and timely information. But she also has a duty to protect patient information from careless policies and practices. Patients would clearly want the physicians who are providing them care to have ready access to their important information, yet they also would not want their information available to anyone who was simply curious.

If Sarah agrees to the suggestions of the physicians, she relinquishes a major portion of her job responsibilities. Consider the following questions:

- What other facts does Sarah need to know to solve this dilemma?
- How might the fact that Sarah reports to the chief information officer (CIO) affect her decision?
- What is the CIO's position regarding this issue?
- Can she obtain the CIO's support to help her with this problem?
- What can Sarah do to enlighten others about this concern?

Currently, residents are only able to view information; however, access to physician passwords can give residents the capability of amending patient information.

- What impact do you suppose this realization might have on physicians?
- Why is it a major concern for Sarah?
- Would it be helpful for Sarah to conduct a literature search to determine if any court cases or similar concerns have arisen regarding breaches of privacy that have occurred because of a lack of appropriate computer safeguards to protect patient information?
- Do you suppose that such information might be of interest to physicians and other administrators?
- Would it be helpful for Sarah to talk with information technology personnel to determine if they can improve the time it takes for residents to acquire a new password when they go on new rotations?
- What other measures might Sarah try in order to increase others' awareness about effective password use and to prevent needless access?

Scenario 14-B: Threat to Integrity of the CDR

Mark Wagner, the director of Health Information Services (HIS) at GHCC, is concerned about the quality of the data being stored in the CDR. He has recently completed both a manual search and a computer search for patient lab values as a part of a quality assessment study. He noticed that several (approximately 12 of 250) lab reports found in the patients' paper medical records were not found in the CDR. He also noticed that most of the discrepancies occurred over a two-month period ending last month. He approached Sarah Jones, the data resource manager, and asked her to investigate.

After examining the collected data, Sarah felt the problem was significant enough to approach her immediate supervisor, the CIO for GHCC. Although the CDR was not the "legal" medical record for GHCC, it was the record used by most nurses and physicians while the patient was in the hospital. The standard operating procedure while a patient was in the hospital was for the clinicians to access the CDR for current lab values. Paper records of lab values were filed in the patient's permanent file in medical records but were not sent to the nursing floors during the patient's hospital stay. Reeducating clinicians to use the CDR to view lab data was viewed as an implementation "success" by the CIO and by the clinical information systems steering committee. The most recent figures for CDR use showed that more than 90% of the medical staff and 94% of the nursing staff accessed the CDR for patient lab data. Sarah's primary concern was that patient care could suffer if lab data were not being uploaded correctly to the CDR. She also wanted to make sure that the appropriate mechanisms were in place to ensure the integrity of the CDR data.

After Sarah presented her concerns about the discrepancies in the lab data, the CIO indicated that he was not concerned about the discrepancies noted. He explained that the CDR had been extensively tested and that he was confident about the integrity of the data housed within the system. He further explained that there had been a problem with the interface between the lab system and the CDR during the period in question. He stated that the problem had been fixed and he saw no reason to investigate any further. When Sarah shared the data from the HIS director, the CIO commented that "everyone knows how unreliable paper records are." He went on to explain why the data from the direct interface were more accurate. He also stated that the percentage of error was not enough to worry about anyway. As Sarah's supervisor, he told her to drop her investigation into the discrepancies. He was particularly concerned about giving the clinicians any more reasons to resist using the current CDR system. He felt there were enough CDR/EHR implementation problems without making problems for this successful area.

Question

1. Is data integrity affected if inaccurate data are not in the legal medical record?

A completed ethical decision-making matrix for the scenario is provided at the end of the chapter.

Is the situation in Scenario 14-B involving missing lab values in the CDR an ethical dilemma for Sarah? It certainly is not as clear-cut as her earlier one (Scenario 14-A). Sarah understands that the paper medical record is currently the facility's legal record. Although the CDR provides the foundation for the facility's eventual EHR, the CDR is not the legal record, because there is no way to authenticate data. Should physicians be relying on a record that is not the legal record? The data collected by Mark Wagner, the HIS director, revealed that close to 5% of the laboratory values that were present in the paper record were not included in the CDR. Should Sarah be concerned about inaccuracy amounting to less than 5%?

This is a concern for Sarah because she knows that many physicians currently use only the CDR and do not review the paper record. She wonders whether they realize that not all of the lab values are present. She also wonders what else may be missing.

The CIO does not seem particularly concerned by these missing data. He is pleased that the physicians are comfortable using the CDR in anticipation of the hospital moving toward the eventual adoption of the EHR. He knows how hard it is for some physicians to consider letting go of the paper record and consulting the CDR, and he does not now want to undermine any confidence they may have built up about the integrity of the CDR. He certainly does not want Sarah to remind the physicians that the paper record is still the legal record, and he does not want her to reveal findings from just this one quality study indicating that the paper record may actually be more complete than the CDR. He knows that some problems may have been created in data integrity when the interface between the lab system and the CDR was not working, but that problem is fixed now, and he does not believe there is any more reason for concern. He also does not feel that 5% missing lab values is significant enough to affect patient care or warrant erosion of physician confidence in the CDR. Consider the following questions:

- Do you believe that physicians would be concerned about patient care or accessibility of accurate, up-to-date laboratory data if they knew the findings of this study?
- Do you believe the problem may now have been solved?
- How would you know?
- Would it be helpful if Sarah suggested a second study to determine if the lab interface problem was now resolved?
- If the results of the second test again demonstrated reliability problems, would you recommend that Sarah confront her superior, the CIO, with the findings?
- Do you believe Sarah will be fulfilling the functions of her job if she ignores this situation?
- Will any of the four ethical principles identified by Beauchamp and Childress (1994) and discussed in Chapter 2 of this book (respect for autonomy, nonmaleficence, beneficence, justice) be violated if this situation is ignored?
- What strategies could Sarah employ to encourage buy-in for improving the accuracy, completeness, and reliability of the data contained in the CDR?

Scenario 14-C: Research Access to Admission/Discharge/Registration Data

Dr. Anne Weatherby heads a cardiac research team at GHCC. She has conducted epidemiological research using nonidentifiable patient information for several years. Her studies have covered a wide range of topics, and she is well known in her field for excellent work. Recently, Dr. Weatherby contacted the CIO at GHCC with a special request. Her current research project requires data to be extracted from the healthcare center's admission, discharge, and registration (ADR) system. After investigating the feasibility of using the ADR system's internal query tools, she determined that these tools were inadequate to provide the multidimensional type of information needed for the research study. It also became apparent that the current hardware configuration (disk space) was inadequate to handle the required data analysis once the data were extracted. The CIO contacted the company who marketed and supported the ADR system to see what the cost of a special data extraction program would be. It was determined that the $20,000 price tag for the special program was more than Dr. Weatherby's team could afford.

As an alternative, the CIO offered Dr. Weatherby the services of his "special" technical team. This team was composed of several graduate students and faculty from a nearby university who had a particular interest in developing Web interfaces and visual integration tools to perform ad hoc queries on large databases. The team had successfully created such an interface to the GHCC payroll system. The CIO was particularly interested in "turning his team loose" on this project because he saw a potential for the project to provide a basis for in-house development of other tools to access clinical databases within GHCC for research purposes.

After attending a meeting in which the CIO and his technical team presented their preliminary findings on the feasibility of creating a Web tool in house, Sarah Jones became very concerned. After leaving the meeting, she drafted a memo to the CIO expressing what she saw as the major issues with allowing the technical team to proceed with development of a Web access tool for the ADR system. The contents of the memo follow:

> We share the goal of eventually having a simple, secure Web-based access to our clinical databases. However, I have some major concerns about opening the access to our ADR system in this manner at the present time.
>
> 1. Putting together the technology to unlock the access to the ADR system may be the simplest part of the process. How are we going to assess the potential impact of this technology on the future of GHCC's clinical information systems?
> 2. Access to clinical data for research purposes raises some issues regarding patient confidentiality. The clinical information systems steering committee has a subcommittee that has been working on the development of specific guidelines to follow when using the CDR and other clinical information systems for research. This subcommittee has spent months discussing patient confidentiality issues with GHCC's designated Institutional Review Board (IRB) and with the compliance officer. How are we going to control the development of "homegrown" Web access tools? What is the potential impact on patient confidentiality? Who will be responsible for oversight of the self-developed tools?
> 3. GHCC just purchased data warehouse tools to be used in conjunction with the CDR. These tools were purchased to allow researchers to extract clinical data in specific data "cubes." An oversight group has been established to work with the researchers and the IRB as requests for research data come in. The ADR system feeds into the CDR, and

much of the information from the ADR can be found there. The data warehouse tools should be available to research teams within a few months. In addition to the data warehouse tools, there are plans to purchase a Web-based report writer for the data warehouse.

My advice is that we at least hold off on the in-house project until we see the new security and confidentiality policies and until the data warehouse tools have been installed and tested. My basic belief, however, is that we should not allow any "homegrown" Web access to clinical databases.

The CIO responded to Sarah by saying that her comments missed a key point—that there were several clinicians and researchers at GHCC who found clinical data to be virtually inaccessible. A generic Web interface would, in his opinion, be a major step in freeing the data for use in research. He further stated that security and confidentiality were always issues but were not of "sufficient importance to impede the development of convenient access to institutional resources." His philosophy was to build the tools and then address security and confidentiality concerns, because if the tools were not technically feasible, "the security was irrelevant." His final word was that the project would proceed and that he would take responsibility for seeing that no patient's confidentiality was violated.

Questions

1. How should Sarah respond to the tensions between control and access?

2. How can Sarah balance the needs of the legitimate users having access with the obligation to protect privacy?

3. Will Sarah be able to protect the information if access is increased?

A completed ethical decision-making matrix for the scenario is provided at the end of the chapter.

Does Scenario 14-C present an ethical dilemma? Let's consider the facts from the perspectives of each of the main stakeholders. This case reflects a difference in priorities surrounding the use and protection of the data housed in the ADR system. The CIO understands the importance of the data for clinical research and is eager to have it available for researchers. He also is amenable to having the team of graduate students and faculty begin to develop Web interface tools for accessing the ADR system. He acknowledges the learning potential for the team and the payoff it could have for the facility in per-

mitting a foundation for the development of other, more sophisticated data extraction tools. He recognizes that these in-house tools could potentially uncover useful data for research purposes and yet be much more cost-efficient than tools purchased from outside vendors. The CIO recognizes his duty to provide access to researchers who may be able to discover breakthroughs in causes of disease or discover more effective treatments. He is confident that he is contributing a service for the benefit of humanity.

Sarah Jones is concerned about the potential impact on patient confidentiality and the potential breach in security of patient data. At this time, policies have not been developed for providing guidance about the use of the information that may be extracted from the databases. She is worried that, without the necessary deliberation about access and control issues from a variety of viewpoints, the potential for breaches in patient confidentiality would be high. She also is very concerned that multiple tools and tool users may be accessing information without adequate and central oversight. Sarah knows that the data housed in the clinical databases can provide very useful information to researchers, but she is concerned primarily about the potential for harm to facility patients without well-planned policies and safeguards. Consider the following questions:

- Do you believe the potential for good is greater than the potential for harm?
- Is the potential for harm greater than the potential for good?
- What could be proposed to help solve this ethical dilemma?
- Would conducting education for the team of graduate students and faculty about the importance of protecting patients' confidentiality be helpful?
- Would signing a statement pledging to protect patient confidentiality impress upon the team the importance of this responsibility?
- Should Sarah consider forming a committee to begin considering and writing policies for protecting patient confidentiality when data are extracted from databases?
- If so, who might be the important stakeholders, and what perspectives would she want represented on the committee? What other strategies might Sarah use?

CONCLUSION

New advanced data management tools are rapidly becoming the norm in healthcare facilities. With these technological advances come some interesting questions regarding the use of patient data. Although the issue of balancing ease of access to patient information versus protecting patient confidentiality is not new, it takes on a new dimension in the information age. Information is much more readily available, and one breach of system security can violate the privacy of many patients. Data integrity concerns are also heightened as more data become available to more people and agencies. The challenge for HIM professionals is to find appropriate ways to ensure that electronically stored patient care information is kept confidential and secure and that the patient information is available to healthcare providers and others with a legitimate need to know about the patient.

Key Terms

- Clinical data repository (CDR)
- Database
- Data mart
- Data resource manager
- Data warehouse
- Electronic health record (EHR)
- Health Insurance Portability and Accountability Act (HIPAA)
- Visual integration tools

Chapter Summary

- A data resource manager is a person who uses technical tools, such as electronic medical record systems, data repositories, and data warehouses, to ensure that the organization's information systems meet the needs of those who provide and manage patient services along the continuum of care and that the organization's data resources are secure, accessible, accurate, and reliable. The skills required to perform the data resource management function include a thorough understanding of health information administration and a working knowledge of the technical aspects of health information systems.

- The Health Information Portability and Accountability Act (HIPAA) affects data resource management with regard to data privacy and security.

- Many data resource management tools are being used in healthcare facilities. Examples of database and data decision tools include databases, clinical data repositories, data warehouses, data marts, data mining tools, and visual integration tools. Other data resource management tools used in health care include electronic health records (EHRs).

- Ethical dilemmas in data resource management involve conflicts between the obligation to ensure ease of access to information for appropriate purposes and the obligation to protect patient information from careless policies and practices.

References

American Health Information Management Association [AHIMA]. (1999). *Vision 2006. Evolving HIM careers.* Chicago: Author.

Beauchamp, T., & Childress, J. (1994). *Principles of biomedical ethics.* New York: Oxford University Press.

Fox, C. S., & Jesse, H. (1999). Electronic health record costs and benefits. In M. A. Hanken, K. Waters, & G. F. Murphy (Eds.), *Electronic health records: Changing the vision.* Philadelphia: W.B. Saunders.

Institute of Medicine. (1991). *The computer based patient record—An essential technology for health care.* Washington, DC: Author.

Institute of Medicine Committee on Data Standards for Patient Safety. (2003). *Key capabilities of an electronic health record system.* Washington, DC: Institute of Medicine.

Rob, P., & Coronel, C. (2002). *Database systems: Design, implementation, and management,* 5th ed. Cambridge, MA: Course Technology.

Russell, L. A., & Patena, K. (2004). Preparing tomorrow's professionals: A new framework for HIM education. *Journal of the American Health Information Management Association,* 75(6), 23–26.

Seliger, R. (2001). *Overview of HL7's CCOW standard.* Retrieved September 23, 2005, from http://www.hl7.org/special/Committees/ccow_sigvi.htm.

The ethical decision-making matrix is a tool to help you organize complex, ethical problems; however, there is no simple fill-in-the-box approach to ethical decision making. The objective is to follow each step of the process and not move from the question directly to what should be done or how to prevent it next time. If you skip steps, you will not fully understand all of the values and options for action. Also, the matrix provided for each scenario in this book is not the only way to examine the problem. You can make an equally compelling ethical argument for a different decision—just be sure to follow all the steps of the matrix.

SCENARIO 14-A: THE PHYSICIANS RESIST A NEW PASSWORD POLICY

Steps	Information	
1. What is the ethical question?	Should Sarah insist on the increased security measures?	
2. What are the facts?	**KNOWN**	**TO BE GATHERED**
	• The CDR does not include electronic signatures. • The EHR will be based on the existing CDR. • 500 passwords have been assigned to access the CDR. • Sarah's proposal was not adopted.	• Would Sarah's allowing the CDR to function as is implicate her in any legal or ethical violation? • What does her boss or supervisor expect her to do? • Does the current system jeopardize security? • Would elimination of the timing out of the computers jeopardize security? • What are the customary practices in such cases? • What is the likely impact on self and family of changing jobs?
3. What are the values? Examine the shared and competing values, obligations, and interests of the stakeholders (i.e., patient, HIM professional, healthcare practitioner(s), administrators, society, and other advocates) involved in order to fully understand the complexity of the ethical problem(s).	**Patient:** Values confidentiality and the security of the medical record; interest in prompt, appropriate care. **HIM professional:** Integrity and accuracy (protect system security); loyalty to employer; avoid harm (continued operation of the system as is could jeopardize security, could implicate Sarah in ethical problems); personal values (promote welfare of self and family by avoiding loss of job). **Healthcare professionals:** Promote welfare of patients through prompt, appropriate care. **Administrators:** Benefit patients and keep from harm; promote welfare of the facility; maximize efficiency without jeopardizing security. **Society:** Promote record security.	

4. What are my options?	• Allow the system to operate as is. • Insist on the implementation of increased security measures.	
5. What should I do?	Insist on the implementation of increased security measures.	
6. What justifies my choice?	**JUSTIFIED**	**NOT JUSTIFIED**
	• Obligation to protect security. • Respect regulatory requirements. • Preserve professional integrity. • Demonstrate loyalty to employer, unless asked to push legal boundaries.	• Allow the system to function as is. • Jeopardize system security for the ease of physicians. • Jeopardize professional integrity. • Violate HIPAA requirements.
7. How can I prevent this ethical problem?	• Determine if system changes are needed. • Learn more about ethics and security issues surrounding EHR systems. • Discuss standards and the values that support them with colleagues. • Evaluate institutional integrity at the job interview and subsequently as ethical problems arise.	

The ethical decision-making matrix is a tool to help you organize complex, ethical problems; however, there is no simple fill-in-the-box approach to ethical decision making. The objective is to follow each step of the process and not move from the question directly to what should be done or how to prevent it next time. If you skip steps, you will not fully understand all of the values and options for action. Also, the matrix provided for each scenario in this book is not the only way to examine the problem. You can make an equally compelling ethical argument for a different decision—just be sure to follow all the steps of the matrix.

SCENARIO 14-B: THREAT TO INTEGRITY OF THE CDR

Steps	Information	
1. What is the ethical question?	Should Sarah drop the investigation?	
2. What are the facts?	**KNOWN**	**TO BE GATHERED**
	• Missing data have been discovered. • The CDR is not the legal record. • The director of HIS asked Sarah to investigate the missing lab values. • Sarah's supervisor has told her to drop the investigation. • There was a period during which there was a problem with the interface.	• Was the problem with the missing data solved? • Would Sarah's dropping the investigation be unethical? • Do the omissions compromise patient care? • What are the customary practices in cases such as this? • What is the likely impact on self and family of changing jobs?
3. What are the values? Examine the shared and competing values, obligations, and interests of the stakeholders (i.e., patient, HIM professional, health-care practitioner(s), administrators, society, and other advocates) involved in order to fully understand the complexity of the ethical problem(s).	**Patient:** Values prompt, appropriate care. **HIM professional:** Integrity, truth, accuracy (ensure accuracy of medical records); loyalty to employer; avoid harm (inaccurate records could result in patient harm); personal values (promote welfare of self and family by avoiding loss of job). **Healthcare professionals:** Promote welfare of patients through accurate documentation and care. **Administrators/IT:** Benefit patients and keep from harm; maximize efficiency without compromising accuracy. **Society:** Promote use of accurate records.	

4. What are my options?	• Drop the investigation. • Conduct a second investigation.	
5. What should I do?	Conduct a second investigation to see if the problem is still occurring.	
6. What justifies my choice?	**JUSTIFIED**	**NOT JUSTIFIED**
	• Obligation to tell the truth. • Support the accuracy of the medical record. • Preserve professional integrity. • Demonstrate loyalty to employer, unless asked to compromise patient care.	• Drop the investigation. • Compromise patient care. • Not fair to physicians who may not know the shortcomings of the CDR. • Compromise professional integrity.
7. How can I prevent this ethical problem?	• Determine is system changes are needed. • Learn more about CDR systems and accuracy issues. • Discuss standards and the values that support them with colleagues. • Evaluate institutional integrity at job interview and subsequently as ethical problems arise.	

The ethical decision-making matrix is a tool to help you organize complex, ethical problems; however, there is no simple fill-in-the-box approach to ethical decision making. The objective is to follow each step of the process and not move from the question directly to what should be done or how to prevent it next time. If you skip steps, you will not fully understand all of the values and options for action. Also, the matrix provided for each scenario in this book is not the only way to examine the problem. You can make an equally compelling ethical argument for a different decision—just be sure to follow all the steps of the matrix.

SCENARIO 14-C: RESEARCH ACCESS TO ADMISSION/DISCHARGE/REGISTRATION DATA

Steps	Information	
1. What is the ethical question?	Should Sarah protest the creation of the Web access interface?	
2. What are the facts?	**KNOWN**	**TO BE GATHERED**
	• The researcher has requested tools for expanded access to clinical data. • The CIO has suggested use of an internal technical team to develop Web access to the clinical database. • GHCC recently purchased data warehouse tools that will be installed soon. • The CIO has taken responsibility for patient confidentiality.	• Would Sarah bear responsibility if there was a violation of patient confidentiality? • Could this new homegrown interface compromise security? • In what way would delayed implementation of a new system impact research? • What is the customary practice in such cases? • What is the likely impact on self and family of changing jobs?
3. What are the values? Examine the shared and competing values, obligations, and interests of the stakeholders (i.e., patient, HIM professional, healthcare practitioner(s), administrators, society, and other advocates) involved in order to fully understand the complexity of the ethical problem(s).	**Patient:** Values confidentiality of medical record; may benefit from research results. **HIM professional:** Integrity, truth (protect confidentiality of records); loyalty to employer; protect welfare of self and family by avoiding loss of job. **Healthcare professionals:** Value ability to conduct research using complete patient data. **Administrators/IT:** Maximize data access without compromising confidentiality. **Society:** Protect confidentiality of patient data.	

4. What are my options?	• Allow the CIO to proceed with the development of a Web access interface. • Protest the creation of the Web access interface.	
5. What should I do?	Protest the creation of the Web access interface.	
6. What justifies my choice?	**JUSTIFIED**	**NOT JUSTIFIED**
	• Obligation to protect security and confidentiality. • Preserve professional integrity. • Demonstrate loyalty to employer, unless asked to push legal or ethical boundaries.	• Allow the CIO to proceed. • Jeopardize patient confidentiality. • Jeopardize professional integrity.
7. How can I prevent this ethical problem?	• Determine if system changes are needed. • Learn more about security and confidentiality issues surrounding Web-based access to clinical databases. • Discuss standards and the values that support them with colleagues. • Evaluate institutional integrity at initial job interview and subsequently as ethical problems arise.	

Learning Objectives

After completing this chapter, the reader should be able to:

- Identify the challenges and key issues regarding the protection of patient information and quality in an integrated delivery system (IDS).
- Identify how the Health Insurance Portability and Accountability Act (HIPAA) affects information protection.
- Define *master patient index (MPI)* and discuss the tasks and ethical issues involved in creating such an index for the IDS.
- Identify the skills and knowledge needed by the health information management (HIM) professional to coordinate HIM efforts across an IDS.

INTEGRATED DELIVERY SYSTEMS

Brenda Olson, MEd, RHIA, CHP
Karen Gallagher Grant, RHIA, CHP

Abstract

Health information management (HIM) professionals must deal with complex issues related to their responsibilities of ensuring the security of electronic information and the privacy and quality of patient information. For HIM professionals working in an integrated delivery system (IDS), the complexities of these issues are multiplied. Privacy, security, and data quality policies and procedures must be developed and monitored for the IDS as a whole, and individual entities may have their own policies and regulations. HIM professionals need to balance the needs of the IDS with the autonomous needs of the individual healthcare entities. This chapter explores the special issues that HIM professionals must consider in carrying out their responsibilities within an IDS and the skills that such tasks require.

Scenario 15-A: Scheduling Clerk Has Access to Clinical Information

Suzy T. has undergone several hospitalizations in Morcity Hospital over the past several years. Morcity Hospital has recently become part of an integrated delivery system (IDS) that includes 40 hospitals, 8 physician clinics, 13 long-term care settings, 1 head injury unit, 20 swing-bed units, and 1 skilled care facility. This is a voluntary IDS; the facilities share information technology and patient demographic information across the continuum. Suzy has just come from her physician's office, where she has been told that she needs to schedule surgery for a hysterectomy. As she leaves the clinic, a staff member informs her that he has access to the hospital's schedule and that Suzy can schedule the surgery right now from the clinic office. Suzy is all for this, but, as she discusses her scheduling needs, the staff member begins to look through her hospital records, which he has downloaded to his workstation. Suzy begins to worry whether the staff member needs to know this information in order to schedule a surgery. After the surgery has been scheduled, she contacts the hospital and is referred to the health information management (HIM) director/ Privacy Officer, Anna Rosen, who listens to her concerns.

Anna has been the HIM director/Privacy Officer for less than a month, but she recognizes that the IDS presents the potential for privacy and security violations. To resolve Suzy's concern, she begins to look through current policies and procedures that address data access for employees at different sites in the IDS. She finds that current policies and procedures cover only issues of data access within individual healthcare entities and do not address issues of data access across the IDS.

Questions

1. How should Anna go about ensuring that policies and procedures address multi-entity use of the data? Who should be involved in writing these policies and procedures? How should it be determined who will have access to what types of information?

2. If Anna receives further complaints from patients in the multi-entity setting, how should these be dealt with?

3. Are policies and procedures in place to allow the sharing of data across the IDS facilities?

A completed ethical decision-making matrix for the scenario is provided at the end of the chapter.

Just a few years ago, only a few **integrated delivery systems (IDSs)** existed. Given the numerous mergers and acquisitions in the healthcare industry and the increasing complexities of reimbursement systems that have occurred over the past few years, these systems are now the norm. HIM professionals who work with data that are shared across multiple sites of care face numerous challenges. HIM professionals who work in an IDS will be involved in all aspects of the healthcare system. They will be required to have an understanding of the entire continuum of care, from physician offices to hospitals to specialized facilities, such as long-term care centers, rehabilitation centers, psychiatric facilities, and hospices. They must be knowledgeable about services, rules, and regulations and patient and provider characteristics. They must know basic HIM functions and understand the flow of health information (AHIMA, 2000; see Figure 15–1).

IDSs can be organized in different ways. IDSs may be corporate (i.e., all facilities are owned by the corporation), noncorporate (i.e., all the facilities are in the network voluntarily), or a combination of both. Also, they may be hospitals only, a combination of hospitals and physician offices, or a broad assortment of healthcare delivery systems, such as home health agencies, physician offices, rehabilitation centers, long-term care settings, subacute settings, skilled nursing facilities, ambulatory care settings, and hospitals.

In any setting, HIM professionals must deal with complex issues related to their responsibilities of ensuring the privacy, security, and data quality of patient information. For HIM professionals working in an IDS, the complexities of these issues are multiplied. Although they will attempt to impose consistency in information policies and procedures across the system, some of the single entities' policies and procedures will remain autonomous. HIM professionals must balance the needs of the IDS with the autonomy of the individual entities. In noncorporate IDSs, the situation can be even more complex, because individual entities have more autonomy than in corporate IDSs because the members of the IDS are not linked by financial incentives.

PRIVACY AND SECURITY ISSUES

The privacy and security of the health record are the responsibility of the HIM department. The security of the electronic health information is the joint responsibility of the HIM and Information Systems departments. Confidential information, or what is now known as **protected health information (PHI),** is information that is private and to which access is restricted. Law protects a patient's right to privacy. Federal and state statutes and regulations protect information, including the patients' personal health information that is collected within healthcare facilities.

As Scenario 15-A shows, the technological innovations that have enabled the employees of linked entities of an IDS to rapidly and easily transmit large amounts of patient information to each other have not necessarily been accompanied by updated and expanded policies that ensure the privacy and security of patient information across the system. Thus, it is extremely important for HIM professionals within IDSs to know who will have access to what information and to take steps to limit that access as necessary through the development of specific policies and procedures. **Health Insurance Portability and Accountability Act (HIPAA)** regulations address this type of access by stating that healthcare facilities must establish minimum necessary criteria for PHI in the privacy subsection and administrative, physical, and technical safeguards in the security subsection. Hospital employees and medical staff members have the right to access information based on their direct involvement in the patient's treatment, which should be determined on a case-by-case basis and in relation to their need to know.

The new standards that have been developed under HIPAA are designed to protect the confidentiality, integrity, and availability of individual health information. HIPAA regulations have been established to help healthcare facilities protect a patient's health information. The privacy standards apply to PHI in any form, whereas the security standards apply only to PHI in electronic form. Fundamentally, the privacy standards give patients more control over their health information and set boundaries on the use and disclosure of health records. They also provide safeguards that must be followed by covered entities so that the privacy of health information is protected.

The security standards require all healthcare organizations to assess risks to their information systems and to take appropriate steps to

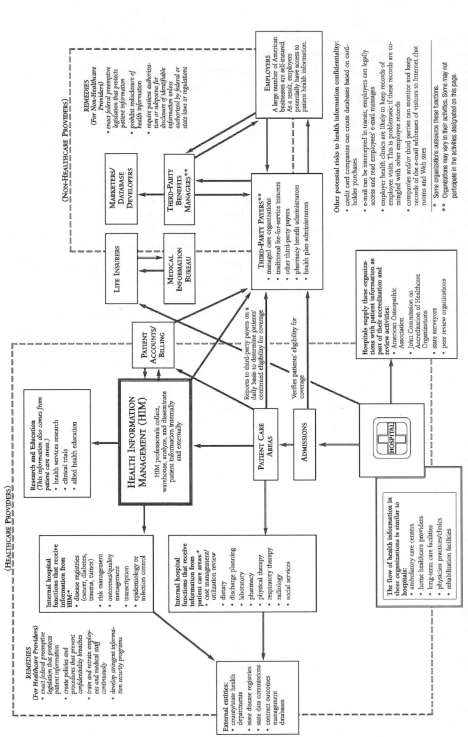

Figure 15–1 Flow of Patient Health Information Inside and Outside the Healthcare Industry. Source: Copyright 2000, American Health Information Management Association, All Rights Reserved.

The American Health Information Management Association (AHIMA) is a national association of 40,000 medical record and health information management (HIM) professionals, who handle hundreds of thousands of medical records each day. Based on the collected experience of its members, AHIMA developed this diagram, which delineates exactly who, both inside and outside the healthcare industry, has access to patient health information. The number of individuals and organizations that have access to these records makes a strong case for federal preemptive confidentiality legislation that protects all patient information equally.

ensure the confidentiality, integrity, and availability of patient information. Security applies to the spectrum of physical, technical, and administrative safeguards that are put in place to protect the integrity, availability, and confidentiality of information. As these regulations are implemented, HIM professionals, while working with the Privacy and Security Officer, will need to address how compliance will be ensured. When the policies and procedures are developed to ensure compliance with the privacy and security standards, the HIM professional will be a major player in ensuring that the IDS complies with the HIPAA privacy and security standards.

Hospital employees cannot disclose PHI without a signed authorization unless the disclosure meets certain criteria as required by law. PHI may be disclosed for the following purposes while applying the minimum necessary standard:

- Public health activities, e.g., to identify dangers to public health that will help avoid disease, injury, or disability; to report births and deaths; to report reactions to drugs and other health products; to report a recall of health products or medications; to tell a person he or she has been exposed to a disease, may get a disease, or could spread the disease; to inform employers about a workplace illness or workplace safety issues; or to report trauma injury to the state.
- Victims of abuse, neglect, or domestic violence, e.g., to a government authority when there is a suspicion that a patient has been abused, neglected, or the victim of violence.
- Health oversight activities, e.g., to provide information to oversight groups as they perform activities to include investigation, inspection, and licensing hospitals.
- Judicial and administrative proceedings, e.g., involvement in a lawsuit or dispute, an order to appear in court, a discovery request, or other legal reason by someone else involved in a dispute.

- Law enforcement purposes, e.g., to respond to a court order, subpoena, warrant, or summons; to find a suspect, fugitive, witness, or missing person; or in emergencies to report a crime.
- Coroners, medical examiners, and funeral directors, e.g., to identify a person who has died or determine the cause of death or to funeral directors so they can carry out their duties.
- Cadaveric organ, eye, or tissue donation, e.g., to people who deal with organ collection, eye or tissue transplants, or to a donation bank.
- Research, e.g., to researchers who want to do scientific research about how well certain drugs or treatments work or to help researchers find the patients they need for their research study.
- Averting serious threats to health or safety, e.g., to someone who may be able to prevent the threat if the health of the public or another individual is at risk.
- Specialized government functions, e.g., to federal authorities for intelligence, counterintelligence, and other situations involving our national safety or to conduct special investigations in order to protect the president or other officials or foreign heads of state.
- Worker's compensation, e.g., for patients so their medical bills can be paid by their employer.
- Marketing and fund-raising, e.g., tell about health benefits or services that may be of interest to a patient, contact a patient to help raise money for the covered entity, or give a patient's information to a foundation to help raise money. Only basic contact information such as name, address, phone number, and the dates the patient was treated at the hospital can be provided.
- Inmates, e.g., give an inmate's PHI to the prison that is providing the health care, to others to protect the health and safety of the inmate and others or for the safety of the prison.

- Facility directories, e.g., limited information about a patient, to include name, room number in the hospital, and the patient's general condition (for example, fair, stable, etc.), which will be available to the public.
- Clergy, e.g., provide patient's religion to a minister, priest, or rabbi.
- Persons (family members, significant others, friends) involved in the patient's care, e.g., provide a patient's PHI to friends or family members that is dependent on how involved they are in the patient's medical care or give PHI to another person who is helping pay for the patient's care.
- Disaster relief, e.g., providing PHI to help coordinate disaster relief activities or to notify family about a patient's condition and location.
- Business associates, e.g., PHI needed by a person, company, or organization to perform a function or activity or provide a service to the covered entity.
- De-identified or limited data set information, e.g., disclosures for research, public health activities, or certain healthcare operations where there is a data use agreement in effect and PHI has been de-identified.

Nonconfidential information may be disclosed to legitimate requesters on a "need-to-know" basis without the patient's authorization. Such information is considered common knowledge, for example, a patient's name and condition, when its disclosure is not prohibited by law or restricted by specific request of the patient or the patient's legal representative.

In voluntary IDSs, it is especially important that HIM professionals gain consensus on the new policies from all of the entities involved in the IDS. Compliance must be monitored without bias. If someone is given inappropriate access, procedures need to be developed to ensure that it does not happen again.

One way to ensure that all employees understand the privacy and security policies for the IDS is to have them sign a confidentiality statement stating that they understand the provisions of the agreement and the consequences of any breach of confidentiality. These consequences must then be enforced so that employees of the IDS realize that the organization is serious about this issue.

Another privacy and security concern in IDSs is whether the patient/consumer should be aware that the information from the single entity is now being used by all of the facilities in the multi-entity setting. Should the patient/consumer be notified of this change as it occurs? Also, is there a need for a signed patient authorization to allow such multi-entity access? If so, what happens if a patient refuses to authorize multi-entity access? These are current concerns, because more and more healthcare entities are being organized or absorbed into IDSs. Under the new HIPAA privacy regulations, patients need to be notified that demographic and clinical information will be shared between IDS facilities. The IDS should determine which entities are part of their affiliated covered entity (ACE) and add those entities to their privacy notice (Miller, 2003; Grant & Adair, 2002). Materials published by AHIMA (1997a, 1997b, 1997f, 1998c) may provide guidance as to the minimum necessary privacy and security standards in IDSs.

DATA QUALITY ISSUES

HIM professionals, in their capacity as data quality managers, have a responsibility to ensure data quality from the point of collection through all of the transactions in which the data are transmitted, combined, analyzed, accessed, and applied. Data quality encompasses such characteristics as accuracy (are the data values correct?), comprehensiveness (are all the data items that are required included?), consistency (are the values of the data the same across applications, and do related items agree?), currency (are the data up to date?), timeliness (are current data available at the intervals when they are needed by users?), clarity of definitions (the same for all applications), granularity (are the attributes and values of data defined at the correct level of detail?), precision (all value ranges are large enough?), and relevance (are the data meaningful to the performance of the process or application for which they are collected?) (see Exhibit 15–1 for AHIMA's list of data quality characteristics with definitions).

The complexities of ensuring data quality are compounded when the data in question are located at several facilities across an IDS. In particular, the features of data consistency and clear definitions are harder to ensure, because different entities employ different definitions of data elements and values and the data are transmitted across facilities,

---

Exhibit 15–1 Characteristics of Data Quality

> **Data accuracy.** Data are the correct values. For example, if a patient's sex is female, this should be accurately recorded.
> **Data.** All data items that are required are included. This may be determined by the comprehensiveness and scope of the application.
> **Data consistency.** The value of the data should be the same across applications (e.g., the patient's medical record number). In addition, related data items should agree (e.g., data are inconsistent when it is documented that a male patient has a hysterectomy).
> **Data currency.** A value of data is up-to-date or current if it is correct for a specific point in time. It is outdated if it is incorrect at a certain point of time but was correct at some preceding time.
> **Data granularity.** The attributes and values of data should be defined at the correct level of detail. For example, granularity for recording outdoor temperatures is different from that for recording patient temperatures. If patient Jane Doe's temperature is 100°, does that mean 99.6° or 100.4°? Appropriate granularity for this application would dictate that the data be recorded to the first decimal point, whereas appropriate granularity for recording outdoor temperatures might not require it.
> **Data precision.** Data values should be just large enough to support the application or process. This would include defining acceptable values or value ranges for each data item.
> **Data relevancy.** The data are meaningful to the performance of the process or application for which they are collected. This includes considerations such as whether the data items can be easily obtained and whether it is legal to collect the data. In addition, establish clear definitions so current and future data users will know what the data mean.
> **Data timeliness.** Timeliness is context dependent and depends on the application and its use. For example, patient census is needed daily to provide sufficient day-to-day operations staffing (i.e., nursing and food service). However, annual or monthly patient census data are needed for facility strategic planning.
>
> *Source:* Reprinted with permission from American Health Information Management Association Data Quality Management Task Force, Data Quality Management Mode, *Journal of American Health Information Management Association,* © June 1998, American Health Information Management Association.

incorporated into new databases, and combined with other data.

Further, the administrative tasks of setting up data collection and monitoring efforts to ensure all of these data quality characteristics are far more complicated in an IDS than in a single entity. In an IDS, decisions must be made for the entire system about how comprehensive the data collection will be; what percentage of data completion will be required; who owns each data element; what will constitute "timeliness," or the intervals at which current data will need to be provided; and whether data will be collected for all patients or, if not, what population of patients will be excluded. The process of designing data collection instruments will be particularly important, because the system must standardize procedures, rules, edits, and processes used by data collectors across all the entities of the IDS and across the continuum of care. Extensive education on data collection must be provided across all entities. Data values must be the same across all applications and systems, and communication of data definitions, along with updates and changes, must be timely and appropriate for all entities.

Within each entity, organization, and department, HIM professionals will be accountable and responsible for coordinating data collection. They will determine what feedback will be provided to data collectors and how that feedback will be communicated. They will ensure data currency and timeliness. They will also serve as project managers for numerous electronic record projects. In this management capacity HIM professionals will document the project status and project progress, changes as a result of a pilot application, improvements after project implementation, changes in data definitions, and other significant information. Further, quality must be monitored across the continuum and arrangements made to ensure data quality. Policies and procedures must be planned and implemented to govern every aspect of data monitoring efforts.

As various multi-entity policies and procedures for data collection and monitoring are addressed and developed, turf issues may well arise. The HIM professional will need to make sure that approved multi-entity procedures do not "step on the toes" of the single entities. How these decisions will be made, whether by corporate staff or a multi-entity committee, must be decided on a case-by-case basis. However, without these policies and procedures, the IDS will not be able to perform the activities that are needed (AHIMA, 1998a, 1998b; Fuller, 1998).

At a higher level, the IDS must ensure that the information systems used by the various facilities in the IDS will carry the necessary information to who needs it, when they need it. If necessary patient information is not transferred, the causes of that failure must be investigated so that similar events will not occur in the future (AHIMA, 2004).

Because more than one facility is involved in an IDS and the cultures within each facility must be managed, and because the regulatory requirements for each entity may differ, data collection and monitoring within an IDS takes significantly more time and effort than it would within a single entity. For example, it may require one month to communicate and effect a change in data collection procedures within one department or facility, but it may require four to five months when multiple facilities are involved. Validating collection instruments and implementing education processes will be similarly affected.

One major task of HIM professionals within single facilities that is more complicated when applied to an IDS is the creation and maintenance of a **master patient index (MPI).** A facility MPI is a master list of all of the facility's patients, along with demographic information, such as gender; date of birth; social security number; medical record number, or other patient ID; address; race and ethnicity; admission and discharge dates; encounter types; and disposition (i.e., intended care setting following discharge). Exhibit 15–2 lists recommended core data el-

Exhibit 15-2 Recommended Core Data Elements for an MPI

Internal patient identification
Person's name
Date of birth
Date of birth qualifier
Gender
Race
Ethnicity
Address
Alias/previous name
Social Security number
Facility identification
Universal patient identifier (when established)
Account number
Admission or encounter date
Discharge or departure date
Encounter or service type
Patient disposition

Source: Reprinted with permission from American Health Information Management Association Master Patient Index (MPI) Task Force, Master Patient (Person) Index (MPI) Recommended Core Data Elements, *Journal of American Health Information Management Association,* © July/August 1997, American Health Information Management Association.

ements of an MPI (AHIMA, 1997d). Some optional additional elements are emergency contacts, allergies/reactions, and problem lists. Some data elements will be text data (e.g., patient address); some will be string data (e.g., social security number); and others will be coded values (e.g., race, gender). Creating and maintaining a facility's MPI involves ensuring consistency in how the data are captured by establishing policies and procedures, monitoring how the data are captured, obtaining missing data elements, resolving inconsistencies, and merging duplicate and overlap entries.

Creating an **enterprise-wide MPI (EMPI)** means merging the MPIs of all of the entities that make up the IDS. All of the tasks regarding facility MPIs must be carried out across facilities. Some of the potential problems involved in this are illustrated in Scenario 15-B.

An accurate MPI is the universal key that accesses patient health information throughout the healthcare organization or enterprise. It directs staff to the location of records. It allows access to computerized patient record files. It permits practitioners to compare previous diagnostic test results with current results (e.g., EKGs, lab values) and reduces the need for duplicate/repeat diagnostic tests. It informs practitioners of historical patient information, such as allergies to medications, other diagnoses, and chronic conditions by connecting this information through the MPI. It reduces the legal risk of the organization by enabling practitioners to make appropriate decisions using complete patient information. In addition, it helps protect a patient's privacy by ensuring that correspondence and billing information are sent to the patient's correct home address and insurance companies.

Laura, in Scenario 15-B, will need to develop system-wide policies and procedures for standardized data collection throughout all of the entities in the IDS. For example, she will need to devise policies and procedures to establish a single set of naming conventions that will address such matters as the use of suffixes, prefixes, aliases, nicknames, and hyphenated names. Clear and consistent conventions and definitions will also be needed for the other elements and for their specific values. System-wide policies and procedures must be in place for resolving inconsistencies in core elements of the same patient across facilities.

Laura also will need to ensure that someone in the IDS will monitor that the policy and procedures are being followed and that the coded data values are the same in all systems that contribute to the collection of data. Once the policy and procedures are in place, data inconsistencies will still occur, and she will need to develop a general guideline for the IDS that will determine which data are the correct data.

Personnel will be needed to resolve inconsistent data elements across facilities, obtain additional patient information as needed, and arrange to have records reviewed at the facilities so that they can be compared. In addition, enterprise MPI staff may need to report enterprise MPI changes to facilities.

Finally, periodic reports will be needed to help staff identify potential duplicate MPI entries, missing core data elements, and inconsistent core data elements for the same patient/person within a facility or across facilities. (For more detailed information on the complexities of developing an enterprise-wide MPI, see AHIMA, 1997c, 1997d, 1997e; Rhodes, 1997).

Scenario 15-B Inconsistencies in the MPI

Laura Bennett is the HIM professional for a corporate IDS that has 3 hospitals, 10 physician clinics, 1 rehabilitation center, and 2 long-term care settings. She is also responsible for the management of patient information that is collected on registration for the MPI.

Laura is currently attempting to create an enterprise-wide MPI (EMPI) for the IDS. As part of this task, she is reviewing the demographic data that are collected at the various entities that make up the IDS. The problem is that each entity has its own naming conventions and procedures, and the naming conventions vary between entities. For instance, one site uses the patient's legal name and another site uses nicknames. At some of the physician clinic sites, some of the children do not have their own separate MPI information, but are included with their parents' information.

Further, even when conventions are the same, the information that is collected from the various entities is not necessarily consistent: for example, one patient's name is spelled differently at multiple sites. Laura is beginning to discover similar inconsistencies in the MPIs' other core elements as well.

Questions

1. Why is it so important for Laura to resolve all of these inconsistencies?

2. What measures will Laura need to take to address the problem?

3. How should she determine which data are correct and which entity's data should be used? What should she do if there is a disagreement as

to which entity's data should be used or whether the data that are used are correct?

4. If Laura were in a voluntary IDS, one with less control over the individual entities, how might her course of action be different?

A completed ethical decision-making matrix for the scenario is provided at the end of the chapter.

REQUIRED SKILLS FOR HIM PROFESSIONALS

HIM professionals who are responsible for the privacy, security, and the quality of patient information across an IDS typically act as data consultants within facilities or enterprises. As such, they should know the available sources of data. They should also be able to facilitate knowledge transfer, standardize data collection processes (including designing data collection instruments), manage projects, and use data creatively to solve problems. They should be able to transform data into actual information as well as present it.

In addition, however, HIM professionals need skills for personal effectiveness. They need to be able to maintain and foster diverse working relationships with others. They also need to be able to use personal influence and facilitation skills to achieve positive results. It is also important that they recognize the differences in the learning and social styles of others and provide processes to meet their needs. They also need to promote the use of data by seizing every opportunity to encourage others to use data by creating meaningful uses for the data.

As HIM professionals in IDSs encounter the complex problems involving information management across multi-entity systems, they discover that they bear more responsibility than their colleagues in single entities and that they are accountable to many different people at each site: administrators, clinicians, staff of the IDS and its individual entities, and the patient/consumer. HIM professionals must exhibit self-accountability to ensure compliance with practice standards. Consequently,

they need to use a decision-making process that helps them define the problem clearly, remove the personality/individualistic characteristics from the issue as they resolve it, explore all possible options and consequences, and negotiate with others. Several approaches they may find useful are problem-solving techniques (Duarte, 1992), conflict-resolution skills (Capozzoli, 1995), the organizational diagnosis process (Manzini, 1988), the opportunity-driven process (Conklin &Weil, 1997), and leadership using an adaptive approach (Heifetz & Laurie, 1999).

CONCLUSION

HIM professionals in an IDS must have a broad knowledge base on collecting and transferring data across the continuum of care. It is important that they understand the healthcare system's entire continuum of care: rules and regulations, patient characteristics, and the various locations and key players that they will be working with.

Clearly, HIM professionals in an IDS must make decisions that have considerable impact on the privacy and security of patient information and the quality of patient care, and in doing so they will be accountable to all parties throughout the system. Therefore, it is important that they be familiar with the issues identified in this chapter and be ready to address them as situations arise.

Key Terms

- Enterprise-wide master patient index (EMPI)
- Health Insurance Portability and Accountability Act (HIPAA)
- Integrated delivery system (IDS)
- Master patient index (MPI)
- Protected health information (PHI)

Chapter Summary

- IDSs may be corporate (i.e., all facilities are owned by the corporation), noncorporate (i.e., all the facilities are in the network voluntarily), or a combination of both. In those that are noncorporate, the individual entities have more autonomy, so they will need to play a larger role in decision making on policies and procedures that the HIM professional may wish to implement across the IDS.
- In any setting, HIM professionals must deal with complex issues related to their responsibilities of ensuring the privacy, security, and quality of patient information. For HIM professionals working in an IDS, the complexities of these issues are multiplied.
- Privacy and security issues in the IDS include the development of system-wide privacy and security policies and procedures and the notification of patients about multi-entity access to their health information. They also include understanding HIPAA and how the laws affect the IDS.
- Data quality issues in the IDS include increased problems with data accuracy and consistency, which affects the accessibility of vital information when data are shared at a system level. The HIM professional must develop system-wide policies and procedures for data collection and ongoing monitoring.
- Data can be made more accessible through the creation of an enterprise master patient index for the IDS as a whole.
- Because HIM professionals working at the IDS level will need to negotiate with numerous individuals and facilities regarding system-wide changes, they will need effective communication and problem-solving skills.

References

American Health Information Management Association [AHIMA]. (1997a). *Faxing safeguards: Guidelines for transmitting patient health information.* Chicago: Author.

American Health Information Management Association [AHIMA]. (1997b). *HIV and confidentiality: Guidelines for managing health information relating to HIV infection.* Chicago: Author.

American Health Information Management Association [AHIMA]. (1997c). Practice Brief: Maintenance of master patient (person) index (MPI)—single site or enterprise. Retrieved October 14, 2005, from http://library.ahima.org/xpedio/groups/public/documents/ahima/pub_bok1_000071.html.

American Health Information Management Association [AHIMA]. (1997d). Practice Brief: Master patient (person) index (MPI) recommended core data elements. *Journal of AHIMA.* Retrieved October 14, 2005, from http://library.ahima.org/xpedio/groups/public/documents/ahima/pub_bok1_000073.html.

American Health Information Management Association [AHIMA]. (1997e). Practice Brief: Merging master patient (person) indexes (MPI). *Journal of AHIMA.* Retrieved October 14, 2005, from http://library.ahima.org/xpedio/groups/public/documents/ahima/pub_bok1_000072.html.

American Health Information Management Association [AHIMA]. (1997f). *Release and disclosure: Guidelines regarding maintenance and disclosure of health information.* Chicago: Author.

American Health Information Management Association [AHIMA], Data Quality Management Task Force. (1998a). Practice Brief: A checklist to assess data quality management efforts. *Journal of AHIMA.* Retrieved October 14, 2005, from http://library.ahima.org/xpedio/groups/public/documents/ahima/pub_bok1_000069.html.

American Health Information Management Association [AHIMA], Data Quality Management Task Force. (1998b). Practice Brief: Data quality management model. *Journal of AHIMA.* Retrieved October 14, 2005, from http://library.

ahima.org/xpedio/groups/public/documents/ ahima/pub_bok1_000066.html.

American Health Information Management Association [AHIMA]. (1998c). *Security and access: Guidelines for managing electronic patient information*. Chicago: Author.

American Health Information Management Association [AHIMA]. (2000). Patient flow of information. Retrieved October 14, 2005, from http:// library.ahima.org/xpedio/groups/public/ documents/ahima/bok1_018217.pdf#page%3D1.

American Health Information Management Association [AHIMA]. (2004). E-HIM strategic initiative: Core data sets. *Journal of AHIMA*. Retrieved October 14, 2005, from http://library.ahima.org/ xpedio/groups/public/documents/ahima/pub_ bok1_023159.html.

Capozzoli, T. K. (1995, December). Conflict resolution: A key ingredient in successful teams. *Supervision, 3.*

Center for Medicare and Medicaid Services. (2000). Privacy regulations. Retrieved December 28, 2003, from http://www.cms.hhs.gov/hipaa2/ regulations/privacy/default.asp.

Conklin, E. J., & Weil, W. (1997). Wicked problems: Naming the pain in organization. *Global Decision Support Systems*. Retrieved October 25, 2005, from http://www.mmmco.be/meetingnetwork/ readingroom/gdss_wicked.html.

Duarte, J. E. (1992, June). Problem-solving techniques for continuous improvement. *CMA—The Management Accounting Magazine.*

Fernandes, L., Yamamoto Tomeck, J. A., & Lenson, C. M. (1998). The role of electronic merges in an integrated delivery system. *Journal of AHIMA* 69(6): 81–88.

Fuller, S. (1998). Practice Brief: Designing a data collection process. *Journal of AHIMA*. Retrieved October 14, 2005, from http://library.ahima.org/ xpedio/groups/public/documents/ahima/pub_ bok1_000067.html.

Grant, K., & Adair, D. (2002). Presentation at the AHIMA Convention; September 23; San Francisco, CA.

Heifetz, R. A., & Laurie, D. L. (1999). *The leader's change handbook: An essential guide to setting direction and taking action*. San Francisco: Jossey-Bass.

Manzini, A. O. (1988). *Organizational diagnosis: A practical approach to company problem solving and growth*. New York: American Management Association.

Miller, J. A. (2003, November). How an integrated delivery system organized, approached, and monitored HIPAA privacy compliance—A case study. *Confidence* 11(11): 4–5. HIPAA Security Rule, Federal Register. Retrieved from http:// www.cms.hhs.gov/hipaa/hipaa2/regulations/ security/ 03-3877.pdf.

Rhodes, H. (1997). Practice Brief: Development of information capture tools. *Journal of AHIMA*. Retrieved October 14, 2005, from http://library. ahima.org/xpedio/groups/public/documents/ ahima/pub_bok1_000086.html.

The ethical decision-making matrix is a tool to help you organize complex, ethical problems; however, there is no simple fill-in-the-box approach to ethical decision making. The objective is to follow each step of the process and not move from the question directly to what should be done or how to prevent it next time. If you skip steps, you will not fully understand all of the values and options for action. Also, the matrix provided for each scenario in this book is not the only way to examine the problem. You can make an equally compelling ethical argument for a different decision—just be sure to follow all the steps of the matrix.

SCENARIO 15-A: SCHEDULING CLERK HAS ACCESS TO CLINICAL INFORMATION

Steps	Information	
1. What is the ethical question?	Should Anna allow the system to operate as it is?	
2. What are the facts?	**KNOWN**	**TO BE GATHERED**
	• The voluntary IDS allows information to be shared across sites. • Suzy has complained about the accessibility of her medical record. • There are policies and procedures at different sites, but not across the IDS.	• Should Anna be involved in writing policies and procedures for use across sites? • What is Anna's responsibility in this case? • How could the current policies negatively affect patients? • What are the customary practices in such cases? • What does Anna's boss or supervisor expect her to do? • What is the likely impact on self and family of changing jobs?
3. What are the values? Examine the shared and competing values, obligations, and interests of the stakeholders (i.e., patient, HIM professional, healthcare practitioner(s), administrators, society, and other advocates) involved in order to fully understand the complexity of the ethical problem(s).	**Patient:** Values confidentiality of the medical record; values accuracy of the medical record. **HIM professional:** Integrity, accuracy (ensure the confidentiality of the medical record by limiting access to patient records); avoid harm (open access to records could threaten security and accuracy); personal values (promote welfare of self and family by avoiding loss of job). **IDS members:** Promote welfare of patients through accurate documentation and preservation of data integrity; promote information sharing without jeopardizing security. **Society:** Protect the confidentiality of medical records.	

4. What are my options?	• Allow the system to operate as is. • Pull together a committee to develop policies and procedures across sites.	
5. What should I do?	Pull together a committee to develop policies and procedures across sites.	
6. What justifies my choice?	**JUSTIFIED**	**NOT JUSTIFIED**
	• Obligation to protect confidentiality and data integrity. • Preserve professional integrity.	• Allow the system to operate as is. • Jeopardize system security. • Not fair to patients who trust in the confidentiality of their records. • Jeopardize professional integrity.
7. How can I prevent this ethical problem?	• Determine if system changes are needed. • Learn more about IDSs and the security issues surrounding them. • Discuss standards and the values that support them with colleagues. • Evaluate institutional integrity at job interview and subsequently as ethical problems arise.	

The ethical decision-making matrix is a tool to help you organize complex, ethical problems; however, there is no simple fill-in-the-box approach to ethical decision making. The objective is to follow each step of the process and not move from the question directly to what should be done or how to prevent it next time. If you skip steps, you will not fully understand all of the values and options for action. Also, the matrix provided for each scenario in this book is not the only way to examine the problem. You can make an equally compelling ethical argument for a different decision—just be sure to follow all the steps of the matrix.

SCENARIO 15-B: INCONSISTENCIES IN THE MPI

Steps	Information	
1. What is the ethical question?	Should Laura work with the data as it is?	
2. What are the facts?	**KNOWN**	**TO BE GATHERED**
	• Each member of the IDS generates an MPI. • Naming conventions are not standard across IDS sites.	• What will be the result of a lack of universal naming conventions? • What naming conventions are the most logical? • What are the customary practices in such cases? • What does her boss or supervisor expect? • What is the likely impact on self and family of changing jobs?
3. What are the values? Examine the shared and competing values, obligations, and interests of the stakeholders (i.e., patient, HIM professional, healthcare practitioner(s), administrators, society, and other advocates) involved in order to fully understand the complexity of the ethical problem(s).	**Patient:** Values accuracy of medical record data. **HIM professional:** Integrity, accuracy (create a system that ensures the continuity and accuracy of data); avoid harm (sharing of inaccurate data could harm the patient). **Healthcare professionals:** Promote the welfare of patients by sharing accurate information. **MPI administrators:** Value ease of entering data without compromising accuracy. **Society:** Values the dissemination of accurate patient information.	

4. What are my options?	• Try to integrate existing data as is. • Create standard naming conventions for use in all MPIs.	
5. What should I do?	Create standard naming conventions for use in all MPIs.	
6. What justifies my choice?	**JUSTIFIED**	**NOT JUSTIFIED**
	• Obligation to disseminate the most accurate information possible. • Preserve professional integrity.	• Try to integrate existing data as is. • Creation of a system that does not make use of the most accurate information available. • Jeopardize professional integrity.
7. How can I prevent this ethical problem?	• Determine if system changes are needed. • Learn more about the creation and maintenance of enterprise-wide MPIs within IDSs. • Discuss standards and the values that support them with colleagues.	

Learning Objectives

After completing this chapter, the reader should be able to:

- Describe the benefits and risks of e-health services.
- Recognize how e-health is changing the nature of health information.
- Discuss some of the ethical considerations and conflicts related to e-health and suggested policies to address them.

E-HEALTH FOR CONSUMERS, PATIENTS, AND CAREGIVERS

Cynthia Baur, PhD
Mary Jo Deering, PhD

Abstract

E-health technologies enable consumers, patients, and caregivers to search for health information and advice, to create and maintain personal health records, and to conduct virtual consultations with their care providers. However, the use of e-health technologies raises a number of ethical issues. Health information management (HIM) professionals will be increasingly involved in these issues as they interact more directly with consumers, patients, and caregivers as partners in health information management. HIM professionals who work for Internet companies and online health information services will face a number of unique challenges as healthcare organizations develop e-health capacities. This chapter explores several of the ethical issues raised by e-health technologies.

Scenario 16-A: Equity and Privacy

Location: The Smith house, Smalltown, USA

Joan Smith, a 40-year-old self-insured owner of a specialty women's clothing store, manages the health of five people: herself; her husband, Jim, who takes daily medication for high blood pressure; their two preteens, one of whom has asthma; and her 65-year-old father, who lives an hour away and who is recovering from his second heart surgery, which occurred three months ago. She can't get in touch with the home care agency nurse who visits her father once a week to find out if her father's primary care physician is receiving the nurse's regular reports on her father's condition. Joan knows that Jim doesn't always remember to take his medicine and that he skipped his last checkup, and he gets irritated every time she reminds him. The daughter with asthma seems to be having more frequent and severe attacks, and Joan is concerned that the doctor isn't doing all that he can. She has thought about switching doctors, but she is overwhelmed at the idea of having to find a different doctor and have her daughter's extensive medical records transferred to a new office.

Joan has a computer and dial-up Internet connection at home. She has used search engines and websites to look for health information to help her with her caregiving demands. She even logged on to an online chat room once. However, Joan's Internet connection is often slow and has disconnected in the middle of her Web searches a few times. Also, she finds many of the websites to be confusing, and she's not sure how reliable some of the information is. She can't talk to her doctor about her use of the Internet to search for medical information, because he told her that he doesn't think it is helpful. He believes that it can even be harmful for patients to look for information on their own.

Location: The Jones house (next door to the Smith house), Smalltown, USA

Glenda Jones also runs her own business, a party-planning company, and manages the health of five people. One difference between Glenda and Joan is that Glenda has a computer with a high-speed Internet connection that she uses for her home business. Glenda is responsible for the health care of the following people: herself; her husband, Doug; their son, Jonathan, who has a learning disability; and Glenda's elderly parents, who live 1,000 miles away. Glenda's parents are in reasonably good health, although she has noticed that her mother is becoming more forgetful than usual.

Last weekend, Glenda logged onto http://www.healthfinder.gov, the federal government's consumer health information website, to look for reliable information about aging, memory loss, and Alzheimer's disease. The site referred her to two organizations that had useful information sheets that she read online and sent by e-mail to her father. Glenda also read the privacy policy before she did her first search on the site, and she was reassured that the site does not collect any information about its users.

Later in the week, Glenda logged on to a commercial website where she has created personal health records for herself and her family. She uses a password to access the records. She needs to update her father's record with the information he e-mailed her from his preoperative visit to the surgeon to discuss his upcoming hip replacement surgery. She plans to review Jonathan's new medications and the doses that the doctor prescribed yesterday and the calendar with the automated reminder system for Jonathan's next visit. She also will double-check the appointment time for the session she has scheduled with a cardiologist. Glenda took an online assessment that suggested she might be at risk for heart disease and should consult a physician.

The first thing Glenda notices on her personal home page is an urgent message from the website. The message informs her that the site detected a security breach and that the site's staff has been working around the clock to assess any damage. The company is also exploring additional security measures. Glenda is encouraged to e-mail any comments or concerns she might have to the site's chief privacy officer. The message concludes with reassurances that the site's operators take the protection of users' privacy very seriously, and they will update their members on new procedures as soon as possible. Glenda is concerned and thinks again about transferring the family's records to her managed care organization, which recently began offering a multifunctional patient portal that includes personal health records connected to doctors' electronic health records. Glenda, however, doesn't even know if such a transfer is possible, and she is worried that if she has to drop or change her insurance coverage because of the cost, she would lose access to the family's online health histories.

Questions

1. You are an HIM professional employed by a clinic whose administration wants to put a sizable amount of effort and funding into communicating with patients and promoting their health and education via the Internet. Do the differences in health care and Internet access like those described in this case between the Smiths and the Joneses raise ethical concerns? What might your input be concerning these differences and policies that might be developed to address them?

2. If you were an HIM professional hired to create either digital personal health records for a commercial website or a patient portal for a managed care organization, what ethical issues would you see with creating proprietary products that do not allow users to transfer their personal health information?

A completed ethical decision-making matrix for the scenario is provided at the end of the chapter.

The circumstances of the two households portrayed in Scenario 16-A represent the present and future of health and health care in the United States. The situation in the Smith household reflects the present for many families with typical health concerns. They confront a complex and fragmented healthcare system that makes it difficult to take actions to maintain wellness, manage illness, and improve health. The situation in the Jones household reflects how e-health can affect consumers, patients, and caregivers and suggests the future of health and health care. Along with many other organizations, The American Health Information Management Association (AHIMA) recognizes that health information is becoming increasingly digitized and defines the future of HIM as "electronic, patient-centered, comprehensive, longitudinal, accessible and credible" (AHIMA E-HIM Task Force, 2003).

The demand for e-health is driven by many factors. As illustrated by the descriptions of the two households in Scenario 16-A, e-health is changing the roles and responsibilities of consumers, patients, caregivers, and the healthcare system. Sometimes out of choice, and sometimes by necessity, consumers, patients, and caregivers are becoming increasingly responsible for the management of their own health (Deering & Baur, 2004). They are taking the initiative in seeking out information and tools to help them with these new demands. Consequently, the role of consumers, patients, and caregivers as critical "information nodes" is becoming more clear. As a result, the HIM process, which used to focus primarily on health professionals as information generators and users, will change so that consumers, patients, and caregivers become critical information generators and users as well.

The AHIMA website (http://www.ahima. org) states that HIM professionals serve the public by managing, analyzing, and utilizing data vital for patient care and making it accessible to healthcare providers when it is needed most. The e-health phenomenon challenges HIM professionals to broaden their understanding of how they will relate to the public, where information will flow from and to, and who will use the information and for what purposes.

Consumer, patient, and caregiver **e-health** refers to digital communication and information technologies that are used by these groups for a variety of personal health purposes, including disease prevention and health promotion, communication, decision making, and health management and improvement. Information is an implicit or explicit component of all these purposes. Consumers, patients, and caregivers use e-health technologies for purposes such as secure messaging, information searches, and risk assessment. Regardless of how or for what purpose these technologies are used, the primary locus of control for the use of these technologies is with the consumers, patients, and caregivers themselves. This use is characterized by active participation and decision making by consumers, patients, and

caregivers to initiate and terminate use as well as to define what is accomplished by using the technology.

Consumers, patients, and caregivers may use e-health technologies to interact with clinical and public health professionals, but not necessarily in ways primarily defined by clinical or public health purposes or needs. Consumers, patients, and caregivers may also choose to keep their use of technology, such as searching the Internet for health information or participating in an online community, separate from their healthcare transactions. This formulation of consumer, patient, and caregiver e-health is consistent with, although not articulated by, the vision of the Personal Health Dimension of the National Health Information Infrastructure (NHII) described by the National Committee on Vital and Health Statistics (NCVHS) (see discussion of the NHII later in this chapter) (U.S. Department of Health and Human Services, 2001). E-health is also a component of what Dr. David Brailer, the National Coordinator for Health Information Technology (HIT), calls the "Nationwide Health Information Network" (Thompson & Brailer, 2004). The Internet and the World Wide Web are currently the most popular channels for e-health activities. Many emerging technologies, such as wireless and wearable applications and smart appliances, also will support the development of e-health for individuals as well as populations (Eng, 2001; 2004). Examples of e-health include:

- Communication between physicians and patients via secure messaging
- Consumers' management of their personal health information on the Web
- Consumers' access to their health records via the Internet
- Websites that furnish information on wellness and prevention, risk assessment, diseases and their management, treatments, and medications
- The purchase of health-related products and services over the Internet

Each of these activities has benefits and risks. For example, consider e-mail communication between physicians and patients. The potential advantages of e-mail communication between patients and healthcare providers includes the elimination of telephone tag and voice mail messages; the ability to attach educational materials or other electronic documents; improved documentation of conversations; and the possibility of an enhanced relationship if used in addition to, rather than as a substitute for, face-to-face communication (AHIMA, 2003).

However, the following risks must also be considered (AHIMA, 2003):

- E-mail can be misdirected, intercepted, or altered without the sender's or receiver's knowledge.
- E-mail can be left visible on unattended screens to be read by unauthorized persons.
- E-mail can be copied, printed, stored, or forwarded without permission—all of which are breaches of confidentiality.
- E-mail is discoverable for legal purposes.
- E-mail may be vulnerable to computer hackers, who can then transmit the information for illegitimate purposes.
- E-mail attachments may introduce viruses.
- Significant misinterpretations may arise due to the poor quality of the written communication or the lack of verbal and nonverbal cues.

Although secure messaging systems and organizational policies can address many of these concerns, human error and misunderstanding of these policies by providers and HIM professionals are always possible. Also, e-mail, by its very nature, creates a detailed trail of communication between providers and patients that did not previously exist and that can be exploited in various ways.

In addition, consider consumers' use of the Web to manage personal health information:

- Healthcare providers can permit consumers to access their own health records via the Internet. Within these records, providers can establish links to

pertinent, reputable reference materials. These reference materials can then serve as tools for consumers to better understand their own health and to make more-informed decisions.
- Consumers can develop their own personal electronic health records. They may use these records to provide new healthcare providers with a complete and accurate medical history, to maintain a comprehensive immunization record, or to store references to relevant disease prevention and health promotion materials.

However, digital health information creates new risks:

- Personal health information may be obtained and used inappropriately by unauthorized individuals or organizations.
- A consumer's health information may be incomplete, incorrect, out-of-date, misinterpreted, entered fraudulently, or altered without detection, resulting in financial or health-related harm to the consumer (AHIMA, 2000).
- Patient-entered data may not be in sync with data in the healthcare organization's electronic health record, which creates confusion and perhaps missed data.

Instances of how individuals can manage their health via the Internet can be multiplied a hundredfold to demonstrate the potential of e-health. For example:

- an elderly cardiac patient who routinely forgot to take his medication now receives automatic daily e-mail reminders and health promotion messages about the importance of healthy eating and regular exercise
- rural residents who previously waited months and traveled hundreds of miles to see specialists already use local telemedicine system nodes to connect monthly with experts for virtual office visits
- a woman newly diagnosed with breast cancer logs on to a chat room on the Internet and instantly finds dozens of women who can provide advice and encouragement as she sorts through her options

- anxious parents of a newborn search the Internet in the middle of the night for one of the many parenting information websites to find out about colic
- a pack-and-a-half-a-day smoker who has thought about quitting for years tries the online decision-support program that her physician recommended and finally takes the first steps to quit
- and a spouse who has primary responsibility for caring for her husband with dementia writes about her loneliness and exhaustion as part of an online community of caregivers who recommend local respite services.

The common factors among all of these examples are that these activities are taking place outside traditional clinical settings; the activities generate relevant and important health information that has not traditionally been part of health information records; and individuals are using nonclinical sources of information, such as websites, to manage their health and make decisions.

As noted earlier, one of the primary risks of e-health relates to the unauthorized collection and use of personal health information. With e-health technologies, personal health information is not confined to a paper medical record at a healthcare facility. It is in a digital format that can be part of Web-based consumer health records, e-mail messages, online chats, and other applications that permit information to be easily stored and shared. These types of information flows raise concerns about violations of confidentiality and the protection of individuals' privacy (Lumpkin, 2000). Electronic networks create a situation of abundance—in the amount of available personal health information and in the number of possible outlets with an interest in having access to that information. As doctor–patient consults move from behind the closed door of a physical office and onto the Internet in the form of telemedicine consults, doctor–patient e-mail, and online advice services, concerns arise that the security of individual online services

may not be adequate to meet a high standard of confidentiality protection. To address these concerns, policies and practices have been implemented in recent years to buttress the privacy and security of online personal health information. The Health Insurance Portability and Accountability Act of 1996 (HIPAA) and the final Privacy Rule that came out of it have led to the application of sophisticated technologies for controlling access to personal health information, including the identification and authentication of individuals authorized to access information, audit trails of those accessing and/or modifying information, and different levels of access to information (U.S. Department of Health and Human Services, 2005).

The application of technology to enhance privacy protections creates the possibility that electronic health records can be as secure, if not more secure, than paper records. Yet, even with the awareness and advances that HIPAA has fostered, federal laws may be inadequate for managing health information flows over the Internet, which is accessed and used internationally. HIM professionals will have to grapple with the challenge of protecting health information in a global environment in which laws vary by country and ethical standards for privacy and security may differ from culture to culture.

E-HEALTH AND THE CHANGING HEALTHCARE SYSTEM

Healthcare trends that emerged in the 1990s have become more pronounced and their impact more clear (Eng, 2001; Institute for the Future, 2003). One of these trends is consumers' responsibility for their own health, including taking action to prevent illness and taking care of minor health problems with self-care. Consumers are expected to take the initiative to find information about health concerns or at least use information provided by clinicians, health educators, and managed care companies (Deering & Baur, 2004).

A second important trend is the lengthening of life spans and the accompanying increase in the prevalence of chronic disease, which places demands on individuals and the healthcare system to find better ways to manage illness over longer periods of time. Slowly, medical activities designed to produce a cure are broadening to include health improvement activities designed to prevent disease or make illness more manageable. These health improvement activities are typically information intensive, require full participation by the patient/consumer, and require documentation beyond what currently occurs.

An additional trend is an increasing emphasis on managing the health of populations and communities, not just individuals. A population focus requires that we know something about not only those who have health insurance and receive medical care, but also about the uninsured and underinsured—which again focuses our attention on the need to have access to information about individuals whose health information is not typically part of a medical record. Outcomes research, which examines the consequences of health treatments and procedures, requires information about large enough groups of people to draw statistically reliable and valid conclusions and provides another impetus to find ways to make sure health information databases are as accurate and complete as possible. Both population health and outcomes research also require de-identified data—that is, data from which personally identifiable information has been removed—before the data may be shared, integrated, and analyzed. Existing medical and public health records are not well designed to capture these types of information, which indicates the need for new methods of HIM.

E-health applications create additional opportunities for change. E-health presents new ideas regarding health, health services, and information management that shift the emphasis to patient-centered care, informed decision making, consumers' management of their own health information, comprehensive health histories, and distributed health services (Deering & Baur, 2004; Harris, 1995). E-health promotes the dispersion of health-care activities from the doctor's office and the hospital to multiple locations, such as the home, and workplace. E-health also encourages the multiplication of sources for health information and the distribution of record-keeping functions among consumers, commercial entities, healthcare providers, and healthcare organizations.

It is unclear, though, if the e-health phenomenon will be a critical force for standardization and interoperability in health information technology (HIT). E-health applications are not inherently interoperable. Many e-health applications are stand-alone products, which limits their value in an environment in which consumers, patients, and caregivers are trying to manage health cross-organizationally and longitudinally.

Noninteroperable and nonstandardized information systems present significant barriers to the sharing of health information. For the same health concern, an individual may visit several different medical specialists. These specialists may not call or write referring physicians about their findings. In addition, they may not have the computer equipment and network infrastructure to send information electronically. Physician offices and healthcare facilities typically have unique record-keeping systems and may only standardize information that is relevant to their own billing system. Also, it is time consuming to collect and copy all relevant patient data to share with other providers. Facilities and individual healthcare providers that want to retain patients have few incentives to allocate resources for creating and adhering to standardized formats that would allow patients to move easily from one practice group or hospital to another.

Existing medical records also leave out a lot of relevant information about an individual's health concerns and activities. Individuals typically only seek medical care for about 20 percent of their health concerns (Sobel, 1987); the rest are managed by the individual with at-home or over-the-counter remedies and advice from family, friends, and other sources of health information.

Patients who visit a physician may also use alternative and complementary medicine, self-care, consumer-oriented health information, over-the-counter and herbal medications, and emotional and spiritual remedies. When these sources are taken into consideration, it becomes clear that typical medical records provide an incomplete picture of an individual's health.

E-health technologies focus attention on the limitations of paper-based records and our understanding of health. Networked, interoperable e-health systems can contribute to the infrastructure so that, if provided the right incentives, medical professionals can harmonize their record systems and exchange patient information easily and rapidly. The systems will also allow consumers, multiple healthcare providers and facilities, insurance companies, and community health professionals to maintain their own records and share information on an as-needed basis. E-health's benefits and potential to improve health and well-being include increased access to health information and support that is personalized and available on demand; more choices for health information, goods, and services; increased security of personal health information; and a bigger "footprint" for dissemination of health information and materials (Eng & Gustafson, 1999; U.S. General Accounting Office, 1996; U.S. Department of Health and Human Services, 2001). These benefits promise to enable patients and health consumers to seek answers to their questions when they need them; to talk to healthcare providers they feel comfortable with; to spend healthcare dollars more efficiently; and to protect their privacy.

E-HEALTH AND NATIONAL POLICY

The potential of health information technology to improve the quality, safety, and efficiency of health care has prompted significant policy initiatives that reinforce consumer, patient, and caregiver e-health trends. The National Committee on Vital and Health Statistics, which advises the Secretary of Health and Human Services on health information policy, published a consensus vision of the National Health Information Infrastructure. It includes a personal health dimension as equal to the provider (healthcare) dimension and the community (public health) dimension. The personal health dimension is a virtual information space that supports "the management of individual wellness and healthcare decision-making. It encompasses data about health status and health care in the format of a personal health record, but also other information and resources relevant to personal health" (U.S. Department of Health and Human Services, 2001). As envisioned by NCHVS, **personal** (electronic) **health records, or PHRs,** are a core component of the NHII, enhancing the ability of individuals to control their own health data and access by healthcare providers to that data.

National policy initiatives building on the NHII concept have elevated consumer and patient e-health. The national plan for promoting HIT, announced in July 2004, sets a goal of personalizing care through technology. Encouraging the use of PHRs is the first strategy listed for achieving this goal (Thompson & Brailer, 2004). In the view of policymakers, secure PHRs could be maintained by patient and his or her physician, insurer, or others, giving the patient unprecedented access and control of the record. This could mean not only better-informed consumers of health care, but also direct patient and caregiver involvement in decision making regarding their care (U.S. Department of Health and Human Services, 2004; AHIMA, 2004).

Connecting for Health, a public–private national collaborative initiative that is mapping out specific steps by which an interconnected healthcare system could be developed and deployed, determined that "a key part of a necessary transformation in healthcare is putting patients' information directly into their own hands, and enabling patients to put often-missing information into the hands of their clinicians" (Markle Foundation, Connecting for Health, 2004). The initiative recommends that PHRs can and should play an important role in helping bridge these information gaps.

Many federal programs are adding components that support the inclusion of e-health applications in the healthcare system. As directed by the Medicare Modernization Act of 2003, the Centers for Medicare and Medicaid Services (CMS) launched Medicare Support Program formerly known as the Chronic Care Improvement Program at the end of 2004. Ten pilot programs offer self-care guidance and support to chronically ill beneficiaries. These programs will help Medicare beneficiaries manage their health and follow their physicians' plans of care and will give them reminders to seek or obtain medical care that they need to reduce their health risks. Although the use of HIT is not mandatory, CMS encourages its use in the pilot projects and views the Medicare Health Support Program as a significant opportunity to demonstrate the value of innovative, integrative information infrastructures and communication technologies. Over several years, the Veterans Administration (VA) has been rolling out a PHR for veterans. The VA launched MyHealth*e*Vet (http://www.myhealth.va.gov/) in 2004 as an Internet tool for personal health management. It permits veterans to voluntarily interact with subsets of their VA electronic health record and, ultimately, manage their own PHR.

There is synergy among these national efforts. All of them are promoting consumer and patient empowerment. They recognize the significance of standards-based approaches to personal health information management so that information can be exchanged accurately and securely. Yet, even when taken together, these national efforts are not likely to achieve their broader goal of ensuring that a patient's information is available to whomever needs it and is authorized to use it. Given the nation's fragmented, public–private healthcare delivery system, the private sector plays a crucial role. Many private health plans and providers are offering personal e-health tools on their Web portals as a means of improving patient services and satisfaction. Some are offering secure messaging (e-mail) to help their patients feel more connected. The benefits of all these private e-health services are tempered by the fact that they are designed to be proprietary;

they do interact with each other; and thus they do not help the consumer when the consumer moves on to another provider, plan, facility, or delivery system.

E-HEALTH AND THE HIM PROFESSIONAL

To participate fully in an information-intensive healthcare system and to maximize the value of self-care, consumers will need to maintain more information about and for themselves apart from sporadic clinical encounters. Consequently, digital personal health records are likely to proliferate outside the boundaries of healthcare organizations and to be set up and managed by individuals, online health services, and companies formed to manage consumer health records. Even though the current system of medical records recognizes that patients "own" their personal health information, the concepts of ownership, control, and levels of permission to access different types of information are evolving in the digital environment. Because the universe of health information records has expanded to include websites and pocket digital devices, the idea of the medical record as a unitary, fixed-location document is already being revisited.

Commercial interest in health information as a source of profit both for traditional medical facilities and for new entrants, such as Web-based information businesses, has been increasing. Even after several years in business, though, the technology entrepreneurs who have been driving much of the development of e-health have yet to develop a consensus on a code of ethics for the field (Baur & Deering, 2001). The commercial sector is interested in health information systems because they perceive great public demand for many different kinds of health information, from online consumer health information services to secure communication systems for electronic health commerce (e-health commerce); that is, commercial health transactions over the Internet. These commercial sites may not fully disclose all of their information practices, especially third-party use of personal information (Goldman, Hudson, & Smith, 2000). Personal information is collected not only explicitly, as in asking for a name and address, but also implicitly with cookies (embedded computer codes to track users' online activities) and online "services," such as surveys and health risk assessments that provide detailed information to the website about individual users, who often are not informed of the uses of their answers. The amount of health activity on the Internet means that HIM professionals may be just as likely to work for an Internet company or HIM firm as for a traditional healthcare institution. This situation brings HIM professionals more directly in contact with patients and consumers and is likely to create new opportunities for HIM professionals to act as advocates for the public's privacy interests.

The HIM professional's changing role points to the evolving nature of the concepts of ownership, control, and permission granting that underlie the management of personal health information. One approach to management is permission based. Permission-based approaches recognize that individuals are the only ones who should permit or deny access to their own personal health information. On a case-by-case basis, an individual is notified of the need to access personal health information, and only uses that the person has explicitly authorized are allowed. Another approach is a paternalistic one in which health professionals decide what constitutes reasonable access and agree to act in the best interests of their patients about questions of access to various types of health information. A third approach frequently used in the current medical record system is an umbrella release, signed by patients to give those who claim a need to know, such as insurance companies, access to personal health information. A fourth approach relies on the development of common, consensual rules to protect confidentiality and facilitate necessary information sharing.

If HIM professionals become involved with the development of e-health systems, they need to be alert to the ethical dilemmas associated with the promotion of technologies' benefits without due consideration of their impact on privacy, confidentiality, and harm to patients. If the systems are not implemented with the necessary safeguards, and if they are consequently unreliable or not secure enough to protect confidential information, they may actually frustrate clinicians and patients alike.

SOME E-HEALTH ETHICAL ISSUES

Choice and Interoperability

Let's return to Scenario 16-A, which was presented at the beginning of the chapter. The Smith and Jones households present a contrast in "meaningful access" for many individuals living in the United States. Although both families have access to health care, a computer, and the Internet, they do not have equal access to all of the e-health resources that are increasingly taken for granted. For instance, differences between dial-up and broadband Internet connections have been identified as part of a new "digital divide."

Yet, many households—approximately 25 percent—in the United States do not have any Internet connection in their home, either because they do not have a computer or they do not find the Internet relevant to their lives (Lebo, 2004). For those who want access but don't have digital devices to connect to the Internet, they must rely on locations such as work, school, or public libraries to gain access (U.S. Department of Commerce, 2002). Several factors potentially limit the use of online health information and support in these settings. Some employers monitor e-mail and the types of sites visited by employees. Access in public settings may be problematic because of privacy and confidentiality concerns, and access may be needed during times when these facilities are unavailable or completely in use. Because of the potentially sensitive nature of health-related uses of the Internet, home access is critical.

Despite the best public policy efforts, some people may never use the Internet at all, for several reasons. First, some individuals may not be technologically literate or may not want to use computers or other digital technologies. It is an important public policy and ethical matter to establish the principle that no one should be denied knowledge about health improvements or left out of the healthcare system because of a reluctance to use e-health technologies. Specifically, some individuals lack general literacy and health literacy. **Health literacy** is defined as "the degree to which individuals have the capacity to obtain, process, and understand basic health information and services needed to make appropriate health decisions" (U.S. Department of Health and Human Services, 2000, pp. 11–20). Even if they have easy access to the Internet in their homes, individuals with limited health literacy are unlikely to feel comfortable using the Internet to look up largely text-based materials that may require well-developed reading skills and a thorough grasp of the healthcare system. Second, some individuals may be unable to find culturally and linguistically appropriate materials on the Internet. Although the number of languages used on the Internet is increasing, the Internet remains primarily an English-language phenomenon. Those who do not know English or who do not feel comfortable using English to communicate are likely to find the Internet less useful.

In addition, there is the danger of creating unrealistic expectations about the positive impact of digital health information systems on health when there are existing inequalities in access to basic healthcare services and information. Therefore, the assumptions and likely consequences of making e-health applications more common and, in some future scenarios, the gold standard, need to be carefully assessed:

- Does excitement about e-health's possibilities obscure multiple access issues for those who don't have regular sources of health care and who have not been early adopters of the Internet?
- How will consumers, patients, and caregivers who are reluctant to use e-health technologies manage their health information in the future?
- Will consumers be expected to document everything about their health, no matter how private they consider it, once we come to expect cradle-to-grave, portable health information systems?
- Do healthcare organizations and professionals have an obligation to promote access to e-health systems to those who can't afford to buy access?
- What are the ethical implications of developing e-health applications that require high technologies to function correctly?

Scenario 16-B: Ensuring Online Quality and Privacy Protections

Vivian uses a commercial health information website with online personal health records to track her family's health histories. The site tries to convey a sense of trustworthiness with its slogans about "information you can trust." Vivian chose the site because she recognized the names of some of the site's sponsors, and she found the chat groups stimulating. However, Vivian doesn't know much about the site's security features or the quality of the site's informational content. The site has "crashed" a few times after she has been logged on, but she has always been able to log back on within a few minutes. She assumes that her personal health records are safe, because, she reasons, the website wouldn't offer the service if they weren't. The ask-a-doc advice sessions always have the name and credentials of the physicians or nurses who participate, and Vivian thinks they must check a lot of the information on the site.

Vivian finds online record keeping far more convenient than keeping paper records, especially when she needs to look up information or visit a new healthcare provider. She assumes that she "owns" her own health information—that she has the final say about which information goes into her record, who has access to which parts of the record, and what they can do with the information. When she registered with the online service, she read the lengthy terms and disclosure statement that were on the website. The statement said that the site wouldn't sell information about Vivian that it collects, but that it would share information with unnamed business partners.

Martin, an HIM professional who has just been hired by the website, has a different reaction to the website's privacy and information-sharing policies. Although he is working on content development—in particular, electronic forms for the collection of consumer health information, rather than on privacy and security issues—specifically, he notices and is disturbed by the privacy policy posted on the company's website.

Questions

1. What ethical questions are raised by e-health services in terms of the quality of the content?

2. If you, as an HIM professional, were to work for such a service, what guidelines might you consult to address these questions? What policies might you develop or advocate?

3. What ethical issues might Martin raise regarding this company's privacy policies?

4. What policy changes might Martin consider to be necessary? How might he advocate for them?

A completed ethical decision-making matrix for the scenario is provided at the end of the chapter.

Vivian is in the same situation as many other online health consumers. She knows a little about the health websites she uses, and she also takes a lot on faith. The commercial health information sites she has surfed rarely provide full information about the identity of those involved in the website and its purposes and policies. The United States currently has a national health objective to improve the quality of health-related World Wide websites—and the ability of a website to provide sufficient protections for personal information is one of the hallmarks of quality. The specific quality elements are drawn from the recommendations of the Science Panel on Interactive Communication and Health and are framed as a matter of disclosure (Eng & Gustafson, 1999). The ob-

jective states that, at a minimum, websites should disclose (1) the identity of the developers and sponsors of the site (and how to contact them) and information about any potential conflicts of interest or biases; (2) the explicit purpose of the site, including any commercial purposes and advertising; (3) the original sources of the content on the site; (4) how the privacy and confidentiality of any personal information collected from users are protected; (5) how the site is evaluated; and (6) how the information is updated (U.S. Department of Health and Human Services, 2000). A process is currently under way to measure the proportion of websites that meet these criteria.

Numerous public and private sector organizations have developed quality criteria and online codes of conduct to help consumers understand the issue of quality and how their personal information is used by health websites. Between July 1996 and September 2000, six separate groups released guidelines, policies, or codes of conduct or ethics for health websites (see Appendix A for a list). Several of these efforts collaborated to work with URAC (http://www.urac.org), an accreditation body, to create standards for the accreditation of health websites. These six frameworks and URAC standards still represent the most widely accepted guidance for information handling on health websites, although none has emerged as dominant or definitive in terms of quality assessments.

As Scenario 16-B shows, websites may not make very clear the trade-offs that individuals face between giving up a little or a lot of control over the uses of their personal information and realizing the benefits, such as ease of access, convenience, and improved organization of personal health information. If the information remains the property of a website or another type of specific for-profit organization, then the primary threats to invasions of privacy are likely to come from commercial entities that share information with affiliates and business partners and use the information to deliver targeted advertising messages. There is also the potential for covert discrimination by employers, insurance providers, and financial services providers who could aggregate pieces of information to build detailed profiles of individual users. Even if legislative and regulatory solutions are developed, a danger is that information that can quickly move from location to location will escape adequate safeguards that existed in the original location to ensure confidentiality and protect privacy. On some websites, consumers cannot tell that when they click on certain icons they've left the site and are actually providing health information to other businesses.

A few of the questions that arise in relation to privacy and the confidentiality of personal health information are:

- Is disclosure of privacy policies sufficient, regardless of the actual provisions of the policy?

- What are the minimum adequate safeguards that a website or similar information agent should offer to protect personal health information?
- Should the default condition be no information sharing without explicit permission from the individual who owns the information or should the party that wants access to the information notify the individual that the information will be shared unless the individual explicitly prohibits it?
- To what extent are appeals to public good, individual health improvement, and access to enhanced services overstated or even manipulative to convince people to provide personal information?

The guidelines for information handling by digital health services include guidelines addressing confidentiality and privacy concerns. For example, AHIMA's Recommendations to Ensure Privacy and Quality of Personal Health Information on the Internet (2000) includes the following tenets:

- Inform consumers about what information is collected, by whom, and how it will be used. The notice-of-information practices should be conspicuously provided in language the layperson can understand.
- Give consumers meaningful opportunities to make choices about what information is collected and how the information will be used. Sites should collect no information without the user's knowledge. Give website consumers the right to opt into or out of specific uses and disclosures of information.
- Notify users on screen when they enter or leave the e-health owner's website.

EMERGING ISSUES

With the heightened national interest in consumer, patient, and caregiver health IT applications (PHRs and other e-health self-management programs), it is becoming clear that the capacity of the technology is far ahead of the policies and practices needed for optimum use of these electronic tools. The problems are most clearly seen in the area of personal health information exchange and consumers' control of their personal health information. The key issues represent "different sides of the patient-control coin," so to speak. On the one hand, patients may not be able to fully limit access to their personal health information that is collected and managed through e-health tools that fall outside official privacy regulations. The HIPAA Privacy Rule does not support individuals' ownership and control of their health records (Gellman, 2004). Moreover, as described in Chapter 3, HIPAA's definition of which healthcare entities and activities are covered encompasses health plans, healthcare clearinghouses, healthcare providers who conduct certain financial and administrative transactions electronically, and government-funded healthcare programs. Websites that collect a significant amount of personal information as a means of customizing their response to the user or companies offering personal health records often do not fall within these categories. Although reputable companies may voluntarily meet or even exceed HIPAA privacy requirements (e.g., see MedicAlert at http://ww.medicalert.org/(nnijkx55dva2xqzz bmvoyqrr)/Main/hippa.aspx), there is no legal basis for influencing, much less sanctioning, unethical companies.

On the other hand, however, even when patients want their information to be exchanged electronically (subject to authorization and security protections) with other providers, for example, because they are changing health providers or plans or seeking second opinions, they are likely to be equally stymied for several reasons. As of mid-decade, electronic health records have not been widely adopted. Those in use are not interoperable—meaning they cannot directly exchange information outside a given healthcare organization. Worse still, from the patient's perspective, physicians continue to view patient data as proprietary and as having a business value, so they are reluctant to exchange it with potential competitors. PHRs are proliferating with even less

assurance that an individual's information can—or will—be exchanged with other programs or across healthcare organizations. Although standards development efforts are focusing on interoperability for institutional electronic health records, the work needed for personal health information to move securely and seamlessly lags behind. Many online PHR providers would like to be able to offer their customers the ability to send their information to authorized healthcare providers, but the providers are not able to receive it, and many are reluctant to receive it because of concerns about the integrity of the data they themselves collected initially.

Another very sensitive issue is that of accurately identifying patients across multiple healthcare providers and plans. National policy rejects the notion of a unique identifier for every individual (U.S. Department of Health and Human Services, 2001). Technical experts maintain that it is neither necessary nor beneficial (Markle Foundation, Connecting for Health, 2004). Alternative technical means of being able to confirm that John Jones is or is not the same as J. Jones have been demonstrated (Markle Foundation, Connecting for Health, 2004). Still, consensus has not been reached on the best means of accomplishing this accurate linkage. Demonstrations of different mechanisms are taking place under federal grants.

CONCLUSION

With proper safeguards, e-health technologies can create significant opportunities to find health information; do more self-help and self-care; create and maintain personal health records; consult with remote healthcare providers; transact healthcare-related business; and purchase health-related goods and services electronically (e-health commerce).

Although there is still great optimism about e-health's benefits, lingering ethical issues regarding the use of e-health technologies have been raised. These issues include the potential harm from the use of digital media to disseminate inaccurate and biased information to large numbers of individuals; to obtain unauthorized access to personal health information; to engage in fraudulent and illegal sales of health services and products; to provide inappropriate or low-quality services; and to interfere with established doctor–patient relationships. In addition, many e-health services do not have integrated evaluation mechanisms for outcome or performance measures. These concerns indicate that public discussion among relevant stakeholders is urgently needed to find appropriate measures and policies to improve information quality; define rules of access to and security for personal health information; continue to monitor and halt illegal online sales; alert individuals to the guidelines for high-quality, appropriate care; and improve the provider–patient relationship.

Of specific concern to the HIM profession is the changing nature of health information. This change is manifest in definitions of what constitutes health information, in concepts of ownership and control of personal health information, and in new challenges with respect to ensuring the quality of health information being created by disparate individuals and enterprises. Health information is no longer just the encounter data that reside in institutional medical records, but an array of information on, for example, prevention, wellness, previous health experiences, alternative and complementary medicine, and over-the-counter remedies, in addition to the clinical data that are created by doctors' visits, hospitalizations, and lab tests. All these different bits of personal health information may be contained in multiple locations with

appropriate security features that will allow permission-based information sharing. Second, concerns about violations of privacy rights and the confidentiality of health information will continue to influence policy debates about who owns or controls health information and who should have access to which information. Even if individuals are the presumed owners of their information, the reality is that current information-handling practices give individuals few concrete ways to control the movement of their information among multiple parties.

Addressing these concerns will require open discussion and the development of international standards. HIM professionals will need to actively participate in these discussions and in standards development. Additionally, they will need to stay abreast of applicable guidelines and regulations and develop a framework that they can use to work through the ethical dilemmas they may face along the way.

Key Terms

- **E-health**
- **Health literacy**
- **Personal health records (PHRs)**

The opinions expressed in this chapter are solely those of the authors, and the authors assume sole responsibility for any errors or misrepresentations. Statements in the chapter do not necessarily represent the official position of the U.S. Department of Health and Human Services or any other federal department or agency.

Chapter Summary

- Expanding e-health technologies are creating new opportunities to provide health services to populations that previously have not had access to health care. These technologies also enable people to locate personalized health information; do more self-help and self-care; create and maintain personal health records; consult with remote healthcare providers; transact healthcare-related business; and purchase health-related goods and services electronically. However, e-health technologies also raise serious ethical issues, including the potential harm from their use to disseminate inaccurate and biased information; to obtain unauthorized access to personal health information; to engage in fraudulent and illegal sales of health services and products; to provide inappropriate or low-quality services; and to interfere with established doctor–patient relationships.

- As more and more healthcare organizations develop e-health capacities, HIM professionals will be increasingly involved in issues concerning consumer, patient, and caregiver access to health information, the quality of the information provided, and the confidentiality of users' health information. Further, some HIM professionals now work for Internet companies or HIM firms rather than for traditional healthcare institutions, which may result in new responsibilities and obligations.

- At present, guidelines and standards to ensure information quality, data integrity, and the interoperability of e-health applications are inadequate. This is an important area in which HIM professionals can promote discussion and be advocates for consumer, patient, and caregiver rights.

References

American Health Information Management Association [AHIMA]. (2000). *AHIMA's recommendations to ensure privacy and quality of personal health information on the Internet*. Retrieved November 5, 2004, from http://www.ahima.org/xpedio/groups/public/documents/ahima/bok1_016155.pdf.

American Health Information Management Association [AHIMA]. (2003). *Email as a provider–patient electronic communication medium and its impact on the electronic health record* (AHIMA Practice Brief). Retrieved November 5, 2004, from http://library.ahima.org/xpedio/groups/public/documents/ahima/pub_bok1_022164.html.

American Health Information Management Association [AHIMA]. (2004). *Maintaining a personal health record*. Retrieved October 15, 2004, from http://www.myphr.com/maintaining/index.asp.

American Health Information Management Association [AHIMA] e-HIM Task Force. (2003). *A vision of the e-HIM future*. Retrieved November 5, 2004, from http://www.ahima.org/infocenter/ehim/.

Baur, C., & Deering, M. J. (2001). E-health. In L. B. Harman (Ed.), *Ethical challenges in the management of health information,* pp. 255–270. Gaithersburg, MD: Aspen.

Deering, M. J., & Baur, C. (2004). They can't do it alone: Information tools for consumers and patients in healthcare reform. Unpublished paper.

Eng, T. R. (2001). *The eHealth landscape: A terrain map of emerging information and communication technologies in health and health care*. Princeton, NJ: The Robert Wood Johnson Foundation.

Eng, T. R. (2004). Population health technologies: Emerging innovations for the health of the public. *American Journal of Preventive Medicine* 26(3), 237–242.

Eng, T. R., & Gustafson, D. (Eds.). (1999). *Wired for health and well-being: The emergence of interactive health communication*. Washington, DC: U.S. Government Printing Office.

Gellman, R. (2004, June 23). When HIPAA meets NHII: A new dimension for privacy. Presentation to U.S. Department of Health and Human Services Data Council Privacy Committee, Washington, DC.

Goldman, J., Hudson, Z., & Smith, R. M. (2000). *Privacy: Report on the privacy policies and practices of health Web sites*. Retrieved November 5, 2004, from http://www.chcf.org/documents/ihealth/privacyexecsummary.pdf.

Harris, L. (Ed.). (1995). *Health and the new media*. Mahwah, NJ: Lawrence Erlbaum.

Institute for the Future. (2003). *Engaged consumers in health and healthcare*. Retrieved November 5, 2004, from http://www.iftf.org/features/library.html.

Lebo, H. (2004). *The digital future report: Surveying the digital future year four*. Retrieved November 5, 2004, from http://www.digitalcenter.org/pages/current_report.asp?intGlobalId = 19.

Lumpkin, J. R. (2000). *Letter to the Assistant Secretary for Planning and Evaluation, U.S. Department of Health and Human Services, with recommendations on the notice of proposed rule-making for standards for privacy of individually identifiable health information.* Retrieved November 5, 2004, from http://www.ncvhs.hhs.gov/000202lt.htm.

Markle Foundation, Connecting for Health. (2004). Connecting Americans to their health care. Retrieved November 5, 2004, from http://connectingforhealth.org/resources/wg_eis_final_report_0704.pdf.

Sobel, D. S. (1987). Self-care in health: Information to empower people. In A. H. Levy & B. Williams (Eds.), *Proceedings of the American Association for Medical Systems and Informatics, 87,* 12–15. San Francisco: Congress.

Thompson, T. G., & Brailer, D. (2004). The decade of health information technology: Delivering consumer-centric and information-rich health care. Washington, DC: U.S. Department of Health and Human Services. Retrieved September 2, 2005, from http:// www.hhs.gov/healthit/documents/hitframework. pdf.

U.S. Department of Commerce, National Telecommunications and Information Administration. (2002). *A nation online: How Americans are expanding their use of the Internet.* Retrieved November 5, 2004, from http://www.ntia.doc.gov/ntiahome/dn/index.html.

U.S. Department of Health and Human Services. (2000). *Healthy people 2010.* Washington, DC: U.S. Government Printing Office.

U.S. Department of Health and Human Services. (2001). Information for health: A strategy for building the National Health Information Infrastructure. Report and recommendations from the National Committee on Vital and Health Statistics. Retrieved November 5, 2004, from http://ncvhs.hhs.gov/reptrecs.htm.

U.S. Department of Health and Human Services. (2004). *HHS fact sheet—HIT report at a glance.* Retrieved November 5, 2004, from http://www.hhs.gov/news/press/2004pres/20040721.html.

U.S. Department of Health and Human Services. (2005). *Office for civil rights: Medical privacy—national standards to protect the privacy of personal health information.* Retrieved September 12, 2005, from http://www.hhs.gov/ocr/hipaa/.

U.S. General Accounting Office. (1996). *Consumer health informatics: Emerging issues.* (GAO Publication No. GAO/AIMD-96-86). Washington, DC: U.S. Government Printing Office.

Appendix 16-A: Examples of Guidelines, Policies, and Codes of Conduct or Ethics for Health Websites

1. The Health on the Net (HON) Code of Conduct appeared in July 1996 (http://www.hon.ch/HONcode/Conduct.html). It is currently in use on several thousand health websites.
2. Guidelines for medical and health information sites on the Internet, created by the American Medical Association (AMA), appeared in March 2000 and are being applied to AMA websites (http://www.ama-assn.org/ama/pub/category/1905.html).
3. Ethical principles for offering Internet health services to consumers, created by Health Internet Ethics (Hi-Ethics), appeared in May 2000 (http://www.hiethics.org/Principles/index.asp). The Hi-Ethics Principles were formulated by 20 for-profit and nonprofit health websites.
4. The International e-Health Code of Ethics, created by the e-Health Ethics Initiative, appeared in May 2000 (http://www.ihealthcoalition.org/ethics/ethics.html). This code was formulated by a cross section of health and healthcare stakeholders.
5. AHIMA's Recommendations to Ensure Privacy and Quality of Personal Health Information on the Internet appeared in September 2000 (http://www.ahima.org/xpedio/groups/public/documents/ahima/bok1_016155.pdf).

The ethical decision-making matrix is a tool to help you organize complex, ethical problems; however, there is no simple fill-in-the-box approach to ethical decision making. The objective is to follow each step of the process and not move from the question directly to what should be done or how to prevent it next time. If you skip steps, you will not fully understand all of the values and options for action. Also, the matrix provided for each scenario in this book is not the only way to examine the problem. You can make an equally compelling ethical argument for a different decision—just be sure to follow all the steps of the matrix.

SCENARIO 16-A: EQUITY AND PRIVACY

Steps	Information	
1. What is the ethical question?	How could the differences in Internet access create ethical problems?	
2. What are the facts?	**KNOWN**	**TO BE GATHERED**
	<ul><li>Internet access can facilitate the dissemination of healthcare information.</li><li>Some families have Internet access.</li><li>Some families do not have Internet access.</li></ul>	<ul><li>Will patients who have Internet access receive better care/more attention than those who do not?</li><li>Is it unethical to provide a service that all patients cannot take part in?</li><li>How does her boss or supervisor expect her to resolve the conflict?</li><li>What are the customary practices in such cases?</li><li>What is the likely impact on self and family on changing jobs?</li></ul>
3. What are the values? Examine the shared and competing values, obligations, and interests of the stakeholders (i.e., patient, HIM professional, healthcare practitioner(s), administrators, society, and other advocates) involved in order to fully understand the complexity of the ethical problem(s).	**Patient:** Values the best care available. **HIM professional:** Integrity, accuracy (create systems to provide the best care possible); avoid harm (security violations could harm patients). **Healthcare professionals:** Promote welfare of patients by providing best possible care without jeopardizing security; fairness in providing equal care for all. **Society:** Values increased patient care capacity.	

4. What are my options?	• Do not offer Internet service because not all patients have Internet access. • Offer Internet service.	
5. What should I do?	Offer Internet service.	
6. What justifies my choice?	**JUSTIFIED**	**NOT JUSTIFIED**
	• Obligation to offer the best possible care while taking steps to preserve security. • Preserve professional integrity.	• Do not offer Internet service. • Limit the care available for all because some don't have access. • Not fair to those who have Internet access. • Jeopardize professional integrity.
7. How can I prevent this ethical problem?	• Determine if system changes are needed. • Discuss standards and the values that support them with colleagues. • Learn more about e-health systems in clinical settings.	

The ethical decision-making matrix is a tool to help you organize complex, ethical problems; however, there is no simple fill-in-the-box approach to ethical decision making. The objective is to follow each step of the process and not move from the question directly to what should be done or how to prevent it next time. If you skip steps, you will not fully understand all of the values and options for action. Also, the matrix provided for each scenario in this book is not the only way to examine the problem. You can make an equally compelling ethical argument for a different decision—just be sure to follow all the steps of the matrix.

SCENARIO16-B: ENSURING ONLINE QUALITY AND PRIVACY PROTECTIONS

Steps	Information	
1. What is the ethical question?	What are some ethical issues surrounding online health information?	
2. What are the facts?	**KNOWN**	**TO BE GATHERED**
	• Information on the Web is not considered secure unless protected by security programs. • Sites are not required to protect health information stored online.	• Could patients use health information obtained online to self-diagnose? • Could patients' confidentiality be violated when storing records online? • Are there any guarantees of the accuracy of the information posted on the Web? • What are the customary guidelines in such cases?
3. What are the values? Examine the shared and competing values, obligations, and interests of the stakeholders (i.e., patient, HIM professional, healthcare practitioner(s), administrators, society, and other advocates) involved in order to fully understand the complexity of the ethical problem(s).	**Patients/site users:** Value accurate information; value security of health information posted on Web. **HIM professional:** Integrity, accuracy, reliability (protect quality, accuracy, and security of information posted on the Web); provide information on who runs the site; avoid harm (warn users about the dangers of self-diagnosis); personal values (promote welfare of self and family by avoiding loss of job). **Site administrators:** Benefit patients/users; ensure security and accuracy of data posted on site. **Society:** Values security and accuracy of information posted on the Web.	

4. What are my options?	• Post information on site without regard for accuracy of the content and the security of the information posted. • Follow the guidelines of the U.S. national health objective when posting information online.	
5. What should I do?	Follow the guidelines of recognized authorities for security and ethical tenets for e-health systems.	
6. What justifies my choice?	**JUSTIFIED**	**NOT JUSTIFIED**
	• Obligation to ensure the accuracy and security of data on the site. • Preserve professional integrity. • Protect patients/users by warning about the dangers of self-diagnosis.	• Post information without regard for security and accuracy. • Jeopardize patient health by providing potentially inaccurate information. • Jeopardize patient record security. • Possible conflict of interest by not disclosing who created and operates the site.
7. How can I prevent this ethical problem?	• Determine if system changes are needed. • Learn more about ethical issues surrounding online health information. • Discuss standards and the values that support them with colleagues. • Evaluate institutional integrity at job interview and subsequently thereafter as ethical problems arise.	

E-HIM: Information Technology and Information Exchange

Meryl Bloomrosen, MBA, RHIA

Learning Objectives

After completing this chapter the reader should be able to:

- Identify recent and on-going public and private sector initiatives in health information technology (HIT) and health information exchange (HIE).
- Illustrate and understand the role of ethics in designing, developing, and implementing electronic health information management (HIM) policies and processes that involve multiple stakeholders across many organizations.
- Identify potential ethical issues facing healthcare and information management professionals resulting from the migration to and implementation of health information technologies and systems.

Abstract

Healthcare information technology (HIT) has been identified as essential for making the healthcare system safer and more efficient. Such HIT systems include electronic medical records, electronic prescribing, bedside bar coding, computerized physician order entry (CPOE), and clinical decision support systems (CDSSs). These systems are widely viewed as being central to reducing errors and improving quality. Interest is growing in electronic medical records, computerized order entry, and other technology-enabled components of an electronic health record (EHR). Healthcare and health information management (HIM) professionals are critical to the ongoing success of these efforts. More widespread adoption of HIT and health information exchange (HIE) will help ensure the delivery of health care based on timely, relevant, accurate, and complete information. HIM professionals need to examine closely the potential ethical implications that will arise from the continued implementation of HIT and HIE.

INTRODUCTION

It has long been recognized that providers need data in order to treat their patients and to choose among treatment modalities; payers require data to verify eligibility for treatment and to determine the medical necessity for care; researchers need data to determine the outcomes of projects; and regulators and policy makers require data to make decisions that will ensure the public's health and the well-being of patients and consumers. The ability to capture, manage, and take advantage of computerized data and information also is essential to continuously improve health services research and public policy.

Healthcare decisions rely on ready access to clear, concise, and up-to-date information—information that is increasingly complex and highly dynamic. In addition, the healthcare industry faces increasing levels of competition, continued legislative and regulatory burdens, and competing demands for better quality, lower costs, and increased access to services. Anticipated industry changes in the next few years include revisions and updates to reimbursement and payment systems; ongoing and more widespread implementation of pay-for-performance methods (there are various approaches to encourage improved quality of care in all healthcare settings where patients receive their healthcare services, including physicians' offices and ambulatory care facilities, hospitals, nursing homes, home healthcare agencies, and dialysis facilities); provision of pharmaceutical benefits for Medicare beneficiaries; deployment of messaging and content standards; implementation and evaluation of increasingly diverse health information technologies, including the deployment of clinical decision support systems (CDSSs) and the increasing use of technology in all aspects of healthcare delivery.

The movement toward the electronic health record (EHR) and electronic health record management (EHRM) is expanding the roles and responsibilities of health information management (HIM) practitioners (AHIMA e-HIM Task Force 2003, 2004). The purpose of this chapter is to identify some of the ethical challenges and considerations facing practitioners in an increasingly paperless healthcare environment.

Managing EHRs

According to AHIMA, **electronic health information management (eHIM™)** is "the process by which electronic (e.g., digital) health records are created or received and preserved for evidentiary (e.g., legal or business) purposes" (AHIMA e-HIM Task Force, 2003, 2004). AHIMA further states that eHIM requires decision making and planning throughout the entire life cycle of the EHR—from planning, processing, distributing, maintaining, storing, and retrieving the health record until it reaches its ultimate disposition, such as archiving or destruction. Decision making includes, but is not limited to, what EHRs to keep and for how long, the assignment of authorities and responsibilities, the design and administration of the process, and the audit and review of the processes.

Roles and Responsibilities of HIM Professionals

As the traditional custodian of the paper medical record and medical record systems, HIM professionals are trained to ensure the quality, privacy, and integrity of the EHR. Today, the EHR can, and often does, reside in several different information systems. Increasingly, HIM professionals must ensure that information management standards are consistently applied across these various systems in order to maintain the level of integrity necessary for the healthcare organization's records. The transition from a paper-based health record to an EHR environment will need to be addressed and managed on many different levels: administratively, financially, culturally, organizationally, and ethically (AHIMA e-HIM Work Group on Health Information in a Hybrid Environment, 2003; Amatayakul, Brandt, Callahan Dennis, Didear-Folck, Frawley,

Grant, et al., 2001; Burrington-Brown & Hughes, 2003; Hughes, 2003).

The transition from a paper-based medical record to an EHR certainly presents some new challenges for HIM professionals to apply their knowledge, skills, and experience in the ethical management of electronic health information. One of AHIMA's areas of strategic focus is electronic health information management (e-HIM). AHIMA has the following goals with regard to electronic health information management (AHIMA, 2004):

- Promote the migration from paper to an electronic health information infrastructure
- Reinvent how institutional and personal health information and records are managed
- Deliver measurable cost and quality results from improved information management

AHIMA's (2003) report, "A Vision of the e-HIM™ Future," states that in the future, health information management will be electronic, patient centered, comprehensive, longitudinal, accessible, and credible. AHIMA has commissioned a number of volunteer work groups to develop practice standards for areas that play an integral role in the transition from paper to EHRs (AHIMA E-HIM Task Force, 2003).

Public and Private Sector Activities

Numerous stakeholders, including patients, caregivers, providers, clinicians, employers, purchasers, and policymakers, believe that health information technology (HIT) will help improve the quality of care and ensure patient safety. HIT has been identified as essential in transforming the healthcare system and in making it safer, more efficient, and more cost-effective.

Public Sector

For many years, the federal government has supported research into medical informatics and the use of computers in clinical practice (Agency for Healthcare Research and Qual-

ity, 1999a, 1999b, 2001, 2002, 2003a, 2003b). Public sector involvement in HIT has been long-standing. A considerable amount of momentum has been building around the need for investment to catalyze the creation of an interconnected, electronic health information infrastructure and the information technology (IT) that will support it—to realize the quality, safety, and efficiency gains that can only be achieved through the use of IT. The federal government has played a leadership role in fostering the development of data standards and encouraging investments to identify and speed the adoption of new technologies throughout the healthcare system.

Efforts to date include the formation of the Consolidated Health Informatics Initiative (CHI) and support for the National Health Information Infrastructure (NHII), an idea noted in an Institute of Medicine (IOM) report on computer-based patient records in 1991 and then elaborated upon in a National Committee on Vital and Health Statistics report (2001) "Information for Health: A Strategy for Building the National Health Information Infrastructure." The concept has since been endorsed by a variety of public and private sector organizations. The broad goal is to deliver reliable data in a secure and private format to patients, clinicians, and providers when and where they need it so that they can use this information to make informed decisions about health and health care.

The government's commitment to addressing healthcare quality and the IT that underlies it is significant. A number of federal efforts, including those listed below, have focused on the development of an interconnected, electronic health information infrastructure (U.S. Department of Health and Human Services, 2005):

- The National Committee on Vital and Health Statistics (NCVHS) Work Group on the NHII and Subcommittees on Standards and Security and Privacy and Security are charged to monitor and make recommendations to the full committee on health data standards and security, primarily related to implementation of the Administrative Simplification provisions of P.L. 104-191 and other related legislation.

The government funds various programmatic activities and grant programs administered by the U.S. Department of Health and Human Services (DHHS) operating divisions, such as the Agency for Healthcare Research and Quality (AHRQ) and the Centers for Medicare and Medicaid Services (CMS). These initiatives range from support for standards development to demonstrations of interoperable health information systems.

- The Consolidated Health Informatics Initiative (CHI) is a government-wide initiative charged with establishing a portfolio of existing clinical vocabularies and messaging standards that will enable federal agencies to build interoperable federal health data systems.
- The Health Resources and Services Administration (HRSA) established the Office for the Advancement of Telehealth (OAT) to serve as a leader in telehealth, a focal point for HRSA's telehealth activities and a catalyst for the wider adoption of advanced technologies in the provision of healthcare services and education. **Telehealth** is the use of electronic information and telecommunications technologies to support long-distance clinical health care, patient and professional health-related education, and public health and health administration.
- The IOM and its Committee on Enhancing Federal Healthcare Quality Programs have released a number of reports relevant to HIT (IOM, 2002a, 2002b, 2002c, 2003a, 2003b, 2003c).
- The President's Information Technology Advisory Committee (PITAC) is a federal advisory committee that provides the president, Congress, and federal agencies involved in information technology

research and development (IT R&D) with expert, independent advice on maintaining America's preeminence in advanced information technologies.

- In 2004, the **Office of the National Coordinator for Health Information Technology (ONCHIT)** within the DHHS was established. ONCHIT provides leadership for the development and nationwide implementation of an interoperable health information technology infrastructure to improve the quality and efficiency of health care and the ability of consumers to manage their care and safety.

In July 2003, DHHS asked the IOM and Health Level-7 (HL-7)[1] to design a functional model and standard for the EHR, and their efforts are continuing.[2] In July 2003, DHHS

---

1. HL-7 is an accredited ANSI standard organization that produces the HL-7 messaging standard. It is the accepted messaging standard for communicating clinical data. It is supported by every major medical informatics system vendor in the United States. The goal of HL-7 is to provide a comprehensive framework and related standards for the exchange, integration, sharing, and retrieval of electronic health information that supports clinical practice and the management, delivery, and evaluation of health services.

2. CHI is a collaborative effort between the Department of Health and Human Services, the Veterans Affairs/Veterans Health Administration, the Department of Defense, and other federal agencies to adopt government-wide health information standards. The first set of CHI standards were announced on March 21, 2003, and include Health Level-7 (HL-7) messaging standards; Logical Observation Identifier Name Codes (LOINC) to standardize the electronic exchange of clinical laboratory results; National Council on Prescription Drug Programs (NCPDP) standards for retail pharmacy transactions; Institute of Electrical and Electronics Engineers 1073 (IEEE 1073) standards that allow for healthcare providers to plug medical devices into information and computer systems; Digital Imaging and Communications in Medicine (DICOM) standards that enable the retrieval and transfer of images and associated diagnostic information.

also announced that the agency had signed an agreement with the College of American Pathologists (CAP) to license the College's standardized medical vocabulary system and make it available without charge throughout the United States.

A number of additional initiatives have gained considerable momentum to improve the quality, safety, and efficiency of the nation's healthcare system. In September 2004, the Agency for Health Research and Quality (AHRQ) awarded more than 100 planning, implementation, and demonstration grants to further implementation of the electronic health record throughout the United States. The grant program included $14 million in new implementation grants for small community and rural hospital settings; $7 million in planning grants to help communities and organizations develop their health IT infrastructure; and $10 million in grants to demonstrate the clinical, organizational, and/or financial value of health IT.

On July 21, 2004, during the Secretarial Summit on Health Information Technology (HIT), the Office of the National Health Information Technology Coordinator unveiled the nation's first strategic framework to develop EHRs and other forms of HIT and to advance the adoption of HIT. The framework report, entitled "The Decade of Health Information Technology: Delivering Consumer-Centric and Information-Rich Health Care," highlights four major collaborative goals that the public and private sectors can work toward together and provides strategies for achieving these goals. The framework for strategic action also describes the concept of the **regional health information organization (RHIO)** (Thompson & Brailer, 2004), which is critical to achieving nationwide linking of disparate healthcare information systems to allow patients, physicians, hospitals, public health agencies, and other authorized users across the nation to share clinical information in real time under stringent security, privacy, and other protections. All of this is in an effort to achieve President George W. Bush's goal of widespread adoption of interoperable electronic health records (EHR) within 10 years.

The Medicare Prescription Drug, Improvement, and Modernization Act of 2003 enacted into law contained a Commission on Systemic Interoperability, which will develop a comprehensive strategy, time lines, and priorities for the adoption and implementation of HIT standards. The commission is to submit a report to the DHHS Secretary and Congress describing the strategy and analyzing its effects no later than October 31, 2005. In October 2003, the General Accounting Office (GAO, 2003) released a report called "Information Technology. Benefits Realized for Selected Health Care Functions." The GAO identified cost savings and other benefits realized by several healthcare organizations that have implemented IT, both in providing clinical health care and in the administrative functions associated with healthcare delivery.

Other initiatives seek to provide consumers access to customized health information. This is reflected in CMS's plans for a Medicare Beneficiary Portal, which will provide secure health information via the Internet. This portal will be hosted by a private company under contract with CMS. Authorized Medicare beneficiaries will have access to their medical information online or by calling 1-800-MEDICARE. Initially, the portal will provide access to fee-for-service claims information, which includes claim types, dates of service, and procedures. CMS plans to expand the portal to include prevention information in the form of reminders to beneficiaries to schedule their Medicare-covered preventive healthcare services. Through the **Doctor's Office Quality—Information Technology (DOQ-IT)** project, CMS is encouraging the adoption and effective use of IT by physicians' offices to improve quality and safety for Medicare beneficiaries, as well as all Americans. DOQ-IT seeks to accomplish this by promoting greater availability of high-quality affordable HIT by providing assistance to physician offices in adopting and using such technology (DOQ-IT, DHHS, Centers for

Medicare and Medicaid Services). DOQ-IT is a national initiative that promotes the adoption of electronic health records (EHRs) and information technology (IT) in small to medium-sized physician offices. The program aims to help physicians increase access to patient information, decision support, and reference data, as well as to improve patient–clinician communications.

Through the VistA-Office EHR project, CMS is working with Veterans Health Affairs (VHA) to transfer HIT to the private sector. CMS is funding and collaborating with VHA and other key federal agencies on the development of a VistA-Office EHR version of the VHA's hospital VistA system for use in clinics and physician offices. An overriding goal of VistA-Office EHR is to stimulate the broader adoption and effective use of EHRs by making a robust, flexible EHR product available in the public domain (Centers for Medicare and Medicaid Services, 2005).

Private Sector

Numerous private sector organizations and stakeholders, including practicing clinicians, payers, purchasers, researchers, healthcare providers, IT suppliers, IT managers, accrediting groups, public health organizations, professional and trade associations, manufacturers, and public sector partners, are involved in initiatives to advance the adoption of information standards for healthcare.

Certification of HIT Products EHRs, and even specific components such as decision support software, are unique among clinical tools in that they do not need to meet minimal standards to be used to deliver care. To increase uptake of EHRs and to reduce the risk of product implementation failure, the federal government is exploring ways to work with the private sector to develop minimal product standards for EHR functionality, interoperability, and security. A private sector ambulatory EHR certification task force (the Certification Commission for Healthcare Information Technology [CCHIT]) is determin-

ing the feasibility of certification of EHR products based on functionality, security, and interoperability. AHIMA, the Healthcare Information and Management Systems Society (HIMSS), and the National Alliance for Health Information Technology (Alliance) formed the Certification Commission for Healthcare Information Technology in July 2004.

Community-Based Health Information Exchange The eHealth Initiative (eHI) and its foundation (the Foundation for eHealth Initiative) are independent, nonprofit organizations that share the same mission: to drive improvement in the quality, safety, and efficiency of healthcare through information and IT. The foundation has funded several strategic demonstration projects to evaluate and demonstrate the impact of IT on health care and to further the development of strategies and tools for accelerating the adoption of IT and electronic connectivity.

Continuity of Care Record The Continuity of Care Record (CCR) is being developed by the American Academy of Family Practitioners (AAFP), the Massachusetts Medical Society (MMS), the American Medical Association (AMA), the American Academy of Pediatrics (AAP), the Healthcare Information and Management Systems Society (HIMSS), and the American Health Care Association (AHCA) in conjunction with the standards-development organization ASTM International. The Continuity of Care Record (CCR) was developed in response to the need to organize and make transportable a set of basic information about a patient's health care that is accessible to clinicians and patients. It is intended to foster and improve continuity of care, reduce medical errors, and ensure a minimum standard of secure health information transportability.

Physicians' Electronic Health Record Coalition In July 2004, 14 medical organizations announced the creation of the Physicians' Electronic Health Record Coalition (PEHRC). This coalition will assist physicians, particularly those in small and medium-sized ambulatory care medical practice, to acquire and use affordable, standards-based EHRs and other HIT to improve quality, enhance patient safety, and increase efficiency (AAFP, 2004).

Connecting for Health Connecting for Health (CFH) is a public–private collaborative that was formed to address barriers to the development of an interconnected health information infrastructure. The first phase of the collaborative's work resulted in the adoption of an initial set of data standards, the development of case studies on privacy and security, and consensus on the definition of electronic personal health record (PHR). Connecting for Health also has developed an incremental road map, the goal of which is to lay out the near-term actions necessary to achieve electronic connectivity.

Health Information Exchange

Efforts to implement HIT vary in their strategy and operational status. Although the evidence supporting the benefits of HIT applications is substantial and growing, additional evidence points to the benefits of **health information exchange (HIE).** HIE is a concept that has evolved over time. It encompasses diverse definitions, approaches, and methods, but generally involves the ability to mobilize clinical information and permit authorized access across multiple providers and locations. The ability to exchange information within and across systems seamlessly within a community is still seen as desirable and is in fact viewed as essential to quality healthcare delivery in the long term. HIE enables improvements in quality, safety, and efficiency.

A growing number of communities and regions have coalesced to implement HIE to address joint challenges and to gain the economies of scale, simplicity of technology deployment, and longitudinal presentation of the patient experience that come from operating an interoperable HIE system. Establishing HIE entities certainly presents a host of technical, regulatory, financial, and practical challenges.

Attempts to communicate patient information across multiple entities are not new. Prior efforts that have come and gone were known by various names, such as regional data networks, community health management information systems (CHMIS), integrated delivery networks (IDNs), and community health information networks (CHINs). Today, the reasons for forming or participating in community-based HIE vary and include the sharing of real-time patient data in a community-wide effort to avoid expensive duplication of services. During the development of such systems, issues of program focus and technology selection will arise, followed by concerns about information privacy and the HIE's role in quality of care. As communities move to develop and implement these new HIE models and national health experts champion regional health information exchanges, more needs to be learned as to how these efforts will evolve and what existing and perceived legal and ethical barriers exist.

Ethical Challenges

Without a doubt, implementing a HIT presents several tactical, technical, and operational challenges, and numerous decisions will affect how a HIE entity or collaborative will function. Decisions must be made as to what data should be included, what technical infrastructure should be used, who will own the data, what organization or group of organizations should lead the exchange development effort, what types of information will be shared, and how patient confidentiality will be ensured. In addition, complex legal, organizational, funding, and control issues will arise. Concerns about information privacy and security, legal and liability issues related to quality of care, ownership and governance, and community readiness also need to be addressed. Other issues include difficulties in technology selection, definitional and operational challenges, and the need for clearly defined organizational goals or program focus.

Given this level of complexity and the dynamic nature of the healthcare industry, a number of potential ethical challenges and decision points will arise. To a large extent, the ethical challenges facing healthcare and HIM professionals in the paperless setting are similar to those in the more traditional paper-based setting. Ethical challenges include the following:

- Achieving billing and coding compliance
- Adhering to medical privacy and research requirements
- Ensuring data validity
- Ensuring patient confidentiality
- Ensuring patient safety
- Avoiding conflicts of interest
- Developing and maintaining information and systems security
- Exchanging information within and across jurisdictions
- Executing technical and clinical service contracts
- Handling release of information
- Implementing and managing telehealth applications
- Maintaining and documenting compliance with HIPAA and state privacy rules
- Maintaining the legal electronic medical record
- Making amendments to records and health information
- Obtaining consent for the use or disclosure of individually identifiable health information
- Outsourcing information systems, transcription, and release of information
- Protecting against fraud and abuse
- Providing patient access

Additional personal and professional ethical challenges as the industry migrates to and achieves electronic health information management will likely emerge. These challenges will likely involve the following types of issues:

- Adhering to updated federal self-referral and anti-kickback protections related to

providing information technology and tools to physicians. Efforts are under way to explore safe harbors or exceptions to these laws, which could accelerate EHR adoption.

- Ensuring that high-quality data are used to make accurate payments for use of the EHR. Programs are under way that will reward providers and physicians for investing in information systems and care management tools.
- Coding and billing processes are evolving as payers evaluate reimbursing for services delivered electronically, such as online or video consultation, through the use of new codes or modifiers.
- Ensuring that high-quality data are used to make accurate payments under various "pay-for-performance," "pay for use," and "pay-for-quality" programs that recognize and reward quality care.[3]

---

3. Various public and private programs link provider incentives or bonuses to performance and/or quality measures. The new Medicare Prescription Drug Improvement and Modernization Act of 2003 (MMA) established two new programs—the Voluntary Chronic Care Improvement Program and the Care Management Performance pilot program—to further explore the potential of disease management techniques. The Voluntary Chronic Care Improvement Program will provide guidance to beneficiaries with chronic diseases who could be responsive to disease management interventions. The goal will be to improve beneficiary self-care and to provide physicians and other providers with the technological support to manage clinical information about the patient.

The Care Management Performance Demonstration will establish a pay-for-performance 3-year pilot with physicians to promote the adoption and use of health information technology to improve quality and reduce avoidable hospitalizations for chronically ill patients. Doctors who meet or exceed performance standards (set by CMS) will receive a bonus payment for managing the care of eligible Medicare beneficiaries. The pilot must show that it does not cost Medicare more than the program would have spent on the beneficiary otherwise.

- Mandating appropriate certification of HIT products. The federal government is exploring ways to work with the private sector to develop minimal product standards for EHR functionality, interoperability, and security.[4]
- Ensuring protection of PHI as communication between patient and practitioner via e-mail and telecommunications becomes more widespread. Providers, clinicians, practitioners, and HIM professionals need to be aware of the clinical, financial, legal, and ethical implications of communications conducted in these new ways.
- Electronic health information management raises potential medico-legal concerns, including establishment of the physician–patient relationship, malpractice liability, consumer-directed health care, offshore outsourcing of services, and regulatory compliance.
- Automated clinical applications, such as evidence-based medicine (EBM), electronic prescribing, and clinical decision support, clinician reminders, and case management will play an increasingly important role as tools for delivering health care (Gupta, 2003; Hudson, Oglesby, Mongan, & Kraus, 1992; Lydon-Rochelle & Holt, 2004; Slowther, Ford, & Schofield, 2004; Stoelwinder, 2001; Weber, 1997; Weiss, 2004; Whitehead & Novak, 2003).

The following scenario is offered as a potential future issue, rather than a formal scenario. Therefore, it does not have a decision-making matrix. It is offered as a framework for discussion.

---

4. AHIMA, the Healthcare Information and Management Systems Society (HIMSS), and the National Alliance for Health Information Technology (Alliance) formed the Certification Commission for Healthcare Information Technology in July 2004.

Scenario 17-A: The HIM Professional's Role in eHIM

You are an HIM professional who has been hired as a project manager by a newly organized regional consortium formed to implement data exchange within the community. The goals of the consortium are to improve health outcomes, deliver healthcare services more cost-effectively, implement provider access to patient records and decision support at the point of care, enable sharing of information among health professionals, ensure safeguards to guard patient confidentiality, and limit access only to authorized users. Integration of evidence-based decision support will enhance patient safety and care outcomes by reducing errors, fraud, and duplication of treatment.

Three of the hospital systems are in varying stages of deploying different EHR products. The fourth hospital system continues to maintain a legacy HIT system. A legacy system is typically an old and large system that remains in operation within an organization. Often, these systems are poorly documented or structured (Tilley, 1999; Warren, 2000).

The consortium will solicit provider input to ensure usability and functionality. Financial incentives will be offered for participation in the system and improved patient outcomes. Because one of the overall goals is to ensure the long-term viability of the system, an appropriate organizational and governance structure needs to be established. The consortium is exploring financial incentives for providers who demonstrate improved health outcomes using HIT.

The consortium is composed of the following:

Doctors: 2,500
Pharmacies: 35 (4 large chains)
Laboratories: 2 national plus 5 hospital-based ambulatory labs
Hospitals: 20 (grouped into 4 systems, including 2 rural hospitals)
Managed care plans: 2 different plans

Questions

1. How do you proceed?

2. What are the challenges (strategic, tactical, operational, legal, technical, financial, cultural, and ethical) regarding systems implementation?

3. What strategies do you use to implement HIT systems?

4. How will patient safety be ensured?

5. How will organizational productivity be improved?

6. How will efficiency be improved?

7. What about clinical decision support systems?

8. How will adverse events be reported?

9. What are the possible ethical challenges in managing health information in this context?

10. What steps do you take to ensure personal, professional, and organizational integrity?

11. How do you go about analyzing the situation and proposing the most ethical courses of action?

CONCLUSION

The increasing prevalence of HIT and HIE raises new questions for the healthcare industry regarding electronic health information management. It is becoming increasingly apparent that HIT and HIE can provide savings, contribute to greater patient safety, enhance patient care, allow for increased delivery systems efficiencies, and achieve clinical and business process improvements (GAO, 2003). In particular, applications such as electronic medical records, order entry, clinical decision support, electronic prescribing, clinical reminders, patient portals, and bedside bar coding have been identified and promoted as vital to facilitate a safer and more efficient healthcare system. It is anticipated that patients will benefit from the comprehensive adoption of HIT and HIE and the ability to share data within and across sites of care and among clinicians. Ultimately, other stakeholders, such as employers, payers, and regulators, will benefit from the ability to share and exchange data.

Ultimately, more widespread adoption of HIT and HIE will likely diminish duplicative information gathering and will help ensure delivery of health care based on timely, relevant, accurate, and complete information. HIM professionals need to examine closely the potential ethical challenges that will arise from the continued movement toward HIT and HIE across organizations, communities, and stakeholders.

The 1980s presented numerous challenges to HIM professionals with regards to coding and documentation and prospective payment and reimbursement. New methods for financing and managing healthcare organizations raised concerns regarding how these changes would affect the ethics of patient care.

The 1990s presented additional challenges with regard to the public reporting of comparative patient- and provider-level data. Some were concerned about the impact of HIPAA on the availability of medical records. Today, there are even more practical and ethical questions about participation in research and the validity of studies, as HIPAA rules present new challenges for those who are involved in the release of health information. Pay-for-performance programs present yet additional challenges regarding the accurate and timely reporting and interpretation of data.

Most patient–provider electronic communications, especially those containing protected health information, are subject to the same storage, retention, retrieval, medicolegal, privacy, security, and confidentiality provisions as any other patient-identifiable health information. The implications of health information management should be included in any discussions of professional, personal, and organizational ethics. Healthcare delivery and management operations and decisions that will be made regarding automation, information technology, and information exchange are riddled with ethical questions. How we handle these questions will ultimately impact patients, clinicians, providers, consumers, payors, employers, and communities.

Key Terms

- Clinical decision support systems (CDSSs)
- Doctor's Office Quality—Information Technology (DOQ-IT)
- Electronic health information management (eHIM™)
- Health information exchange (HIE)
- Office of the National Coordinator for Health Information Technology (ONCHIT)
- Regional health information organizations (RHIOs)
- Telehealth

Chapter Summary

- The movement toward the electronic health record (EHR) and electronic health record management (EHRM) is expanding the roles and responsibilities of HIM practitioners.

- Because patients receive care from multiple providers over an increasingly dispersed geographic area, collecting, coordinating, and accessing relevant, meaningful, and timely information have been and continue to be a challenge.

- The transition from a paper-based health record to an EHR environment must be addressed and managed on many different levels: administratively, financially, culturally, organizationally, and ethically.

- The transition from a paper-based medical record to an EHR presents challenges for HIM professionals to apply their knowledge, skills, and experience in the ethical management of electronic health information.

- A number of public and private sector initiatives involving HIT and HIE are under way to improve the quality, safety, and efficiency of the nation's healthcare system.

- As communities move to develop and implement HIE, more needs to be learned as to how these efforts will evolve and what existing and perceived legal and ethical barriers exist to community collaboration and health information exchange.

- Given the increasing level of complexity and the dynamic nature of the healthcare industry, a number of potential new ethical challenges and decision points are emerging. To a large extent, the ethical challenges facing healthcare and HIM professionals in the paperless setting are similar to those in the more traditional paper-based setting.

References

Agency for Healthcare Research and Quality [AHRQ]. (1999a). *Healthcare informatics standards activities of selected federal agencies (a compendium)*. Rockville, MD: Author.

Agency for Healthcare Research and Quality [AHRQ]. (1999b). *Summary report: Current healthcare informatics standards activities of federal agencies*. Rockville, MD: Author.

Agency for Healthcare Research and Quality [AHRQ]. (2001). *Patient safety reporting systems and research in HHS*. Fact Sheet. Rockville, MD: Author.

Agency for Healthcare Research and Quality [AHRQ]. (2002). Bioterrorism preparedness and response: Use of information technologies and decision support systems. *Summary, Evidence Report/Technology Assessment,* Number 59. Rockville, MD: Author. Retrieved October 31, 2005, from http://www.ahrq.gov/data/informatics/ informatria.htm.

Agency for Healthcare Research and Quality [AHRQ]. (2003a). Case study finds computerized ICU information system care can significantly reduce time spent by nurses on documentation. Press Release, October 10. Rockville, MD: Author.

Agency for Healthcare Research and Quality [AHRQ]. (2003b). *Expert panel meeting: Health information technology. Meeting Summary.* Rockville, MD: Author.

American Academy of Family Practitioners [AAFP]. (2004). Premier medical organizations announce formation of Physicians Electronic Health Record Coalition. Press Release, July 22. Washington, DC: Author.

American Health Information Management Association [AHIMA]. (2003). A vision of the e-HIM future: A report from the AHIMA E-HIM Task Force. Retrieved June 2005 from http://library.ahima.org/xpedio/groups/public/documents/ahima/pub_bok1_020835.html.

American Health Information Management Association [AHIMA] e-HIM Task Force. (2003). HIM professionals vital in transition to e-HIM. *AHIMA Advantage, 7*(6), 1, 3–4.

American Health Information Management Association [AHIMA] e-HIM Task Force. (2004). The strategic importance of electronic health records management. *Journal of AHIMA, 75*(9), 80A–80B.

American Health Information Management Association [AHIMA] e-HIM Work Group on Health Information in a Hybrid Environment. (2003). The complete medical record in a hybrid electronic health record environment. Retrieved October 31, 2005, from http://library.ahima.org/xpedio/groups/public/documents/ahima/pub_bok1_022142.html.

American Health Information Management Association [AHIMA] e-HIM Work Group on the Legal Health Record. (2005, September). Update: Guidelines for defining the legal health record for disclosure purposes. *Journal of AHIMA, 76*(8), 64A–G.

American Health Information Management Association [AHIMA] e-HIM Work Group on Defining the Legal Health Record. (2005, October). The legal process and electronic health records. *Journal of AHIMA, 76*(9), 96A–D. [expanded online version]

Burrington-Brown, J., & Hughes, G. (2003). Provider-patient e-mail security. *AHIMA Practice Brief*. Retrieved June 2005 from http://library.ahima.org/xpedio/groups/public/documents/ahima/bok1_019873.html.

Centers for Medicare and Medicaid Services. (2005). Physician focused quality initiative. Retrieved October 31, 2005, from http://www.cms.hhs.gov/quality/pfqi.asp.

General Accounting Office [GAO]. (2003). *Information technology. Benefits realized for selected health care functions*. Washington, DC: Author.

General Accounting Office [GAO]. (2004). *HHS's efforts to promote health information technology and legal barriers to its adoption HHS's health information technology efforts*. GAO-04-991R. Washington, DC: Author.

Gupta, M. (2003). A critical appraisal of evidence-based medicine: Some ethical considerations. *Journal of Evaluative Clinical Practice, 9*(2), 111–121.

Hudson, T., Oglesby, D. K., Jr., Mongan, J. J., & Kraus, I. (1992). Administrative ethics in the 1990s: CEOs confront payment, access dilemmas. *Hospitals, 66*(1), 20–28.

Hughes, G. (2003). Defining the designated record set. *AHIMA Practice Brief. Journal of AHIMA, 74*(1), 64A–64D.

Institute of Medicine [IOM]. (2002a). *Report: Fostering rapid advances in health care: Learning from system demonstrations*. Health Care Finance and Delivery Systems, Janet M. Corrigan, Ann Greiner, Shari M. Erickson, eds. Washington, DC: Committee on Rapid Advance Demonstration Projects.

Institute of Medicine [IOM]. (2002b). *Report: The future of the public's health in the 21st century*. Washington, DC: Committee on Assuring the Health of the Public in the 21st Century.

Institute of Medicine [IOM]. (2002c). *Report: Who will keep the public healthy: Educating public health professionals for the 21st century*. Kristine Gebbie, Linda Rosenstock, and Lyla M. Hernandez, eds. Washington, DC: Committee on Educating Public Health Professionals in the 21st Century.

Institute of Medicine [IOM]. (2003a). *Letter Report: Key capabilities of an electronic health record system*. Washington, DC: Committee on Data Standards for Patient Safety.

Institute of Medicine [IOM]. (2003b). *Report: Patient safety: Achieving a new standard of care*. Philip Aspden, Janet M. Corrigan, Julie Wolcott, Shari M. Erickson, eds. Washington, DC: Committee on Data Standards for Patient Safety.

Institute of Medicine [IOM]. (2003c). *Report: Priority areas for national action: Transforming healthcare quality*. Karen Adams & Janet M. Corrigan, eds. Washington, DC: Committee on Identifying Priority Areas for Quality Improvement.

Lydon-Rochelle, M., & Holt, V. L. (2004). HIPAA transition: Challenges of a multisite medical records validation study of maternally linked birth records. *Journal of Maternal and Child Health, 8*(1), 35–38.

National Committee on Vital and Health Statistics [NCVHS]. (2001). *Information for health: A strategy for building the national health information infrastructure*. Washington, DC: Workgroup on National Health Information Infrastructure.

Slowther, A., Ford, S., & Schofield, T. (2004). Ethics of evidence based medicine in the primary care setting. *Journal of Medical Ethics, 30*(2), 151–155.

Stoelwinder, J. U. (2001). EBM in healthcare: Management and policy. *Medical Journal of Australia, 174*(12), 644–646.

Thompson, T. G., & Brailer, D. J. (2004). *The decade of health information technology: Delivering consumer-centric and information-rich health care framework for strategic action.* Washington, DC: U.S. Department of Health and Human Services.

Tilley, S. (1999). The net effects of product lines SEI interactive. Retrieved June 2005 from http://interactive.sei.cmu.edu.

Warren, I. (2000). *The renaissance of legacy systems.* New York: Springer Verlag.

Weber, L. J. (1997). Taking on organizational ethics. To do so, ethics committees must first prepare themselves. *Health Progress, 78*(3), 20–23, 32.

Weiss, N. (2004). E-mail consultation: Clinical, financial, legal, and ethical implications. *Surgical Neurology, 61*(5), 455–459.

Whitehead, A. W., & Novak, K. F. (2003). A model for assessing the ethical environment in academic dentistry. *Dental Education, 67*(10), 1113–1121.

Selected Resources

Abdelhak, M., Grostick, S., Hanken, M. A., & Jacobs, E. B., eds. (2001). *Health Information.* 2d ed. Management of a Strategic Resource (2001) Philadephia: WB Saunders.

Agency for Healthcare Research and Quality [AHRQ]. (1999). *Healthcare informatics standards activities of selected federal agencies (a compendium).* Rockville, MD: AHRQ.

Agency for Healthcare Research and Quality [AHRQ]. (2001). *Patient safety reporting systems and research in HHS. Fact Sheet.* Rockville, MD: AHRQ.

Agency for Healthcare Research and Quality [AHRQ]. (2002). Bioterrorism preparedness and response: Use of information technologies and decision support systems. *Evidence Report/Technology Assessment, 59.*

Agency for Healthcare Research and Quality [AHRQ]. (2002). Medical informatics for better and safer health care [summary]. *Research in Action, 6.* AHRQ Publication Number 02-0031, June 2002. Rockville, MD. Retrieved October 31, 2005, from http://www.ahrq.gov/data/informatics/informatria.htm.

Agency for Healthcare Research and Quality [AHRQ]. (2003). Case study finds computerized ICU information system care can significantly reduce time spent by nurses on documentation. Press Release, October 10. Rockville, MD: AHRQ.

Agency for Healthcare Research and Quality [AHRQ]. (2003). Expert panel meeting: Health information technology: Meeting summary. Retrieved June 2005 from http://www.ahrq.gov/data/hitmeet.htm.

Alliance of Community Health Plans Foundation. [ACHPF]. (2003). *Promoting prevention through information technology.* Washington, DC: ACHPF.

Amatayakul, M. (1999). *The role of health information managers in CPR projects.* Chicago: AHIMA.

Amatayakul, M. (2004). *Electronic health records: A practical guide for professionals and organizations.* Chicago: AHIMA.

American Health Information Management Association [AHIMA]. (1999). Correcting and amending entries in a computerized patient record admissibility of medical records. Practice Brief. Retrieved June 2005 from http://library.ahima.org/xpedio/groups/public/documents/ahima/pub_bok1_0000451.html.

American Health Information Management Association [AHIMA]. (2003). The complete medical record in a hybrid EHR environment: Part I: Managing the transition. Practice Brief. Retrieved June 2005 from http://library.ahima.org/xpedio/groups/public/documents/ahima/pub_bok1_021581.html.

American Health Information Management Association [AHIMA]. (2003). The complete medical record in a hybrid EHR environment: Part II: Managing access and disclosure. Practice Brief. Retrieved June 2005 from http://library.ahima.org/xpedio/groups/public/documents/ahima/pub_bok1_021582.html.

American Health Information Management Association [AHIMA]. (2003). The complete medical record in a hybrid EHR environment: Part III: Authorship of and printing the health record. Practice Brief. Retrieved June 2005 from http://library.ahima.org/xpedio/groups/public/documents/ahima/pub_bok1_021583.html.

American Health Information Management Association [AHIMA]. (2003). Electronic document management as a component of the electronic health record. Practice Brief. Retrieved June 2005 from http://library.ahima.org/xpedio/groups/public/documents/ahima/pub_bok1_021594.html.

American Health Information Management Association [AHIMA]. (2003). E-mail as a provider–patient electronic communication medium and its impact on the electronic health record. Practice Brief. Retrieved June 2005 from http://library.ahima.org/xpedio/groups/public/documents/ahima/pub_bok1_021593.html.

American Health Information Management Association [AHIMA]. (2003). Implementing electronic signatures. Practice Brief. Retrieved June 2005 from http://library.ahima.org/xpedio/groups/public/documents/ahima/pub_bok1_021585.html.

American Health Information Management Association [AHIMA]. (2004). Building an enterprise master person index. Practice Brief. Retrieved June 2005 from http://library.ahima.org/xpedio/groups/public/documents/ahima/pub_bok1_022283.html.

Appleby, C. (1995). The trouble with CHINs (community health information networks). *Hospital Health Network, 69*(9), 42–44.

Ball, M., Garets, D. E., & Handler, T. (2003). Leveraging IT to improve patient safety. *Methods of Information in Medicine, 42*(5), 503–508.

Bates, D. W., & Gawande, A. A. (2003). Improving patient safety with information technology. *New England Journal of Medicine, 348*(25), 2526–2534.

Baxter, C., Levin, R., Legaspi, M. M., Bailey, B. E., & Brown, C. L. (2002). Community health-center-led networks: Cooperating to compete. *Journal of Healthcare Management, 47*(6), 376–389.

BNA's Healthcare. (1993). Wisconsin health information network offers model for regional alliances. *Electronic Data Report, 1*(11), 107.

Boland, P., White, K., Wieners, W., & Peabody, J. (2003). A boost to service and quality. *Healthcare Informatics*. Retrieved October 31, 2005, from http://www.healthcare-informatics.com/issues/2003/10_03/partnerships.htm.

Brailer, D. J. & Terasawa, E. L. (2003). *Use and adoption of computer-based patient records*. Oakland: CA: California Healthcare Foundation.

Briggs, B. (2003). CPOE order from chaos. *Health Data Management, 11*(2), 45–48.

Buller-Close, K., Schriger, D. L., & Baraff, L. J. (2003). Heterogeneous effect of an emergency department expert charting system. *Annals of Emergency Medicine, 41*(5), 644–652.

California Healthcare Foundation. (2003). *A primer on physician order entry*. Oakland, CA: First Consulting Group.

California Healthcare Foundation. (2003). *Digital hospitals move off the drawing board*. Oakland, CA: First Consulting Group

Community Health Information Networks. (1995). The SunHealth Alliance and First Consulting Group. Boston, Massachusetts.

Comprehensive Guide to Electronic Health Records. (2000). New York: Faulkner & Gray.

Corn, M., Rudzinski, K., & Cahn, M. (2002). Bridging the gap in medical informatics and health services research: Workshop results and next steps. *Journal of the American Medical Informatics Association, 9*(2), 140–143.

Coye, M. J., & Bernstein, W. S. (2003). Perspective: Improving America's health care system by investing in information technology. *Health Affairs, 22*(4), 56–58.

Davenport, R. L., & Zimmerman, J. (1995). Technological considerations in the CHIN (community health information network) design process. *Healthcare Information Management, 9*(2), 29–34.

Dick, R. S., Steen, E. B., & Detmer, D. E., eds. (1997). *National Academy of Sciences, Institute of Medicine, Committee on Improving the Patient Record. The computer-based patient record: An essential technology for health care* (rev. ed.). Washington, DC: National Academy Press.

Fitzmaurice, J. M., Adams, K., & Eisenberg, J. (2002). Three decades of research on computer applications in health care: Medical informatics support at AHRQ. *Journal of the American Medical Informatics Association, 9*(2), 144–160.

Flaks, J. A., & Porter, A. T. (1998). Community health information networks: A strategic view. *Journal of Oncology Management, 7*(6), 18–20.

Furukawa, M. (1997). Models for evolving community health information networks. *Topics in Health Information Management, 17*(4), 11–19.

General Accounting Office [GAO]. (2003). *Information technology. Benefits realized for selected health care functions*. GAO-04-224. Washington, DC: GAO

General Accounting Office [GAO]. (2004). *HHS's efforts to promote health information technology and legal barriers to its adoption*. GAO-04-991R. Washington, DC: GAO.

Glaser, J. (2003). When IT excellence goes the distance. *Healthcare Financial Management, 57*(9), 102–104, 106, 108.

Goldsmith, J., Blumenthal, D., & Rishel, W. (2003). Federal health information policy: A case of arrested development. *Health Affairs, 22*(4), 44–55.

Gupta, M. (2003). A critical appraisal of evidence-based medicine: Some ethical considerations. *Journal of Evaluative Clinical Practice, 9*(2), 111–121.

Hopkins, D. S., Oswald, N., McCaffrey, K., Bressler, S., Davidson, N., & Vela, L. (2000). CALINX (California Information Exchange): A multi-stakeholder statewide initiative to improve healthcare information flows. *Journal of Healthcare Information Management, 14*(4), 41–52.

Hudson, T., Oglesby, D. K., Jr., Mongan, J. J., & Kraus, I. (1992). Administrative ethics in the 1990s: CEOs confront payment, access dilemmas. *Hospitals, 66*(1), 20–28.

Institute of Medicine [IOM]. (2000). To err is human: Building a safer health system. Kohn, L. T., Corrigan, J. M., & Donaldson, M. S. eds., *Committee on Quality of Health Care in America*. Washington, DC: National Academy Press.

Institute of Medicine [IOM]. (2002). *Fostering rapid advances in health care: Learning from system demonstrations*. In J. M. Corrigan, A. Greiner, S. M. Erickson (Eds.), Committee on Rapid Advance Demonstration Projects: Health Care Finance and Delivery Systems. Washington, DC: National Academy Press.

Institute of Medicine [IOM]. (2002). *The future of the public's health in the 21st century*. Committee for the Study of the Future of Public Health; Division of Health Care Services. Washington, DC: National Academy Press.

Institute of Medicine [IOM]. (2002). *Who will keep the public healthy: Educating public health professionals for the 21st century*. In K. Gebbie, L. Rosenstock, and L. M. Hernandez (Eds.), Committee on Educating Public Health Professionals for the 21st Century. Washington, DC: National Academy Press.

Institute of Medicine [IOM]. (2003). *Key capabilities of an electronic health record system. Letter Report, Committee on Data Standards for Patient Safety*. Committee on Data Standards for Patient Safety. Washington, DC: National Academy Press.

Institute of Medicine [IOM]. (2003). *Patient safety: Achieving a new standard of care*. Philip Aspden, Janet M. Corrigan, Julie Wolcott, Shari M. Erickson (Eds.), Committee on Data Standards for Patient Safety. Washington, DC: National Academy Press.

Institute of Medicine [IOM]. (2003). *Priority areas for national action: Transforming health care quality*. In K. Adams & J. M. Corrigan (Eds.), Committee on Identifying Priority Areas for Quality Improvement. Washington, DC: National Academy Press.

Journal of Management Information Systems. (2000). Special Issue: Impacts of Information Technology Investment on Organizational Performance. *Journal of Management Information Systems, 16*(4).

Kennedy, R. (1995). Building the CHIN (community health information network) organization. *Healthcare Information Management, 9*(2), 21–28.

Krohn, R. W. (1997). Success factors of risk based specialty networks. *Medical Group Management Journal, 44*(2), 28, 30, 32–34.

Lassila, K. S., Pemble, K. R., DuPont, L. A., & Cheng, R. H. (1997). Assessing the impact of community health information networks: A multisite field study of the Wisconsin Health Information Network. *Topics in Health Information Management, 18*(2), 64–76.

Lorenzi, N. M. (2003). Strategies for creating successful local health information infrastructure initiatives. Report under contract 03EASPE00722.

Lumpkin, J. R. (2001). Air, water, places, and data—public health in the information age. *Journal of Public Health Management Practice, 7*(6), 22–30.

Lydon-Rochelle, M., & Holt, V. L. (2004). HIPAA transition: Challenges of a multisite medical records validation study of maternally linked birth records. *Matern Child Health Journal, 8*(1), 35–38.

MacDonald, K., & Metzger, J. (2004). First Consulting Group, Connecting communities: Strategies for physician portals and regional data sharing—including results from a recent survey by the College of Healthcare Information Management Executives (CHIME). Prepared for the California HealthCare Foundation (CHCF) by First Consulting Group (FCG).

Massachusetts Technology Collaborative. (2003). Advanced technologies to lower health care costs and improve quality. Innovation Outlook Series. Boston: Massachusetts Technology Collaborative.

McClurg, J. (2002). Putting your ASP on the line. Business service providers let healthcare organizations concentrate on healthcare. *Healthcare Information, 19*(5), 72.

Mercer, K., Roach, G., & Leonard, K. (1996). The missing piece of the long-term care reform puzzle: The Community Health Information Network. *Health Law Canada, 16*(4), 114–120.

Murphy, G., Hanken, M. A., & Waters, K. (1999). *Electronic health records: Changing the vision.* Philadelphia: W.B. Saunders.

National Action Agenda for the National Health Information Infrastructure. (2003). *Recommendations of the financial incentives track.* Retrieved June 2005 from http://aspe.hhs.gov/sp/nhii/.

National Committee on Vital and Health Statistics. (2001). *Information for health: A strategy for building the national health information infrastructure.* Washington, DC: DHHS.

National Electronic Disease Surveillance System Working Group. (2001). National electronic disease surveillance system (NEDSS): A standards-based approach to connect public health and clinical medicine. *Journal of Public Health Management and Practice, 7*(6), 43–50.

Noss, B., & Zall, R. J. (2002). A review of CHIN initiatives: What works and why. *Journal of Healthcare Information Management, 16*(2), 35–39.

Ortiz, E., & Clancy, C. M. (2003). Use of information technology to improve the quality of healthcare in the United States. *Health Services Research, 38*(2), xi–xii.

Ortiz, E., Meyer, G., & Burstin, H. (2001). The role of clinical informatics in the Agency for Healthcare Research and Quality's efforts to improve patient safety. *Proceedings of the AMIA Annual Fall Symposium,* 508–512. Philadelphia: Hanley & Belfus.

Payton, F. C., & Ginzberg, M. J. (2001). Interorganizational health care systems implementations: An exploratory study of early electronic commerce initiatives. *Health Care Management Review, 26*(2), 20–32.

Petry, J. M., & Chandler, M. M. (1995). Assessing your CHIN (community health information network) readiness. *Healthcare Information Management, 9*(2), 15–20.

Rabunski, J. S., & Weil, J. P. (1995). Fitting the CHIN (community health information network) to the customer: Three case studies. *Healthcare Information Management, 9*(2), 53–60.

Rosenstein, A. H. (1999). Measuring the benefit of performance improvement and decision support. *American Journal of Medical Quality, 14*(6), 262–269.

Rybowski, L., & Rubin, R. (1998). *Building an infrastructure for community health information: lessons from the frontier.* Seattle, WA: Foundation for Health Care Quality.

Sederholm, K. (2002). Centralized health data. A multiplatform problem is solved. *Healthcare Information, 19*(3), 48.

Shingles, R. B., Shaman, H. J., Kongstvedt, P. R., & Hohner, J. H. (2001). Next phase of medical management systems: Automating administrative transaction to integrate payors and providers. *Journal of Healthcare Information Management, 15*(3), 223–235.

Slowther, A., Ford, S., & Schofield, T. (2004). Ethics of evidence based medicine in the primary care setting. *Journal of Medical Ethics, 30*(2), 151–155.

Stoelwinder, J. U. (2001). EBM in healthcare: Management and policy. *Medical Journal of Australia, 174*(12), 644–646.

U.S. Department of Health and Human Services. (2005). Office of the national coordinator for health information technology (ONC): Directory of federal HIT programs. Retrieved October 31, 2005, from http://www.os.dhhs.gov/healthit/federalprojectlist.html#intitiativestable.

Warren, I. (2000). *The renaissance of legacy systems.* New York: Springer Verlag.

Weaver, C. G. (1995). CHINs: Making the important decisions. *Healthcare Financial Management, 49*(6), 58–60, 62, 64–65.

Weaver, C. G. (1999). CHINs: Infrastructure for the future. *Trustee,* American Hospital Publishing, Inc. Vol. 465.

Weber, L. J. (1997). Taking on organizational ethics. To do so, ethics committees must first prepare themselves. *Health Progress, 78*(3), 20–23, 32.

Weiner, B. J., Alexander, J. A., & Zuckerman, H. S. (2000). Strategies for effective management participation in community health partnerships. *Health Care Management Review, 25*(3), 48–66.

Whitehead, A. W., & Novak, K. F. (2003). A model for assessing the ethical environment in academic dentistry. *Dental Education, 67*(10), 1113–1121.

Part IV

MANAGEMENT OF SENSITIVE HEALTH INFORMATION

The protection of all health information is important; however, health information involving genetics, adoption, and behavioral issues requires special consideration. These topics are addressed in Part IV. Chapter 18 discusses access to and misuse of genetic information and the federal and state laws pertaining to genetic information. Chapter 19 explores traditional assumptions regarding access to health information for adoption. It analyzes the implications of the adoption model of access to familial information in relationship to the larger issue of familial access to information, regardless of adoption status. Chapter 20 focuses on highly sensitive health information, such as information on drug and alcohol abuse, sexually transmitted diseases, and behavioral conditions. This chapter also discusses how to balance requests from law enforcement officials while protecting patient privacy. Issues related to substance abuse treatment, health information and the law, sexually transmitted diseases, employees and children, workers' compensation cases, and children's protective services also are analyzed.

18

GENETIC INFORMATION

Barbara P. Fuller, JD, RHIA
Kathy L. Hudson, PhD

Learning Objectives

After completing this chapter, the reader should be able to:

- Comprehend the sensitivity of genetic information and the possible uses and misuses of this information.
- Discuss the state and federal laws that may limit access to genetic information by health insurers and employers.
- Understand why protecting genetic information requires providing a high level of protection for all medical information.
- Appreciate the role of the health information management (HIM) professional in ensuring the privacy of genetic information.

Abstract

Rapid advances in genetics research and the emerging applications to medical practice have heightened public concerns about who will have access to genetic information and how it will be used. This chapter discusses the misuse of genetic information and the federal and state laws that have begun to address it by prohibiting health insurance and employment discrimination on the basis of genetic information and prohibiting health insurers and employers from requesting or requiring genetic information. The chapter also discusses the responsibility of HIM professionals to protect the privacy and confidentiality of genetic information and to ensure compliance with federal and state laws.

The views expressed are those of the authors. No official endorsement by the NIH or the Department of Health and Human Services is intended or should be inferred.

Scenario 18-A: Genetic Privacy

Catherine Greene, an HIM professional in a large teaching hospital, receives a request from a local business for medical information on Mrs. Jones. Mrs. Jones has applied for a job with the business, and the business has made her a job offer pending a medical clearance. The request for medical information is accompanied by an authorization that is signed and dated by Mrs. Jones; it meets all of the criteria for authorizations for release of medical information.

Mrs. Jones has been very healthy and has had only one brief hospital stay that was the result of minor injuries sustained in a car accident. However, during this hospital stay, her attending physician documented a family history of breast cancer. The physician also documented that Mrs. Jones had participated in a genetics research protocol and that a genetic test had indicated an alteration in the BRCA1 gene. This particular genetic test is an indication that Mrs. Jones has a predisposition to breast cancer; that is, she has a higher chance of developing breast cancer than someone with a negative test result. This test result is not a definitive predictor of breast cancer.

Due to concerns that employers could make discriminatory hiring and personnel decisions based on an individual's genetic makeup, the state legislature has recently enacted genetic privacy and antidiscrimination legislation. This legislation prohibits employers from discriminating on the basis of genetic information and prohibits employers from obtaining genetic information regarding an employee or prospective employee. Mrs. Jones's prospective employer has not specifically requested genetic information, but the family history and history of a positive genetic test is contained within the medical record.

Question

1. What should Catherine do?

A completed ethical decision-making matrix for the scenario is provided at the end of the chapter.

THE ISSUE OF GENETIC INFORMATION

The number of genetic technologies has increased tenfold over the last decade, dramatically increasing the amount of **genetic information** that can be determined. Genetic information can be the results of an individual's genetic tests, the genetic tests of family members of the individual, or the occurrence of a disease or disorder in family members of the individual. The Human Genome Project has given us the technology to decipher what were once an individual's most personal and intimate "family secrets"; that is, the information contained in our DNA. The instructions encrypted in our genes affect nearly every function the human body carries out, from fighting infection to thinking. Research to understand those instructions offers the promise of better health, because it gives researchers and clinicians critical information to work out therapies or other strategies to prevent or treat a disease. In addition, **genetic testing** can alert individuals to a heightened risk of some health problems and the need to screen for them more frequently and thoroughly and to take more preventive measures.

Often, however, individuals are reluctant to participate in genetic research and testing because they feel they cannot be sure of the privacy of the genetic information that will be obtained from them and placed in their medical records or in research records. Consider, for example, a healthy 38-year-old man who is considered at risk to develop colorectal cancer because of his family history: Two of his brothers, an aunt, and his grandfather have been diagnosed with a type of colon cancer that is known to have a genetic component [hereditary nonpolyposis colorectal cancer (HNPCC)], and two of them have undergone genetic testing that showed a genetic predisposition to HNPCC. This individual has been undergoing biannual colonoscopies as a way of detecting polyps before they turn into cancerous lesions. Testing could be useful to him: If he were to test positive, he would continue the biannual colonoscopies, because he would know he was at heightened risk for HNPCC, but if he were to test negative, he would only have to have less invasive, and less frequent, sigmoidoscopies, because he would have the same risk as the general population. However, he declines to be tested, opting instead for the frequent colonoscopies, because he knows that any test results will be placed in his medical record and will be subject to release to his health insurer. He is afraid that if he tested positive, he could lose his health insurance, even though testing positive merely would indicate a predisposition to colon cancer, not a certainty of colon cancer.

Concerns like these are actually common among U.S. citizens. A survey by the Genetics and Public Policy Center at Johns Hopkins University found that 80 percent of those surveyed did not want their insurers to have access to their genetic information, and 92 percent did not want their employers to have access to their genetic information (Hudson, 2004). Further, potential study volunteers are concerned that the genetic information obtained from them in research projects will not be kept confidential (Cooley, 1996). For example, one-third of the women invited to participate in a study of women with a breast cancer gene mutation refused to participate because they feared discrimination or a loss of privacy (Kolata, 1997).

Several publicized incidents have shown that there is a legitimate basis for such concerns. For instance, in the early 1970s, some insurance companies denied coverage and charged higher rates to African Americans who were carriers of the gene for sickle cell anemia, even though these African Americans themselves were not at risk for developing the disease (Hudson, Rothenberg, Andrews, Kahn, & Collins, 1995, p. 391). In addition, according to the American Medical Association's Council on Ethical and Judicial Affairs (1991), "Some companies may have restricted employment opportunities for individuals who carry the sickle cell trait, even though no scientific basis for the restrictions existed" (see also Reinhardt, 1978; Omenn, 1982).

More recently, other studies have demonstrated similar instances of genetic discrimination against healthy people with a genetic alteration that predisposes them or their children to a later illness (Geller, Alper, Billings, Barash, Beckwith, & Natowicz, 1996), even though having such a genetic alteration is not an indication that the disease will ever manifest during this individual's lifetime (Task Force, 1998). A young, healthy woman with outstanding performance evaluations was fired from her job after her employer learned she had tested positive for the genetic alteration that predisposes to Huntington disease. Another company performed secret genetic testing for a possible predisposition to carpal tunnel syndrome, presumably with the intent to deny worker's compensation benefits for claims regarding work-related carpal tunnel syndrome (*Brotherhood of Maintenance of Way Employees v. Burlington Northern Santa Fe R. Co.,* 2001). Another individual was screened and learned that he was a carrier of a single misspelled gene for Gaucher's disease. His carrier status indicated that he might pass this mutation to his children, but that he would never develop Gaucher's disease himself. He revealed this information when applying for a job and was denied the job because of his genetic status, even though it had no bearing on his present or future ability to perform a job. In other instances, a health problem may be considered more serious and intractable if it is discovered to have a genetic component. For example, one woman with "bad knees" who worked for a healthcare company was fired shortly after her boss told her he had learned from a fellow coworker that there was a genetic basis for her orthopedic problem. If an individual's genetic information is known by a health insurer or an employer, the individual often cannot determine if the loss of health insurance coverage or the loss of an employment opportunity was based on his or her genetic information or on some other factor.

Some states have legislation prohibiting the discriminatory use of genetic information, but some of these laws do not restrict access to genetic information. People are concerned about access to their information by others, regardless of whether the information will be used for specific economic or social harm. For example, the discovery and disclosure of genetic information often have harmful implications for family relationships: The siblings of a young woman who tested positive for Huntington disease cut off their relationship with her because they had chosen not to be tested and could not cope with the prospect that they might also test positive (because they had a 50 percent chance of inheriting the genetic alteration). Although medical record privacy protections are afforded by the Health Insurance Portability and Accountability Act Privacy Rule **(HIPAA Privacy Rule)** and privacy and confidentiality laws in each state, clearly many people do not trust their effectiveness in preventing unauthorized access to this information.

The power and potential of genetic testing cannot be realized if individuals are afraid to be tested. Further, genetic research, which requires the participation of large numbers of volunteers, cannot fulfill its promise if potential volunteers are dissuaded from participation because of concerns about the confidentiality of their genetic information and possible discriminatory uses of that information. The prevention of discrimination and the protection of privacy and confidentiality of genetic information should be considered the absolute prerequisites for an environment in which individuals feel free to participate in genetic testing.

THE RELATIONSHIP BETWEEN GENETIC INFORMATION AND GENERIC MEDICAL INFORMATION

Genetic information is potentially predictive, and its disclosure can cause significant psychosocial and economic harm. It is considered by many to be more personal, more sensitive, and more likely to result in stigmatization and discrimination than some other types of health-related information, and it already has a history of misuse. Like mental health, HIV status, and substance abuse information, it is a category of information with higher levels of public sensitivity. These special features of genetic information have suggested that there might be a scientific, moral, political, and/or pragmatic reason for affording extra protections for genetic information as distinct from other health-related information.

However, because virtually all disease has some genetic basis, the emerging consensus among genetics professionals, industry and citizen groups, and policymakers is that genetic information cannot reasonably be maintained separately from the rest of the medical record (Genome Action Coalition, 1997; Pharmaceutical Research, 1997). Dr. Francis Collins (1996), director of the National Human Genome Research Institute, stated, "Genetics is part of the tapestry of medical information. . . . It is often difficult to decide whether you are looking at something that is genetic or is not" (p. 183).

Segregation would create a system of incomplete medical information and would interfere with optimal health care. Consequently, the best way to ensure the highest level of protection for genetic information is to ensure uniform high standards for the protection of all health information and to enact antidiscrimination legislation to prevent misuse of genetic information. The HIPAA Privacy Rule does offer the same level of protection for genetic information as for almost all other health information.

WHAT DO WE MEAN BY PRIVACY OF MEDICAL INFORMATION?

The terms *privacy* and *confidentiality* have been defined in many diverse ways, ranging from the spiritual to the philosophical to the practical. Among the early legal analyses of privacy rights was Judge Thomas Cooley's (1888) *A Treatise on the Law of Torts,* which suggested that the "right to one's person may be said to be a right of complete immunity: to be let alone" (p. 29).

In contrast to privacy, which historically has been used to refer to protection against unwanted access to the person or to one's personal property, *confidentiality* refers to the protection against unwanted access to information about a person or a group: "Confidentiality pertains to the treatment of information that an individual has disclosed in a relationship of trust and with the expectation that it will not be divulged to others in ways that are inconsistent with the understanding of the original disclosure without permission" (Office for Protection from Research Risks, 1993, p. 27). To some extent, there has been a blurring between the concepts of privacy and confidentiality because both refer to protections from unwanted intrusion. In this chapter, however, *privacy* refers to the right of an individual not to divulge his or her genetic information, whereas *confidentiality* refers to the necessity to obtain an individual's authorization in order to access his or her genetic information.

Individuals seeking health care should anticipate that information from their medical record will be shared with a wide range of third parties, including healthcare providers, health insurers, life insurers, courts, employers, social service agencies, and others with a business, personal, clinical, or social interest in the health status of the individual. Although the HIPAA Privacy Rule and state medical record confidentiality laws restrict access to medical records to those with signed authorizations, court order, or other limited circumstances, the laws do not otherwise attempt to prohibit access as long as the conditions for access are met (Health Insurance Portability and Accountability Act Privacy Rule, 2002). In addition to the HIPAA Privacy Rule, federal laws that also address the privacy and confidentiality of medical records are specific to a few federally funded programs [e.g., 42 U.S.C.A. §3789g(a), 42 U.S.C.A. §299; Public Health Service Act §308(d)], the Privacy Act of 1974 (P.L. 93-579, 93rd Cong., S. 3418), and unique categories of records such as the records of substance abuse patients [Public Health Service Act §301(d)].

RESEARCH RECORDS

Unlike medical records, research records contain experimental data and analysis necessary to test a hypothesis. Research records from studies involving human subjects include information provided by the research subject, such as individual and family medical history, name and other identifying information, personal lifestyle, and symptoms. For example, in a research study attempting to identify genes that play a role in a hereditary form of Parkinson's disease, the research records would include detailed information on the participants' family members, including whether they had been diagnosed with Parkinson's disease.

Unlike individuals seeking health care, individuals participating in healthcare research but not receiving health care as part of the research do not anticipate that information from their research record will be shared with others. When healthcare research protocols involve the actual delivery of health care, the research information placed in the individual's record is accessible, as is all other medical record information. However, when a health research protocol does not involve the delivery of health care, the research information is maintained solely to assist the research project, is kept in the researcher's scientific files, and is not placed in the participant's medical record (Mayo Clinic, 1998). Individuals who volunteer to participate in healthcare research protocols that will not provide direct impact on their health are participating for the good of society and not to gain a direct benefit for themselves. Consequently, the social purposes of research justify more stringent privacy protections to protect the research participant from third-party access and use of clinical findings from the research. This principle is reflected in the HIPAA Privacy Rule.

It is also recognized that research information, by its very nature, cannot automatically be considered clinically valid, as is the case with clinical data used in healthcare delivery. Research is designed to explore unanswered questions and requires scientific verification to ensure the reliability and validity of the results. Some research findings are never validated, and individual research results are sometimes difficult, if not impossible, to interpret or use in a meaningful way. Data may be derived from experimental tests or procedures that are not clinically and/or analytically valid (Task Force, 1997)[1] or that were generated in a laboratory without certification under the Clinical Laboratory Improvement Amendments of 1988 (P.L. 100-572).[2] CLIA is a federal law designed to enhance the quality of laboratory testing for patients and requires the regulation of any facility that performs tests for the purpose of providing information for the diagnosis of human beings. Generally, CLIA does not apply to facilities that conduct laboratory testing only for the purpose of research.

THE MISUSE OF GENETIC INFORMATION AND DISCRIMINATION

A wide variety of individuals and organizations may desire access to an individual's genetic test results. For example, insurers would like genetic information to determine possible risk factors for use in underwriting ("Genetic Profiles," 1998). They consider genetic information to offer the likelihood of identifying potential health problems. However, insurers also call for the "appropriate use of genetic information and continued protection of the privacy of individual information" ("Genetic Profiles," 1998, p. 86).

Employers may be hesitant to employ those with a genetic predisposition to a debilitating disease such as colorectal cancer or breast cancer. They may fear that these individuals will spend fewer years in the workforce or that they will cause increased health insurance premiums (American Medical Association, 1991). Consequently, employers may seek genetic information to identify such at-risk employees or potential employees (American Medical Association, 1991). The U.S. military uses genetic information to deny medical benefits to retirees who have an illness with a known genetic basis [10 U.S.C.A. §1207a(a) (1999)]. Recent reforms restricting use of genetic information in

---

1. The Task Force on Genetic Testing defined *clinical validity* as the probability that a person with a disease, or who will get a disease, will have a positive test result. It defined analytical validity as the probability that a test will detect an analyte when it is present in a specimen.

---

2. CLIA applies to laboratories that examine human specimens for the diagnosis, prevention, or treatment of any disease or impairment of, or the assessment of the health of, human beings.

group health insurance [enacted by the Health Insurance Portability and Accountability Act of 1996; 104 P.L. No. 104-191, 701, 110 Stat., 1936 (1996)] have, if anything, created increased incentive for employers to use this information when hiring or firing employees in order to minimize risks that may increase healthcare costs.

In many states, health insurers, employers, or both are prohibited from requiring genetic testing and/or inquiring into the results of tests or obtaining genetic information.[3] The legislatures in these states have recognized that a genetic test is only an aid to be utilized in predicting an individual's future health, not a definitive indicator of an individual's health. Many factors may play a role in whether a genetic predisposition ever manifests in the disease itself. Further, the ability, or inability, to perform a job function today cannot be determined by a predictive genetic test, because there is no scientific evidence to substantiate a relationship between unexpressed genetic factors and an individual's inability to perform his or her job functions (American Medical Association, 1991; National Action Plan, 1996).

Even if employers do not themselves require genetic testing of prospective employees, they have access to the medical records of their employees and prospective employees and thus to any existing genetic information (Rothstein, 1992). Once a job offer has been made, an employer may require the individual to undergo a medical clearance, including the collection of all the individual's medical records. If the individual refuses to sign an authorization for release of information deemed necessary for the medical clearance, the employer does not have to proceed with the hiring process.

In addition to insurers and employers, family members or the courts may obtain an individual's genetic information: "Some argue that family members should have automatic

access to genetic test results if they too may have a high risk of a significant disorder and if prevention or treatment is available" (Human Genome Organization, quoted in Wadman, 1998, p. 826). Courts of law are increasingly getting and using genetic test results in cases ranging from child custody (Rothstein, 1994–1995) to third-party liability (Rothstein, 1996). The outcome of a child custody dispute may hinge on whether one parent has a predisposition to a debilitating condition (Rothstein, 1994–1995). For example, during one custody battle, the husband requested that his ex-wife be tested for the Huntington disease gene. The ex-wife had a 50 percent chance of developing Huntington disease because her mother had been diagnosed with and died from this fatal disease. The man thought that if his ex-wife tested positive, he would have a better chance of gaining custody of the children (Rothstein, 1994–1995). The outcome of a third-party liability case may hinge on whether the plaintiff has a predisposition to a life-threatening condition. A defendant in a civil suit may seek the plaintiff's genetic information in an attempt to reduce a monetary award based on life expectancy or lost income (Rothstein, 1996).

FEDERAL LEGISLATIVE PROTECTIONS

In 2002, the U.S. Department of Health and Human Services issued the HIPAA Privacy Rule, as mandated by the Health Insurance Portability and Accountability Act of 1996. The Privacy Rule protects the privacy of individually identifiable health information by establishing conditions for its use and disclosure by health plans, healthcare clearinghouses, and certain healthcare providers.

In addition to the HIPAA Privacy Rule, there are federal laws that address the privacy and confidentiality of medical records.[4]

3. See http://www.genome.gov, accessed September 4, 2004. See also Hudson et al. (1995) and Rothenberg et al. (1997).

4. For example, 42 U.S.C.A. §3789g(a); 42 U.S.C.A. §299; Public Health Service Act §§301(d) and 308(d); and P.L. 93-579, 93rd Congress, S. 3418 (1974).

The Federal Privacy Act of 1974 (P.L. 93-579, 93rd Congress, S. 3418; from here on in referred to as the Act) safeguards health records and other records held by federal agencies retrievable by personal identifiers. The stated purpose of the Act is to provide safeguards for an individual against invasions of personal privacy, but the Act specifies many instances where disclosures without the consent of the individual are allowable. This statute also provides for individuals to access and correct or amend information pertaining to them in medical records held by federal agencies that conduct research.

The HIPAA Privacy Rule protects the confidentiality of individually identifiable health information. It generally addresses the responsibilities of those maintaining health information, describes who can have access to an individual's medical information, and outlines the process for obtaining access. It includes protections for data generated by healthcare providers and payers, including research information utilized in the course of healthcare delivery. Recognizing the critical role of information from medical records in biomedical, public health, and epidemiology research, it also provides guidance on steps to be taken in providing researchers access to medical information and balances the privacy interests of the individual with the societal need for research.

The HIPAA Privacy Rule encompasses individually identifiable health information transmitted or maintained in electronic form by healthcare providers, health plans, and healthcare clearinghouses. The regulations also are designed to include the information generated from research studies when the research information is included in the medical record or is used to make decisions about an individual's healthcare delivery.

On February 8, 2000, President Clinton signed an executive order [Exec. Order No. 13,145, 65; Fed. Reg. 6,877 (2000)] that provides the following safeguards: Federal employers are prohibited from requiring or requesting genetic tests as a condition of being hired or receiving benefits; federal employers are prohibited from using protected genetic information to deprive employees of advancement opportunities; and strong privacy protections are provided for any genetic information used for medical treatment or research. For instance, the executive order prohibits any federal employment department from requesting, requiring, collecting, or purchasing protected genetic information with respect to an employee or information about a request for or the receipt of genetic services by an employee [§1-202(c)]. In announcing the executive order, President Clinton (2000) expressed hope that it would "set an example and pose a challenge for every employer in America" to adopt a policy not to discriminate on the basis of protected genetic information, "because . . . no employer should ever review your genetic records along with your resume." The implications of the executive order are that genetic information will not be collected or used by federal agencies and that the ability to do a job should be judged on just that—the ability to do the job.

STATE LEGISLATIVE PROTECTIONS

Each state has a medical record confidentiality statute designed to offer privacy and confidentiality protection for medical information obtained in the course of healthcare delivery (Health Privacy Project, 2000; Tomes, 1996). When these state laws offer a higher level of privacy and confidentiality protection than that offered by the HIPAA Privacy Rule, the provisions in the state laws prevail. However, if the state laws provide less privacy and confidentiality protection than that offered by the HIPAA Privacy Rule, the HIPAA Privacy Rule prevails. The level of protection afforded to medical information varies widely from state to state, but all state statutes are designed to provide access to medical records only if authorized by the individual or as otherwise provided by law (Health Privacy Project, 2000; Tomes, 1996).

Further, access to genetic information is specifically addressed in many of the state laws that prohibit genetic discrimination by insurers or employers.[5] These laws generally include privacy protections for genetic information that prohibit insurers and/or employers from requesting or requiring genetic information and that consequently prohibit them from obtaining an individual's genetic information, whether that information is contained in a medical record or a research record (Rothenberg, Fuller, Rothstein, Duster, Ellis Kahn, Cunningham, et al., 1997; Rothenberg, 1995; Hudson et al., 1995). For instance, Wisconsin's health insurance anti-discrimination law [Wisc. Stat. Ann. §631.89 (West 1998)] prohibits insurers from requiring or requesting "directly or indirectly any individual to reveal whether the individual or a member of the individual's family has obtained a genetic test or what the results of the test, if obtained by the individual or a member of the individual's family, were."

LEGISLATION ON RESEARCH RECORD PRIVACY

The HIPAA Privacy Rule establishes the conditions under which covered entities can use or disclose protected health information, including for research. Not all researchers have to comply with the Privacy Rule (if they are not a covered entity, e.g., a health plan, a healthcare clearinghouse, or a healthcare provider). However, a new layer of privacy protection for research volunteers may be afforded by the Privacy Rule as it introduced new ways in which covered entities must handle protected health information, including that for research (Department of Health and Human Services, 2003).

Generally, research is not mentioned in state medical record confidentiality statutes, and then only as an exception to the need for

authorization to receive medical information, not as a distinct type of information to be protected.[6] For example, the Maryland statute regarding the confidentiality of medical records provides that a healthcare provider may disclose a medical record without the authorization of the individual if it is for "research purposes, subject to the applicable requirements of an institutional review board" (Maryland, Health-General Code §4-305). Thus, the generation of experimental data by a research protocol is not specifically addressed by most state laws. Minnesota and New Hampshire are exceptions. In 1996, Minnesota enacted legislation restricting the release of medical records to researchers (MN St. §144.335). This restriction requires the healthcare provider to disclose to patients currently being treated that their health records may be released and that the patient may object, in which case the records will not be released (MN St. §144.335). New Hampshire has enacted a statute designed to protect the confidentiality of medical and/or scientific data obtained via research authorized by the Commissioner of Health and Human Services [NH Rev. Stat. Ann. §126-A:11 (Supp. 1996)].

Access to genetics research information is indirectly prohibited in some state health insurance or employment genetic antidiscrimination laws (Rothenberg et al., 1997; Rothenberg, 1995; Hudson et al., 1995). These laws generally prohibit insurers and/or employers from requesting or requiring genetic information and, consequently, prohibit them

---

5. See N.H. Stat. Ann. §§141-H:1 and 3 (Michie Butterworth, 1995); Wis. Stat. §631.89 (1991).

6. New Hampshire is an exception. New Hampshire has enacted a statute designed to protect the confidentiality of medical and/or scientific data obtained during research authorized by the Commissioner of Health and Human Services. The statute states that these data may be used solely for medical or scientific purposes and this information shall not be "admissible as evidence in any action of any kind in any court or before any tribunal, board, agency or person" [N.H. Rev. Stat. Ann. §126-a:11 (Supp. 1996)].

from obtaining an individual's genetic information, whether the information is contained in a medical record or a research record (Rothenberg et al., 1997; Rothenberg, 1995; Hudson et al., 1995).

The regulatory framework for the protection of individuals who participate in research is the **Common Rule** (45 C.F.R. 46). The Common Rule is used by federal agencies that conduct, support, or regulate research. It deals with issues such as the rights of research participants, informed consent, institutional review boards (IRBs), and several other matters. This framework was based on a report of the National Commission for the Protection of Human Subjects in Research that addressed basic ethical principles to protect human research subjects (U.S. National Commission, 1979). Both the report and subsequent regulations concentrated on concerns regarding the violations of body integrity and did not comprehensively address the privacy and confidentiality of the information resulting from research on human subjects. The Common Rule requires that all human subjects research supported, conducted, or regulated by federal agencies be reviewed by an IRB (45 C.F.R. 46.107). IRBs are responsible for ensuring that consent is informed and voluntary, that risks to the participant are minimized, and that the participant's rights and welfare are protected (45 C.F.R. 46). These regulations apply to the vast majority of biomedical research conducted in the United States. IRBs also consider whether the proposed informed consent contains "a statement describing the extent, if any, to which confidentiality of records identifying the subject will be maintained" [45 C.F.R. 46.116(a)(5)]. A guidebook for IRBs developed by the Office for Protection from Research Risks (1993) provides guidance on issues of privacy and confidentiality, but otherwise there are no specific mandates or requirements for even the most basic levels of privacy and confidentiality protections.

Several federal statutes protect research data specific to particular types of studies. The most comprehensive level of protection for research data is for research conducted on crimes [42 U.S.C.A. §3789g(a)], healthcare outcomes and medical liability (42 U.S.C.A. §299), and the efficiency and quality of health services [Public Health Service Act, §308(d)]. These statutes prohibit the use of the research information for any purpose other than the purpose for which it was supplied, thus protecting it from use in court, access by families, and access or use by anyone or anything other than the original research project. Because these categories are considered extremely sensitive, the statutory protections are intended to provide an environment conducive to research. The Privacy Act, described earlier, also applies to research records held by government agencies.

Under the Public Health Service Act, certificates of confidentiality are provided as a method to confer privacy protection on persons participating in biomedical, behavioral, clinical, or other research [§301(d)]. A certificate provides a legal defense protecting a researcher from compelled disclosure of names or other identifying information as a result of a subpoena or court order (Gostin, 1995). The protection afforded by a **certificate of confidentiality** is available on a project-by-project basis upon application to the Assistant Secretary of Health or the appropriate designee (National Institutes of Health, 1997). This protection is available for federal and federally funded research activities as well as for research activities with no federal funding (Secretary of Health and Human Services, 1989). According to the Interim Policy Statement regarding the granting of the certificates, the certificates are to be "granted sparingly" (Secretary of Health and Human Services, 1989). The project must involve research of a sensitive nature, including information that if released "could reasonably be damaging to an individual's financial standing, employability, or reputation within the community" or that "could reasonably lead to social stigmatization or discrimination" (Secretary of Health and Human Services, 1989). Even though participation in a research protocol for a condition such as schizophrenia, AIDS, or alcoholism is not an indication of whether the individual has or does not have the condition, the participation can be sufficient to create an atmosphere of suspicion and distrust. The certificates can be a critical device for the protection of genetics research data (Earley & Strong, 1995). In the absence of a certificate of confidentiality, the researcher has an obligation to disclose research information when compelled by subpoena or court order (Fanning, 1997).

The protection of the certificate of confidentiality has been upheld by the New York Court of Appeals (*People v. Newman,* 1973). The doctor in charge of the methadone treatment program in New York City refused to comply with a grand jury subpoena to provide pictures of persons undergoing methadone treatment. The Supreme Court of New York found the doctor in contempt, but on appeal to the Court of Appeals of New York (New York's highest court), the contempt verdict was reversed based on the protection afforded by the certificate of confidentiality. This case was appealed to the United States Supreme Court, but the Court refused to hear it.

Certificates of confidentiality provide a legal defense for researchers from compelled disclosure of names or other identifying information about research participants as a result of a subpoena or court order (Earley & Strong, 1995), but they do not provide legal protection from compelled disclosure for research participants. Thus, individual research participants may be compelled to disclose their research information.

ETHICAL ISSUES FOR THE HIM PROFESSIONAL

HIM professionals need to comply with federal and state legislation concerning genetic information. To do this, they should be conversant with concepts such as the Common Rule, certificates of confidentiality, the HIPAA Privacy Rule, state laws regarding medical record privacy and confidentiality, and whether the laws in their state are preempted

by or supercede the HIPAA Privacy Rule. However, as the scenario that opened this chapter suggests, they also have a broader role: They can be the key to ensuring that these concepts are used to protect the privacy and confidentiality of the individual.

The state laws protecting individuals from genetic discrimination by health insurers and/or employers may have provisions prohibiting health insurers from requesting genetic information or requiring applicants to provide genetic information. But these provisions do not necessarily keep requesters from gaining this information when the request is merely for the medical record and not specifically for the genetic information contained in it. In the opening scenario, does Catherine have a responsibility to screen information before it is released to ensure the protection of Mrs. Jones's privacy? When Mrs. Jones signed the authorization for release of her medical information, she may not have even been aware that her medical records contained genetic information; if she was aware, she may not have considered the possible consequences of having that information fall into the hands of her employer.

CONCLUSION

HIM professionals must be guided first and foremost by the ethical imperative to protect the privacy and confidentiality of patients. Thus, it is their responsibility to ensure that release-of-information practices adhere not only to the letter, but also to the spirit of the law. It is not sufficient for HIM professionals to rely on the ethics and legal expertise of insurers and employers. They must connect expertise and ethical decision making to protect the privacy and confidentiality of patients. These principles hold regardless of the type of medical information but are particularly important when the medical information is potentially predictive, has implications for family members, and may result in stigmatization and discrimination (Fuller & Hudson, 2001).

Key Terms

- Certificate of confidentiality
- Common Rule
- Genetic information
- Genetic testing
- HIPAA Privacy Rule

Chapter Summary

- Genetic research and testing can give researchers, clinicians, and patients a means to prevent, treat, or screen for a disease. Often, however, individuals are reluctant to participate in genetic research and testing because they believe they cannot be sure of the privacy of the genetic information that will be obtained from them and placed in their medical records or in research records.
- Insurers and employers may seek genetic information to identify at-risk individuals and deny them employment or insurance coverage, fire them, or raise their insurance premiums. Genetic information may also be sought in custody battles or in cases of third-party liability. Even when this information is not used to discriminate, individuals may be concerned about its disclosure because of its possibility of causing psychosocial harm, such as harm to family relationships.
- It is difficult to provide special protections for genetic information as a category, because it cannot be clearly separated from other medical information. Therefore, the best way to protect genetic information is to strengthen privacy/confidentiality protections for medical information in general and to enact antidiscrimination legislation.
- The HIPAA Privacy Rule provides a basic level of privacy and confidentiality protection for protected health information. The Privacy Rule does not preempt state laws (including genetic antidiscrimination laws) that offer a higher level of privacy protection.
- The generation of experimental data by a research protocol is not specifically addressed by most state laws.
- HIM professionals have the responsibility to ensure that their practices are guided by state and federal laws and regulations to protect genetic information and by the ethical imperative to protect the privacy and confidentiality of patients.

References

American Medical Association, Council on Ethical and Judicial Affairs. (1991). Use of genetic testing by employers. *Journal of the American Medical Association, 266,* 1827.

Brotherhood of Maintenance of Way Employees v. Burlington Northern Santa Fe R. Co., No. CO1-4012 MWB, 2001 WL 788738 (N.D.Iowa, Apr. 27, 2001).

Clinton, W. (2000, February 8). Remarks at the announcement of the executive order to prohibit discrimination in federal employment based on genetic information. Transcript.

Collins, F. S. (1996, October 4). Remarks before the first meeting of the National Bioethics Advisory Commission, Bethesda, MD.

Cooley, G. (1996, December 23). Flunk the test and lose your insurance. *Newsweek,* 48–50.

Cooley, T. C. (1888). *A treatise on the law of torts,* 2d ed. Chicago: Callaghan.

Earley, C. L., & Strong, L. C. (1995). Certificates of confidentiality: A valuable tool for protecting genetic data. *American Journal of Human Genetics, 57,* 727–731.

Fanning, J. P. (1997, June 9). *Protecting research subjects with certificates of confidentiality.* In-house document prepared for Planning Meeting, Privacy and Confidentiality in Genetics Research, National Institutes of Health. Bethesda, MD: Author.

Fuller, B. P., & Hudson, K. L. (2001). Genetic information. In L. B. Harman (Ed.), *Ethical challenges in the management of health information*, pp. 273–284. Gaithersburg, MD: Aspen.

Geller, L. N., Alper, J. S., Billings, P. R., Barash, C. I., Beckwith, J., & Natowicz, M. R. (1996). Individual, family, and societal dimensions of genetic discrimination: A case study analysis. *Science and Engineering Ethics, 2*(1), 71–88.

Genetic profiles headed for CD-ROM. (1998, September). *Best's Review,* 86.

Genome Action Coalition. (1997). *Statement of principles.* Retrieved April 2, 2001, from http://www.tgac.org.

Gostin, L. O. (1995). Health information privacy. *Cornell Law Review, 80,* 451, 505.

Health Insurance Portability and Accountability Act. (1996). 104 Public Law No. 104–191, 701, 110 Stat 1936.

Health Privacy Project. (2000). *The state of health privacy: An uneven terrain.* Retrieved September 4, 2004, from http://www.healthprivacy.org/resources.

Hudson, K. (2004). Genetic non-discrimination: Examining the implications for workers and employers. Hearing before the Employer-Employee Relations Subcommittee for House Education and the Workforce Committee, 108th Congress, 2nd Session. Statement of Kathy Hudson, Director, Genetics and Public Policy Center.

Hudson, K. L., Rothenberg, K. H., Andrews, L. B., Kahn, M. J. E., & Collins, F. S. (1995). Genetic discrimination and health insurance: An urgent need for reform. *Science, 270,* 391–393.

Kolata, G. (1997, January 4). Advent of testing for breast cancer genes leads to fears of disclosure and discrimination. *New York Times,* C-1, C-3.

Mayo Clinic. (1998, May 5). *IRB policy regarding genetic research.* In-house document. Rochester, MN: Author.

National Action Plan on Breast Cancer and the NIH-DOE Working Group on Ethical, Legal and Social Implications of Human Genome Research. (1996). *Recommendations on genetic information and the workplace.* Bethesda, MD: National Institutes of Health.

National Institutes of Health. (1997, June 13). Minutes of certificate of confidentiality meeting. Bethesda, MD: Author.

Office for Protection from Research Risks. (1993). Protecting human research subjects. Washington, DC: U.S. Government Printing Office.

Omenn, G. S. (1982). Predictive identification of hypersusceptible individuals. *Journal of Occupational Medicine, 24,* 369.

People v. Newman, 345 N.Y.S.2d 502 (1973), 414 U.S. 1163 (1973)(cert denied).

Pharmaceutical Research and Manufacturers of America. (1997). *Principles for maintaining confidentiality of patient-identifiable medical information.* Retrieved February 13, 2004, from http://www.phrma.org .

Reinhardt, C. F. (1978). Chemical hypersusceptibility. *Journal of Occupational Medicine, 20,* 319.

Rothenberg, K. (1995). Genetic information and health insurance: State legislative approaches. *Journal of Law, Medicine and Ethics, 23,* 312–319.

Rothenberg, K., Fuller, B. P., Rothstein, M. A., Duster, T., Ellis Kahn, M. J., Cunningham, R., et al. (1997). Genetic information and the workplace: Legislative approaches and policy challenges. *Science, 275,* 1755–1757.

Rothstein, M. A. (1992). Genetic discrimination in employment and the Americans with Disabilities Act. *Houston Law Review, 29*(38), 23.

Rothstein, M. A. (1994–1995). The use of genetic information for nonmedical purposes. *Journal of Law and Health, 9,* 109.

Rothstein, M. A. (1996). Preventing the discovery of plaintiff genetic profiles by defendants seeking to limit damages in personal injury litigation. *Indiana Law Journal, 71,* 877.

Secretary of Health and Human Services. (1989, May 22). *Protection of identity: Research subjects.* Interim Policy Statement. Washington, DC: Department of Health and Human Services.

Task Force on Genetic Testing. (1998). *Promoting safe and effective genetic testing in the United States.* Baltimore: Johns Hopkins University Press.

Tomes, J. P. (1996). *Compliance guide to electronic health records.* New York: Faulkner & Gray.

U.S. National Commission for the Protection of Human Subjects of Biomedical Research. (1979). The Belmont Report: Ethical principles for the protection of human subjects. *Federal Register, 44,* 23192–23197.

Wadman, M. (1998). Genome panel defends researchers'—and families'—interests. *Nature, 391,* 826.

The ethical decision-making matrix is a tool to help you organize complex, ethical problems; however, there is no simple fill-in-the-box approach to ethical decision making. The objective is to follow each step of the process and not move from the question directly to what should be done or how to prevent it next time. If you skip steps, you will not fully understand all of the values and options for action. Also, the matrix provided for each scenario in this book is not the only way to examine the problem. You can make an equally compelling ethical argument for a different decision—just be sure to follow all the steps of the matrix.

SCENARIO 18-A: GENETIC PRIVACY

Steps	Information	
1. What is the ethical question?	Should Catherine release the genetic information to the employer?	
2. What are the facts?	**KNOWN**	**TO BE GATHERED**
	• The local business has requested Mrs. Jones's medical record. • There is information in the record from a genetic test. • State legislature has passed legislation that prohibits employers from obtaining genetic information.	• Would Catherine's sending the entire record break the law? • Is there any reason Catherine would have to include the genetic information in the record? • What is the customary practice in such cases? • What does Catherine's boss or supervisor expect her to do? • What is the likely impact on self and family of changing jobs?
3. What are the values? Examine the shared and competing values, obligations, and interests of the stakeholders (i.e., patient, HIM professional, healthcare practitioner(s), administrators, society, and other advocates) involved in order to fully understand the complexity of the ethical problem(s).	**Patient:** Values confidentiality of the medical record; has an interest in getting the job. **HIM professional:** Integrity; comply with laws, regulations, and policies; avoid harm (disclosing genetic information could cause patient to lose job offer); protect medical and social information. **Employer:** Wants as much accurate medical information as possible without violating the law. **Society:** Protect genetic information on medical records.	

4. What are my options?	• Send the entire record to the employer. • Omit the genetic test information for the information transmitted to the employer.	
5. What should I do?	Omit the information on the genetic test in the information transmitted to the employer.	
6. What justifies my choice?	**JUSTIFIED**	**NOT JUSTIFIED**
	• Obey the law. • Protect patient confidentiality. • Preserve professional integrity.	• Send entire record. • Break the law. • Break confidentiality. • Jeopardize professional integrity.
7. How can I prevent this ethical problem?	• Determine if system changes are needed. • Learn more about issues surrounding legislation and the release of genetic medical information. • Discuss standards and the values that support them with colleagues.	

ADOPTION INFORMATION

Martha L. Jones, PhD, LSW

Learning Objectives

After completing this chapter, the reader should be able to:

- Identify the historical roots of current ethical issues in adoption.
- Identify current ethical issues related to adoption situations that health information management (HIM) professionals may be confronted with.
- Identify implications of ethical issues for adoption as they relate to other emerging areas for HIM decision making.
- Identify possible responses to ethical dilemmas for HIM professionals in adoption situations.

Abstract

Adoption is an arena in which traditional assumptions regarding access to health information among relatives are being reconsidered. Previous reliance on legal secrecy in these relationships is being challenged as more importance is being placed on the right of individuals to know their biological heritage. Further, families in which children are not biologically related to one or either parent are increasingly being created by new reproductive technologies. Although these families are not currently considered adoptive, their creation raises ethical issues regarding access to familial information that are similar to the issues raised by adoption. Health information management (HIM) professionals will be increasingly confronted with issues related to access to medical information, and adoption provides a useful framework for considering them.

Scenario 19-A: Seeking Information Many Years Later

Anna and Bob Snyder are the adoptive parents of Charlie, a lively nine-year-old boy who has been with them since he was three days old. The Snyders are fairly well known and well respected in this medium-sized community. Anna volunteers with church activities and helps with various community fund-raising projects. Bob is a school principal and is considered one of the leaders in this upscale community of professionals.

Both Anna and Bob are very open about their adoption experience. After struggling for years with infertility, they finally heard, through friends, of this baby that was to be born and given up for adoption. The birth mother, Carolee, was young and looking for help. Her family doctor, Sam Gruen, knew the Snyders socially and arranged for the adoption to be done discreetly and quickly. Anna remembers meeting Carolee at the local fast-food restaurant and trying to make a good impression on the young woman so that she would let them adopt her baby. They all agreed with Dr. Gruen's suggestion that they not learn too much about each other—just first names and some general things about shared values.

Although Carolee had come late for prenatal care, there appeared to be no problems with the pregnancy, and Charlie was born strong and healthy. The Snyders were thrilled to bring him home and held their breath until the legal work was complete so that he was totally theirs. Until the adoption decree was signed, they worried that Carolee might change her mind and want Charlie back, but they never thought about needing to know more than they did about her social and health history.

Dr. Gruen knew little about Carolee's background. She came from the "poor part of town," never did very well in school, and always seemed rather quiet to him. He was surprised to hear of the pregnancy, but because she appeared healthy and was sure that she didn't want to keep the baby, he thought it was a great opportunity for the Snyders. Carolee never volunteered much information about the baby's father, Derek, and Dr. Gruen didn't push the subject—the young man seemed willing to go along with adoption, and no one wanted to have anything go wrong.

The Snyders are now seeking more information on Carolee and Derek's medical history. Dr. Gruen has passed away, and his records are now part of a large healthcare center with connections to the hospital where Charlie was born.

The request for more information comes after a stressful childhood. Charlie has always had trouble in school, with difficulty concentrating and following instructions. These problems are becoming more pronounced as he gets older, and Bob is beginning to think that there might be some hereditary factors at work. For the past couple of years, Anna and Bob have talked about trying to find out more about Charlie's extended family history, but now they believe that it is crucial to learn more about his parentage.

In addition to the learning disability, Charlie has developed a serious medical condition that could well be life-threatening, although a final diagnosis has not yet been established. The physical symptoms are somewhat confusing to the specialists involved, and they are asking for more complete background information to help them with the diagnosis. The Snyders want to have access to medical records for Charlie's birth mother and father and then possibly for other extended family members. Because it is now likely that Charlie will need a transplant in the future, it seems imperative that they know as much as possible about who might be a donor for him.

The Snyders also argue that Carolee needs to know about Charlie's condition, because if she has other children, they might be at risk. The same holds true for Charlie's birth father and any of his relatives. There is also some concern that something may have occurred during Carolee's pregnancy that might explain Charlie's condition. The Snyders are convinced that her medical records might show some possible drug use or other prenatal experience that could shed light on their son's health.

You are the HIM professional responsible for the records. A review of the records shows that Carolee had one abortion before her pregnancy with Charlie and was successfully treated for a venereal disease during the pregnancy. She has married and given birth to two other children who live in a nearby community. Both of those children appear to be healthy. Records for Derek are sparse, but there does appear to be some neurological disorders and a history of drug abuse. However, among Derek's records is a blood test from several years ago, and you notice that his blood type is such that it is possible he is not Charlie's biological father.

Questions

1. Does this constitute an ethical issue? What are the core values involved here?

2. Do you have sufficient information with which to make a decision regarding the release of any information?

3. Is the information about Charlie's prenatal care, including his mother's treatment for venereal disease, his information or hers?

4. What is your personal belief regarding which, if any, information should be shared, and with whom?

5. What does your professional code of ethics tell you with regard to addressing this set of requests for information?

6. Does the Snyders' request constitute a true need to know?

7. Does the birth mother have a right to have her medical records kept private even when doing so could threaten her biological child's life?

A completed ethical decision-making matrix for the scenario is provided at the end of the chapter.

The ethical issues related to the appropriate sharing of health information are extremely important when brought into the arena of adoption. At first glance, the choice to examine adoption may seem to be focusing on a small minority population and to raise issues that, though interesting, are limited in application. However, adoption will affect a larger population than is commonly recognized as reproductive technologies and the availability of genetic information increase in both use and importance. Adoptions can become a platform for discussion of emerging issues of family, parenthood, and identity—issues related to the right to and need for access to health information. HIM professionals will increasingly be participating in decisions as to when and if health information about biologically related individuals may be shared.

This chapter first presents a brief history of adoption, including some of the basic terms and themes that have influenced social and family relationships surrounding the adoption experience. An overview of some of the long-standing and emerging ethical issues in adoption is provided to assist the reader in anticipating and putting into context both current and future adoption-related issues facing the HIM professional. The **adoption triad**—the key individuals involved in adoption, namely, the person who is adopted, the biological parents of that individual, and the parent(s) who adopted—is also discussed.

The chapter also discusses the ethical issues that HIM professionals may encounter regarding adoption, beginning with the scenario that opened this chapter and two additional scenarios. Each scenario is presented from the perspective of one party to the adoption and is meant to generate discussion and to highlight the dilemmas inherent in these relationships. Readers are encouraged to take multiple views of each story and to identify ways to approach resolutions in real-life situations. Discussion of these scenarios illustrates ways of addressing the issues. For example, can you make equally compelling arguments to release or not to release the information to the biological mother in Scenario 19-C?

The final section of this chapter identifies some emerging issues with regard to the impact of reproductive technologies. Families created through artificial insemination, donor eggs, and other technologies are not currently considered adoptive families. However, I will argue that some of the ethical dilemmas already being considered in the world of adoption will affect those families created through reproductive technologies.

ADOPTION: HISTORICAL AND EMERGING ETHICAL ISSUES

It is estimated that between 2% and 4% of families in the United States have adopted a child (Moorman & Hernandez, 1989; Mosher & Bachrach, 1996). Although some adoptions are by relatives or stepparents to a child, most appear to be adoption of a child into a family not biologically related to that child (National Adoption Information Clearinghouse, 2004). Although the total number of adopted individuals in this country is not known, estimates from a number of years ago range from as few as 1 million to as many as 5 million. Adoptions appear to be increasing (National Adoption Information Clearinghouse, 2004). Certainly the open discussion of adoption is on the rise. The demand for information about family and health background for people affected by adoption is one surrounded by much emotion and increasing political advocacy. HIM professionals will increasingly be confronted by the individuals and families impacted by adoption.

The closed nature of these proceedings has led them to be referred to as **closed adoptions** and reflect a number of legal and social issues. Adoption in the United States has an interesting legal and social history that is useful to help frame some of the issues being addressed in this chapter. The following background is meant to give a broad overview of some of the themes that emerge in discussions about adoption, ethics, rights, and needs.

Adoption is a legal status in which the parental rights and responsibilities of one set of parents are legally terminated and a new parental relationship is established by law. The **adoptive parents** are then granted the full rights and responsibilities as the parents of the person being adopted (the **adoptee**). The original birth certificate for the adoptee is changed to reflect this new legal status. Traditionally, all records related to the adoption are sealed, and none of the parties are allowed access to the records without special court approval. In some states, the original birth certificate is sealed and not made available to any party to the adoption.

The legality and secrecy surrounding adoption reflect several social issues. The strong legal base is generally thought to have roots in English laws of inheritance brought to this country. In situations where there was no heir, a legal provision to pass on property and wealth was provided through adoption law. This remains a strong component of current adoption law, in which an adoptee is eligible, for example, for social security, insurance, and other benefits of the adoptive parent just as fully as any child born to the family. The provision of adoption allowed for orphans to become legal heirs to families without children, and until recently "Orphans Court" was the jurisdiction for most adoption cases.

The secrecy has other roots as well. The inability to conceive a child has long been viewed as a loss to the couple experiencing infertility. At times, such couples feel stigmatized due to their childlessness. Likewise, unwed parenthood has a long history of being viewed as unacceptable, with children born "out of wedlock" being labeled as "bastards." The dictionary definition of *bastard* is "a person born of unmarried parents; an illegitimate child." Such terminology certainly speaks to the historical nature of stigma attached to children born to single mothers. Adoption became a way in which both the infertile couple and the unwed parents could be "helped." Homes for unwed mothers were established where a pregnant woman could go away from her community until her child was born and then return with some cover story about where she was for a year. The adoptive family joined in the secrecy, sometimes even faking a pregnancy and coming home with their new baby after a short trip. During the mid-twentieth century, this form of adoption became very common.

Adoption agencies during these years supported such practices. Families were selected on the basis of their proof of infertility, children were matched with families to look as much like the adoptive parents as possible, and secrecy was paramount. The unwed mother wanted assurance of privacy, and agencies promised that no one would come around later to disclose this past indiscretion. Adoptive families wanted the assurance that the birth family would not come looking to disrupt their legally constructed family, either by trying to take the child back or by wanting to be involved in the life of the child.

Significant changes began with the combined introduction of birth control pills and the sexual revolution of the 1960s. Unplanned pregnancies were both not as necessary and not as stigmatized. This combined set of circumstances drove down the number of children available for adoption just as the concept of adopting as an acceptable way to build a family was catching on. By the late 1970s, families wanting to adopt began to actively advocate for the adoption of children not previously considered for adoption. Over the next 20 years, children with different racial backgrounds, those with physical and emotional challenges, and older children all became potential adoptees. Language changed from labeling children as "unadoptable" to "hard to place" to labeling them as having "special needs" and finally simply as "waiting" for adoption. The term *older child,* which at one point meant age 2 years or older, has changed to 12 to 18 years, and sibling groups of all sizes are now regularly placed for adoption.

Children are no longer matched to look like their adoptive parents, and transracial adoptions have become routine. Adoptions from Korea, China, and South America have contributed to a very different appearance of many American families by the early twenty-first century. Many Caucasian families began adopting Korean orphans, and now it is common to see white families with children of Korean, Chinese, or African American heritage. Although some families still travel to Russia, Poland, or other eastern European countries to adopt a child of similar racial heritage to themselves, there is a growing subculture of multiethnic families created through adoption.

The emphasis on secrecy in adoptions is being challenged at many levels. Obviously, with significant numbers of children who are of a totally different race from their adoptive parents, there is no pretense that the child was born into the family. From a psychological perspective, there has been growing evidence that birth parents and adoptees have increasingly wanted to meet each other to share stories and to know what happened. Healthcare and medical research have added to the discussions regarding more openness or **open adoptions** as individuals increasingly believe that who they are is based to a significant extent on their genetic heritage.

The current state of adoption reflects the full range of this history. The long history of secrecy, for example, helps to explain the very difficult task of trying to identify the total number of individuals affected by adoption. What we do know, however, is that for each person who has been adopted, at least three other individuals are directly affected: a set of birth parents and at least one adoptive parent. Beyond this are siblings, grandparents, cousins, and other relatives—all of whom may at some point feel a need to explore the previously well-kept secret of adoption. A good test of the extent of adoption's impact is to bring the subject up at random social events to see how many people will identify having some connection to an adoption.

The long history of secrecy in adoptions is based on an ethical stance that would argue for the right of birth parents who decide to place a child for adoption to have a guarantee that their privacy will be maintained. Conventional wisdom in the adoption field has also maintained that families need this guarantee of future privacy for adoptions to be most beneficial to all concerned. Indeed, some activists continue to argue that failure to guarantee secrecy will result in decisions to seek abortion rather than adoption in situations of unplanned pregnancies.

There is, however, a growing school of thought that openness among the members of the adoption triad is more beneficial to all. The most conservative arguments for openness are based on a belief that adoptees and adoptive parents need to know about the health history of birth parents. With the growing emphasis in the medical community on the role of hereditary and genetic factors in physical, mental, and even emotional health, the adoptee is at an obvious disadvantage when seeking health care. Even when birth parents provided what they thought was full information on family health

history prior to the adoption, new information is always unfolding. Health problems in a family may emerge, may be differently diagnosed, or may make more sense as a pattern as medical and genetic research links previously unconnected phenomena.

Consider, for example, a situation with regard to the prevalence of breast cancer in families. In an adoptive situation, the birth parents might not have even known to disclose a history of breast cancer in family members. When you live with the family you are genetically related to, you know about new cases of such a disease and may also become involved in searching out other cases in the family tree. However, in the case of a closed adoption, there is no way to know whether this newly recognized health threat is one to be concerned about.

There is an increasing recognition that adoptees need to know about health information. Attempts to maintain the privacy of both parties while providing nonidentifying health information are resulting in the establishment of certain health information registries. Birth parents can provide ongoing health information updates for the adoptee's use, and vice versa. Privacy is maintained for each party to the extent that names are not exchanged and the information shared is voluntary and self-reported.

The limitations of such registries are fairly obvious. At a minimum, reporting is based on the active registration of information. Often even competent adults are not fully aware of the implications of some potentially significant medical or other health information. Also, individuals often do not really understand the specifics of their own diagnoses. In the area of mental health, there are even greater challenges, because a mental illness may itself preclude the individual from accurately reporting such vital information.

The argument that one has a right to know one's own biological heritage is quite compelling. Those who are not adopted take for granted simple things like knowing who else in the family has ears like theirs or who has red hair, or even how often the men have drinking problems. When we prepare for the births of our children we generally have relatively easy access to information about risk factors in our family history. This access to information is not readily available to the adult adoptee (nor to an individual conceived through sperm or egg donation). One might easily argue that the *need* to know can be translated into a *right* to know. Political action may well lead to the establishment of legal rights to have access to certain information that has previously been considered off limits.

Although the history of adoption may have emphasized privacy, there is a growing movement toward more openness. Members of this school of thought argue that the secrecy of records violates the rights of adoptees to know who they really are. They stress the importance of having access to original birth certificates and ultimately the right to make contact with birth parents. This increasingly active group believes that adult adoptees should be able to have access to information about their biological and social heritage and see it as a civil right. They argue that most birth parents are, in fact, willing and eager to be found and to know about the child they relinquished for adoption. This is a difficult proposition to document empirically due to the current laws regarding privacy, thus leaving much of the debate in the arena of personal conviction and experience.

This possible changing of the rules regarding what one has a right to know from healthcare records directly affects the decisions HIM professionals will be called upon to make. A request for personal records seems simple on the face of it. Few would argue that an adult, or even the adoptive parents of a minor, should have access to healthcare records regarding the adoptee's birth. However, the need to know more about the health of the birth mother is the first step in opening information that would not necessarily be available to a third party.

Did the mother have any illnesses during pregnancy or take any medications that might be significant to understanding current or future health of the adoptee? Who should make the decision as to which information in the birth mother's background should be shared as part of a child's birth history and which kept confidential? Once the door is open to knowing the birth mother's health history, it is a small step to wanting to know something about the father—perhaps not so directly as with particular birth information, but certainly for potential hereditary patterns.

The previously unquestioned need for privacy is now being challenged by strongly held feelings of a need, or even right, to know. Much of the rhetoric for these arguments is rooted in the perceived need to know the health history of blood relatives. These issues are being addressed through the growth of activist organizations, legal challenges, and even changes in adoption laws. HIM professionals will be at the center of many of the issues that previously were totally in the realm of adoption agencies and the courts.

WHO'S WHO IN ADOPTION: SOME EXPLANATIONS OF TERMINOLOGY

Every profession has its own jargon, and adoption is no different. As noted previously, certain terms have changed in meaning over the years, and new terminology has replaced old concepts. Social pressures have encouraged the change of some terms to be more sensitive to the feelings of individuals involved in adoption, and this has led to other changes in usage for some words. A complete listing of terms is provided in the Key Terms at the end of this chapter, but the following section discusses some of the terms currently in use, some of which have historical significance and may be used by individuals in the field of adoption in ways that differ from the ways in which these same terms are used in general conversation.

A few comments about terminology seem important in the context of this chapter. Adoption is a social and legal phenomenon. The words used to describe relationships between members of the adoption triad represent this social context more than the purely legal or scientific relationships. The historically simple question of who are one's father and mother was changed when laws established the bonds of parenthood between unrelated children and adults. Words have evolved to clarify and sanction the new forms of relationships, and they have grown largely out of the social context.

Let's begin with the apparently simple terms *mother* and *father*. For many years, the term **natural mother** was used to refer to the woman who gave birth to a child given up for adoption. Adoptive mothers took issue with this term, arguing that by inference they were "unnatural" mothers. Thus, the terms **biological mother** and more recently **birth mother** became the vogue. However, as we look at new reproductive technologies, these terms may need to be reconsidered in order to be technically accurate. When there is a donor egg, is the donor the biological mother? When there is a second gestational carrier of that egg, is she then the actual birth mother? For those managing health information records, the question of what information about either mother is essential for the child to know about his or her relevant birth history becomes quite a challenge. Were there, for example, health issues during the pregnancy, such as excessive drinking or drug abuse? Likewise, are there genetic issues with the egg donor that are relevant to the birth record history that a child might actually need to know?

Definitions of *fatherhood* are similarly blurred. The adoption field has used such terms as **legal father** (i.e., the man married to the mother when the child was born/conceived), **natural father, biological father, birth father,** and finally **putative,** or **alleged, father.**

The last term refers to the man who is presumed to be the father. Recent advances in DNA testing have made it possible to eliminate the guesswork as to who is the biological father of a child, but many of the social and legal issues remain. Adoption deals with terminating the rights and responsibilities of all "fathers" who have legal claim or responsibility for a child. Recently, individuals fathered by sperm donors have become active in questioning their relationship to their biological father, even raising questions about legal and financial responsibility.

A couple of other terms that are being used in the adoption field are of significance to the HIM professional. First is the concept of **"full disclosure,"** an imprecisely defined term that has been increasingly used in both law and policy. As adoptees and adoptive parents become more concerned about the genetic and biological roots of physical, mental, and emotional health, more emphasis has been placed on the obligation of adoptive professionals to ensure the full disclosure of relevant background information. What is relevant information and how much is sufficient is not clear. Professionals in HIM may well be called upon to help define these legal and ethical boundaries.

Finally, the term **wrongful adoption** is increasingly being used. Families have brought suit against medical and adoption professionals for withholding or providing misleading information about real or potential problems with the child being adopted. The idea that information in the health history of relatives of a child is essential to the adopting parents is gaining more importance. There are some significant challenges to existing assumptions about people's right to privacy if they must share everything in order to place a child for adoption. It seems likely that this same demand for information, and potential legal action for failure to fully disclose, will extend to situations in which children are created through reproductive technologies with donor eggs, sperm, and gestational carriers.

ETHICAL ISSUES FOR HIM PROFESSIONALS

The scenario that opened this chapter and the additional scenarios presented in this section, all from the perspectives of different parties in the adoption triad, raise many possible issues for discussion. Current movements for greater openness of records make it likely that any member of the adoption triad may attempt to gain information through HIM professionals. It is important to recognize that multiple ethical dilemmas can arise from situations that may initially appear rather simple. In particular, definitions of rights and needs may be quite different depending on the personal or professional positions of the people who assert them. Likewise, attempts must be made to determine which of the four core principles of principle-based ethics—respect for autonomy (self-determination), nonmaleficence (not harming), beneficence (promoting good), and justice (fairness) (Beauchamp & Childress, 1994; see Chapter 2 of this book)—is affected by the decisions of the HIM professional and may be open to significant differences in interpretation. All members of the adoption triad may seek information about each other.

Adoptive Parents Seek Information on Their Adopted Child

Review Scenario 19-A and the questions that follow it at the beginning of this chapter. The questions and the discussion here are meant as a starting point for informed talk about the issues involved. Readers are encouraged to take multiple views of the case and to consider similar situations that the HIM professional might face.

It would appear that one could keep the Snyders' case from presenting an ethical dilemma by narrowly limiting the scope of the inquiry. The Snyders could easily have access to Charlie's medical records, but this would not address their request. The situation presents ethical considerations on many levels for the HIM professional.

The Snyders are not able to make fully informed medical decisions regarding their adoptive son's health care without information from the healthcare records of his biological parents. This raises the core principle of self-determination and the value of allowing individuals to make decisions regarding their health care (and their children's) with full information at their disposal. Withholding of information by the HIM professional could be viewed as interfering with the family's right to self-determination.

The next core principle has to do with not causing harm. The Snyders are arguing that failure to share information will cause harm because they will not be able to obtain the proper diagnosis and treatment for their son without it. Beyond this, they believe that the information will be beneficial. The family certainly believes that they need the information, even though they may not have the formal right to information about Charlie's birth relatives.

The formal rights to privacy that are granted by adoption law and rules of confidentiality with regard to personal healthcare records conflict with the Snyders' request. It is possible that the health history of the mother and her family would have no useful impact on the care and treatment of this child. It is also possible that releasing this information would violate Carolee's trust in the healthcare institution, hurt her current marriage and extended-family relationships, and open up an emotionally painful relationship with Charlie and the Snyders. The Snyders are a prominent family and they may be able to exert various forms of pressure on Carolee or members of her extended family to be subject to tests for transplant compatibility or other involvement. If there turns out to be no correlation whatsoever with Charlie's problems and his mother and the rest of her family, disclosure will produce no benefit, only harm.

If it turns out that the individual named as the father of this child is not in fact biologically related, there could be significant negative repercussions. One possible impact could be that the adoption of Charlie by the Snyders might be considered nonbinding, with legal action to set aside the adoption in favor of the actual biological father, who did not have the chance to exercise his rights previously. In short, there could be any number of significant social and legal consequences to opening information that might or might not produce a positive result.

What makes this an interesting ethical dilemma for the HIM professional is that there is no simple answer. It does help to know what the specific laws, rules, and rights are, but this is just a start. The questions of who needs to know what and whether know-ing would be beneficial are very difficult to answer definitively. As with all ethical dilemmas, we need to look at personal and professional value systems and professional standards and recognize conflicting positions.

The HIM professional is the guardian of information that may not be available to adoptees in other ways. The perceived need to know such information about biological relatives who are not otherwise available can make for a very strong and emotional argument to disclose that information. HIM professionals need to continue talking about the implications for disclosure and the ethics of maintaining privacy versus sharing. For the adoptee looking for information, the HIM professional may be one of the only available resources. It is important to recognize the potential ethical implications of various actions.

Scenario 19-B: An Adoptee Seeks Information on Her Biological Family

Francine is an adult adoptee in her late 20s who has recently married. She says that she grew up in a very loving family, but that for many years she has had questions about her birth parents. "It's not that I don't love my adoptive family," says Francine, "but I wonder about my roots—who I came from, what my kids might inherit, things like that." At this point in her life, she is feeling a stronger desire to search out more information about her family background.

Francine brings up a couple of specific things that she wonders about. First, her husband's family is very involved in genealogy, so she obviously feels awkward when those discussions come up. She cannot really refer to her adoptive family tree as her own, though she is legally related to them. As she and her husband, Tom, begin planning to have children, she recognizes that it is important to know more about what she brings as traits and risk factors. Tom's family does have some history of genetic risks. Francine feels it is very important that she be able to find out her birth family's history. The information could determine whether she will decide to get pregnant and the degree of risk involved for their child.

Also, Francine has questions about her racial background that have never been fully addressed. She thinks that by gaining access to some of her birth parents' medical history she will get some of the answers that she knows are missing. Although raised by a white family of German and English background, Francine clearly has some heritage of darker skin. Her parents have always been a little vague about this heritage—maybe Native American, Mediterranean, or African American. Now that she is thinking of having children, this lack of specificity has become more crucial. Francine has some serious question as to what her children might look like depending upon what her racial mix truly is.

Francine has gone to the court where her adoption took place for permission to see her adoption records. After getting a court order authorizing the agency that did the adoption to provide her with information, she has reviewed the records that the agency kept. Her next step is to come to you, the keeper of medical records for her birth parents. She is asking for as much information as possible, not only about her parents, but also about other relatives, so that she can see if there are risk factors for several potential conditions that she knows run in her husband's family, including a risk for cystic fibrosis. She is also specifically interested to find out the racial heritage of her immediate and extended birth relatives.

Questions

1. Does this constitute an ethical issue? What are the core values involved here?

2. Is there a difference between seeking information about genetic risks versus racial characteristics?

3. Do you have sufficient information with which to make a decision regarding the release of any information?

4. If Francine weren't adopted but were asking for similar information about relatives, would you think that the request should be treated any differently?

5. What is your personal belief regarding what should be made available to this woman?

6. What does your professional code of ethics tell you with regard to addressing this set of requests for information?

7. Does Francine's request constitute a true need to know?

8. How does a court order authorizing the release of the adoption records affect your decision?

A completed ethical decision-making matrix for the scenario is provided at the end of the chapter.

The ethical issues in Scenario 19-B again point to questions of how far the HIM professional can go in disclosure of information. The actual legal right to Francine's medical information has been clearly determined through the court, but the HIM professional still needs to address the question of where to draw the line as to how much information to provide.

The emotional issue of not knowing who one is genetically related to is one that the HIM professional may find quite compelling. Each of the four core principles might well be interpreted to value open sharing of information, because the only way to guarantee autonomy and self-determination is with good knowledge. However, once again we are faced with the ethical dilemma regarding the right of one member of the adoption triad to privacy versus the rights of those who want to know.

This case is less compelling than the first with regard to the immediate need to know based on a specific medical concern. Francine's interest in knowing her heritage is driven more by curiosity than by something that can be strongly shown as immediate necessity. Still, if there is some important background that opening of medical records could show, would that not be potentially beneficial to this woman and her future children?

If one accepts this premise, the implications become quite significant. Suppose, for example, that Francine was not adopted but was conceived through artificial insemina-

tion. Would she not still find it important to know about the health history of this unknown father, and then beyond this to any other children he had after her birth? In both situations, Francine does not have the option of either observing her parents' health or asking relevant questions. The HIM professional may be the keeper of information vital to her own health and to that of her children.

Scenario 19-C: A Birth Mother Seeks Information on Her Biological Son

Marlene Baxter is a 45-year-old woman who was recently admitted to a healthcare facility in a neighboring community. She is in urgent need of a transplant and initially said that there were no living relatives to check for a possible match. Now that her situation is worsening, she tells her physician that as a teen she gave birth to a baby boy and subsequently placed him for adoption. Her family did not know of this, and she had kept the secret all these years. However, now that she is so ill, she has been thinking of him as a possible donor.

Marlene would like to know if her son is alive and could be a donor and if he might be at risk for developing the same illness that now threatens her life. She believes that if his health records could be checked, and if someone could contact him to give him appropriate warnings, he could be tested and could take appropriate precautions.

Marlene's husband is emphatic that every step must be taken to locate a donor organ to save his wife. He was surprised to learn about this child's existence and sees it as a great opportunity to possibly locate a donor. Mr. Baxter is convinced that if this son knew of his birth mother's situation he would be eager to participate in her treatment. He wants the records checked to see if the young man might be a possible match. If not, then he wouldn't need to be contacted.

The Baxters make their request to you, the HIM professional for the facility that has records of the birth and subsequent medical care of this young man. You review the material available and see that the young man is generally healthy, but you have no way of knowing whether he is even a potential match for his birth mother. Because the Baxters seem to know the name of this young man, you assume that this may be an open adoption, but you do not know exactly what the relationship is. The Baxters insist that Marlene, as his mother, should have some rights with regard to knowledge pertaining to her son.

Time is running out. You are being pressured by the hospital administrator and Marlene's physician, both of whom are friends of the Baxters. They want you to check the medical records and give the information to all of the parties. There is a strong sense of urgency that this woman's one last chance for the treatment she needs rests with you and your quick sharing of information.

Questions

1. Does this constitute an ethical issue? What are the core values involved here?

2. Do you have sufficient information with which to make a decision regarding release of any information?

3. What do you personally believe is right to do in this case?

4. What does your professional code of ethics tell you with regard to addressing this request for information?

5. Does the request for information have any validity?

A completed ethical decision-making matrix for the scenario is provided at the end of the chapter.

Once again we have a situation in which there appears to be a medically compelling reason to share information that might otherwise have been kept private. It is important in this scenario to recognize the concern about the right of the son to privacy as provided legally through the adoption. The young man in question may not want to have contact or interaction with this woman. Perhaps an intermediary, such as a social worker or adoption professional, should be the one to make contact and to share appropriate information.

In the larger context, the issue of birth parents' making use of HIM professionals to locate and initiate contact with the children they gave up for adoption should be examined. The same situation could arise with children conceived through egg donation or artificial insemination. If the biological parents of any of these children begin to seek them out, there will be more challenges to the HIM professional to make wise and ethical decisions regarding sharing or not sharing family information.

FUTURE ISSUES

The previous scenarios represent fairly typical situations that may be brought to HIM professionals by members of the adoption triad. Issues that might ordinarily be discussed among family members, such as risks for certain illnesses or conditions, cannot occur when there is no contact between the parties. This lack of basic information about one's identity can be highly emotional for adoptees, who may argue that this is a right they are denied—a right to basic information about who they are.

Adoptive parents may advocate for access to information when their adopted child begins to exhibit suspicious symptoms. Without a strong family medical history, they often feel handicapped in helping to diagnose a problem. Even when an adoption agency was diligent in collecting information at the time of the adoption, new advances in the healthcare field now require data that was not asked about before. In areas such as mental illness, an early diagnosis might be better made with information about other family members.

Other arguments, however, emphasize the need to recognize the privacy rights of individuals. There is fear in some areas that although the request may be framed in terms of the need to know medical information, the adoptee or birth parent is really trying to get identifying information in order to contact his or her parent or child. The contact could be upsetting, could become harassment, or could otherwise be very difficult for extended family members. The innocent sharing of some piece of information might just be the clue needed to locate someone who did not want to be found and exposed.

Another emerging issue has to do with how much of a parent's background might be used to stigmatize a child for whom adoption is the plan. What if there is a history of mental illness and alcohol abuse? If the full extent of the problem is not understood by the birth parents, should the healthcare industry be responsible for providing information? Is it wrong not to inform adoptive parents that a child is at high risk to become schizophrenic? However, if possible families are told, will the child not get adopted and instead end up in the foster care system for his or her whole life?

This balance between the right to privacy and the need or right to know family background is not easily resolved, but we can expect that it will increasingly need to be dealt with. The adoption community is already identifying the ethical issues and becoming vocal about articulating some of them. These issues provide a starting point for looking at future ethical issues related to family health histories and the sharing of that information. Recent changes to more openness are partially informed by generations of individuals involved in adoption who are reporting that secrecy is not the best approach. The growing importance of genetic research emphasizes the role of "nature" over "nurture" as a significant factor in who we are. Adoptive parents and adoptees are increasingly demanding information on biological family members to complete the picture of identity.

The laws regarding individuals' parental rights and responsibilities toward a child who is not born to them are part of adoption law, and much of the ethical discussion regarding these legally created families is in the field of adoption. However, an increasing number of families are being created through various reproductive technologies

that have not been subject to these legal and social debates.

The use of artificial insemination has followed some of the same secrecy patterns as adoption has. Couples dealing with infertility have gone for medical treatments, including artificial insemination. Families have rarely talked about the specifics of the procedure, and children have been raised as if they were the children of both parents. A term does not even exist for children to use to identify themselves as the children of their mother and an anonymous father who donated sperm. The use of sperm donors has broadened to become a fairly common practice for single and lesbian women.

The greater openness about sperm donation is leading to more discussion of rights, needs, and ethical decisions. Children conceived through artificial insemination are beginning to ask some of the same questions as adoptees. The questions about health history are the first to arise and these may lead to other questions regarding the responsibilities of the men who technically fathered these children. Likewise, the men who donated sperm are becoming aware that they may have children to whom they owe some responsibility, at least for the sharing of health information. For some donors, several children may be involved.

More recently, we have begun to see the use of egg donation as a technology to assist the infertile couple. The possibility now exists to conceive a child from a donated egg and a donated sperm and even have the child carried to term by a third person, or gestational carrier. The child might then be raised by the couple who paid for the procedures; however, the child would have no biological tie to either of the parents.

The ethical issues with regard to the sharing of health information become even more complex when we consider the implications of these new technologies. If we have established guidelines for access to medical and other health records for adoptees, then they should also apply to this newer group of individuals. The health background of the biological father, the biological mother, and the gestational carrier may all be significant for understanding the health risks for a child.

We cannot separate dialogue about health information from the social implications. Adoption establishes a legal family bond between individuals who are not genetically related. The questions of rights for birth parents, adoptees, and adoptive parents with regard to information about one another can be dealt with by the most strict interpretation of rights—that is, legally. But families created through artificial insemination, egg donation, or a combination of such technologies are currently less clearly defined from a legal standpoint.

In the scenarios presented earlier, there was a common theme that the biological ties between two individuals might be important to both at certain times. Might it not be argued that an egg donor's medical history could be crucial to the diagnosis and treatment of the son created through that donation, who is now ill? Furthermore, should the egg donor be given information about her son's illness, either for her own need to know or for her to be considered for a transplant of some sort?

However, shouldn't there be some guarantee of privacy and protection from intrusion by others who believe that biological ties supersede all others? If a man donates sperm with the guarantee that he will have no further responsibility, shouldn't that be respected? If the donation of sperm or eggs means the loss of privacy regarding all medical and health information, is this not exceeding the terms of any reasonable agreement?

Several significant issues are raised about health information and its management as we examine adoption and some of these emerging family relationships. First is the question of identity. To the extent that individuals believe that their identity is solely or primarily based on biology, they will consider access to health records crucial. The le-

gal rights to access are based on policy and law, so that as more emphasis is placed on the genetic basis of identity, it is likely that there will be increased demand for family background information through access to health records. Adoptees do not have the same access to daily information about biological family background as others do, so they may need to rely on other sources, such as records. The growing population of individuals conceived through donor eggs and sperm will also need to rely on health records, because the specific individuals are not available to them for information.

Second, the right to privacy of one's own health information in the situations we have been discussing here seems to be challenged. In the more traditional family setting, one might not be told of a parent's or sibling's health history, but there is at least the opportunity to observe some of it. However, if the adoptee can claim a right to know health information of a parent, why would that same argument not begin to extend to others as well? The opening of health information to others has many implications for work, insurance, and family interactions. This population of individuals who have very limited access to personal family history may challenge the very structure of privacy built into our healthcare system. If an adoptee can get otherwise private information about a birth relative, then why not another adult whose parent refuses to share something that might be considered important to know? If information can be accessed on a parent, then why not on a sibling or other relative?

Finally, the role of the HIM professional can be pivotal in helping to create forums for the discussion of these ethical concerns. The decisions as to what may be disclosed, to whom, and under what circumstances rest with the HIM profession. These decisions have social as well as personal impact. Recognition of the ethical principles and the competing arguments for and against various actions can be useful in framing the interdisciplinary dialogues that need to occur. Access to family health information is one area in which those affected by adoption may help to initiate with the HIM professionals some of the discourse needed to plan for future guidelines.

In summary, the HIM professional of the future will be faced with ethical challenges regarding adoption and reproductive technologies. Specifically, the issues will revolve around the degree of openness of individual health histories and where the boundaries lie with regard to sharing family information. Adoption law and practice provide some beginning frameworks for the questions that will need to be addressed as reproductive technologies increasingly change the way we define self and family. As with all ethical dilemmas, there are no simple answers, but awareness of the issues involved can help to inform and improve the ways in which we decide how and when to share health information.

Key Terms

- Adoptee
- Adoption
- Adoption triad
- Adoptive parent
- Biological father
- Biological mother
- Birth father
- Birth mother
- Closed adoption
- Full disclosure
- Legal father
- Natural father
- Natural mother
- Open adoption
- Putative, or alleged, father
- Wrongful adoption

Chapter Summary

- The legal and social concept of adoption establishes bonds of a parent–child relationship between individuals not related biologically to one another.
- Traditionally, adoption records have been kept secret so that adoptees would not seek out and invade the privacy of their birth parents and so that birth parents would not try to take their child back or to become involved in his or her life.
- Today, the emphasis on secrecy in adoptions is being increasingly challenged. An increasing emphasis on the importance of genetic factors in mental and physical health and in the formation of identity has caused many adoptees and adoptive parents to seek access to health information about the adoptee's birth relatives. Adoption laws are being challenged and revised.
- Ethically, decisions on what information on birth relatives should be made available involve balancing the birth relatives' rights to privacy with the rights of adoptees to make informed decisions regarding their own health care and the rights of adoptive parents to make such decisions on their adopted children's behalf. They also involve considering the possible harms and benefits of information sharing and the extent of the need to know. HIM professionals will need to actively participate in the decisions regarding what is considered full disclosure of health information concerning adopted persons.

- The creation of families by new reproductive technologies is raising issues regarding access to relatives' health information that are similar to the issues raised by adoption. For example, the health background of a sperm donor, an egg donor, and/or a gestational carrier may all be significant for understanding the health risks of a child, and families may seek to access this information. HIM professionals can play an important role in discussing and framing policies on these issues and exploring their ethical implications.
- Access to health information for biological parents by adoptees raises the question of access to parental information by all children.

References

Beauchamp, T. L., & Childress, J. F. (2001). *Principles of biomedical ethics.* New York: Oxford University Press.

Moorman, J. E., & Hernandez, D. J. (1989). Married-couple families with step, adopted, and biological children. *Demography, 26*(2), 267–277.

Mosher, W. D., & Bachrach, C. A. (1996). Understanding U.S. fertility: Continuity and change in the National Survey of Family Growth. *Family Planning Perspective, 28*(1), 4–12.

National Adoption Information Clearinghouse. (2004). *How many children were adopted in 2000 and 2001?* Washington, DC: Author.

The ethical decision-making matrix is a tool to help you organize complex, ethical problems; however, there is no simple fill-in-the-box approach to ethical decision making. The objective is to follow each step of the process and not move from the question directly to what should be done or how to prevent it next time. If you skip steps, you will not fully understand all of the values and options for action. Also, the matrix provided for each scenario in this book is not the only way to examine the problem. You can make an equally compelling ethical argument for a different decision—just be sure to follow all the steps of the matrix.

SCENARIO 19-A: SEEKING INFORMATION MANY YEARS LATER

Steps	Information	
1. What is the ethical question?	Should you disclose the information to Charlie's adoptive parents?	
2. What are the facts?	**KNOWN**	**TO BE GATHERED**
	• Charlie is having health problems that could be related to his birth parents' histories. • Derek may not be Charlie's father. • The Snyders have requested access to the medical records. • The Snyders have much power and influence in the community. • Carolee has since married and given birth to two other children.	• Would your giving the information to the adoptive parents be illegal? • Could you give only limited medical information that would be of relevance? • Would not sharing the information cause Charlie harm? • What is the customary practice in such cases? • What does your boss or supervisor expect you to do? • What is the likely impact on self and family of changing jobs?
3. What are the values? Examine the shared and competing values, obligations, and interests of the stakeholders (i.e., patient, HIM professional, healthcare practitioner(s), administrators, society, and other advocates) involved in order to fully understand the complexity of the ethical problem(s).	**Patient:** Could come to harm whether or not information is disclosed. **Adoptive parents:** If information is released, parents could find out that Derek is not Charlie's father; Charlie's health could be harmed if the information is not released. **Biological parents:** Could have personal issues as a result of information release; may want to help Charlie by releasing the information. **HIM professional:** Values patient care; values confidentiality; avoid harm (to patient, to adoptive parents, to biological parents); fairness (follow rules and obey the law); loyalty to employer; personal values (promote welfare of self and family by avoiding loss of job). **Society:** Preserve child's health; respect confidentiality.	

4. What are my options?	• Do not disclose the information. • Disclose the information.	
5. What should I do?	Do not disclose the information.	
6. What justifies my choice?	**JUSTIFIED**	**NOT JUSTIFIED**
	• Obey the law. • Protect confidentiality. • Preserve professional integrity. • Demonstrate loyalty to employer.	• Disclose information. • Jeopardize current lives of biological parents. • Jeopardize validity of the adoption. • Break the law. • Disclosure undermines adoption system. • Jeopardize professional integrity.
7. How can I prevent this ethical problem?	• Determine if system changes are needed. • Learn more about issues surrounding adoption and health records. • Discuss standards and the values that support them with colleagues.	

The ethical decision-making matrix is a tool to help you organize complex, ethical problems; however, there is no simple fill-in-the-box approach to ethical decision making. The objective is to follow each step of the process and not move from the question directly to what should be done or how to prevent it next time. If you skip steps, you will not fully understand all of the values and options for action. Also, the matrix provided for each scenario in this book is not the only way to examine the problem. You can make an equally compelling ethical argument for a different decision—just be sure to follow all the steps of the matrix.

SCENARIO19-B: AN ADOPTEE SEEKS INFORMATION ON HER BIOLOGICAL FAMILY

Steps	Information	
1. What is the ethical question?	Should you release the information to Francine?	
2. What are the facts?	**KNOWN**	**TO BE GATHERED**
	• Francine has received a court order for access to her records. • Francine wants information about medical histories and racial heritage of her birth parents and extended family.	• Is provision of this information illegal? • Can you provide medical and racial information without jeopardizing confidentiality? • Does the release authorization include medical information? • What are the customary practices in such cases? • What does your boss or supervisor expect you to do? • What is the likely impact on self and family of changing jobs?
3. What are the values? Examine the shared and competing values, obligations, and interests of the stakeholders (i.e., patient, HIM professional, healthcare practitioner(s), administrators, society, and other advocates) involved in order to fully understand the complexity of the ethical problem(s).	**Patient:** Values access to information on medical history and racial heritage. **HIM professional:** Truth, integrity, accuracy (disclose accurate information); protect confidentiality of records; fairness (follow rules and obey the law); loyalty to employer; avoid harm (Francine's children may be harmed if they have illness as a result of their genetic history); personal values (promote welfare of self and family by avoiding loss of job). **Birth family:** Values confidentiality of medical records; may want to help Francine by disclosing the information. **Society:** Promote health of unborn children; promote confidentiality of medical records.	

4. What are my options?	• Release the information to Francine. • Do not release the information to Francine.	
5. What should I do?	Release the information to Francine, if the release authorization covers medical records.	
6. What justifies my choice?	**JUSTIFIED**	**NOT JUSTIFIED**
	• Protect unborn children. • Obey the release authorization. • Preserve professional integrity.	• Do not release information though authorization covers it. • Do not obey release authorization. • Jeopardize health of unborn children. • Jeopardize professional integrity.
7. How can I prevent this ethical problem?	• Determine if system changes are needed. • Learn more about issues surrounding adoption and the confidentiality of medial records. • Discuss standards and the values that support them with colleagues.	

The ethical decision-making matrix is a tool to help you organize complex, ethical problems; however, there is no simple fill-in-the-box approach to ethical decision making. The objective is to follow each step of the process and not move from the question directly to what should be done or how to prevent it next time. If you skip steps, you will not fully understand all of the values and options for action. Also, the matrix provided for each scenario in this book is not the only way to examine the problem. You can make an equally compelling ethical argument for a different decision—just be sure to follow all the steps of the matrix.

SCENARIO 19-C: A BIRTH MOTHER SEEKS INFORMATION ON HER BIOLOGICAL SON

Steps	Information	
1. What is the ethical question?	Should you release the information to the Baxters?	
2. What are the facts?	**KNOWN**	**TO BE GATHERED**
	• Marlene gave up a son for adoption and is now in need of a transplant. • The son may be in danger of developing the same illness. • The Baxters and the hospital administrator want you to release the information.	• Was this an open adoption? • Would disclosure be illegal or violate confidentiality? • Could you contact the son and disclose the information? • What will happen to Marlene if you do not release the information? • What does your immediate supervisor expect you to do? • What is the customary practice in such cases? • What is the likely impact on self and family of changing jobs?
3. What are the values? Examine the shared and competing values, obligations, and interests of the stakeholders (i.e., patient, HIM professional, health-care practitioner(s), administrators, society, and other advocates) involved in order to fully understand the complexity of the ethical problem(s).	**Patient:** Could suffer physically if biological son is not contacted. **HIM professional:** Integrity, truth (protect confidentiality of medical record); loyalty to employer; fairness (follow rules equally for all); avoid harm (protect patient's health); personal values (promote welfare of self and family by avoiding loss of job). **Biological son:** Values confidentiality; may want the opportunity to help biological mother. **Administrator:** Values relationship with friends; promotes welfare of facility. **Society:** Protect confidentiality of records.	

4. What are my options?	• Release the information to the Baxters. • Do not release the information to the Baxters.
5. What should I do?	Contact the son and give him the choice of whether or not to contact the biological mother, if it was an open adoption.

6. What justifies my choice?	JUSTIFIED	NOT JUSTIFIED
	• Obligation to protect confidentiality. • Preserve professional integrity. • Follow rules equally for all. • Demonstrate loyalty to employer, unless asked to push legal boundaries.	• Release information to the Baxters. • Violate confidentiality. • Make exceptions for friends of administrator. • Jeopardize professional integrity. • Undermine confidentiality of adoptive records.

7. How can I prevent this ethical problem?	• Determine if system changes are needed. • Learn more about issues surrounding disclosure of adoption records. • Discuss standards and the values that support them with colleagues. • Evaluate institutional integrity at job interview and subsequently as ethical problems arise.

DRUG, ALCOHOL, SEXUAL, AND BEHAVIORAL INFORMATION

Sharon J. Randolph, JD, RHIA
Laurie A. Rinehart-Thompson, JD, RHIA, CHP

Learning Objectives

After completing this chapter, the reader should be able to:

- Describe how legislation addresses the disclosure of sensitive health information regarding substance abuse and treatment, sexually transmitted diseases, and mental health/behavioral disorders.
- Explain the role of the privacy requirements of the Health Insurance Portability and Accountability Act (HIPAA) in the protection of sensitive health information.
- Identify typical ethical dilemmas that health information management (HIM) professionals may encounter in relation to the disclosure of behavioral health information.
- Discuss some of the factors to consider in making decisions about ethical issues in behavioral health.
- Identify possible responses to ethical dilemmas regarding the disclosure of behavioral health information.

Abstract

Certain health information, such as information about substance (i.e., drug and alcohol) abuse and treatment, sexually transmitted diseases, and mental illnesses (also referred to as behavioral or psychiatric illnesses), is highly sensitive and therefore receives special legal protections because its disclosure can have unfortunate legal and stigmatic consequences. The AHIMA Code of Ethics (2004) emphasizes this principle by identifying drug, alcohol, sexual, and behavioral information as sensitive information that requires special attention to prevent misuse. However, this same information that requires special protection may also be requested for law enforcement purposes or for the protection of others. HIM professionals working in the behavioral health and substance abuse/treatment fields are likely to encounter ethical challenges above and beyond those experienced by individuals working in other healthcare settings. This chapter describes several difficult situations that HIM professionals may face and explores the legal and ethical aspects of those situations.

Scenario 20-A: The Arrest Warrant: Is This Person in Your Facility?

You are an HIM professional at a behavioral health facility. Several patients in your facility have mental illnesses, possibly coupled with substance abuse problems, that have led them to commit crimes. A deputy sheriff with jurisdiction over the county in which your facility is located arrives in your department. He informs you that John Jones has been charged in connection with a recent string of burglaries in this county. The deputy further indicates that he has reason to believe Mr. Jones is a patient in your facility. He presents you with an arrest warrant and informs you that it is his duty and obligation to execute it. You know that Mr. Jones is a patient in your facility.

Questions

1. What should you do? What factors do you need to consider in your decision?

2. If Mr. Jones is not a patient in your facility, should you inform the deputy of that fact?

A completed ethical decision-making matrix for the scenario is provided at the end of the chapter.

Health information management (HIM) professionals are faced with changing legislation and technological advancements that have had a major impact on how patient information is created, maintained, preserved, and accessed. This environment precipitates many ethical dilemmas, especially if the information pertains to such highly sensitive topics as drug and alcohol (substance) abuse, sexually transmitted diseases, and mental health (psychiatric or behavioral) disorders.

With the advent of paperless medical records and the implementation of the **Health Insurance Portability and Accountability Act of 1996 (HIPAA)** Privacy Rule in 2003, patients are becoming more aware and informed of their right to the information contained in their medical records and the responsibility of HIM professionals to preserve the confidentiality of that information. HIM professionals need to remain at the forefront of knowledge regarding all types of health information (whether created in hard-copy format or electronically), particularly highly sensitive information. This type of health information and the ethical responsibilities related to it are discussed in this chapter.

SUBSTANCE ABUSE TREATMENT, HEALTH INFORMATION, AND THE LAW

HIM professionals must be aware that state and federal legislation has been passed that specifically addresses the confidential nature of certain medical information, above and beyond statutes addressing health information generally, and that such legislation stipulates specific disclosure conditions and requirements. Federal law places great emphasis on the confidentiality of substance abuse treatment information. Two federal statutes mandate confidentiality of the identity, diagnosis, prognosis, and treatment of any patient for substance abuse: the Federal Drug Abuse Prevention, Treatment, and Rehabilitation Act (42 U.S.C. §290dd-3) and the Comprehensive Alcohol Abuse and Alcoholism Prevention, Treatment and Rehabilitation Act (42 U.S.C. §290ee-3). In the federal statutes, *drug and alcohol abuse records* are defined as records of the identity, diagnosis, prognosis, or treatment of any patient that are maintained in connection with the performance of any program or activity relating to substance abuse education, prevention, training, treatment, rehabilitation, or research that is conducted, regulated, or directly or indirectly assisted by any department or agency of the United States. The U.S. Department of Health and Human Services (2003) interprets these regulations to apply to (1) an individual or entity (other than a general medical facility) that provides drug or alcohol abuse diagnosis, treatment, or referral for treatment; (2) an identified unit within a general medical facility that provides drug and alcohol abuse diagnosis, treatment, or referral for treatment; or (3) medical personnel or other staff in a general medical facility whose primary function is the provision of drug or alcohol abuse diagnosis, treatment, or referral for treatment.

The regulation further stipulates that disclosure is authorized to the extent that a patient consents in writing. In the absence of written consent, disclosure is authorized (1) to medical personnel to the extent necessary to meet a bona fide medical emergency; (2) to qualified personnel for the purpose of conducting scientific research, management audits, financial audits, or program evaluation (but such personnel may not identify, directly or indirectly, any individual patient in any report of such research, audit, or evaluation or otherwise disclose patient identities in any manner); or (3) if authorized by a court order. Violators of these federal statutes can receive a criminal penalty.

ETHICAL CHALLENGES IN BEHAVIORAL HEALTH AND SUBSTANCE ABUSE TREATMENT

HIM professionals working in the behavioral health and substance abuse treatment fields are very likely to encounter complex requests for information that present ethical challenges above and beyond those experienced by individuals working in other healthcare settings. These challenges involve the types of information that are considered confiden-

tial and worthy of heightened protection and the types of individuals who are requesting that highly protected information. It has been a universally accepted health information principle that the identity of a patient and verification of that patient's hospitalization are nonconfidential information (Brandt, 1997). HIPAA has not vastly changed that principle, with the exception that an individual must be afforded the opportunity to agree or object before that basic information can be shared [45 CFR 164.510(a)]. However, a broad exception has historically been carved out for the protection of behavioral health and substance abuse treatment information, including patient identification.

It is important to note that the special protection granted to behavioral health and substance abuse treatment information does not stem from HIPAA, which protects behavioral health and substance abuse treatment health information in the same manner and to the same extent as all other health information. Rather, state laws (for behavioral health information) and the aforementioned federal laws (for substance abuse treatment information) are what provide additional protection for these highly sensitive types of information. The very fact of an individual's status as a patient in a behavioral health or substance abuse treatment facility is associated with a powerful and unfortunate stigmatization that continues to influence that individual's life. Once someone is identified as a recipient of behavioral health or substance abuse treatment services, our society tends to develop limited, and often negative, perceptions about that individual's intellectual capabilities, educability, employability, social skills, ability to be a good neighbor, propensity for violence, and ability to lead a productive life. Therefore, the most basic patient information must be treated with the highest degree of confidentiality and sensitivity.

Ethical issues also arise regarding the types of requesters that are likely to be encountered. In the behavioral health and substance abuse treatment fields, it is not uncommon for a patient who is being treated to also be sought out by law enforcement as the suspected perpetrator of an unlawful act. It is important to recognize that many individuals with mental illness have never committed criminal acts and to steer away from the widely held misconception, mentioned earlier, that individuals with mental illness are prone to violence by virtue of their illnesses. It is also important to realize, however, that mental illness may cause some of its victims to commit criminal acts. One research study that tracked individuals during their first year after discharge from acute behavioral health facilities (Steadman, Mulvey, Monahan, Clark Robbins, Appelbaum, Grisso, et al., 1998) found no significant difference in the prevalence of violence between the former patients and others living in the same neighborhoods. The study indicated that with or without mental illness, those with substance abuse problems are more likely to commit violent acts. As a result, individuals experiencing substance abuse are much more likely to become the subjects of law enforcement investigations or public safety efforts. When they are admitted to behavioral health facilities, a perceived conflict of interest regarding the accessibility of information about them may very well arise.

Although the basic tenet ingrained in HIM professionals is that behavioral health and substance abuse treatment information is to be handled with the utmost sensitivity, compelling circumstances may cause law enforcement officials to seek the very information that HIM professionals are taught to diligently protect. The HIM professional is therefore confronted with a dilemma on two levels: (1) potential conflicts between laws and (2) ethical considerations.

Before discussing conflicts between laws, it is important for the reader to understand the role of the HIPAA Privacy Rule with regard to the types of information discussed in this chapter. As stated earlier, HIPAA provides no additional protections for behavioral health or substance abuse treatment information beyond what it provides for any type of protected health information. Further, HIPAA provides twelve situations—commonly referred to as **public interest and benefit activities**—whereby a covered entity may disclose protected health information without an individual's authorization (45 CFR 164.512) (Exhibit 20–1). Disclosure of pro-

Exhibit 20–1 Public Interest and Benefit Activities Where Patient Authorization Is Not Required (45 CFR 164.512)

1. Required by law
2. Public health activities
3. Victims of abuse, neglect, or domestic violence
4. Health oversight activities
5. Judicial and administrative proceedings
6. Law enforcement purposes
7. Decedents
8. Cadaveric organ, eye, or tissue donation
9. Research
10. Serious threat to health or safety
11. Essential government functions
12. Workers' compensation

tected health information for law enforcement purposes is one of those twelve "public interest and benefit" activities that may not require an individual's authorization [45 CFR 164.512(f)]. However, HIM professionals must recognize that HIPAA limits such law enforcement disclosure to only six allowable circumstances [45 CFR 164.512(f)]:

1. As required by law (including court orders, court-ordered warrants, subpoenas)
2. To identify or locate a suspect, fugitive, material witness, or missing person
3. To provide information about a victim or suspected victim of a crime
4. To alert law enforcement of a person's death
5. When a covered entity believes that protected health information is evidence of a crime on the premises
6. By a covered healthcare provider in off-premises medical emergencies when necessary to provide law enforcement with information about a crime

Even if one of these circumstances is met, a state law prevails if it provides greater patient privacy protection than that afforded by HIPAA. Although this may seem counterintuitive to the general principle that federal law preempts or supersedes contrary state law, HIPAA is only permissive—not mandatory—as to law enforcement disclosures that are permitted without patient authorization. State law has the ability to provide greater privacy protections than those provided by HIPAA.

Against this backdrop, one must consider carefully the potential conflicts between laws. A law enforcement official who is seeking information about a behavioral health or substance abuse patient often has a valid reason for seeking this information. Additionally, the official may present a copy of a statute that firmly convinces the HIM professional that the law requires him or her to comply with the official's request. Those with knowledge of statutes protecting such patient information, however, realize that the statute presented by the information-seeking law enforcement offi-

cial is not the only law governing a situation. Statutes requiring the protection of patient information are generally equal (if not greater, as in the case of federal law protecting substance abuse treatment information) in their force and effect. Fortunately for the HIM professional, conflicts between laws can, and should, be referred to legal professionals for resolution.

The HIM professional is also faced with a difficult ethical tension that forces an uneasy balancing act between the two critical interests of (1) protecting the most highly sensitive medical information (while possibly facing a hostile, armed law enforcement officer voicing the threat of arrest or contempt) and (2) doing what justice seemingly requires. We have been taught since childhood, by parents and other influential figures, to go by our sense of justice in our life experiences and do what is morally "fair," "equitable," and "right." When two laws conflict, one requiring disclosure and one prohibiting it, it is only natural that the HIM professional will begin to contemplate ethical considerations and questions about justice. Is it "fair" and "right" to protect information about someone who has committed a crime against an innocent person? Is it "fair" and "right" to protect information about someone who potentially poses a physical danger to another human being? In contrast, is it "fair" and "right" to release information, even for what seems to be a valid reason, about an individual who is receiving treatment for a diagnosis that automatically subjects him or her to unfair societal prejudices? Is it "fair" and "right" to share such intensely private, and often embarrassing, information about this individual? Beyond an analysis of the laws governing the confidentiality of behavioral health and substance abuse treatment information, these are questions and dilemmas that will always confront the HIM professional working in the behavioral health and substance abuse treatment fields (Hughes, 2002; Office for Civil Rights, HHS, 2002; Public Health Service, HHS, 2001).

Law Enforcement Requests Patient-Identifying Information

In Scenario 20-A, which opened this chapter, you were asked to imagine a situation in which you, as an HIM professional at a behavioral health facility, were confronted by a law enforcement official who requested patient-identifying information for the execution of an arrest warrant. The following are some factors that you would need to consider. The confidentiality of behavioral health information is uniformly provided for by individual state statutes, which must be read in conjunction with HIPAA. Although HIPAA delineates law enforcement circumstances where an individual's protected health information (PHI), including the fact of admission, may be disclosed, the limitations provided by state law must be referred to and followed (45 CFR 160.202) if they provide a greater degree of privacy protection.

The Ohio Revised Code (§5122.31), for example, provides that the identity of a behavioral health patient shall be kept confidential and shall not be disclosed unless one or more of several exceptions are met. The release of a patient's identity to a law enforcement official is not included in the list of exceptions. However, in this situation, justice seems to require the HIM professional to "do the right thing" with respect to an individual who has been charged with a series of crimes affecting the safety and security of the citizens in the community. What is the ethical thing to do?

An individual in this situation has several options. First, it is important for you to remind yourself that you are a representative of the facility that is treating Mr. Jones. As such, it is your first obligation to represent that patient's rights by releasing nothing immediately. It is not mandatory that the deputy be provided with an immediate answer, particularly if the individual is not being readied for discharge in the near future. Second, if the state statute provides that patient-identifying information may be released without patient authorization pursuant to a **court order**, which is a legal directive signed by a judge—as also permitted by HIPAA—you may inform the deputy that, with a court order, you will be able to legally comply with his request (a **subpoena** is not synonymous with and does not have the force of a court order, as it is a document initiated by a party in a legal case). Finally, the healthcare facility may decline to provide such information to the deputy but may speak with the patient and the patient's representative (e.g., a family member or the facility client advocate) regarding the arrest warrant and the fact that it may be in the patient's best therapeutic interest to contact the sheriff's department and deal with the issue rather than eluding law enforcement on this matter. Without compromising the patient's confidentiality, you may inform the deputy that, if Mr. Jones is a patient in the facility, he will be informed of the arrest warrant and be advised to turn himself in. In any event, legal counsel for the facility should be consulted for the most appropriate course of action, and the state statute affecting the facility should be followed. If the deputy is uncooperative and threatens immediate arrest if the information he is seeking is not revealed, you should try to agree on a mutual period of time in which you can contact your legal counsel for guidance.

The basic principle that the HIM professional must bear in mind in this situation is that Mr. Jones is a patient in this facility because of a behavioral health diagnosis that may or may not have led to the burglaries for which he is charged. In either case, it is your obligation to protect Mr. Jones's confidentiality to the furthest degree possible, while still respecting the important responsibilities of the law enforcement community.

Now suppose that Mr. Jones is not a patient in your facility. Should you inform the deputy of that fact? This situation asks whether stating that an individual is not a behavioral health patient (if this is true) rises to the same level of disclosure as admitting that an individual is a patient. Are you breaching the patient's confidentiality by stating that he is not a patient? Generally, truthfully stating that an individual is not a patient in one's behavioral health facility is not a problem. However, a confidentiality problem would be created if you expressed any familiarity with

Mr. Jones or provided any information regarding prior admissions. If these factors are not disclosed, then revealing that he is not a patient does not breach your legal and ethical obligations to either the patient or the facility for which you work.

Scenario 20-B: Safety of a Citizen versus Privacy of a Patient

The sheriff's deputy has told you, the HIM professional, that Robert Smith is in your facility but that he needs you to confirm this fact and also agree to inform the sheriff's department when Mr. Smith is discharged. The deputy tells you that he has received a call from Mr. Smith's former girlfriend, who states that she is afraid of Mr. Smith. Mr. Smith has a diagnosis of schizophrenia and a history of violent behavior due to his mental illness and history of alcohol abuse. The former girlfriend informed the deputy that Mr. Smith was admitted to your facility last week. She wants the sheriff's department to let her know when Mr. Smith is discharged. According to the former girlfriend, Mr. Smith has made no specific threats toward her. However, he assaulted her severely several months ago, was convicted, and served two months in jail.

Questions

1. Should you confirm Mr. Smith's status as a patient in your facility, since the deputy already knows this fact?

2. Should you agree, in the interest of the woman's safety, to let the sheriff's department know when Mr. Smith is discharged?

A completed ethical decision-making matrix for the scenario is provided at the end of the chapter.

Law Enforcement Requests Patient Information for Public Safety Reasons

With regard to Scenario 20-B, consider the following. This situation presents an ethical dilemma that involves balancing two compelling interests: (1) protecting the confidentiality of a behavioral health/substance abuse patient (which is your first obligation as an employee of this facility) and (2) protecting

the physical safety of an individual. As with Scenario 20-A, the facility should not be pressured to provide an immediate response if Mr. Smith is not being readied for discharge. If the deputy is informed that an immediate response cannot be provided but that you will look into what information you can legally provide, the deputy will know that you are willing to assist to the extent permitted by law. The deputy may be informed that such information can be released pursuant to a court order, provided that the state statute allows the release of information under that circumstance. Also, as with the previous scenario, HIPAA's disclosure for "public interest and benefit activities"—although permissive only—must be considered and read in conjunction with existing state law. In this situation, the HIPAA "public interest and benefit activity" that is most applicable is disclosure for the prevention or lessening of a serious threat to health or safety [45 CFR 164.512(j)], because the six allowable law enforcement disclosures discussed earlier in this chapter do not apply to this situation.

On the basis of the facts the deputy has provided, it does not appear that a specific threat has been made to the former girlfriend or that a "duty to warn" obligation has been initiated. A **duty to warn** is a legal responsibility of a treatment provider to breach patient confidentiality to inform an identifiable person that he or she is in imminent danger. However, legal counsel should be consulted and the applicable state statute (if one exists in your state) should be referred to regarding this matter. In the absence of a "duty to warn" statute in your state, common law will most likely provide the parameters for such a duty (e.g., the California Supreme Court landmark case of *Tarasoff v. Regents of University of California*, 1976).

Further, this situation is clearly a clinical issue that requires the expertise and involvement of the patient's clinicians. It would be appropriate to contact the patient's clinicians or treatment team regarding the request. Those individuals may have additional information regarding the patient's relationship with the former girlfriend. They will be able to determine whether there is a need to clinically address this issue with the patient during treatment, and they can conclude whether there is a duty to warn the former girlfriend upon the patient's discharge from the facility. If the patient is to be discharged on the date that the deputy requests the information, immediate notification to and consultation by the patient's clinicians and the facility's legal counsel are necessary. If a clinical assessment reveals imminent danger to the former girlfriend upon the patient's discharge, steps can be taken to delay the patient's discharge (by court order if necessary). Alternatively, if discharge cannot be delayed and the potential for danger is severe, a "duty to warn" should be in effect that will override the patient's confidentiality.

As an HIM professional, your first obligation is to protect the patient's confidentiality. Although the deputy appears to already know that Mr. Smith is a patient in the facility, it is important not to be fooled by potential bluffing. Further, it is not your responsibility to decide whether the safety of the former girlfriend outweighs the patient's right to have his confidentiality protected. It is your responsibility to refer the situation to the appropriate personnel. This scenario presents a complex matter that should be referred to and explored by those treating Mr. Smith, along with guidance from legal counsel.

Scenario 20-C: Patient Confesses to a Psychiatrist

Sam Clark came to the behavioral health facility a week ago as a voluntary admission. During a session with his psychiatrist, he admitted that he committed a crime about six months ago for which he was never charged due to insufficient evidence. He stated that he broke into an elderly man's home at night and took $2,000 in cash. When the man woke up and came into the kitchen, where Mr. Clark was taking the cash, Mr. Clark grabbed the bat that he had brought with him and swung at the man. After knocking the man to the ground, Mr. Clark fled. According to newspaper reports, the man suffered a broken shoulder and has since recovered.

> Gillian, an HIM staff member, is reviewing Mr. Clark's medical records when she sees the documentation containing his confession. In her state, where her facility is located, Mr. Clark's crimes are felonies.

Question

1. What should Gillian do?

A completed ethical decision-making matrix for the scenario is provided at the end of the chapter.

A Behavioral Health Patient Confesses to a Staff Member That He Has Committed a Crime

With regard to Scenario 20-C, consider the following. Generally, states have **felony-reporting statutes** that dictate the conditions under which a person who knows about a felony-level crime must report it to law enforcement authorities. (Note that HIPAA's "public interest and benefit activities" provision would therefore permit such disclosures as "required by law.") Felony-reporting statutes may include categories of professionals for which the reporting of felonies to law enforcement officials is permitted rather than required. For example, Ohio statute provides that the admission of a felony by a patient to a physician, a patient to a psychologist, or a client to an attorney is a **privileged communication** [Ohio Rev. Code §2921.22(G)]. Therefore, the professional to whom the admission has been made may or may not choose to report the admitted crime to authorities. There are often exceptions to this privilege, such as gunshot and stab wounds, which all individuals with knowledge are required to report [Ohio Rev. Code §2921.22(B)]. But Mr. Clark's crimes do not fall under those exceptions. Consequently, the psychiatrist in this scenario is not obliged to report, though he may choose to do so, and would, further, be in compliance with the HIPAA "public interest and disclosure" provision that allows disclosure for law enforcement purposes by identifying a suspect [45 CFR 164.512(f)].

What about Gillian, the HIM professional who discovers this information in the patient's record? First, she should not be expected to know all the laws on reporting of crimes, and as an employee and agent of the behavioral health facility, she should not have to make this decision by herself. In situations like these, HIM professionals should always first consult with the facility's legal counsel to look at the particular situation, analyze the specific language of the statute, and contact other legal professionals, as necessary, to discuss the matter (possibly as a hypothetical), thus reaching a decision and providing legal guidance that is within the limits of the governing statute. If the HIM professional is advised by legal counsel not to report, yet believes that such nonreporting is contrary to statute, it is important to relay those concerns to the facility's legal counsel and then engage legal counsel in discussion with the facility's administration in order to comply with the obligation as an employee and agent of the facility. The HIM professional also has an obligation to abide, as a state citizen, by the governing statute.

Generally speaking, HIM professionals do not constitute one of the categories of professionals that are exempt from being required to report felonies to law enforcement officials. However, because in this situation Gillian gained her information secondhand (i.e., by reading the medical record and learning that the patient made an admission to another person as opposed to actually hearing the patient admit to committing the crime), under no circumstance should she take it upon herself to report it externally. This exemplifies the importance of consulting with in-house legal counsel.

Scenario 20-D: Patient Confesses to the Nurse's Aide

Mr. Baker is a voluntary admission in a behavioral health facility. He reports to a nurse's aide that he has a drug stash at his home. In that state, possession of this particular drug is a misdemeanor. The nurse's aide documents the patient's confession in the patient's medical record. When Andrea, the HIM staff member, analyzes records for completeness, she reads the confession.

Question

1. What should Andrea do?

A completed ethical decision-making matrix for the scenario is provided at the end of the chapter.

As a general rule, there is no privileged communication between patients and nurses or nurse's aides. In this case, if the patient had admitted to committing a felony, the nurse's aide would generally, by law, have been required to report the admission. Having obtained the information as an agent of the behavioral health facility, however, the nurse's aide should not report the crime directly to law enforcement officials. The facility's legal counsel should be consulted and should direct the reporting process according to the specific statute relating to the reporting of crimes in the state where the facility is located.

With regard to the particular set of facts in Scenario 20-D, the patient's confession was in reference to a misdemeanor. Therefore, a felony-reporting statute would not apply. However, neither the nurse's aide nor the health information analyst can be presumed to know whether an admitted crime is a misdemeanor or felony. In this case, the nurse's aide was aware of the crime because the patient directly confessed to him or her. The HIM staff member became aware because she read the confession in the patient's medical record. Although both obtained knowledge of the crime by different means, the result was that both had knowledge of it by being agents of the facility. This results in an obligation to report it internally only. HIM staff should be instructed to notify their supervisor if they detect information of this nature.

In this instance, once notified by a staff member, the supervisor should consult with legal counsel. Although the first priority of HIM professionals is to maintain the confidentiality of patient information, this does not mean that the information cannot be brought to the attention of appropriate individuals within the facility. On the contrary, it should be brought to their attention. Further, at the time the admission was made to the nurse's aide, that employee should have notified his or her supervisor so that legal counsel could have been consulted in a more timely manner. It appears that additional training for direct-care staff is warranted as a result of this situation.

In determining whether an admitted crime should be reported in a situation where such reporting is not required, facility personnel should consider several factors—with legal counsel involvement, of course. Besides the severity of the crime (e.g., felony or misdemeanor), other factors include the type of crime (e.g., violent or nonviolent) and whether there was a victim. Ethical considerations (fairness and justice), public safety, and the patient's treatment and recovery must also be considered. In the absence of a statute that compels reporting in a particular situation, facility personnel must balance the patient's treatment and recovery needs against ethical considerations and in light of HIPAA's permissive disclosure for six law enforcement purposes, although none of those circumstances appear to apply to this scenario. Balancing these factors is often not a simple task.

Protecting Information About a Patient's Admission to a Behavioral Health Unit of a General Hospital

A different type of ethical dilemma can present itself when a facility provides general medical services but also has a behavioral health or substance abuse unit. It can sometimes be difficult to separate the two. If a patient has entered a hospital but is admitted to the substance abuse unit, how do you protect the information that concerns the patient's presence in the special unit?

Scenario 20-E: Verifying Admission Can Violate Privacy

You are the director of the health information department in a general hospital with a recently opened behavioral health unit. Your department handles all telephone requests for patient information. Per hospital policy, nonconfidential information about patients is given when a caller requests it and a patient has agreed to its release. This is a generally pleasant task because your staff gets to share general information, potential visitors of patient room numbers. An individual calls your department and identifies himself as Ray Ralston, a manager at ABC Corporation. He states that he is concerned about one of his employees who has not reported to work for two days. He asks whether this employee, Mary Martin, is in your facility. As your staff member reviews the patient list, she discovers that Mary Martin was recently admitted to the new behavioral health unit.

Question

1. What should your staff member tell the caller?

A completed ethical decision-making matrix for the scenario is provided at the end of the chapter.

The HIPAA Privacy Rule speaks specifically to facility directories, which contain patient contact information for individuals who request it. If formally or informally permitted to do so by the patient or the patient's representative, a provider may disclose the individual's name (i.e., fact of admission), condition, and location in the facility to those who ask for the patient by name [45 CFR 164.510(a)]. Fortunately, the HIPAA facility directory provision has made this situation easier for providers because instead of basic information being automatically considered nonconfidential, as in the past, providers must now ensure that it is acceptable to all patients, regardless of diagnosis, for this information to be released.

With regard to Scenario 20-E, your staff member's first obligation is to protect Mary Martin's confidentiality as a patient in a behavioral health unit. Although Mr. Ralston has expressed a valid reason for wanting to know if Ms. Martin has been admitted, his concern does not outweigh the facility's responsibility to protect this sensitive information about Ms. Martin. The most prudent course of action, so as not to disclose the fact of a behavioral health patient's admission and not to violate any existing state confidentiality laws with respect to this category of patients, is for a facility to develop a policy whereby behavioral health patients are automatically excluded from the facility directory. By not including their names in a facility directory, this sensitive information would never be disclosed and the facility would avoid the risk of wrongful disclosure.

Alternatively, if the facility has chosen to ask its behavioral health patients if they wish to be included in the facility directory and they agree, it should be clearly explained and documented that such disclosure could ultimately result in a requester knowing about an individual's status as a behavioral health patient. Such an approach should be taken extremely cautiously, particularly if the patient may not fully realize the impact of authorization because of the nature of his or her illness. Therefore, such an approach is not advised.

In any event, it is important that your staff member respond in a manner that will raise the least amount of suspicion in the caller's mind as to whether an individual is receiving behavioral health treatment. Further, it is important, when developing procedures, to realize that withholding information in a suspicious manner breaches an individual's confidentiality nearly as much as actually providing it. Perhaps staff members handling the telephone requests in this situation should be provided with a clear and definite script (examples are provided as follows). Further, simply not providing a staff member with a list of patients in the behavioral health unit is a way of exempting him or her from dealing with potentially uncomfortable and difficult situations in which these patients' confidentiality may be placed at risk.

Following is a possible script for the HIM employee who does not have access to the list of patients in the behavioral health unit:

> **Caller:** Can you tell me if Mary Martin is still in the hospital, and what her room number is? I'd like to visit her this evening.
>
> **HIM employee:** I'm sorry, but Ms. Martin's name does not appear in our facility directory.

Generally, this should be sufficient to answer the caller's question without raising suspicion. The employee has been truthful and has not been tempted to provide more information, because he or she has not been given access to the list of patients in the behavioral health unit. At the same time, the patient's confidentiality has been preserved, and the response has raised either no suspicion or only a minimal amount of suspicion. If the caller inquires about the facility directory, it may be explained as described in the next example.

The following is an example of a script for the HIM employee who has access to the list of patients in the behavioral health unit:

> **Caller:** Can you tell me if Mary Martin is still in the hospital, and what her room number is? I'd like to visit her this evening.
>
> **HIM employee:** I'm sorry, but Ms. Martin's name does not appear in our facility directory.

If this satisfies the caller's question, the employee has carried out his or her responsibility of protecting the patient's confidentiality. However, the response may lead to further questions by the caller:

> **Caller:** What do you mean by "facility directory"?
>
> **HIM employee:** You may be familiar with HIPAA, the new federal patient privacy law that our facility is legally obligated to follow. Because of HIPAA requirements, we include only those patients who want to be included in our directory of patients. The person you are asking about is not in the facility directory, either because she has chosen not to be or because she is not a patient in this facility. Unfortunately, I have no other information to give to you.

It is important to note that this is not a simple situation and that different "scripts" may have varying degrees of effectiveness at different facilities. If you are employed by a facility with special units that require heightened attention to confidentiality, an extensive discussion of release-of-information procedures affecting patients in those units is warranted. This discussion should include the facility directory requirements set forth by HIPAA, a determination of who will handle such requests for patient information, what information that person will be given access to, preparation of responses or scripts, determining what infor- mation can and cannot be released, and staff training.

Requests for Information on Sexually Transmitted Diseases

HIM professionals working in facilities that provide general medical/surgical services can also face ethical challenges when the general medical/surgical record contains information regarding a sexually transmitted disease (STD).

Scenario 20-F: A Prisoner Who May Have AIDS

You are an HIM professional at a county health facility. An injured prisoner is brought to the emergency department for treatment for injuries sustained in a strug- gle with the police while in the process of being arrested. The next day, one of the arresting officers presents himself to your department for a copy of the medical records on the prisoner because he bit the arresting officer during the struggle and told the arresting officer he had AIDS.

Question

1. Do you give the arresting officer a copy of the prisoner's record so that the officer may obtain the necessary treatment if needed?

A completed ethical decision-making matrix for the scenario is provided at the end of the chapter.

An STD is a disease that is suspected or pos- itively diagnosed through laboratory tests for STDs as defined by the state health and safety code statute and the Centers for Disease Con- trol and Prevention (CDC). An STD is an infec- tion, with or without symptoms or clinical manifestations, that may be transmitted from one person to another during, or as a result of, sexual relations between two persons and that may (1) produce a disease in, or otherwise im- pair the health of, either person; or (2) cause an infection or disease in a fetus in utero or a newborn. Some specific diseases that are clas- sified as STDs are HIV infection, AIDS, syphilis, gonorrhea, viral hepatitis B, genital herpes, genital warts, and genital infections from *Chlamydia trachomatis.* Although HIV can be transmitted through nonsexual means, it is still classified as an STD.

Under the HIPAA Privacy Rule, hospitals (covered entities) may disclose protected health information to (1) public health au- thorities by law to collect or receive such information for preventing or controlling disease, injury, or disability and to public health or other government authorities au- thorized to receive reports of child abuse or neglect; (2) individuals who may have con- tracted or been exposed to a communicable disease when notification is authorized by law; and (3) employers, regarding employees, when requested by employers, for informa- tion concerning work-related illness or injury or workplace-related medical surveillance, because such information is needed by the employer to comply with the Occupational Safety and Health Administration (OSHA), the Mine Safety and Health Administration (MHSA), or similar state law [45 C.F.R. section 164.512 (b)]. Although HIPAA delineates public health activities, limitations provided by states law must be referred to and followed (HIPAA preemption requirement—45 C.F.R. section 160.202).

As an HIM professional, your first obligation is to protect the patient's right to privacy and to maintain the confidentiality of patient's protected health information. It can be argued that the arresting officer has a right to the information because it is not confidential,

since the prisoner voluntarily told the officer that he had AIDS. But in compliance with HIPAA privacy regulations regarding release of records containing this type of sensitive information, the record cannot be released to the arresting officer without written authorization from the patient. If the patient refuses to provide a signed authorization to release protected health information, hospital policy and procedure should stipulate that the arresting officer must go through the process of being tested for AIDS exposure in the emergency department or other designated hospital service area. If the hospital has not implemented a specific policy and procedure, the arresting officer *must* obtain written authorization from the patient.

Scenario 20-G: Workers' Compensation Case

A female employee of Company X is admitted to the hospital for severe back strain due to an on-the-job injury. While in the process of taking the patient's history, the patient informs her attending physician that she is experiencing severe pain in her genital area. The attending physician orders a consultation by a gynecologist. After a pelvic examination, the patient is diagnosed with genital herpes and treated appropriately. After the patient is discharged from the hospital, the risk manager of Company X requests a copy of the employee's medical records to approve payment of the hospital bill because this is a workers' compensation case and Company X is self-insured. You, as an HIM professional at the hospital, receive the request.

Question

1. Do you release a copy of the employee's entire medical record to the company's risk manager?

A completed ethical decision-making matrix for the scenario is provided at the end of the chapter.

Requests About Employees and Children

A central aspect of the HIPAA Privacy Rule is the principle of "minimum necessary" use and disclosure. A hospital *must* make reason-

able efforts to use, disclose, and request only the minimum amount of protected health information needed to accomplish the intended purpose of the use, disclosure, or request. The minimum necessary requirement is not applied in any of the following circumstances: (1) disclosure to or request by a healthcare provider for treatment; (2) disclosure to an individual who is the subject of the information (the patient), or the individual's personal representative; (3) use or disclosure made pursuant to an authorization; and (4) use or disclosure that is required by law [45 C.F.R. sections 164.502(b) and 164.514(d)]. In the case of the risk manager, only information relating to the back injury from the medical record is needed to substantiate an on-the-job injury. Omitting portions of the medical record may be very obvious and suspicious to the risk manager.

As the HIM professional processing the request, you may inform the risk manager that, under HIPAA privacy regulations, the portion of the medical record released was the minimum amount needed to accomplish the intended purpose of the request submitted and that a written authorization for release of protected health information from the patient is needed to obtain copies of the entire medical record.

Scenario 20-H: Children's Protective Services

A two-year-old girl was admitted to General Hospital for sexual assault. The alleged attacker was the child's 25-year-old uncle, who lives in the home of the mother. The attack is immediately referred to Children's Protective Services (CPS). During the investigation by a CPS caseworker, the mother states that the uncle is very sexually promiscuous. The mother also states that the uncle is currently being treated for gonorrhea and that he was diagnosed at General Hospital. The CPS caseworker goes to the HIM department at General Hospital and asks you, the HIM professional, for permission to review the records of the patient's uncle.

Question

1. Do you allow the CPS caseworker to review the medical records of the uncle?

A completed ethical decision-making matrix for the scenario is provided at the end of the chapter.

As an HIM professional, you have the ethical obligation to protect the uncle's confidential, protected health information. CPS is investigating this case to determine if they must represent the "best interest of the child" by taking custody of the child from the mother and consenting for appropriate treatment, if the condition exists. In order to preserve the confidentiality of the uncle's protected health information, you should ascertain whether the CPS caseworker has obtained a written authorization from the uncle, allowing CPS access to review his medical records. If a written authorization from the uncle has not been obtained, as standard hospital policy (if state law permits), you may request one to be obtained. If the CPS caseworker objects to the request or the uncle refuses to provide a written authorization, then review the HIPAA Privacy Rule and applicable state laws, along with your hospital counsel, to determine when the hospital is permitted to use and disclose protected health information without an individual's authorization. Under HIPAA privacy regulations, a hospital may disclose protected health information to public health authorities (e.g., local health department) authorized by law to collect or receive such information for preventing or controlling disease, injury, or disability and to public health or other government authorities (e.g., CPS) that are authorized to receive reports of child abuse and neglect [45 C.F.R. section 164.512(b)].

This case may be handled in the following manner: Contact the hospital's Infection Control Nurse or Representative and inquire if the patient (child's uncle) was tested for STD and if so, if the results were reported to the local health department as required by state law (explain why you are inquiring). If a test was performed and the result was positive, you can refer the CPS caseworker to the Infection Control Nurse/Representative for confirmation of a reportable disease. After confirmation that the protected health information may be disclosed without the authorization of the patient, the CPS caseworker should be permitted to review the laboratory test results only of the uncle (applying the HIPAA minimum necessary requirement) in order to make the appropriate decisions in the best interest of the child. If the hospital Infection Control Nurse/Representative does not feel comfortable in providing this information or this is not an option, then consult with your hospital legal counsel for guidance.

CONCLUSION

The scenarios presented in this chapter represent just a few examples of the gray areas associated with the confidentiality and disclosure of highly sensitive protected health information. Effectively safeguarding sensitive protected health information requires strict internal departmental policies and procedures that are customer service oriented and reflect what is in the best interest of the patient. This suggests that departmental staff must be trained adequately on proper and improper disclosure of these types of patient health information. All disclosures of sensitive health information should be reviewed and scrutinized very carefully.

HIM professionals must also consider how they can comply with the state and federal laws (especially HIPAA) when patient information disclosure falls within the gray areas, without compromising their code of professional ethics. As an HIM professional, you have an ethical responsibility to ultimately always act in the best interest of the patient. However, other responsibilities may include the following:

- Using your best judgment when analyzing situations dealing with records classified as "sensitive"
- Staying up-to-date on the most current regulations and statutes regarding confidentiality and disclosure
- Maintaining current health information policies and procedures
- Seeking advice from your facility's legal or corporate counsel when a situation is questionable or when you are in doubt

HIM professionals of the future will be faced with more ethical challenges as general patient information becomes more and more accessible via new technological advances such as the electronic health record (EHR). New ethical issues will evolve concerning highly sensitive protected health information that state and federal legislation, including HIPAA, were designed to protect. Because it is virtually impossible for state and federal patient confidentiality and privacy legislation to keep up with the fast pace of technological advancements, HIM professionals should become more involved in educating the public on the new ethical challenges and become a strong voice of reason to help shape how patient information of the future will be protected, accessed, and disclosed.

Key Terms

- Court order
- Duty to warn
- Felony-reporting statute
- Health Insurance Portability and Accountability Act of 1996 (HIPAA)
- Privileged communication
- Protected health information (PHI)
- Public interest and benefit activities
- Subpoena

Chapter Summary

- Health information regarding substance abuse treatment, sexually transmitted diseases, and behavioral health is considered highly sensitive because of its stigmatizing nature. At the same time, it is often requested for purposes of law enforcement or the protection of others. Consequently, HIM professionals face ethical challenges in determining when this information should be disclosed.
- Special federal and state legislation addresses those conditions under which behavioral health information can or must be disclosed. Such legislation may conflict with other laws, but where it mandates the protection of patient health information, it generally has at least as much force, if not more, than other laws. Conflicts between laws should be referred to legal professionals for resolution.
- The identity of a patient and verification of that patient's hospitalization are nonconfidential information provided that a patient has agreed to disclosure of that information, but in the areas of behavioral health and substance abuse treatment, even patient identification must receive heightened confidentiality protections. HIM directors should institute special procedures to ensure that this information will not be wrongfully disclosed by staff.
- When a law enforcement official requests patient-identifying information from a behavioral health facility for the execution of an arrest warrant, the HIM professional should release nothing except as required by law. In any event, legal counsel should be consulted first.
- When a law enforcement official requests patient-identifying information from a behavioral health facility because of public safety concerns, no immediate response is necessary unless the patient is being readied for discharge. Legal counsel can determine whether the facility has a "duty to warn" persons potentially endangered by the patient that would override confidentiality obligations.
- State laws generally dictate who must report knowledge of a felony to law enforcement and under what conditions. In any case, this information should be reported internally.
- Law enforcement and health/safety provisions, which are included in HIPAA's permissive "public interest and benefit" disclosures, and which are often pertinent to the release of information about behavioral health, substance abuse treatment, and sexual health information, must be read in conjunction with state laws or other federal laws that provide special protections for the confidentiality of these sensitive types of health information.

References

American Health Information Management Association [AHIMA]. (2004). *AHIMA code of ethics.* Chicago: Author.

Brandt, M. (1997). *Release and disclosure: Guidelines regarding maintenance and disclosure of health information.* Chicago: AHIMA.

Haines, P. (2004). Reconciling the privacy rule and substance abuse record confidentiality. *Journal of AHIMA, 75*(10), 60–61.

Hughes, G. (2002). Laws and regulations governing the disclosure of health information. *AHIMA Practice Brief.* Retrieved January 4, 2006, from http://library.ahima.org/xpedio/groups/public/documents/ahima/pub_bok1_016464.html.

Office for Civil Rights, HHS (2002). Standards for Privacy of Individually Identifiable Health Information: Final Rule. *Federal Register* 45 CFR, Parts 160 and 164. 67, (157).

Public Health Service, HHS (2001). Confidentiality of Alcohol and Drug Abuse Records. *Code of Federal Regulations,* 42 CFR, Chapter I, Part 2.

Steadman, H. J., Mulvey, E. P., Monahan, J., Clark Robbins, P., Appelbaum, P. S., Grisso, T., et al. (1998). Violence by people discharged from acute psychiatric inpatient facilities and by others in the same neighborhoods. *Archives in General Psychiatry, 55,* 393–401.

U.S. Department of Health & Human Services. (2003, May). *Summary of the HIPAA Privacy Rule. OCR privacy brief.* Retrieved November 3, 2004, from http://www.hhs.gov/ocr/privacysummary.pdf.

The ethical decision-making matrix is a tool to help you organize complex, ethical problems; however, there is no simple fill-in-the-box approach to ethical decision making. The objective is to follow each step of the process and not move from the question directly to what should be done or how to prevent it next time. If you skip steps, you will not fully understand all of the values and options for action. Also, the matrix provided for each scenario in this book is not the only way to examine the problem. You can make an equally compelling ethical argument for a different decision—just be sure to follow all the steps of the matrix.

SCENARIO 20-A: THE ARREST WARRANT: IS THIS PERSON IN YOUR FACILITY?

Steps	Information	
1. What is the ethical question?	Should you give information to the officer?	
2. What are the facts?	**KNOWN**	**TO BE GATHERED**
	• John Jones is a patient in your facility. • Mr. Jones has been charged with a recent string of burglaries. • The deputy sheriff has a warrant for Mr. Jones's arrest.	• Would the disclosure of information about Mr. Jones be a violation of his confidentiality? • Would not disclosing the information potentially put others in danger? • Does the deputy sheriff require an immediate answer? • Does the state's statute provide that information can be released pursuant to a court order signed by a judge? • Can you inform Mr. Jones of the arrest warrant and give him the option of what to do? • What are the customary practices in such cases? • What does your boss or supervisor expect you to do? • What is the likely impact on self and family of changing jobs?
3. What are the values? Examine the shared and competing values, obligations, and interests of the stakeholders (i.e., patient, HIM professional, health-care practitioner(s), administrators, society, and other advocates) involved in order to fully understand the complexity of the ethical problem(s).	**Patient:** Values confidentiality and privacy of information. **HIM professional:** Truth and integrity (protect patient confidentiality); tell the truth regarding the patient's presence at the facility; fairness (follow the rules and obey the law); avoid harm (failure to disclose information about Mr. Jones could result in perpetration of additional crimes); personal values (promote welfare of self and family by avoiding loss of job). **Deputy sheriff:** Values protection of citizens from crime. **Administrators:** Benefit patients and keep from harm; promote welfare of facility; comply with law enforcement without violating patient rights. **Society:** Promote confidentiality; be protected from crime.	

4. What are my options?	• Disclose information about Mr. Jones. • Do not disclose information about Mr. Jones.
5. What should I do?	• Do not disclose the information about Mr. Jones. • Approach Mr. Jones or have the doctor approach him to tell him about the sheriff's warrant. • Encourage Mr. Jones to contact the sheriff's department.

6. What justifies my choice?	JUSTIFIED	NOT JUSTIFIED
	• Obligation to protect patient confidentiality. • Respect the law. • Preserve professional integrity.	• Disclose information about Mr. Jones. • Make special exception to the rules. • Disclosing information in selected cases undermines the confidentiality system. • Jeopardize professional integrity.

7. How can I prevent this ethical problem?	• Determine if system changes are needed. • Discuss standards and the values that support them with colleagues. • Learn more about issues surrounding confidentiality of patients at behavioral health facilities.

The ethical decision-making matrix is a tool to help you organize complex, ethical problems; however, there is no simple fill-in-the-box approach to ethical decision making. The objective is to follow each step of the process and not move from the question directly to what should be done or how to prevent it next time. If you skip steps, you will not fully understand all of the values and options for action. Also, the matrix provided for each scenario in this book is not the only way to examine the problem. You can make an equally compelling ethical argument for a different decision—just be sure to follow all the steps of the matrix.

SCENARIO 20-B: SAFETY OF A CITIZEN VERSUS PRIVACY OF A PATIENT

Steps	Information	
1. What is the ethical question?	Should you disclose information on Mr. Smith's status?	
2. What are the facts?	**KNOWN**	**TO BE GATHERED**
	• The deputy has told you of Mr. Smith's alleged recent behavior. • The deputy has asked you to confirm Mr. Smith's presence in the facility and to contact him when Mr. Smith is released.	• Would disclosing the information violate Mr. Smith's confidentiality? • Would disclosing the information violate the law? • Would not disclosing the information violate the law? • Would not disclosing the information potentially put Mr. Smith's former girlfriend in danger? • Are you required to provide an immediate response? • Does the state statute allow release of information pursuant to a court order? • Does the state statute include a "duty to warn" obligation? • What are the clinicians' opinions regarding release of the information? • When is Mr. Smith to be discharged? • What are the customary practices in such cases? • What does your boss or supervisor expect you to do? • What is the likely impact on self and family of changing jobs?

3. What are the values? Examine the shared and competing values, obligations, and interests of the stakeholders (i.e., patient, HIM professional, healthcare practitioner(s), administrators, society, and other advocates) involved in order to fully understand the complexity of the ethical problem(s).	**Patient:** Values confidentiality; values opportunity to receive appropriate treatment. **HIM professional:** Truth, integrity (protect patient confidentiality); fairness (follow the rules and obey the law); avoid harm (release of information could hamper Mr. Smith's treatment, failure to release information could put Mr. Smith's former girlfriend in danger); personal values (promote welfare of self and family by avoiding loss of job). **Healthcare professionals:** Promote welfare of patients through providing appropriate care. **Deputy:** Protect former girlfriend and others from harm; follow the rules and obey the law. **Society:** Protect patient confidentiality; protect society from potential harm.
4. What are my options?	• Release information about Mr. Smith. • Do not release information about Mr. Smith.
5. What should I do?	Release the information about Mr. Smith to the deputy, if a "duty to warn" obligation has been initiated and if Mr. Smith's clinicians agree that he may be a threat to others and if Mr. Smith is to be released shortly.

6. What justifies my choice?	**JUSTIFIED**	**NOT JUSTIFIED**
	• Obligation to protect society from potential harm. • Respect the law. • Obligation to tell the truth. • Preserve professional integrity.	• Do not release information about Mr. Smith (if all of the above conditions are present). • Put welfare of others in danger. • Make special exception to the law. • Failure to release information undermines state's "duty to warn" initiative.

7. How can I prevent this ethical problem?	• Determine if system changes are needed. • Discuss standards and the values that support them with colleagues. • Learn more about legal issues surrounding the release of information regarding patients in behavioral health facilities.

The ethical decision-making matrix is a tool to help you organize complex, ethical problems; however, there is no simple fill-in-the-box approach to ethical decision making. The objective is to follow each step of the process and not move from the question directly to what should be done or how to prevent it next time. If you skip steps, you will not fully understand all of the values and options for action. Also, the matrix provided for each scenario in this book is not the only way to examine the problem. You can make an equally compelling ethical argument for a different decision—just be sure to follow all the steps of the matrix.

SCENARIO 20-C: PATIENT CONFESSES TO A PSYCHIATRIST

Steps	Information	
1. What is the ethical question?	Should Gillian release the information about Sam to law enforcement officials?	
2. What are the facts?	**KNOWN**	**TO BE GATHERED**
	• Sam Clark is a patient in the facility. • Sam has admitted to having committed a crime. • The man Sam assaulted and robbed has recovered from his injuries.	• Would releasing this information to authorities violate Sam's confidentiality? • Is Gillian obligated to report this information? • Does the state have a felony-reporting statute? • If there is a statute, is the disclosure of this information permitted or required? • What is the opinion of the facility's legal counsel? • What are the customary practices in such cases? • What does her boss or supervisor expect her to do? • What would be the impact on self and family of changing jobs?
3. What are the values? Examine the shared and competing values, obligations, and interests of the stakeholders (i.e., patient, HIM professional, healthcare practitioner(s), administrators, society, and other advocates) involved in order to fully understand the complexity of the ethical problem(s).	**Patient:** Values confidentiality; values opportunity to receive appropriate treatment. **HIM professional:** Truth and integrity (protect patient confidentiality); tell the truth; fairness (follow the rules and obey the law); avoid harm (disclosure of the information could disrupt Sam's treatment, failure to disclose the information could put others in jeopardy upon Sam's release); personal values (promote welfare of self and family by avoiding loss of job). **Healthcare professionals:** Promote welfare of patients by providing appropriate care. **Law enforcement officials:** Promote welfare of citizens by apprehending criminals. **Society:** Protect patient confidentiality; apprehend and prosecute criminals.	

4. What are my options?	• Release the information about Sam to law enforcement officials. • Do not release the information about Sam to law enforcement officials.	
5. What should I do?	If it is in compliance with state law and if the facility's lawyer is in accord, do not release the information about Sam to law enforcement officials.	
6. What justifies my choice?	**JUSTIFIED**	**NOT JUSTIFIED**
	• Obligation to protect patient confidentiality. • Obligation to ensure patient receives appropriate treatment. • Preserve professional integrity. • Respect the law.	• Release the information to a law enforcement official. • Violate patient's confidentiality. • Make special exception to the state statute. • Deny patient the opportunity to receive appropriate care.
7. How can I prevent this ethical problem?	• Determine if system changes are needed. • Discuss standards and the values that support them with colleagues. • Learn more about state disclosure statutes regarding patients in behavioral health facilities.	

The ethical decision-making matrix is a tool to help you organize complex, ethical problems; however, there is no simple fill-in-the-box approach to ethical decision making. The objective is to follow each step of the process and not move from the question directly to what should be done or how to prevent it next time. If you skip steps, you will not fully understand all of the values and options for action. Also, the matrix provided for each scenario in this book is not the only way to examine the problem. You can make an equally compelling ethical argument for a different decision—just be sure to follow all the steps of the matrix.

SCENARIO 20-D: THE PATIENT CONFESSES TO THE NURSE'S AIDE

Steps	Information	
1. What is the ethical question?	Should Andrea disclose the information about Mr. Baker to appropriate internal sources?	
2. What are the facts?	**KNOWN**	**TO BE GATHERED**
	• Mr. Baker has confessed to having an illegal substance in his home and the medical record includes the documentation. • In that state, possession of the substance is a misdemeanor.	• What does the facility's legal counsel suggest? • Is Andrea required to report the crime externally? • Is Andrea required to report the crime internally? • What are the customary practices in such cases? • What does her boss or supervisor expect her to do? • What is the likely impact on self and family of changing jobs?
3. What are the values? Examine the shared and competing values, obligations, and interests of the stakeholders (i.e., patient, HIM professional, healthcare practitioner(s), administrators, society, and other advocates) involved in order to fully understand the complexity of the ethical problem(s).	**Patient:** Values ability to receive appropriate treatment. **HIM professional:** Truth and integrity (protect patient confidentiality); tell the truth about contents of patient's record; fairness (follow the rules and obey the law); avoid harm (failure to disclose the information to internal sources could jeopardize patient care); personal values (promote welfare of self and family by avoiding loss of job). **Healthcare professionals:** Promote welfare of patient by providing appropriate care. **Legal counsel:** Promote welfare of facility; protect patient confidentiality without violating the law. **Society:** Protect patient confidentiality; protect authority of law enforcement system.	

4. What are my options?	• Report information about Mr. Baker internally. • Report information about Mr. Baker externally. • Do not report the information about Mr. Baker to anyone.
5. What should I do?	Disclose the information about Mr. Baker to appropriate internal sources, if not required by law to disclose information on a misdemeanor externally.

6. What justifies my choice?	JUSTIFIED	NOT JUSTIFIED
	• Obligation to protect patient confidentiality. • Obligation to tell the truth. • Preserve professional integrity. • Follow rules equally for all.	• Do not report the information about Mr. Baker to anyone. • Jeopardize professional integrity. • Jeopardize Mr. Baker's ability to receive appropriate care.

7. How can I prevent this ethical problem?	• Determine if system changes are needed. • Discuss standards and the values that support them with colleagues. • Learn more about issues surrounding disclosure of information on patients in behavioral health facilities.

The ethical decision-making matrix is a tool to help you organize complex, ethical problems; however, there is no simple fill-in-the-box approach to ethical decision making. The objective is to follow each step of the process and not move from the question directly to what should be done or how to prevent it next time. If you skip steps, you will not fully understand all of the values and options for action. Also, the matrix provided for each scenario in this book is not the only way to examine the problem. You can make an equally compelling ethical argument for a different decision—just be sure to follow all the steps of the matrix.

SCENARIO 20-E: VERIFYING ADMISSION CAN VIOLATE PRIVACY

Steps	Information	
1. What is the ethical question?	Should the staff member tell the caller that Mary Martin has been admitted to the behavioral health unit?	
2. What are the facts?	**KNOWN**	**TO BE GATHERED**
	• Mary Martin has been admitted to the behavioral health unit. • The caller wants to know if Mary is a patient in the facility.	• Is the caller really Mary's employer? • Would disclosing the information violate Mary's confidentiality? • Would not disclosing the information violate the employer's rights? • What is the customary practice in such cases? • What is the likely impact on self and family of changing jobs?
3. What are the values? Examine the shared and competing values, obligations, and interests of the stakeholders (i.e., patient, HIM professional, health-care practitioner(s), administrators, society, and other advocates) involved in order to fully understand the complexity of the ethical problem(s).	**Patient:** Values confidentiality; values continued employment. **HIM professional:** Truth, integrity, and accuracy (tell the truth and provide accurate information about patient status); protect patient confidentiality; fairness (follow the rules and obey the law); avoid harm (disclosing the patient's status could result in loss of employment or stigmatization); personal values (protect welfare of self and family by avoiding loss of job). **Employer:** Concern over employee's whereabouts. **Staff member:** Protect patient confidentiality; obligation to tell the truth. **Society:** Protect patient confidentiality.	

4. What are my options?	• Release the information about the patient's admission to the caller. • Tell the caller that the person is not on the published list of inpatients.	
5. What should I do?	Tell the caller that the person is not on the published list of inpatients.	
6. What justifies my choice?	**JUSTIFIED**	**NOT JUSTIFIED**
	• Obligation to protect patient's confidentiality. • Obligation to tell the truth. • Protect professional integrity. • Respect the law.	• Release the information to the caller. • Violate patient confidentiality. • Put patient in jeopardy of job loss or stigmatization. • Jeopardize professional integrity. • Break the law.
7. How can I prevent this ethical problem?	• Determine if system changes are needed, including increased training. • Discuss standards and the values that support them with colleagues, including employees. • Learn more about issues surrounding disclosure of patient admission status.	

The ethical decision-making matrix is a tool to help you organize complex, ethical problems; however, there is no simple fill-in-the-box approach to ethical decision making. The objective is to follow each step of the process and not move from the question directly to what should be done or how to prevent it next time. If you skip steps, you will not fully understand all of the values and options for action. Also, the matrix provided for each scenario in this book is not the only way to examine the problem. You can make an equally compelling ethical argument for a different decision—just be sure to follow all the steps of the matrix.

SCENARIO 20-F: A PRISONER WHO MAY HAVE AIDS

Steps	Information	
1. What is the ethical question?	Should you give the officer a copy of the prisoner's medical record?	
2. What are the facts?	**KNOWN**	**TO BE GATHERED**
	• The officer claims that the prisoner bit him during a struggle and the prisoner claims to have AIDS. • The officer has requested a copy of the prisoner's medical record.	• Is it a violation of the prisoner's confidentiality to provide the officer with a copy of the medical record? • Is it a violation of the prisoner's confidentiality to not provide the record, but reveal whether the patient has AIDS or is HIV positive? • Do you have, or can you obtain, written authorization from the patient? • Has the officer been tested for HIV/AIDS exposure in a designated hospital service area? • What are the customary practices in such cases? • What does your boss or supervisor expect you to do? • What is the likely impact on self and family of changing jobs?
3. What are the values? Examine the shared and competing values, obligations, and interests of the stakeholders (i.e., patient, HIM professional, healthcare practitioner(s), administrators, society, and other advocates) involved in order to fully understand the complexity of the ethical problem(s).	**Prisoner:** Values confidentiality. **HIM professional:** Truth and integrity (tell the truth); protect confidentiality of medical record; fairness (follow the rules and obey the law); avoid harm (failure to reveal the HIV/AIDS status of the prisoner may cause harm to the officer); personal values (protect welfare of self and family by avoiding loss of job). **Officer:** Values personal health; obligation to protect and follow the law. **Society:** Preserve confidentiality.	

4. What are my options?	• Give a copy of the record to the officer. • Do not give a copy of the record to the officer.	
5. What should I do?	Do not give a copy of the record to the officer and recommend that he follow guidelines and seek testing at a designated hospital service area.	
6. What justifies my choice?	**JUSTIFIED**	**NOT JUSTIFIED**
	• Protect confidentiality of medical record. • Follow the rules and obey the law. • Preserve professional integrity.	• Release the medical record to the officer. • Break confidentiality. • Jeopardize professional integrity. • Break the law.
7. How can I prevent this ethical problem?	• Determine if system changes are needed. • Discuss values and the standards that support them with colleagues. • Learn more about issues surrounding the release of information from prisoners' medical records.	

The ethical decision-making matrix is a tool to help you organize complex, ethical problems; however, there is no simple fill-in-the-box approach to ethical decision making. The objective is to follow each step of the process and not move from the question directly to what should be done or how to prevent it next time. If you skip steps, you will not fully understand all of the values and options for action. Also, the matrix provided for each scenario in this book is not the only way to examine the problem. You can make an equally compelling ethical argument for a different decision—just be sure to follow all the steps of the matrix.

SCENARIO 20-G: WORKERS' COMPENSATION CASE

Steps	Information	
1. What is the ethical question?	Should you release a copy of the patient's medical record to the company's risk manager?	
2. What are the facts?	**KNOWN**	**TO BE GATHERED**
	• The patient was admitted for an on-the-job injury. • The patient was treated for an STD. • The company's risk manager has requested a copy of the patient's medical record.	• What are the state's STD regulations? • What are the consequences of omitting portions of the medical report given to the risk manager? • What are the customary practices in such cases? • What does your boss or supervisor expect you to do? • What is the likely impact on self and family of changing jobs?
3. What are the values? Examine the shared and competing values, obligations, and interests of the stakeholders (i.e., patient, HIM professional, healthcare practitioner(s), administrators, society, and other advocates) involved in order to fully understand the complexity of the ethical problem(s).	**Patient:** Values confidentiality; values appropriate processing of workers' compensation claim. **HIM professional:** Truth, accuracy, integrity (tell the truth about patient record); protect patient confidentiality; provide accurate medical information; fairness (follow the rules and obey the law); avoid harm (failure to disclose information could result in delayed processing of claim, disclosure of full information could stigmatize employee); personal values (protect welfare of self and family by avoiding loss of job). **Risk manager:** Values accuracy of medical records; values prompt processing of workers' compensation claim. **Society:** Protect confidentiality; ensure workers' rights to benefits.	

4. What are my options?	• Release all information to the risk manager. • Release limited information to the risk manager.	
5. What should I do?	Release only the information related to the injury.	
6. What justifies my choice?	**JUSTIFIED**	**NOT JUSTIFIED**
	• Obligation to protect patient confidentiality. • Obligation to aid in claims processing by releasing appropriate information. • Obligation to tell the truth. • Respect the law. • Preserve professional integrity.	• Release the entire record to the risk manager. • Violate patient confidentiality. • Break the law. • Jeopardize professional integrity.
7. How can I prevent this ethical problem?	• Determine if system changes are needed. • Discuss standards and the values that support them with colleagues. • Learn more about rules surrounding disclosure of sensitive medical information.	

The ethical decision-making matrix is a tool to help you organize complex, ethical problems; however, there is no simple fill-in-the-box approach to ethical decision making. The objective is to follow each step of the process and not move from the question directly to what should be done or how to prevent it next time. If you skip steps, you will not fully understand all of the values and options for action. Also, the matrix provided for each scenario in this book is not the only way to examine the problem. You can make an equally compelling ethical argument for a different decision—just be sure to follow all the steps of the matrix.

SCENARIO 20-H: CHILDREN'S PROTECTIVE SERVICES

Steps	Information	
1. What is the ethical question?	Should you allow the caseworker to review the uncle's records?	
2. What are the facts?	**KNOWN**	**TO BE GATHERED**
	• The niece has been admitted to the hospital as a result of a sexual assault. • The alleged attacker is the uncle. • The uncle is allegedly being treated for gonorrhea at the hospital. • The caseworker has asked to see the uncle's records.	• Would allowing the caseworker to review the records violate the uncle's confidentiality? • Does the child's best interest supersede the uncle's rights? • What does the hospital's legal counsel advise? • What do the state's health and safety code statues say about such cases? • What does your boss or supervisor expect you to do? • What is the likely impact on self and family of changing jobs?
3. What are the values? Examine the shared and competing values, obligations, and interests of the stakeholders (i.e., patient, HIM professional, healthcare practitioner(s), administrators, society, and other advocates) involved in order to fully understand the complexity of the ethical problem(s).	**Patient/uncle:** Values confidentiality. **Patient/child:** Values receipt of appropriate medical care; values safe environment in which to live. **HIM professional:** Truth, integrity (tell the truth about the contents of the patient's records); protect patient confidentiality; fairness (follow the rules and obey the law); avoid harm (failure to disclose the information could result in harm to the child); personal values (protect welfare of self and family by avoiding loss of job). **Healthcare professionals:** Promote welfare of patient by providing appropriate treatment. **Society:** Protect children from harm; protect confidentiality of medical records.	

4. What are my options?	• Release information to caseworker. • Withhold information from caseworker.	
5. What should I do?	Allow caseworker to review uncle's medical record, if hospital legal counsel agrees.	
6. What justifies my choice?	**JUSTIFIED**	**NOT JUSTIFIED**
	• Protect best interests of child. • Obligation to tell the truth. • Preserve professional integrity. • Follow legal guidelines.	• Withhold information from caseworker. • Preserve confidentiality but jeopardize health of child. • Jeopardize professional integrity.
7. How can I prevent this ethical problem?	• Determine if system changes are needed. • Discuss standards and the values that support them with colleagues. • Learn more about issues surrounding state health and safety codes and patient nondisclosure issues.	

ROLES

Part V presents ethical implications for the HIM manager who is responsible for daily operational decisions; the entrepreneur who can serve as an internal or external consultant; the HIM professional as advocate; and the intricacies of vendor relationships.

Chapter 21 discusses the complexities of balancing daily operational issues with ethical decision making when dealing with employees. The importance of moral development and awareness and issues related to socialization, rationalization, and equity are reviewed. The implications of moral muteness and the failure of ethical leadership are discussed.

Chapter 22 discusses the health information entrepreneur, focusing on business practices and professional ethics. This chapter discusses the ethical dilemmas typically encountered in consulting and contracting, along with principles and practice standards for resolving problems.

Chapter 23 explores the complexity of dealing with vendors, including issues related to vendors who are friends, gifts, and the ethical considerations for the RFP process. Negotiation and the enhancement of vendor relationships are analyzed.

Chapter 24 discusses the health information professional's role as advocate, defining *advocacy* as "ethics in action." HIM professionals have many opportunities to advocate for patients, peers, staff, employers, themselves, the community-at-large, and society as a whole. This chapter explores the tensions, risks, and personal and professional benefits of the advocate's role.

MANAGEMENT

Cathy A. Flite, MEd, RHIA
Sharon L. Laquer, MS, RHIA

Learning Objectives

After completing this chapter, the reader should be able to:

- Discuss factors that challenge managers' ability to increase moral awareness for themselves and their employees.
- Understand the stages of moral development and the importance of applying values when making management decisions.
- Discuss ethical issues associated with the orientation of new employees, including rationalization, socialization, and equity.
- Discuss work environment factors that contribute to the acceptance of unethical behaviors.

Abstract

This chapter explores some of the ethical issues facing health information managers (HIM) and discusses the importance of moral awareness, rationalization, socialization, moral muteness, and the consequences of ethical failures. This chapter will explore stages of moral development as a guide for managerial decision making and review some reasons why ethical management decisions are not always congruent with departmental and organizational policy. This chapter focuses on the professional values that challenge managers to increase moral awareness and nurture an ethical work environment.

Scenario 21-A.1 and 21-A.2: Lateness and Absenteeism

Gerri Randolph was hired through a welfare-to-work initiative at Memorial Medical Center. She is a divorced mother with four small children under the age of six. During her first month of employment, Gerri was absent from work on three separate occasions and reported to work late several times.

The employee handbook states that the probationary period is a time for the employee to adjust to the organization, and the employer must quickly socialize the employee. It also states expectations for punctuality and attendance. According to Memorial Medical Center, employees who do not fit or adhere to the policies may have their employment terminated at any time during the probationary period.

Alarmed by the pattern of lateness and absenteeism, Gerri's supervisor, Mitch Malloy, approached her to discuss the situation. Gerri explained her childcare issues and lack of social support to Mitch. Mitch noted that the quality and quantity of her work were exceptional for a new employee, and because of this he decided not to fire her, although that would have been allowed during the three-month probationary period. Mitch warned Gerri that continuing this pattern would lead to termination, because the organization has a very strict attendance policy, which states that "three or more absences during the probationary period is grounds for suspension and even termination."

Gerri did not come to work the next day so Mitch fired her.

Questions

1. Did Mitch do the right thing by following the hospital's policy?

2. Did Mitch fail to consider the ethical implications of trying to balance policies with the reality of a working mother trying to take care of her family?

3. Was he aware that this was an ethical conundrum?

4. Did he consider all stakeholders in this case? Who are the stakeholders?

5. What responsibility does the manager have to society and the employer to keep people employed?

6. Should a mother of small children be terminated this quickly, requiring her to find another job, go back on welfare, and lose health benefits for her family?

A Completed ethical decision-making matrices for the scenario are provided at the end of the chapter.

MORAL DEVELOPMENT AND MORAL AWARENESS

Health information management (HIM) professionals are responsible for the daily operations that support the information management system. They must constantly ensure that the "bottom line" is met with regard to the budget and performance standards, assuring quality operations in a fast-paced environment (LaTour & Eichenwald, 2002; Abdelhak, Grostick, Hanken, & Jacobs, 2001). Managers must make many decisions, including the following ones, that relate to human resource management:

- Should you terminate an employee who is always late?
- You've been asked to cut the personnel budget. Who should you lay off?
- An employee is very pleasant and well liked, but incompetent. What should you do?
- Employees are stealing supplies and equipment because their children need them for school. How can you stop this practice?

Although the environment is changing as systems move to the electronic health record (EHR), what remains constant is that the manager is faced with daily ethical decisions as a result of the continuous operational decisions that must be made. Does the manager have to remain neutral and unattached to people in the organization in order to make these difficult decisions? Managers have been educated to make difficult decisions when facing employee situations, but do they consider all the stakeholders? Do they fail to consider the employee as a stakeholder because the expectation of the manager is to be loyal to the company and follow policy? Some managers may not think twice about firing Gerri and assume that for the good of the organization she should be fired, because they are following the organization's policies and procedures. Others may consider a larger issue, such as putting an employee back into the unemployment or welfare lines or whether firing an employee would be in the best interests of the employee, the organization, and society at large. Mitch can be guided in his decision making if he understands the stages of moral development and factors that challenge his ability to increase his moral awareness.

The situation presented in the opening scenario presents two opposing perspectives when making employment decisions. The first perspective comes from the responsibility that the organization has to the individual. In the scenario, Mitch hired a welfare-to-work employee with limited work experience, and this individual needs assistance with integrating work and family life. The objective for the employer in hiring a welfare-to-work employee is twofold. Hiring a welfare recipient not only supports society's goals, but it may also lower employee turnover rates and increase employee retention for the organization. A lower employee turnover rate may be an outcome of hiring a welfare recipient, because that person may recognize that if he or she quits or loses his or her job, getting back into the welfare system may be difficult. The fear of losing healthcare benefits as well as economic support for their family may keep welfare recipients from changing jobs, and thus increases employee retention. Overall, it has been reported that welfare worker employee retention rates are lower than the national workforce averages (Holzer, Stoll, & Wissoker, 2004).

The organization also has a responsibility to provide quality healthcare services for society through a commitment to hire and retain skilled workers. If an employee is not present to do the work, then this latter responsibility cannot be met. What are the responsibilities of the manager to help this employee in the personal aspects of her life, in addition to ensuring that performance standards are met?

When making a decision, a manager has to understand the laws, rules, and regulations that affect employment decisions. In this scenario, it would be important for Mitch to have a basic understanding of welfare reform. In 1996, the Personal Responsibility and Work Opportunity Reconciliation Act (PRWORA, Public Law 104-193) replaced the Aid to Families with Dependent Children (AFDC) system. This was the end of the federal welfare program and the beginning of an emphasis on work and self-support for families. PRWORA established the Temporary Assistance for Needy Families (TANF) program, which allows states to administer welfare programs and provide assistance and work initiatives for five years (US Department of Health and Human Services, 2005a). The original law expired in 2002, and since that time Congress has passed many extensions to the TANF program. A reauthorization passed on September 30, 2004, allowed some state TANF programs to operate until March 31, 2005 (US Department of Health and Human Services, 2005b). Although the federal Welfare-to-Work Program ended, the larger social issue of moving people out of poverty and into sustainable employment will remain an issue in our society and impact employers and managers such as Mitch.

Mitch was well aware that he was hiring a back-to-work welfare recipient. This was an opportunity for the organization to reach out to the community and put a welfare recipient on a different path. During this transition period from welfare to work, issues such as child care and transportation are common (Holzer, Stoll, & Wissoker, 2004). During the probationary period, employees may need additional support from the organization to make them successful in sustaining employment and this support may come in the form of additional education, training, or even assistance with child care or transportation. Mitch was well aware of this commitment to the welfare-to-work program. New employees, including "back-to-work" employees, often need educational sessions on the importance of a work ethic (interpersonal skills, time and attendance, collaboration) and a commitment to meeting technical standards, such as scanning documents accurately.

However, managers are responsible for advancing the organization's goals—this sometimes means firing an employee who is absent and late for work, even if the employee is a welfare-to-work employee. Considering the employee's interests first and still complying with the organization's policies is not always possible. The organization has a responsibility to make fiscally sound decisions and provide quality healthcare services to the community. What is the manager's or the organization's responsibility to society, if any? Some may argue that mothers on welfare, need employment and have special issues. Others may argue that all em-

ployees bring a unique set of circumstances into the workplace and that the manager cannot begin to make individual rules for each employee. A busy manager might say, "I don't have time to worry about the personal lives of all of my employees—I have to get the work done!" This perspective may encourage managers to make and follow stringent uniform policies. This viewpoint may be unacceptable for those who prefer to consider the individual rights of the employee or for those who take into account the impact of their decision on the rest of the society. Another consideration is society's need to provide for economic and health opportunities to individuals. In any case, the polarity in the discussion of this case is extremely important, and the competing obligations, interests, and values of the different stakeholders must be considered when making an ethical decision.

An understanding of this scenario would not be complete without some discussion of the manager's stage of moral development. Lawrence Kohlberg's **stages of moral development** are used as a guide for the following discussion. Lawrence Kohlberg's contributions to the study of morality include a recognition that cognitive moral reasoning takes place among individuals and he provides a theory on moral development (Pritchard, 1999). The research explored how individuals develop and respond to ethical situations. The moral development is a learning process in which an individual gains greater insight into decision making or framing moral decisions (Pritchard, 1999). Kohlberg focused on the progression of the moral growth and development of individuals and not merely changes in morality but "moral improvement" (p. 397). This theory of moral development is based on three levels: the preconventional, conventional, and postconventional levels (Kohlberg, 1981). Each level is composed of two stages. See Table 21–1 to see how Kohlberg's stages of moral development apply to the opening scenario.

The first level of moral development consists of stages 1 and 2, which are collectively known as the *preconventional level*. At this level, moral development is defined in terms of avoidance of punishment and self-interest. In stage 1, the individual is not as concerned with societal rules; the individual is concerned with avoiding punishment. Generally, this is the stage at which most children and teenagers are at; they have not yet learned societal norms, but they do know how to avoid immoral behavior because of punishment. Mitch wants to avoid punishment; moreover, he is concerned with obeying the rules of the organization and performing his managerial duties. Therefore, Mitch's level of moral development is consistent with stage 2.

The second level, which includes stages 3 and 4, is referred to as the *conventional development level*. At this level, individuals are concerned with the norms of society and what the group thinks is moral. As the name implies, most people attain this level of development, which is why it is referred to as *conventional*. The person exhibits loyalty and commitment to groups, and the groups follow the conventions of society. Adults who operate at this second level of moral development adopt behaviors that are consistent with good or expected behaviors. At this stage (conventional) Mitch's professional values and responsibilities to his employer and customers are very important. Furthermore, an adult operating at this second stage would consider one's professional responsibility to follow the rules of the organization.

As individuals mature in their moral development their perspectives change from one level to the next. For example, when Mitch was functioning at the conventional level he believes that good employees should follow the institution's policies. He feels that he is expected to fire Gerri. Even though Gerri explained her childcare issues and lack of social support to Mitch, he is more concerned with the institution's rules.

Stages 5 and 6 are referred to as the *post-conventional level*. At this level, the individual is able to separate individual views from societal views on moral behavior. There is a strong concern for society as well as the individual. An important distinction in the post-conventional level is that the individual not only understands the laws and rules governing the situation but must evaluate them— the rules may be biased or unfair (Pritchard, 1999). Mitch is not at this stage. If Mitch had questioned the organization's policy or had considered whether it was legal to fire Gerri and had decided not to fire her because it would better serve society if she maintained her job, he would be placed at this stage. Gerri's rights to contribute to society and add value to the workplace are important, but Mitch never considered them. Mitch could have fought the policy and not have fired Gerri, but at no time did he consider this option, so he rightfully would be considered as behaving at level 2. Individuals acting at level 3 recognize different values for both individuals and society. Keep in mind that the decision to fire Gerri can be viewed as a moral behavior; however, the process by which an individual reaches that decision is important.

Moral development can be advanced by increasing one's moral awareness. Managers can stay at stage 4, but Kohlberg wants managers to consider perspectives at a higher level. Managers operating at higher stages may come to the same conclusions, but they will take into account values beyond obedience, punishment, and social norms. The ethical decision-making matrices in all of the chapters of this book assume that the HIM professional will consider stages 5 and 6.

Before we discuss moral awareness, it is important to note that Kohlberg approaches moral development with the underpinning of justice, individualism, success, rights, and fairness. Carol Gilligan (1982) conducted research that contributed to an understanding of the feminine perspectives of compassion, caring, and social responsibilities. Gilligan

Table 21–1 Kohlberg's Stages of Moral Development

Level	Stage	Decision: Should Mitch fire Gerri? *Mitch's thoughts are in italics* Explanation follows
Level 1: Preconventional	Stage 1 Punishment/obedience	Fire: *If I don't fire Gerri, I may be fired.*
		Mitch's decision *to fire* Gerri is based on avoidance of punishment. If Mitch does not fire Gerri, he could be reprimanded for not following the organization's policy.
		Don't Fire: *I don't want to be reprimanded for not following the probationary period policy, after all Gerri has sixty days to get her act together!*
		Mitch's decision *not to fire* Gerri is based on a fear of punishment.
	Stage 2 Self-interest	Fire: *This action will look good on my evaluation; if I fire Gerri, my boss will know that I'm a tough manager; I follow the rules and perhaps my boss will give me a raise or promote me.*
		Mitch has learned self-interest and follows the rules.
		Don't Fire: *There is so much work to get done and I must run this department! Who will do the work if I fire her? I don't have the time to recruit and hire for this position.*
		Mitch's decision *not to fire* is based on self-interest and he follows the rules only when they suit his immediate self-interest.
Level 2: Conventional	Stage 3 Affiliation to society and group and family expectation	Fire: *My staff will know that I'm a fair manager and that I follow the rules.*
		Mitch is trying to conform to the expectations of the manager's mantra—remain unattached and impersonal while following the rules or norms of the organization. He is considering what others expect of him.
		Don't Fire: *My staff is expecting me to do the right thing and keeping this employee is the right thing.*
		Mitch's decision *not to fire* is based on expectations of others, which override self-interest. Kolhberg refers to this as following the "Golden Rule" (Kolhberg, 1981, p. 176).
	Stage 4 Law and order	Fire: *I'm firing Gerri because it is company policy, and it wouldn't be fair to other employees in the department if I treated this employee as if her problems were more important than everyone else's. I don't want other employees to get angry with me.*
		Mitch fires Gerri based on the law and keeping order. He understands that the rules in the organization must be followed in order to maintain harmony within the organization.

Table 21–1 continued

Level	Stage	Decision: Should Mitch fire Gerri? *Mitch's thoughts are in italics* Explanation follows
		Don't Fire: *It is company policy to grant employees a probationary period of sixty days.*
		Mitch *does not fire* Gerri based on the law (probationary policy) and keeping order. He understands that the rules in the organization allow Gerri sixty days and he can maintain harmony within the department and the organization.
Level 3: Postconventional	Stage 5 Legal or social contract	Fire: *I'm firing Gerri because the rules of this organization call for it. Legally, I can fire her because of the policies in the employee handbook. I have an obligation to keep only qualified employees.*
		Mitch considered the polarities in this situation and after thoughtful consideration, makes the decision based on what society values—he has a contract to hire and retain competent employees.
		Don't Fire: *Gerri has a right to work—she is a welfare-to-work employee and is producing high-quality work!*
		Mitch decided *not to fire* Gerri. He placed a high value on the quality and quantity of Gerri's work and decided that it is in the best interest of the organization, department, and Gerri.
	Stage 6 Universal ethics	Fire: *I'm firing Gerri* not *because it is policy, but because it is the ethical action, even though that requires courage on my part.*
		There is strong concern for society and individual rights, and Mitch looks for a more global or universal solution in making his decision. His decision may be in direct conflict with societal laws or the organization's policies. He would engage ethical principles of fairness, justice, and beneficence. It is in the best interests of the department *to fire* Gerri.
		Don't Fire: *I have an obligation to society that is higher than my obligation to my employer. According to my personal/religious and professional values, I want to give Gerri a chance to succeed. I can't just be fair to those employees who have a good family support system and economic stability.*
		Mitch does have the option of not firing the employee, based on the perspectives of both the individual and society. This level follows the "universal principles of justice" (Kohlberg, 1981, p.176).

Source: Adapted from L. Kohlberg. (1981). *Essays in moral development.* New York: Harper and Row.

noted that Kohlberg's model reflects a bias in gender and showed the male perspective only, and her research demonstrated that those with feminine perspectives, regardless of gender, based the decisions on caring and relationships, not justice and individualism. Gilligan developed an orientation to ethics that reflects moral development from the feminine perspective (Little, 1998). Gilligan made many contributions to the study of morality but most importantly offered a perspective that had been missing from the preliminary research on moral development.

The notion of caring, emotional involvement, and relationships are the hallmarks of this perspective. Caring includes an understanding that we have a responsibility to others and this responsibility includes not hurting others (Gilligan, 1993). Gilligan's research found that women engage in relationships and offer contextual thinking. But a decision based solely on caring or emotions is inadequate; Gilligan clarifies values that include personal integrity, which captures a deep understanding of others, one self, and our relationships (Gilligan, 1993, p.167).

When making management decisions, the HIM professional will need to engage the perspectives of justice and fairness, as described by Kohlberg, and the perspectives of caring and compassion, as described by Gilligan. Both perspectives are needed when resolving complex ethical problems, such as teaching and orienting the "back to work" mother with family issues.

See the ethical decision-making matrices at the end of this chapter for compelling ethical arguments to both fire and not fire Gerri.

MORAL AWARENESS

Moral awareness, which is sometimes referred to as *ethical sensitivity* or **moral intensity,** refers to an individual's ability to recognize that a situation has moral implications (Trevino & Brown, 2004). Generally, managers are acutely aware of certain moral situations, such as fraud and abuse, because they can clearly relate to them as having legal or moral conse-

quences for their organizations. Such situations are obvious and have a high moral intensity. But what about the situation in Scenario 21-A? How would you describe Mitch's moral awareness?

Clearly, the opening scenario highlights the importance of the manager's moral development. Mitch is not immoral, even if he makes his decision based on level 1 moral development. However, he could progress in his role as a manager if he moved beyond the minimum criteria of moral development. The goal of moral awareness for managers requires them to take a deeper look into each situation and reflect on their own personal moral understanding of the situation. Simultaneously, managers must understand the situation, identify the moral implications of the situation, and most importantly make decisions. Moral awareness in many situations is akin to driving a car—we don't need to read the driver's manual every time we drive. The act of driving requires us to have an understanding of the rules and a heightened expectation of what might occur. Knowing what we ought to do in certain situations is the basis for moral awareness. Moreover, moral awareness is not only critical in today's business world, but it is a skill taught in most disciplines.

An understanding of a manager's level of moral development will enable an exploration of the interplay of the level of moral development and decisions made in everyday managerial situations.

When faced with ambiguous situations, managers may find it easier to rely on the organization's rules (staying at level 2). When should the comfort level with these rules cease to exist or present tension for the manager? Does the manager have the mindfulness or the awareness to identify and analyze his or her responsibility in moral terms? Does the manager have the time to identify and analyze his or her responsibility in moral terms? Managers working in health care must make many complex decisions in a fast-paced environment. Moral awareness can be seen as the first step in ethical decision making (Trevino & Brown, 2004; Glover, 2001).

Scenario 21-B: National Convention Misadventures

Tom Golden, the HIM director at University Medical Center (UMC), Southern Division, and his newly hired assistant director, Nancy Jordan, attended the American Health Information Management Association (AHIMA) national conference last fall. UMC, like most healthcare organizations, is under tremendous pressure to cut costs and remain financially sound as an organization. However, UMC strongly values continuing education, and while most expense categories in the organization have been cut, continuing education expenses continue to increase.

The rationale for increasing support for education stems from the medical center's vision to move UMC to the top of the healthcare industry. The medical center wants to be more technologically advanced than its competitors. In order to achieve this goal, the organization promotes a learning environment and encourages continuing education. Tom, like most of the directors at UMC, is aware of the mission and takes full advantage of the continuing education package. All of the expenses related to attending the conference (i.e., travel, food, lodging, conference registration) are reimbursed by UMC.

This year the AHIMA conference was held in San Francisco, and this was Tom's first trip to the West Coast. Tom was delighted that he got budgetary approval for both him and his assistant to attend the conference. Tom and Nancy both checked in on Sunday evening and were planning to attend the conference for three days. Nancy was excited because this was her first AHIMA conference, and she was looking forward to the educational sessions.

Tom asked Nancy to join him in sightseeing the San Francisco area on Monday, immediately after the keynote speaker. Nancy stated she had plans to attend three afternoon educational sessions, but that she could print out the PowerPoint slides and miss the presentations. Nancy was not forced to do this, but she believed that no harm would result from a few hours away from the convention.

During the course of Monday evening, Tom introduced Nancy to many of the vendors at the individual receptions, which were sponsored by the vendors. They both got the opportunity to eat and drink and to discuss products with the vendors that evening. Tom pointed out to Nancy the value in meeting vendors and establishing good relationships with them, because it is a good way to find out about new products and technologies. The vendors provided Tom and Nancy with numerous sales pitches and provided product information. Tom and Nancy also received complimentary dinner, art, and theater passes for the city for Tuesday.

They had such a fabulous time visiting the city that they decided to finish the sightseeing tour on Tuesday, so Tom and Nancy used the gift passes they received from the vendors. At the end of the day, Nancy asked Tom if they would be attending sessions on the last day. Nancy really wanted to attend more educational sessions, because she had worked in many other healthcare organizations that had never provided continuing education support, so she was very appreciative of being allowed to attend the convention. She also needed the continuing education credits in order to maintain her credentials.

Tom told Nancy that mangers at UMC routinely bring their families and enjoy vacation and business at conferences and continuing education sessions. He stated, "Of course we will stop in at an educational session." The last day of the conference offered three educational sessions. Tom and Nancy went to breakfast with a group of vendors and attended two of the sessions.

Tom felt really good about attending the conference, because he got the opportunity to attend a couple of educational sessions, the vendor exhibits, and the opening keynote address. In addition, he retrieved information from the vendor exhibits to read on the flight home, so he felt satisfied. Tom thought that even though they spent much time sight-seeing and dining with vendors, they could catch up on the conference materials on the plane ride home. Nancy, however, had serious doubts as to whether reading the conference proceedings would edify her as much as attending the actual sessions in San Francisco.

Nancy wanted to ask why they had spent so much time sight-seeing, but she remained quiet because she felt it would affect her relationship with her new boss. After some consideration on the plane ride home, she agreed with Tom. Nancy had a change of mind, she enjoyed the opportunity to visit San Francisco, meet vendors, and converse with HIM professionals at the conference. She was quite pleased that UMC had afforded her the opportunity to get away from the office and mix business with pleasure.

Tom was persistent in his instruction to Nancy and made sure that she accepted the company's social norms, as he described them. He felt confident that she would not raise any concerns with his supervisors when they returned to work, based on what she said during the plane ride home.

Questions

1. How appropriate was Tom's decision to sightsee instead of attending educational sessions?

2. Do you know whether Tom is telling the truth that "everyone" mixes business with pleasure? Is this the social norm for the medical center?

3. Should Nancy have questioned the practice of mixing business with pleasure?

4. What were the potential consequences to Nancy, if she had decided to attend the sessions and not sightsee with Tom?

5. Should Nancy say anything when she returns from the convention? Who would she speak with?

A completed ethical decision-making matrix for the scenario is provided at the end of the chapter.

ORIENTATION OF NEW EMPLOYEES

Employees may be introduced to unethical behaviors either gradually or suddenly in the organization (Anand, Ashforth, & Joshi, 2004). Although most organizations provide a code of ethics, a mission statement, policies, and training programs on ethics, employees quickly learn through socialization the rules and culture of the organization and adapt to the culture, even if it involves some unethical behaviors. New employees learn from the actions of their managers, not from the words in the code of ethics or employee handbook.

In Scenario 21-B, Nancy was introduced to unethical behaviors as a new employee. The processes of socialization, rationalization, and equity are important when trying to understand the complexities of orienting the new employee to the organization's culture and values.

Socialization is the process by which employees learn the norms and acceptable behaviors of the group (Anand et al., 2004). The new employee learns to adapt, accept, and gradually fit into the customs of the organization. The new employee can learn more than the politics of the organization through socialization. It is the mechanism by which the new employee learns acceptable behaviors, even if they are unethical ones. Organizations can socialize new employees by providing orientation programs, job training, and formal policies and procedures.

The process of socialization is very powerful. It has an impact on the employee while he or she is employed and even long after he or she leaves the organization. Socialization occurs as a result of behavior modification. Because the socialization process can change an individual, it is important for organizations to discuss their values during the application or hiring process in order to avoid a misunderstanding of values. What values and socialization lessons will the new employee bring to the new job? Is the new employee's existing work ethic compatible with the organization's? For some employees, the work ethic might be "I do as little as possible to get paid." For others, it might be "I'll do everything I can because I really want this job, like this organization, and want to do quality work."

In Scenario 21-B, the HIM manager supposedly hired Nancy because she was an ethical person with a good work ethic; however, Nancy's values began to erode because Tom did not support ethical behavior; that is, attending the educational sessions versus sightseeing. If Nancy had expressed her concerns, would Tom have found a way to terminate her employment? Nancy was introduced to unethical behavior and decided not to take any chances, so she decided to conform and accept the values, as told to her by Tom.

It is important for organizations to realize that all employees will not welcome the organization's values. What happens when an employee does not accept the organization's values? Employees who resist the socialization process have a tendency to leave the organization, resulting in high turnover. Even worse, they may decide to stay in the organization and demonstrate a poor work ethic—inadequate performance, low morale, or a failure to commit to the organization.

Individual behaviors or practices can start to erode the organization's ethics and gradually become business as usual (Anand et al., 2004). Unethical practices in UMC could erode the organization's ethics and become normal practice. Tom suggested that all the managers at UMC routinely bring their families and enjoy vacation and business at continuing education sessions. Tom considers this kind of activity as the normal course of business, resulting in an "everybody does it" rationale for the behaviors.

Rationalization occurs when an employee seeks to justify unethical behaviors (Anand et al., 2004). A common theme and reason for rationalization includes the belief that the organization owes the employee or that the employee deserves a perk, such as paid educational sessions, pencils and pens, or arriving late at work but still expecting to get paid for the whole day. Rationalization has been attributed as an explanation as to why some seemingly ethical people commit unethical acts or behaviors. Employees rationalize behaviors in many different ways, but the perception of fairness or equity is a common reason for justifying unethical behaviors.

Equity means that the employee perceives fairness in relationships. When employees feel that they are not compensated appropriately or that others in the organization have more commensurable goods, feelings of inequity can overshadow ethical decisions. This is commonly seen when employees feel that they are not hurting the department by stealing office supplies or surfing the Internet for hours during work time. In Scenario 21-B, the sight-seeing was considered a perk for working hard the rest of the year. Tom may have included the sight-seeing activities as part of the educational expenses because he felt that he deserved it for working hard all year. Tom and Nancy used both rationalization and equity as reasons to justify their behaviors at the convention.

As mentioned earlier, although most organizations provide a code of ethics, a mission statement, and policies and training programs on ethics, employees quickly learn the rules and culture of the organization and adapt to the culture even if it involves some unethical behaviors. How can an organization develop a moral code or moral character in management?

Scenario 21-C: Avoiding an Employee Who Will Be Fired

Carol Wright is an outstanding manager. She has worked for C&S Pharmaceuticals for 15 years. She has received five promotions and is currently responsible for abstracting and quality operations. Carol has been quick to identify personnel problems and provides educational and instructional support to her staff.

Carol supervises Joan, who is often absent or late for work. When she does come to work, she makes many mistakes, but she always seems to meet work standards prior to her performance reviews. Various forms of motivation, education, and administrative support have been offered to Joan in the past. This week, Joan failed to show up for three days, without notifying the office. The company policy states that if an employee does not show up for work for three consecutive days without notifying the office by the end of the third business day (5:00 PM), the employee's employment shall be terminated.

On the third day, some managers may be anxiously waiting for the employee to call and explain the absence, but this was not the case with Carol. Carol had recognized that this employee was nonproductive, noncompliant, and met the criteria for job abandonment. Carol was prepared to terminate Joan, because she repeatedly demonstrated a clear disregard for the policy related to reporting to work. Carol no longer had any patience for Joan's behaviors. Carol was confident that the employee was not going to comply with the policy and this would be an easy termination. So, she completed the termination paperwork, based on job abandonment, at 3:00 PM and left it on her desk for the 5:00 PM submission to human resources. At 4:30 PM, Carol's secretary told her that Joan was on the telephone, but Carol did not accept the call. The paperwork was sent to human resources at 5:00 PM, and Joan's employment was terminated the next day.

Questions

1. Should Carol have taken the call from Joan?

2. Did Carol act with integrity when she knowingly did not answer the call from Joan?

3. Were there steps that could have been followed to prevent this situation from occurring?

4. What are Joan's responsibilities to her employer?

5. Should Joan have been fired?

6. What if Carol had taken the call and had found out that this was a legitimate absence and that Joan had been in an accident?

7. Should the grounds for termination be based on performance or failure to call in on time?

A completed ethical decision-making matrix for the scenario is provided at the end of the chapter.

THE CODE OF ETHICS IS NOT ENOUGH: ACTIONS SPEAK LOUDER THAN WORDS

Organizations need to understand why an employee code of ethics, a mission statement, and policies are not enough to discourage or prevent unethical behavior. Although "an increasing number of companies have adopted codes of ethics, these codes are not sufficient" (Anand et al., 2004, p. 49); organizations must nurture an ethical environment. Anand and colleagues (2004) suggest that employees and managers need access to resources and an environment in which they can openly discuss ethical situations when they arise.

Unethical behaviors can permeate an entire organization, but they can be stopped. What can happen when employees notice that the behaviors of their managers or other employees are unethical? What should an individual do at that point? Will employees be supported if they raise an ethical problem or will they be called a whistle-blower and alienated from the rest of the group?

Anonymous hotlines and codes of ethics should be available for employees and managers so that they can receive guidance once they recognize moral situations. They need to be educated not only in identifying ethical situations with severe consequences (e.g., fraud and abuse), but also those situations that are not easily identified or that have less

serious consequences (e.g., stealing supplies). Organizations need to establish a culture of ethics that will raise the level of moral awareness throughout the organization. Developing a moral culture is challenging. It should start at the top of the organization (e.g., the board of trustees) and work down to involve all managers. Managers can be role models by communicating and exhibiting the ethical values and standards in the organization (Trevino & Brown, 2004).

WHEN LEADERSHIP FAILS

Three themes resonate for managers when making decisions that are not congruent with company policy: "performance-based judgment calls," "social norms," and "faulty rules" (Veiga, Golden, & Dechant, 2004, p. 86). These three themes appeal to the wide range of things that managers must consider during the decision-making process; for example, social responsibility and expectations for organizational performance. Managers clearly have a responsibility to make sure that department goals are congruent with organizational goals, and this is generally achieved by monitoring and maintaining high-quality work performance.

The first theme, "performance-based judgment calls," applies to Scenario 21-C in the sense that the organization cannot expect to obtain adequate performance levels with this type of employee—one who is inconsistent, produces poor quality work, and is routinely absent. Even though Joan called the office before 5:00 PM on the third day, she is harmful to this organization, and she does not add value to the organization. "Performance-based judgment calls are managerial decisions to bend the rules because, in so doing, company or individual performance will be enhanced" (Veiga et al., 2004, p. 85). The organization's rule is *not to fire Joan,* because she notified the department within the specified time frame; however; Carol is bending the rule (and firing her), because she knows that the company will be better served without Carol.

When Carol fired Joan, she had reached a point where she recognized that no matter what she did, Joan was not going to add value to the company. Therefore, Carol "bent the rules" and made a judgment call, which implied that calling in 30 minutes before the deadline was still grounds for termination. Carol concluded that a temporary worker or overtime given to other employees would benefit and add value to the organization more than Joan's continuous failure to perform. In Scenario 21-C, Carol felt that the organization would clearly not benefit from retaining Joan. In fact, one might argue that the manager waited too long to process the paperwork for termination.

The second theme for bending the rules is a "faulty rule." A "faulty rule" refers to "company policies that are ambiguous, out-of-date, or simply wrong in the eyes of the manager and can lead to rule bending" (Veiga et al., 2004, p. 86). Carol may have thought that the employee was given ample time to call in and explain the absence and that it is wrong to call on the last day at the last possible time. Carol may feel that in today's high technological environment there is no excuse for failing to communicate in a timely fashion. Simply stated, she may believe that the policy is outdated, because employees have access to e-mail, cellular phones, and voice mail. Although the rule states that the employee has until 5:00 PM on the third day, Carol disagreed. Is it Carol's obligation to initiate a change in organizational policy?

The third theme, "social norms," supports that "no one expects strict adherence to the rules" (Veiga et al., 2004, p. 87). This theme suggests that the social norms of the organization may include the manager's flexibility or discretion to decide on what rules to follow. Managers have a responsibility to consistently adhere to the rules and raise questions when the rules are ambiguous in organization—they are not exempt from following rules. There might also be a time and place for the mantra "rules are made to be broken." Regardless of what reason the manager may have for not answering the telephone, the question remains: Should the manager have accepted the call at 4:30 PM? Does the manager have a greater responsibility to the organization or to the employee? How does Carol balance the competing interests and obligations of both? As Carol struggles to make a decision, she needs to balance the good of the organization with the good of the individual employee. What is the role of the employee in this situation? Did the employee have any obligation or responsibility to the manager or the organization? What are those obligations?

Did Carol behave in an ethical way when she failed to answer the telephone, or did she make the correct decision in the best interest of her department? Did she act with integrity? The rigidity of answering the questions in terms of policy and procedures does not offer the full answer. The policy states that the employee can call before 5:00 PM on third day, which Joan did. Was Carol wrong in not answering the phone at 4:30 PM? Carol could be a moral person with a high level of moral awareness who made a decision that was unethical. You might conclude from this case that the manager made an ethical decision because she only has a social obligation to the organization and does not need to consider the needs of the employee. What professional values could have been engaged on the part of the manager to assist her with the decision?

Scenario 21-D: Failure to Document Poor Work Performance for a Friendly Employee

Samuel has worked for the Memorial Center Hospital for 23 years. He believes in the concept of seniority and thinks that loyalty to an organization is worth a yearly 5% increase in pay, regardless of his work performance. Over the past 23 years, Samuel had many promotions. He was promoted from incomplete file clerk to senior analyst and then to coder. At the time of his promotion from senior analyst to coder, the physicians had been complaining because Samuel was inaccurate with record assignments. They were happy with his promotion to the coding area. The promotion occurred at a time when shortages and turnovers were occurring in the coding area. Samuel has not been able to meet performance standards for several years, but nothing has been done because of his longevity with the organization and his friendliness.

From Samuel's perspective, he reports to work every day on time and never misses a day of work. In fact, he has had perfect attendance for the last 15 years. He attends every mandatory training session and even some additional training courses at the hospital. When Samuel first started to work, he assisted a patient in retrieving her medical records from five healthcare providers prior to her move to Florida. Samuel was honored with the "employee of the month" award for his efforts in assisting this patient. Samuel knows that everyone in the organization likes him. It is clear that Samuel offers many fine attributes to the organization, such as punctuality, attendance, commitment, and motivation to learn.

Over the past several years, the management team in the HIM department has changed, but the coding staff has remained stable. Samuel is now 51 years old, and his new manager, a young graduate who just received her RHIA credential, is requiring him to accurately assign the appropriate ICD-9-CM and CPT codes to the medical records and to meet quantitative performance standards. He has received written communication from his manager that his merit pay is in jeopardy. Samuel has raised questions concerning the discrepancy in his current appraisal with that of his past appraisals, because his past performance appraisals were stellar. He expresses concern that age discrimination might be a factor in his recent appraisal.

Questions

1. Given Samuel's age, should the new manager evaluate him at a lower performance standard?

2. Did the managers make good decisions in the past with regard to Samuel's performance and promotions?

3. What should be done with Samuel now?

4. Can Samuel make a claim of age discrimination?

5. Is it enough to show up for work but not contribute to the organization's core performance values?

A completed ethical decision-making matrix for the scenario is provided at the end of the chapter.

A dilemma faced by many managers is dealing with long-term employees who have *not* received honest feedback in the past. Take Samuel, for example: He was promoted to a coding position because of a need to fill a vacancy rather than because of his meritorious performance. He moved throughout the department several times with promotions because he was pleasant, not because he was competent. It would appear that he received each promotion so that the current manager would not have to deal with Samuel's poor performance; no one wanted to fire Samuel. The promotions and job changes over the years enabled managers to say "it's not my problem any more, it's someone else's."

Samuel's manager is concerned with his work performance, but she is also concerned that no other manager has been honest with this employee. In terms of moral obligation, did the previous management team promote this employee because of loyalty and not performance? Ethically, did the management team have a responsibility to both the organization and the employee to provide constructive feedback? Samuel's manager is now faced with a potential age discrimination issue because the previous documentation in Samuel's personnel records reflects superior work performance.

MORAL MUTENESS

Rating an employee's performance is a systematic way for an organization to acknowledge performance and confirm organizational goals. **Moral muteness** is a manager's inability to discuss situations in terms of what is right and wrong (Bird & Waters, 1989). Managers can be mute because it is an easier path and it enables them to avoid conflict (as least for the short term). Are managers mute because they don't understand the issue or because they are afraid to speak? Managers remain morally mute in organizations for a variety of reasons. They may want to avoid interpersonal conflicts, as suggested in Scenario 21-D. They may also shy away from making difficult decisions that require an accurate reflection of appropriate standards and/or behaviors. Some managers may have a problem confronting their employees or they may lack the interpersonal skills needed to provide constructive feedback to employees (Bird & Waters, 1989).

Whatever the case, managers have a responsibility to both the organization and the employee to provide appropriate feedback on performance. They must act with integrity and tell the truth, noting both positive and negative performance standards and behaviors. Otherwise, the manager who ultimately tells the truth could be charged with discrimination by the employee who says "everyone else liked my work but you are picking on me" (because of my age, gender, race, or the like).

Managers have an obligation to provide honest feedback to employees. More importantly, managers need to act with behaviors that are fair and consistent to all employees. They cannot shy away from their responsibility even if the employee is over 40 years old and well liked by all. It should be noted that in this scenario the manager did provide training and continuing education. Managers need to have courage and make decisions based on professional values, accepting responsibility for their duties, even if the decision may result in the denial of merit pay. Excellence can only be provided when managers plan, evaluate, and provide honest feedback to employees on their performance.

CONCLUSION

Many factors may challenge a manager's ability to increase moral awareness. Many situations or decisions can challenge the manager's professional values (AHIMA, 2004). It is important to recognize that most managers have a strong affinity to follow the rules and adhere to lines of authority. Because of this, they may be challenged in recognizing situations that have a higher moral intensity. Managers have an obligation to consider the consequences or impact of their decisions on the individual, the organization, and society (Walton, 1988).

HIM professionals and the organizations that they work for will be better off if there is moral awareness on the part of all employees. It is insufficient to merely hand out a code of ethics or a compliance plan. These resources must be enhanced through formal educational programs so that managers and employees can learn to make ethical decisions. Organizations that allow managers to freely question policies and discuss areas of tension are better prepared to raise the moral awareness of their employees and managers (Anand et al., 2004). The work environment must promote and allow managers to initiate discussions about ethical behaviors.

Moral development, socialization, rationalization, moral muteness, and ethical failures have been explored as a basis for helping the HIM managers who must deal with daily operational decisions. Organizations can begin to raise moral awareness by providing proper socialization so that employees will learn the norms and acceptable behaviors that reflect ethical behavior.

Professional values, including honesty and integrity and providing services to many stakeholders, are important. Building on these values can offer tremendous guidance in directing organizations to be morally successful. Successful organizations can offer training, education, and work environments that are mindful of professional values. Such organizations will raise the ethical awareness of their employees, and their efforts will improve the quality of the services provided in the healthcare delivery system.

Key Terms

- Equity
- Moral awareness
- Moral intensity
- Moral muteness
- Rationalization
- Socialization
- Stages of moral development

Chapter Summary

- HIM managers are responsible for the daily operations of the information system. They have social and ethical responsibilities in the workplace and are challenged by fast-paced operational activities. The workplace is changing, but what remains constant is that managers are faced with making ethical decisions each day.
- HIM managers, along with other healthcare managers, must understand the different orientations to moral decision making and moral development, moral awareness, rationalization, socialization, moral muteness, and ethical failures as guides for making decisions.
- Mangers experience real tension between deciding what is right for the individual, the organization, and society. Organizations need to understand the tension for management and how the organizational culture impacts routine behaviors. The management challenge is to increase moral awareness and nurture an ethical environment.

References

Abdelhak, M., Grostick, S., Hanken, M. A., & Jacobs, E. (Eds.). (2000). *Health information: Management of a strategic resource*, 2d ed. Philadelphia: W.B. Saunders.

American Health Information Management Association [AHIMA]. (2004). *AHIMA code of ethics*. Chicago: Author.

Anand, V., Ashforth, B. E., & Joshi, M. (2004). Business as usual: The acceptance and perpetuation of corruption in organizations. *Academy of Management Executive, 18*(2), 39–53.

Bird, F. B., & Waters, J. A. (1989). The moral muteness of managers. *California Management Review, 32*(1), 73–87.

Gilligan, C. (1993). *In a different voice*. Cambridge, MA: Harvard University Press.

Glover, J. J. (2001). Ethical decision-making guidelines and tools. In L. B. Harman (Ed.), *Ethical challenges in the management of health information*, pp. 25–38. Gaithersburg, MD: Aspen.

Holzer, H. J., Stoll, M. A., & Wissoker, D. (2004). Job performance and retention among welfare recipients. *Social Service Review, 78*, 343–369.

Kohlberg, L. (1981). *The philosophy of moral development: Essays on moral development*, Vol 1. New York: Harper and Row.

Latour, K. M., & Eichenwald, S. (Eds.). (2002). *Health information management: Concepts, principles and practice*. Chicago: American Health Information Management Association.

Little, M. O. (1998). Care: From theory to orientation and back. *Journal of Medicine and Philosophy, 23*(2), 190–209.

Pritchard, M. S. (1999). Kohlbergian contributions to educational programs for the moral development of professionals. *Educational Psychology Review, 11*(4), 395–409.

Trevino, L. K., & Brown, M. E. (2004). Managing to be ethical: Debunking five business ethics myths. *Academy of Management Executive, 18*(2), 69–78.

US Department of Health and Human Services. (2005a). Office of Family Assistance. Retrieved October 17, 2005, from http://www.acf.dhhs.gov/programs/ofa/.

US Department of Health and Human Services. (2005b). Office of Family Assistance: Table 12:11. Retrieved October 17, 2005, from http://www.acf.hhs.gov/programs/ofa/annualreport5/1211.htm.

US Department of Labor: Employee and Training Administration. (2005). Welfare to work highlights. Retrieved October 11, 2005, from http://www.doleta.gov/wtw/.

Veiga, J., Golden, T., & Dechant, K. (2004). Why managers bend company rules. *Academy of Management Executive, 18*(2), 69–78.

Walton, C. (1988). *The moral manager*. Cambridge, MA: Ballinger Publishing Company.

The ethical decision-making matrix is a tool to help you organize complex, ethical problems; however, there is no simple fill-in-the-box approach to ethical decision making. The objective is to follow each step of the process and not move from the question directly to what should be done or how to prevent it next time. If you skip steps, you will not fully understand all of the values and options for action. Also, the matrix provided for each scenario in this book is not the only way to examine the problem. You can make an equally compelling ethical argument for a different decision—just be sure to follow all the steps of the matrix.

SCENARIO 21-A.1: LATENESS AND ABSENTEEISM

Steps	Information	
1. What is the ethical question?	Should Mitch fire Gerri for lateness and absenteeism in the probationary period?	
2. What are the facts?	**KNOWN**	**TO BE GATHERED**
	• Gerri Randolph, a divorced single mother with four small children, was hired as a welfare-to-work employee. • During her first month of employment, Gerri was absent three times and late several times. • The quantity and quality of her work were exceptional for a new employee. • Employees can be terminated during a three-month probationary period. • Mitch Malloy, Gerri's supervisor, discussed the problem with Gerri, warned her of the strict attendance policy, and decided to fire her.	• What responsibility does Mitch have to society to keep people employed? • What are the implications to Gerri and society of terminating Gerri, going back on welfare, and losing health benefits for her family? • Does Mitch understand his stage in moral development and awareness? • Should Mitch follow the policy, indicating unquestioned loyalty to the employer? • Are performance standards the only criteria for employee evaluation? • Does Mitch have obligations to help an employee resolve personal problems? • Can Mitch get assistance with moving to higher stages of moral development?
3. What are the values? Examine the shared and competing values, obligations, and interests of the stakeholders (i.e., patient, HIM professional, healthcare practitioner(s), administrators, society, and other advocates) involved in order to fully understand the complexity of the ethical problem(s).	**Employee:** Employment that allows her to take care of her family and provide health benefits; contribute to society. **HIM professional:** Support organizational goals (including firing of employees, if necessary); consider individual rights and problems of employees; comply with laws, regulations, and policies. **Employer:** Support societal goals for welfare reform; provide quality health care through hiring and retention of skilled workers; make fiscally sound decisions; treat employees fairly. **Society:** Follow welfare program rules that give citizens assistance with employment.	

4. What are my options?	• Fire Gerri during the probationary period. • Do not fire Gerri during the probationary period.	
5. What should I do?	Fire Gerri.	
6. What justifies my choice?	**JUSTIFIED**	**NOT JUSTIFIED**
	• Obligation to follow organizational policies. • Treat all employees fairly, based on performance standards.	• Ignore performance standards. • Treat employees differently and unfairly. • Apply societal goals rather than organizational goals.
7. How can I prevent this ethical problem?	• Collect additional information after hiring that might help a new employee deal with the transition from welfare to work. • Provide training on life management, work ethic, and technical health information skills. • Provide information on employee assistance programs to help the new employee deal with issues of transportation and child care. • Seek educational assistance in learning more about making ethical decisions based on a higher level of moral development.	

The ethical decision-making matrix is a tool to help you organize complex, ethical problems; however, there is no simple fill-in-the-box approach to ethical decision making. The objective is to follow each step of the process and not move from the question directly to what should be done or how to prevent it next time. If you skip steps, you will not fully understand all of the values and options for action. Also, the matrix provided for each scenario in this book is not the only way to examine the problem. You can make an equally compelling ethical argument for a different decision—just be sure to follow all the steps of the matrix.

SCENARIO 21-A.2: LATENESS AND ABSENTEEISM

Steps	Information	
1. What is the ethical question?	Should Mitch fire Gerri for lateness and absenteeism in the probationary period?	
2. What are the facts?	**KNOWN**	**TO BE GATHERED**
	• Gerri Randolph, a divorced single mother with four small children, was hired as a welfare-to-work employee. • During her first month of employment, Gerri was absent three times and late several times. • The quantity and quality of her work were exceptional for a new employee. • Employees can be terminated during a three-month probationary period. • Mitch Malloy, Gerri's supervisor, discussed the problem with Gerri, warned her of the strict attendance policy, and decided not to fire her.	• Does Mitch have a full understanding of the welfare acts that affect employees? • What responsibility does Mitch have to society to keep people employed? • What are the implications to Gerri and society of terminating Gerri, going back on welfare, and losing health benefits for her family? • Does Mitch understand his stage in moral development and awareness? • Should Mitch follow the policy, indicating unquestioned loyalty to the employer? • Are performance standards the only criteria for employee evaluation? • Does Mitch have obligations to help an employee resolve personal problems? • Can Mitch get assistance with moving to higher stages of moral development?

3. What are the values? Examine the shared and competing values, obligations, and interests of the stakeholders (i.e., patient, HIM professional, healthcare practitioner(s), administrators, society, and other advocates) involved in order to fully understand the complexity of the ethical problem(s).	**Employee:** Employment that allows her to take care of her family and provide health benefits; contribute to society. **HIM professional:** Support organizational goals (including firing of employees, if necessary); consider individual rights and problems of employees; comply with laws, regulations, and policies. **Employer:** Support societal goals for welfare reform; provide quality health care through hiring and retention of skilled workers; make fiscally sound decisions; treat employees fairly. **Society:** Follow welfare program rules that give citizens assistance with employment.
4. What are my options?	• Fire Gerri during the probationary period. • Do not fire Gerri during the probationary period.
5. What should I do?	Do not fire Gerri.

6. What justifies my choice?	**JUSTIFIED**	**NOT JUSTIFIED**
	• Refer Gerri to those who can provide assistance with home problems, because she is still in the first month of probation and has two more months to demonstrate competency and the ability to meet time and attendance standards. • Develop a performance-based contract with Gerri with defined goals toward resolving home problems to be reviewed for outcomes at the end of the second and third months of probation. • Support societal laws that facilitate employment for citizens who need welfare. Learn more about higher stages of moral development and apply them in this situation.	• Applying time and attendance standards during the probationary period without any consideration of the individual who has been hired; knowing, yet ignoring, that her quantity and quality of work are exceptional and that the employee has problems with child care. • Avoiding decisions that require a high level of moral development and awareness. • Applying organizational goals at the expense of societal goals.

7. How can I prevent this ethical problem?	• Collect additional information after hiring that might help a new employee deal with the transition from welfare to work. • Provide training on life management, work ethic, and technical health information skills. • Provide information on employee assistance programs to help the new employee deal with issues of transportation and child care. • Seek educational assistance in learning more about making ethical decisions based on a higher level of moral development.

The ethical decision-making matrix is a tool to help you organize complex, ethical problems; however, there is no simple fill-in-the-box approach to ethical decision making. The objective is to follow each step of the process and not move from the question directly to what should be done or how to prevent it next time. If you skip steps, you will not fully understand all of the values and options for action. Also, the matrix provided for each scenario in this book is not the only way to examine the problem. You can make an equally compelling ethical argument for a different decision—just be sure to follow all the steps of the matrix.

SCENARIO 21-B: NATIONAL CONVENTION MISADVENTURES

Steps	Information	
1. What is the ethical question?	Should Tom and Nancy accept the gifts from the vendors and sightsee or attend the HIM educational sessions?	
2. What are the facts?	**KNOWN**	**TO BE GATHERED**
	• Tom attends the convention with new employee, Nancy (her first). • Continuing education (CE) expenses will be reimbursed by the employer. • They went sight-seeing instead of attending educational sessions. • Vendors sponsored social events. • Nancy needs CE credits to maintain credentials.	• Is it the norm for business and family vacations to occur with full reimbursement? • It is acceptable to socialize new employees in this way? • What are the medical center's policies regarding gifts from vendors? • Is it acceptable to read materials rather than attend sessions? • Should Nancy talk with others regarding what happened? • What might be the consequences for Nancy if she raises questions about what happened at the convention? • Could she be fired?
3. What are the values? Examine the shared and competing values, obligations, and interests of the stakeholders (i.e., patient, HIM professional, healthcare practitioner(s), administrators, society, and other advocates) involved in order to fully understand the complexity of the ethical problem(s).	**Employees:** Be socialized appropriately; take advantage of continuing education opportunities; follow organizational norms of behavior and adapt to the cultural norms; develop professional values. **HIM professional:** Honesty and integrity; bring honor to self and colleagues; sustain work ethic; follow policies of employer; receive appropriate compensation. **Employer:** Provide orientation programs to socialize new employees; offer continuing education opportunities; want recognition as being an excellent and technologically advanced organization; develop employees' work ethic. **Society:** Competent, ethical employees; appropriate utilization of financial resources.	

4. What are my options?	• Accept gifts and sightsee. • Attend the HIM educational sessions.	
5. What should I do?	Attend HIM educational sessions.	
6. What justifies my choice?	**JUSTIFIED**	**NOT JUSTIFIED**
	• The employer sponsors educational sessions to support employee competency and organizational excellence. • Employer trusts employees to use financial resources appropriately. • New employees should be socialized to develop an honorable work ethic.	• Taking gifts from vendors instead of attending educational sessions. • Misusing money from employer that is intended for educational purposes. • Socializing new employees to a poor work ethic.
7. How can I prevent this ethical problem?	• Clarify policies and normative behaviors about accepting gifts from vendors before attending educational sessions. • Develop an organizational culture that allows new employees to ask questions about practices that could be in violation of personal values and/or work ethic norms.	

The ethical decision-making matrix is a tool to help you organize complex, ethical problems; however, there is no simple fill-in-the-box approach to ethical decision making. The objective is to follow each step of the process and not move from the question directly to what should be done or how to prevent it next time. If you skip steps, you will not fully understand all of the values and options for action. Also, the matrix provided for each scenario in this book is not the only way to examine the problem. You can make an equally compelling ethical argument for a different decision—just be sure to follow all the steps of the matrix.

SCENARIO 21-C: AVOIDING AN EMPLOYEE WHO WILL BE FIRED

Steps	Information	
1. What is the ethical question?	Should Carol refuse to answer the telephone and terminate Joan's employment?	
2. What are the facts?	**KNOWN**	**TO BE GATHERED**
	• Carol is an outstanding manager who pays attention to personnel problems and the educational needs of employees. • Joan is absent or late most of the time. • Joan does not meet performance standards. • Joan failed to report for work for three days; she is eligible for termination at end of the third day at 5:00 PM. • Carol completed the termination paperwork and did not accept the call from the employee at 4:30 PM. • Termination paperwork was filed the next day and Joan was terminated.	• What are the organizational norms for responding to this situation? • Should Carol have taken the call from Joan? • What advice would human resources provide? • What are the obligations to the employer, knowing that this is a poor-performance employee? • Should a manager knowingly keep an employee who does not meet the organization's standards? • What is the reason that Joan waited until the end of the day before calling Carol? Was it an emergency? • Should the policy for termination be enforced, even though the employee technically called in on time? • Can the manager make "performance-based judgment calls"?
3. What are the values? Examine the shared and competing values, obligations, and interests of the stakeholders (i.e., patient, HIM professional, healthcare practitioner(s), administrators, society, and other advocates) involved in order to fully understand the complexity of the ethical problem(s).	**Employee:** Keep a job and take care of family. **Manager:** Keep employees who meet performance standards and who adhere to time and attendance policies; treat all employees fairly and consistently; act with honesty and integrity; know and follow human resource policies; seek consultation, when appropriate. **HIM professional:** Honesty and integrity; follows employment laws, organizational policies, and rules; manages an HIM organization that has competent employees who follow the rules to support patient care. **Healthcare professionals:** HIM employees that are competent and at work to support patient care through a quality health information system. **Administrators:** Competent employees who follow the rules; rules applied fairly and appropriately for all employees. **Society:** Employees should be paid to provide appropriate services and terminated if they do not.	

4. What are my options?	<ul><li>Decide in advance to terminate the employee and refuse to take the call.</li><li>Take the call and follow rules and regulations appropriately.</li></ul>	
5. What should I do?	Take the call from Joan and follow the organization's policies, as appropriate.	
6. What justifies my choice?	**JUSTIFIED**	**NOT JUSTIFIED**
	<ul><li>Do not fire Joan because she followed the rule to notify the department before the end of the third day.</li></ul>	<ul><li>Use the themes of performance-based judgment calls, social norms, and faulty rules to justify termination.</li><li>Rationalize that the employer will be better served without this employee.</li><li>Put employee needs before needs of the organization.</li></ul>
7. How can I prevent this ethical problem?	<ul><li>Develop continuing education programs for managers that can explore employee situations that do not fall in the "this is right and that is wrong" category for decision making.</li><li>Establish increased organizational accountability for employees for following performance, time, and attendance standards that support the complexities faced by both the employee and the manager.</li></ul>	

The ethical decision-making matrix is a tool to help you organize complex, ethical problems; however, there is no simple fill-in-the-box approach to ethical decision making. The objective is to follow each step of the process and not move from the question directly to what should be done or how to prevent it next time. If you skip steps, you will not fully understand all of the values and options for action. Also, the matrix provided for each scenario in this book is not the only way to examine the problem. You can make an equally compelling ethical argument for a different decision—just be sure to follow all the steps of the matrix.

SCENARIO 21-D: FAILURE TO DOCUMENT POOR WORK PERFORMANCE FOR A FRIENDLY EMPLOYEE

Steps	Information	
1. What is the ethical question?	Should Samuel be fired for failure to meet work performance standards?	
2. What are the facts?	**KNOWN**	**TO BE GATHERED**
	• Samuel has worked for the organization for 23 years. • Samuel has demonstrated excellence for attendance, commitment, and motivation and wants to be rewarded for seniority, regardless of work performance. • He was promoted in past for being pleasant, not competent. • A new HIM manager requires Samuel to meet quantity and quality performance standards. • Samuel implies that he will pursue an age discrimination lawsuit.	• What are the norms for responding to such situations? • Can performance standards be lowered for older employees? • What are the laws and policies for age discrimination? What advice would human resources provide? • What are the obligations to the employer, knowing that this is a poor-performance employee? • Should a manager knowingly keep an employee who doesn't meet the standards?
3. What are the values? Examine the shared and competing values, obligations, and interests of the stakeholders (i.e., patient, HIM professional, healthcare practitioner(s), administrators, society, and other advocates) involved in order to fully understand the complexity of the ethical problem(s).	**Employee:** Stay employed and be rewarded for dedication and longevity. **Manager:** Keep employees who meet performance standards; know how to avoid age discrimination issues; treat all employees fairly and consistently; act with honesty and integrity; know and follow human resource policies; seek consultation, when appropriate. **HIM professional:** Honesty and integrity; follows employment laws, organizational policies, and rules; manages HIM system that has competent employees who follow the rules to support patient care. **Healthcare professionals:** HIM employees who are competent and work to support patient care through a quality health information system. **Administrators:** Competent employees who follow the rules; rules applied fairly and appropriately for all employees; managers who will deal with interpersonal problems appropriately, acting with integrity and telling the truth. **Society:** Employees should be paid to provide appropriate services and terminated if they do not.	

4. What are my options?	• Terminate Samuel for failure to meet performance standards. • Keep a long-term employee who meets other standards, such as time and attendance standards and attending educational sessions, and who is pleasant.	
5. What should I do?	Terminate Samuel for failure to meet performance standards.	
6. What justifies my choice?	**JUSTIFIED**	**NOT JUSTIFIED**
	• Obligation to give employees honest feedback regarding performance standards. • Apply same standards to all employees.	• Facilitate an organizational culture that supports employees who do not meet performance standards. • Treat employees inconsistently because of employee characteristics.
7. How can I prevent this ethical problem?	• Develop continuing education programs for managers that can explore employee situations that do not fall in the "this is right and that is wrong" category for decision making. • Establish increased organizational accountability for employees for following performance standards that support the complexities faced by both the employee and the manager.	

ENTREPRENEURSHIP

Marie Gardenier, MBA, RHIA, CHPS

Learning Objectives

After completing this chapter, the reader should be able to:

- Understand concepts and trends in entrepreneurship and intrapreneurship within health information management (HIM).
- Describe the principles and issues of general business ethics that apply to entrepreneurial relationships.
- Describe current and future ethical dilemmas that may be faced by HIM entrepreneurs.

Abstract

Entrepreneurship and intrapreneurship are growing trends among health information management (HIM) professionals. Although both offer exciting opportunities, they also involve unique ethical challenges. To deal with these challenges, HIM professionals need to know about business ethics as well as the code of ethics for the HIM profession. This chapter describes ethical dilemmas typically encountered in consulting and contracting and discusses principles and practice standards by which they may be resolved.

Scenario 22-A: Competing Constituencies

Val Lewis, RHIA, is an independent health information management (HIM) consultant. She arrives at a client for her regularly scheduled consulting visit. Her client, the R&R Retirement Village, is a life-care retirement community that offers residential and healthcare services to its members. Its parent company, R&R Corporation, owns and operates 20 life-care communities in several states.

Val has been engaged by R&R Retirement Village for the last three years to monitor the collection and use of patient information at the Village's skilled nursing facility. Val provides professional advice and counsel on record-processing activities and monitors the facility's compliance with state and federal regulations, JCAHO standards, and HIM professional practice standards. She makes quarterly visits to the facility, reviewing samples of records for adequate documentation and assessing the status of the facility's patient information department operation. At the conclusion of each visit, Val submits a written report of her findings to Larry Christianson, R&R's vice president for healthcare services. These reports include the results of her documentation review, comments on patient record operations, and an inventory of the status of incomplete records. Val's reports have always been accepted by Larry without question, and her invoices are paid on a timely basis.

Val is conducting her twelfth visit to the R&R Retirement Village. Up to this point, her experience with the client has been positive. She has a good working relationship with Sarah Beal, the part-time clerk who performs most of the day-to-day record-processing activities. Sarah also supervises several volunteers who assist with filing and other functions.

Today, Val begins her visit with an open patient-record review. While on the nursing unit, she receives a telephone call from Larry who tells her that the date for the JCAHO accreditation survey has been set and will occur in three months. He asks her if she will join the facility's survey preparation team. He would like her to act as R&R's HIM representative during the survey and devote additional time over the next three months to help the facility prepare for the event. Larry indicates that he has great confidence in Val's abilities and believes she would be an asset to the team as it finishes its preparation and undergoes this important survey. Val tells him that she would be happy to help the facility through the survey. She presumes that she will provide value by bolstering their information management expertise and taking some pressure off the rest of the management team.

When Val returns to the patient record department, she tells Sarah about her discussion with Larry and her upcoming role in the JCAHO survey. Sarah thinks this is a splendid idea and is glad to have Val's expertise for the survey. Until now, Sarah has been involved in the preparation efforts, and this is her first experience with a JCAHO survey.

Later in the day, while Val is preparing the incomplete record inventory, Sarah comes to her to review the numbers with Val. As they review the inventory together, Sarah tells Val, "Now that you are involved with the survey, there is something I want to share with you. When we began preparing for the survey, Larry asked to meet with me about the incomplete record volumes. He said he needed my assistance to submit some paperwork prior to the survey. He showed me a form that asked for the total number of incomplete and delinquent medical records over the last 12 months." Val says she is familiar with that form. "Well," Sarah continues, "Larry asked me to complete the form for his signature. He told me to include only records that were missing reports or notes, not records awaiting signatures. He asked me to take your incomplete record inventories, deduct the records missing signatures only, and fill in the form with the adjusted numbers. I didn't think it was right, but I did what I was told."

Sarah then pulls out her JCAHO file and shows Val the completed form, with Larry's signature at the bottom. Val sees that the numbers reported on the form do not match the totals she has been submitting on her reports and immediately calls Larry to clarify the situation. Val tells Larry that she has the JCAHO file and asks him about the differences in the reported statistics. Larry indicates, "There is no mistake." He says that he feels a patient record is substantially complete as long as all the needed documents are present. The lack of a signature is not materially important, and therefore does not warrant reporting as an incomplete record.

Val responds that his numbers are inconsistent with the data that are being reported internally to the patient record committee and that state regulations require every entry in a patient record to be authenticated. Larry replies, a bit impatiently, that he is aware of both of these facts and will take full responsibility for the numbers reported at the JCAHO survey. "Believe me," he says, "this will not be a problem. Look, we need to keep these numbers reasonable. Also, I know what the surveyors are focusing on this year, and this will not be a significant part of our survey." He makes it clear to Val that he expects her to support his reporting approach when it comes time to update the numbers at the time of the survey.

On occasion, Val also works with the facility's medical director, Dr. Lawrence Harper, who chairs the utilization management/patient record committee. Dr. Harper has sought Val's counsel on behalf of the committee on specific patient record issues, and she considers calling Dr. Harper to see if he knows what is going on, but she hesitates. After all, she does not know Dr. Harper well, and calling him could create additional problems with Larry.

Val leaves the facility knowing that his approach to reporting the survey data is not in strict compliance with the reporting requirements.

Questions

1. Are there other areas where data were being "fudged"?

2. Should Val withdraw her verbal agreement to participate in the survey, or is she overreacting?

3. What ethical issues does Val face in her role as consultant and what values should she consider before deciding what to do?

4. What competing constituencies does Val need to consider? What duties does Val owe to each group?

5. Is this situation better analyzed by weighing the consequences of each potential course of action?

6. What risks does Val face if she pursues the issue with Dr. Harper?

7. Does this situation offer Val an opportunity to act as a voice for truth and honest reporting?

8. Is this important within the larger context of the goals of the organization?

9. Do you see a clear course of action that Val can take?

A completed ethical decision-making matrix for the scenario is provided at the end of the chapter.

ENTREPRENEURSHIP IN HEALTH INFORMATION MANAGEMENT

Entrepreneurship is a growing trend among HIM professionals. The interest among individuals to establish new businesses, to work independently, and to become an entrepreneur is part of an American phenomenon that began to emerge in the 1970s. From 1994 to 1996, more than 800,000 new businesses were incorporated in the United States, and the number continues to increase. When you include sole proprietorships and partnerships, the annual total exceeds 1.3 million new businesses per year (Glauser, 1998). Through the 1970s, conventional wisdom held that big business created most new jobs. Currently, small businesses (businesses comprising 20 or fewer employees) are reportedly creating two out of every three new jobs in the current U.S. economy (Glauser, 1998). Many of these jobs have surfaced as entrepreneurs have conceived of a new business, started the new enterprise, and enlisted people to share in their dream. Many of these businesses are started in the owner's home.

In the healthcare industry, sweeping economic reforms and increased competition have spawned new models for delivering, managing, and paying for health care. Many traditional employee-based organizations have reduced their staffs and services (an action commonly referred to as *downsizing*). To maintain flexibility while still meeting demands for services, these organizations are relying on professional service firms to perform functions that were previously the responsibility of the organization's employees. Employing external firms to perform these functions, or *outsourcing,* has become common in hospital departments, such as nursing, dietary, and housekeeping. Healthcare organizations are now outsourcing such diverse operations as information technology, laboratory services, and health information management. Although most HIM professionals are still employed in established healthcare organizations, increasing numbers are opting to join small service companies or contracting independently as professional service providers. Many more supplement full-time, traditional jobs with part-time, contract-based work in consulting, coding, or medical transcription.

HIM entrepreneurs may be found working in the same practice domains as other, more traditionally employed HIM professionals. Although some may think of these professionals mainly as consultants, many are **independent contractors (ICs)** that provide traditional HIM services, such as data classification and analysis, transcription, release of information, and health record management, under contractual arrangements with clients. A consultant gives advice. An independent contractor gives advice and then performs the HIM functions based on that advice.

The independent contractor relationship is commonly referred to as an "outsourcing" relationship. The only difference between independent contractors and employees is the method by which their compensation for services is accounted for and channeled. The independent contractor is paid as an expense under negotiated contract terms, whereas the employee is compensated through a payroll system, according to an established wage rate and benefit plan. When functioning as an independent contractor, the HIM professional can expect to confront many of the same ethical issues as the employed practitioner. In contrast, the consultant may encounter some unique challenges not found in other HIM practice roles.

Global economic, technological, and industry trends favor increased entrepreneurial growth, as technology provides more workplace flexibility and as organizations seek to become leaner, more agile, and more successful at leveraging their most valuable assets—their knowledge workers.

Defining the Entrepreneur

Although some describe an entrepreneur in terms of character traits, others maintain that entrepreneurs are characterized by what they do. Although a psychological model of entrepreneurship has not yet been supported by research, Timmons, Smollen, and Dingee (1990) suggested that entrepreneurs share some of the following attitudes and behaviors:

- They work hard and are driven by intense commitment and perseverance.
- They strive for integrity.
- They burn with a competitive desire to excel and win.
- They are often dissatisfied with the status quo and seek opportunities to improve situations they encounter.
- They use failure as a tool for learning and reject the obsession with perfection in favor of effectiveness.
- They believe they can personally make an enormous difference in the outcome of their ventures and their lives.

In 1993, similar themes emerged from testimony given by the first 21 inductees to Babson College's Academy of Distinguished Entrepreneurs. All 21 inductees described three attributes as the principal reasons for their successes: (1) the ability to respond positively to challenges and learn from mistakes,

(2) a willingness to take personal initiative, and (3) ongoing perseverance and determination (Timmons et al., 1990).

Notice that some of the values contain the following traits and behaviors: commitment (loyalty), integrity, and beneficence (the desire to do good). These are some of the same values that underpin ethical decision making. It is a myth that entrepreneurs are motivated by money. Making money is rarely the primary motivator for the entrepreneur. What motivates successful entrepreneurs more than money are things such as the excitement and challenge of innovating or starting new enterprises, the freedom of being one's own boss, the chance to be creative, and the opportunity to help others.

With a solid foundation of skills and behaviors, the HIM entrepreneur seeks to change the current environment through the strategic use of the following tactics:

- Listening to the conversations of others (people will talk about what needs to be improved)
- Being alert for discussions about procedures that don't work to serve customers/patients
- Volunteering for projects that will improve quality or productivity
- Asking potential clients about their satisfaction with current service providers

Once identified, each opportunity can then be analyzed in terms of its possibilities. Experts suggest keeping an eye on both the real world and the world of possibilities. First, does the opportunity represent an unfilled need? Perhaps a job isn't being done or a service needs to be provided. For example, the roles of information privacy and security managers have only recently been created by the growth of electronic health record technologies and regulatory imperatives such as the Health Insurance Portability and Accountability Act (HIPAA). This important legislation has created brand new roles and functions within healthcare organizations, along with opportunities for HIM entrepreneurs. The HIM entrepreneur should gather information about what services are needed, assess and acquire the qualifications needed to provide them, and then set out to deliver the needed goods.

Another way to innovate is to re-create something that has been lost. Is there a quality or an aspect of an existing service that was once valued but that has been lost or deemphasized? If so, there may be a market for a newly differentiated product. An example may be the personalized transcription services often enjoyed by physicians when they employed their own personal typists versus the anonymous, long-distance services that are now the norm in a highly consolidated transcription marketplace.

A third approach to analyzing opportunities is to enhance the commonplace; in other words, to take a common, unimaginative service and make it outstanding. Adding new features to an existing product or service and enhancing its quality is an example of this approach. Even though a hospital's current coding performance may meet organizational standards, the HIM entrepreneur may set out to exceed current expectations by creating ways to increase reimbursement for the facility based on improved coding quality. The entrepreneur may then go about realizing that possibility by identifying vulnerable codes or DRGs, enlisting physicians to improve their documentation, improving coding education programs, hiring specialized staff to code difficult cases, or electing to establish a professional service firm to deliver these services on a contract basis.

ENTREPRENEUR VERSUS INTRAPRENEUR

Intrapreneur is a term that describes an internal entrepreneur. Although at first glance the term may appear to contradict itself, it describes a common phenomenon in organizational life. Intrapreneurs are people who work as employees in traditional organizations. They may differ from other workers in their attitude, approach, and goals. Like en-

trepreneurs, intrapreneurs are focused on creating innovative products, services, and work methods. They often work independently or in organized teams and are involved in rethinking current products, services, and organizational structures.

In its strategic statement on professional development entitled "e-HIM: A Vision of the e-HIM Future," the American Health Information Management Association (AHIMA, 2003) codified and promoted intrapreneurial efforts in health information management by encouraging professionals and industry leaders to champion change and rethink HIM roles and functions for the twenty-first century, noting that creating new roles, functions, and work methods is critical to success in volatile environments such as health care. The "skunkworks" teams made famous by organizations such as 3M and Hewlett-Packard in the 1970s are early examples of bands of intrapreneurs who were credited with creating such well-known innovations as the Post-It Note and the mass-market personal computer.

Understanding the role of the intrapreneur in championing change from within an organization is critical, because most HIM professionals with entrepreneurial skills and aspirations will not, for a variety of reasons, venture into independent enterprises. Many will continue to work in traditional, employee-based roles and will be essential to innovating HIM practices within their healthcare organizations. If they choose to be internal change agents, they will face many of the same challenges as their independent colleagues and will have the opportunity to reap the same rewards. Given the increasingly dynamic, competitive employment marketplace facing all workers today, career management advisors recommend that every worker think of him- or herself as an independent entity offering a unique service. Some argue that workers should approach personal career management as a business enterprise.

The scope and velocity of change inherent in today's healthcare environment demand a commitment from each HIM professional to develop and nurture his or her entrepreneurial skills. The core competency on which many practicing professionals were educated—managing paper-based patient records—is being radically transformed by the transition to electronic health information. In addition, managed care, consumerism, clinical breakthroughs, and other trends are all converging to change the HIM landscape. Whether working inside or outside traditional workplaces, HIM professionals will need to operate as change agents as they seek to carry out their professional duties and achieve career success and fulfillment. Entrepreneurial skills will play an important role in the future of every HIM professional, regardless of the work setting.

BUSINESS ETHICS: CONCEPTS AND PRINCIPLES

HIM professionals who choose an entrepreneurial path will interact with other professionals in new ways. As entrepreneurs, they will practice their profession within the context of the world of business. They may have established a business entity or may be part of a business that delivers professional services to others. The business entity may take one of many forms, such as a sole proprietorship (single-person firm), a partnership, or a corporation. Regardless of its form, practicing HIM through a business entity invokes an additional layer of ethical considerations related to general business activities and business relationships. HIM entrepreneurs should be aware of these challenges and the principles of business ethics so that they can recognize and resolve ethical issues as they occur in the course of doing business.

Business ethics is a specialized study of moral right and wrong. To understand the concept of business ethics, it is important to remember that businesses exist within the larger context of society. A society consists of people who have common ends and whose activities are organized by a system of insti-

tutions designed to achieve these ends. Societies, in large part, seek to sustain themselves for the good of all by invoking shared beliefs about values and duties. This is often called *societal morality.*

Societal morality is expressed through formal institutions such as the government and religious hierarchies. However, studies have shown that even in liberal societies in which authorities have a limited impact on how their citizens deal with one another, people will encourage behavior that contributes to the common good. This "group wisdom" often takes the form of commonly accepted cultural conventions or norms of behavior that are largely enforced voluntarily by members of the group. These conventions, which are generally executed without a great deal of thought or effort, have been shown to play not only an important role in everyday social life, but also on a society's economic life and on the way companies do business (Surowiecki, 2004).

General ethics is the activity of examining a society's moral standards and asking how these standards apply to individual lives and circumstances. Business enterprises are the primary economic institutions through which people in modern societies accomplish the tasks of producing and distributing goods and services. They provide the fundamental structures within which the members of society combine and distribute their resources for the good of society as a whole. Business and the free-market system can be justified insofar as they provide prosperity, both for those people involved in the business and for those who live in the society in which the business operates. As such, business is a cooperative enterprise with rules and expectations established by society. The rules of business exchange reflect the societal morality. Without fixed rules and commonly accepted norms of behavior, business could not be conducted, and the society's economic foundation would collapse.

Business ethics is the study of a society's moral standards as they are applied to the activities and relationships created by business transactions. As this description suggests, business ethics encompasses a wide variety of topics. Velasquez (2002) organized these issues into three categories: systemic, corporate, and individual issues.

Systemic issues in business ethics are ethical questions raised about the economic, political, legal, and other social systems within which businesses operate. These include questions about the morality of capitalism or of the laws, regulations, and social practices that govern business activities. Individual issues in business ethics are ethical questions raised about a particular individual or individuals employed by a business enterprise. These include questions about the ethical basis of the decisions, actions, or the character of the individual employee.

Corporate issues in business ethics are ethical questions raised about a particular company, including questions about the morality of an enterprise's policies, business practices, or organizational behavior. Solomon (1997) identified five key ethical principles that every corporation should follow in serving its varied constituencies: fairness to employees, quality to consumers, dependability to suppliers, trustworthiness to superiors, and responsibility to the community (see Table 22–1).

Keeping these ethical values in mind, let us highlight three contexts within which ethical

Table 22–1 Five Keys to Corporate Ethics

Constituency	Ethical Value
Employees	Fairness
Consumers	Quality
Suppliers	Dependability
Superiors	Trustworthiness
Community	Responsibility

Source: Reprinted with permission from R. C. Solomon, *It's a Good Business: Ethics and Free Enterprise for the New Millennium,* ©1997, Rowman & Littlefield.

issues may arise between an HIM business enterprise and its consumer constituency.

Contracts

Most activity between business enterprises and their customers is governed by contractual agreements. Whether expressed (written) or implied, a **contract** is a codified set of mutual expectations that carries the weight of law. Contracts create special rights and duties between people. Contracts provide a way of ensuring that individuals keep their word, and this in turn makes it possible for businesses to operate in society. The system of rules that underlies contractual rights and duties has been traditionally interpreted as including several moral underpinnings:

- Both of the parties to a contract must have full knowledge of the nature of the agreement they are entering.
- Neither party to a contract must intentionally misrepresent the facts of the contractual situation to the other party.
- Neither party to the contract must be forced to enter the contract under duress or coercion.
- The contract must not bind the parties to an immoral act.

Contracts that violate one or more of these four conditions have traditionally been considered void (Velasquez, 1998). A special moral duty is recognized for the party providing the product or service stipulated in the contract. This duty, referred to as **due care,** obligates the seller to take special "care" to ensure that the customer's interests are not harmed by the products or services offered. This obligation is based on the idea that customers and sellers do not meet as equals in most sales transactions. Most often, the seller has significantly greater knowledge and expertise about the item being sold than does the buyer. Because customers must rely on the greater expertise of the seller about the product being sold, the seller has a duty to deliver a product that lives up to the express and implied claims about it. The buyer has a right to expect the product to live up to the promises made by the seller. The seller has a further duty to exercise due care to prevent the buyer and others from being injured by the product or service being sold. This due care obligation is also referred to as an *ethic of care* and is especially important in relationships in which the buyer or consumer is dependent or vulnerable, such as when the product or service is of a highly technical nature or the consumer is a patient or a child. The ethic of care for the HIM entrepreneur includes obligations such as protection of patient privacy.

An extension of the ethic of care is the expectation of fairness in all business transactions. Indeed, the notion of fairness in business exchanges is central to the conduct of business. Without the recognition that all parties to a contract are operating in good faith, individuals would be unlikely to participate in business transactions, and the free enterprise system would come to a halt. Business is made possible because of the rules or expectations established by society about how transactions will occur, and contracts are the means for spelling out those expectations for specific transactions. These ethical principles are well understood as part of the ethics of professions and professional practices. In view of this, Solomon (1997) encourages people to think about all business as a practice and businesspeople as professionals when applying ethics to business activities.

Advertising

All business enterprises must advertise to be successful. The most valuable product or service will remain unsold unless potential consumers are aware of its existence. Therefore, every business enterprise must invest some of its resources in creating awareness of its product. *Advertising* can be defined as a certain kind of communication between a seller and potential buyers. It is distinguished from other forms of communication by one key feature. Unlike other communications, advertising is intended to induce its audience to buy the seller's product, generally either by creating a desire for the product or by creating a belief in the consumer that the product is a means of satisfying some desire the buyer already has. As a result, advertising always contains some measure of bias. Indeed, the most common criticism of advertising concerns the deceptive nature of advertisements.

Deceptive advertising can take several forms. An advertisement may misrepresent the nature of the product, imply product "guarantees" when no guarantees are truly offered, quote misleading prices, or fail to disclose known defects in a product while misleadingly disparaging a competitor's goods. Ethical traditions have long condemned deception in advertising on the grounds that it violates consumers' rights to choose. "Truth in advertising" is a commonly acknowledged maxim. However, it is also generally accepted, perhaps somewhat cynically, that advertising is usually biased and misleading. Some consider all advertising to be a lie because it always tells only one side of the story. Further, although lying is understood to be morally wrong, "truth" and "falsehood" often are defined subjectively, with some "lies" considered more offensive than others.

Solomon (1997) offers a "hierarchy of lying" and suggests that lies carry an increasing offensiveness as one moves down the hierarchy (p. 113). According to Solomon, the least offensive form of lying is "telling less than the whole truth"; the most offensive form involves "stating vicious falsehoods." In the middle of the hierarchy are efforts to tell a biased truth, to give misleading information, or to state obvious falsehoods.

It is nearly impossible to tell the whole truth when advertising a product or service. Nonetheless, giving misleading information or telling obvious falsehoods is always wrong and, in the long run, counterproductive to a business's success. Although in the short term these tactics may pay off in additional sales, in the long run lies are a bad business risk. First, lies involve an enormous amount of effort, which increases over time. As past political events have shown, the cost of a cover-up always far exceeds the damage done by the initial lie itself, even if the cover-up is successful. Second, and more importantly, every lie diminishes trust. Not only does lying undermine others' faith in the liar, but, more subtly, telling a lie diminishes one's trust in others (i.e., "If I lie, everyone else must be lying to me as well"). Does this mean that one must never lie? Perhaps not. But ethicists suggest that it does mean that it is never right to tell a lie—that telling a lie always requires extra thought and some very good reasons to show that a violation of the truth should be tolerated. If lying were generally accepted, business activity would quickly be undermined by the dissolution of trust between parties.

Although the exact nature of truth in advertising may be controversial, advertising in general must not only be based on fact but also be believable and trustworthy. To be ethical, it must strive to meet the same moral standards as all communication between individuals; that is, to be truthful.

The Profit Motive

Those who object to applying ethical standards to business practices often use the profit motive to advance this argument. They contend that in a free-market society the pursuit of profit is the businessperson's paramount objective. To that end, individuals involved in businesses should not sidetrack their energies or resources into "doing good works," but rather should single-mindedly pursue the firm's financial interests. In the end, they argue, market forces will ensure that members of society are served in the most socially beneficial way. This argument is based on a few flawed assumptions.

The first flawed assumption is that a perfectly free market really exists anywhere on earth. Although the concept is widely used, most economists agree that in real life a variety of factors may be found in every economic market, even in free-market systems, that constrain the choices and actions of the participants, making the "totally free market" useful only as economic theory. The second flawed assumption is that businesses, and businesspeople, work primarily for financial profit. Although generating profits is certainly an important goal of any business, many business analysts agree that financial rewards are not the primary motivator for most businesses or business owners. Earlier in this chapter, we saw that most entrepreneurs are motivated by factors other than profit. To believe in the supremacy of the profit motive is to take a narrow view of the reason businesses exist. Businesses exist and are justified, not by the profits they produce, but by the extent to which they provide value to society. Although profits are part of the equation, they are more of a means than an end unto themselves.

The discussion becomes even more complex in the business of health care. Although most healthcare businesses are deemed "not-for-profit" enterprises whose mission is the improvement of community health, they nonetheless are required to act in pursuit of operating profits—hence the truism, "no money, no mission." In addition, the prosperity achieved in the healthcare sector over the past 20 years has promoted the entrance of more and more for-profit firms into the healthcare delivery business. These for-profit enterprises have a duty to their shareholders to place profits first—ahead of the traditional medical mission. Indeed, the decision by Tenet Healthcare in 2004 to close the Medical College Hospital in Philadelphia, Pennsylvania, in the face of significant multiyear losses could be construed as an example of a sound business decision (to stem a sustained loss of profit) that trumped the competing and compelling duty to provide medical services to an underserved urban community.

In the end, profits are important as measures of a business's success, in comparison to its competitors, and money is a means to purchase goods and other intangible items, such as power, prestige, and status. But businesses are successful insofar as they promote prosperity and well-being for members of society, both those who are involved in the business's activities and those who live in the society in general. Not everyone in the world agrees on what constitutes "well-being," but business forms the core of U.S. society not because of its profit-making potential but because of the general belief that business promotes a prosperous, free, and just society.

Corporate Responsibility

As described earlier, corporate issues in business ethics relate to the morality of a company's activities, taken as a whole, as they relate to its stakeholders. Working through an ethical issue always includes an assignment of responsibility. Who is responsible for acting appropriately? The legal rules that govern corporations enable us to say that corporations act as "individuals" with legal standing separate from the individuals who work on their behalf. Further, the individual members of the company act within organizational roles and according to corporate policies and culture. As a result, some argue that the corporate entity itself should bear moral responsibility for the actions of its members.

However, a business is a collection of individuals—individuals acting together for a shared purpose—and individuals are the source of all ethical and unethical behaviors. Therefore, others say it follows that the individual members should be seen as the primary bearers of moral responsibility. In truth, the responsibility for acting ethically in a business organization is shared between the corporate entity and the individual members. Velasquez (2002) asserts that individuals bear the primary moral responsibility because they are free to choose whether to comply or even change an organization's rules and objectives.

A recent spate of corporate scandals has elevated the issue of corporate responsibility in the public's consciousness. After filing the largest bankruptcy claim in U.S. history, Enron became the subject of an enormous public scandal and legal investigation. At the heart of Enron's troubles were questions of individual and corporate responsibility for unethical business actions that tragically impacted the lives of its employees, shareholders, customers, and the U.S. energy industry. In Enron's wake came similar business ethics scandals involving companies such as Tyco, WorldCom, and Adelphia (McLean & Elkind, 2003).

Debates as to what constitutes "illegal" versus "unethical" business activities in these cases and who bears responsibility for the actions of these organizations are expected to continue for years to come. Some of the defendants in these cases hold forth the position that individuals at the top of the corporate hierarchy hold only narrow responsibility for the acts of others. They stake their defense on claims that they fulfilled their ethical obligations by relying on assertions of propriety from other professionals (such as accountants and lawyers) and avoided explicitly illegal actions.

The Case for Ethics in Business

In addition to applying a narrow scope of individual ethical responsibility, other arguments are sometimes used to discount the importance of ethics in business. Business ethicist Richard de George called these arguments the "myth of amoral business" (Solomon, 1997, p. 21). According to the myth, business and ethics don't mix. People in business are not necessarily immoral, but they are amoral; that is, they are not concerned with morals. Moralizing is out of place in business. Companies act in accordance with Darwinian theory, with only "the fittest" enterprises surviving over the long term.

To be sure, anecdotal stories are available about businesses and businesspeople who have succeeded by using unscrupulous tactics. Also, businesses that do not meet moderate thresholds of success perish every day in America. However, many other businesses manage to survive without being the "fittest" in their industry. Further, although attempts to correlate profitability with ethical behavior have shown mixed results, no studies have found a negative correlation that would indicate that ethics is a drain on profits. Other studies have looked at how socially responsible firms perform on the stock market and have concluded that ethical companies provide higher returns than other companies. The amoral rhetoric of business is destructive in itself, because it feeds public suspicion of business and easily becomes part of the condemnation of business (Velasquez, 2002).

To be successful, most businesses and businesspeople adhere to some standard of ethics. Business is a cooperative activity; its very existence requires ethical behavior. This is especially obvious in service businesses, where a service provided by one individual to another is at the heart of each business transaction. This results in a more intimate and direct relationship between seller and buyer than is obvious when manufactured goods are involved. When healthcare services are involved, the stakes are raised to a higher level, given the expectations placed by society on the actions of caregivers and health professionals.

Apart from its contributions to society, ethical behavior should also be considered a good business strategy. Although studies that have examined whether profitability is correlated with ethical behavior have had mixed results, together they suggest that, by and large, ethical practices do not put a drain on profits and that they seem to contribute to profitability over the long term (Velasquez, 2002). Businesses that act unscrupulously or deceptively may in fact gain profit from these actions. However, the success will be short-lived. In markets of some size or competition, unethical practices will eventually be discovered, and those businesses will ultimately fail.

More importantly, business should be thought of as an ethos, a way of life. It is a way of life that is ethical at its very foundation. Business needs ethics to survive. At the core of business ethics are the societal values of fairness, truthfulness, and trust. The single value that sums up and ties these values together is the value of integrity. Integrity implies a wholeness of being and defines the character of both businesspeople and business entities. Businesses that operate with integrity are ethical businesses. Ethical businesses are more likely to achieve their goals of individual success and to contribute to the overall prosperity of society.

THE INTERSECTION OF THE ETHICS AND HIM ENTREPRENEURSHIP

Like other HIM professionals, the entrepreneur will confront ethical issues that challenge personal and professional decision making. As a member of the healthcare team, the HIM professional works in the increasingly complex system of healthcare delivery and information management. HIM professionals are often at "ground zero" of the explosion of information technology and clinical knowledge and are challenged daily with balancing competing interests and dwindling resources. How does the entrepreneur's experience differ from that of the traditional HIM professional? How is it similar?

In some ways, the entrepreneur's ethical challenges are likely to mirror those of the traditional HIM professional. After all, the HIM entrepreneur and the traditional professional are guided by and responsible to a common professional code of ethics and set of practice standards. Their personal moral values are likely to be similar, because like-minded people are generally drawn to the same profession. In addition, the day-to-day ethical challenges of patient confidentiality, data integrity, and other information management functions are inherent in HIM practice.

Despite these similarities, the entrepreneur's experience is distinctive in two ways. First, the very nature of the entrepreneur, namely, the penchant to "push the envelope" in pursuit of innovation, invites more frequent and probably more complex encounters with ethical issues in the workplace. The environment in which the entrepreneur works is likely to be less structured, less predictable, and more volatile than the workplace of the more tradition-minded HIM professional. Whether working from within or outside of a healthcare organization, the entrepreneur will seek out professional challenges and be driven toward projects that defy conventional wisdom and that threaten the status quo. For example, as a consultant, the entrepreneur may ask difficult questions to determine why patient record information is not available when needed for continuity of care. As an interim or full-time HIM department manager, the entrepreneur may be redesigning work processes and reallocating resources to bring new solutions to solve operational problems related to record completion and billing delays. As a system implementation specialist or project manager, the HIM entrepreneur may be installing beta versions of EHR technologies for medical information processing.

In any one of these scenarios, the entrepreneur is likely to be found on the front lines of innovation (the "bleeding edge," as it is sometimes called). While there, one is far more likely to be pricked by the horns of difficult ethical dilemmas than when in a more traditional professional role. Ethical dilemmas will surface under these circumstances for a number of reasons. Chiefly, these dilemmas arise from attempts by the HIM professional to act as a change agent within an organization. Attempts to implement new ideas to solve old problems inevitably create conflict and resistance. No matter how eager an organization seems to be to fix an identified problem, it will always, to some extent, resist needed changes. Conflicts will erupt, and the individual in the role of change agent will often be called upon to lead people through difficult decision-making and implementation tasks involving cultural changes and conflicting ethics and values.

Similarly, when new technologies emerge, they bring with them the ability to perform work in new ways. The rate of development of these technologies always outpaces our ability to manage their implementation. This includes resolving dilemmas associated with how and when to use (or not to use) the new technology and its new function. A good example of this is the growing family of EHR technologies, which are being used to transform traditional paper-based patient records into digital resources. These technologies, and their capabilities for rapid and simultaneous access to information, have vaulted patient consumerism and issues of information privacy and security to the status of national priorities. These issues, rife with ethical concerns and conflicts, are as yet unresolved, even as the technologies continue to be developed and implemented at a rapid pace.

Another way to look at the entrepreneur's special ethical challenges is to categorize them as function-based versus relationship-based issues. Function-based ethical issues are issues encountered by the HIM professional that arise from the performance of HIM functions; that is, from the specific areas of HIM practice. These issues, which are described throughout this text, may come up in a wide variety of circumstances. They may involve, for example, decisions to release patient information, to edit physician dictation, or to code medical information. In addition, the HIM entrepreneur will face special function-based ethical challenges when working in the role of consultant. Some of these include providing expert advice, delivering recommendations that are difficult to hear or implement, managing conflicts of interest, and working in a collaborative role with clients.

Relationship-based issues are those that arise from the relationship between the HIM entrepreneur and the primary recipient of the HIM services, namely, the client. These issues can arise regardless of the role or service being performed. Some of these issues involve social isolation, contract negotiations, unrealistic client expectations, the discovery of sensitive information about a client or competitor, the management of the relationship with the client, and assertion of one's rights as an independent contractor.

Function-Based Issues for the Consultant

Here we will examine several different types of issues and discuss how they can be described in terms of ethical thought, identify the values that may be involved, and articulate ideas for analysis and action.

First, what is a consultant? A **consultant** is someone hired to apply special expertise to a situation in order to solve a problem or accomplish a defined objective. HIM professionals can be found providing consultative services on a broad array of topics in many different settings, from evaluating the quality of coding in an integrated delivery system to monitoring HIM operations and documentation quality in a small skilled-nursing facility.

A consultant is in a position to exert influence over an individual, a group, or an organization, but by definition this person has no direct power to make changes or implement programs. The recipient of the advice provided by the consultant is the client. The consulting event, typically referred to as an *engagement,* may be short term, such as a review of a specific problem, or long term, such as an engagement for quarterly HIM department and record reviews.

Each consulting engagement will have similar phases: contracting, data collection and analysis, feedback, and a decision on needed actions. The work product of each engagement is typically a report. This report is usually written and contains the consultant's evaluation, findings, and recommendations for action. Once an individual is hired to take direct responsibility for an operation or a project, he or she begins acting as an independent contractor, with direct control over certain actions and individuals. For example, a consultant may be called upon to evaluate the organizational design of an HIM department to determine if operational efficiency can be improved. If, after making recommendations for redesigns, the consultant is hired to implement the design, that person is now functioning as an independent contractor providing project management services.

This distinction between consultant and independent contractor is important because the consultant needs to function differently from the independent contractor and, as a result, may face some unique ethical challenges. Typically, consultants work with their clients in one of two ways: in the role of expert or in the role of collaborator. The choice of role depends largely on the nature of the task, the resources available from the client, and the consultant's own style and preference. In each of these roles, the consultant may encounter different ethical challenges.

The Expert Role

Suppose that you are an HIM consultant who has been engaged by Regional Medical Center to evaluate the hospital's HIM department and recommend technologies to improve efficiencies and reduce operating costs. This kind of engagement is typical. Consultants are often engaged to provide special expertise that is not otherwise available to a client in order to solve a particular problem or to ensure that activities are in compliance with accepted standards. In this role, you accept responsibility for up-to-date knowledge of HIM strategies and available technologies. You also commit to an understanding of not only what is available, but also what is realistically possible in relation to improving HIM operations.

In return, the client takes a passive role and accepts that the advice given will be accurate and helpful. Accepting the role of expert can present a number of ethical challenges. First, you should be prudent about promoting yourself or accepting the mantle of "expert" conferred by others. An *expert* is defined as "a person who has special skill or knowledge in some particular field" (Stein, 1975, p. 465). This is a higher standard than simply knowing more about the subject than the client. It requires a command of the current body of available knowledge as well as the ability to apply it properly to the current situation. In the face of the rapid growth of knowledge and changes inherent in the HIM and healthcare fields, maintaining command over the entire body of HIM knowledge is a difficult, if not impossible, task.

Before accepting an engagement to provide expert advice, you should be confident that you deserve the title of "expert." You should be confident in your command of the knowledge and skills required to meet the client's needs. How much knowledge do you need to be considered knowledgeable? The answer is rarely clear-cut. As a result, you must look to your professional integrity to inform your answer. Indeed, the current AHIMA Code of Ethics (2004) directs all HIM professionals to truthfully and accurately represent their professional credentials, education, and experience.

Along with the ambiguity of the situation, competitive and economic pressures may entice you to exaggerate your experience or expertise. It is always difficult to turn away an interested client. As a result, it is not unknown for a consultant to say, "I'll land the client today and figure out how to do the engagement tomorrow." Although this approach may work in the short term, it is a dangerous strategy. First, the risk of failure is high. Second, the amount of energy and anxiety created to avert failure and ensure success may be draining on you and may affect relations with the client. There is nothing wrong with learning on an engagement or using it to further expand your skills and understanding. Indeed, this is the hallmark of continued professional growth and should be a goal for every engagement. However, before submitting a proposal for this engagement, you should honestly examine your current skills and expertise.

Your commitment to the values of truthfulness, integrity, and loyalty to serve the interests of the client will guide you to objectively determine if you are competent to act as an "expert" in this situation. If, after careful consideration, you are uncertain about your firm's ability to render "expertise" to this client, you should refuse the engagement. A potential client will not be disappointed if you offer a referral to a more suitable individual or firm, along with an honest explanation for your action. This action will, in the end, nurture a relationship of trust, enhance rather than detract from your professional reputation, and increase the likelihood that the customer will consider your firm for future work.

Delivering a Difficult Message

Once hired, your first duty is to analyze and diagnose the situation at hand. This may include gathering data, interviewing people, and observing events. Once facts have been obtained and analyzed, it is time to report the findings and conclusions to the client. If you have been observant during your data gathering, you will probably have some notion of what the client believes is happening before you present your findings. If this is a problem to be solved, you will have solicited feedback from many sources (if your fact gathering has been thorough) as to the possible sources of the problem. In the end, sometimes your analysis and conclusions will conflict with the client's expectations. You may have obtained information and drawn conclusions that the client will find difficult to hear. For example, more money may have to be spent to fix a problem in an area where management wants to decrease funding. Worse yet, you may have uncovered information involving unethical or incompetent behavior among trusted staff. For example, say that you discover that a correspondence manager fails to log reportable disclosures of patient information as required by HIPAA when the workload becomes excessive in the hopes that odds are slim that a patient will notice if he or she requests an accounting of these disclosures from the facility.

It is difficult to deliver information that will not be easily received. From an ethical perspective, you may feel tension between your desire to be truthful and your desire to please the client. Focusing on the objective of the engagement, you may ask yourself, "Is the information I have learned germane to the problem I've been called in to address? Or is it peripheral to the scope of the engagement? Do I need to report everything I know? Should I tailor my recommendations to match what the client is expecting or desiring to hear?" Certainly, if illegal activities are discovered, your duty to report is clear. But in most cases the answer is less obvious. What if there is evidence of incompetence involving a well-known HIM colleague? This dilemma can be analyzed in terms of your duties as the consultant to your client. You have a duty to tell the truth and to apply your expertise in a full and complete way, no matter what the consequences may be. Telling clients only what they want to hear is how consultants have earned the pejorative reputation as people who "borrow your watch to tell you the time." A more utilitarian approach to analyzing the problem will look for the course of action that will accomplish the best possible result for all involved. For example, if you tell the whole truth, including information that the client is not willing to hear, then you may be dismissed and none of your recommendations heeded. If, however, your conclusions are tempered, tailored, or edited for the client's ear, there may be a better chance for at least some of the recommended improvements to be adopted and for some good to be accomplished as a result.

This situation may be further complicated if you must report your findings to a committee or workgroup, where a mix of expectations, perspectives, and agendas is in play. Often these agendas and expectations are not only varied but also in conflict with one another. In this situation it is especially important for you to know who the "primary" client is (i.e., the one established during the contracting phase) and to be clear about the engagement objectives. Within this context, you will examine values such as truth-telling, loyalty, and fairness to determine the best course of action. If you are a mature and skillful consultant, you will seek ways to shape rather than distort your report, creating a message that the client can hear and trust, even if the message is difficult to accept.

Advice Not Taken

Consultants may become frustrated when a situation is carefully analyzed, sound conclusions are reached, and recommendations are offered that are accepted and then promptly ignored by the client. Consultants are often envied because they can offer advice and "walk away," but in reality the inability to implement needed changes and take control of a problem situation is discouraging to the HIM consultant who cares about the client. In the role of advisor, the consultant does not have the authority to implement recommendations.

The consultant must rely on the client to convert recommendations into action. Often, for a variety of reasons, clients fail to effectively carry through sound recommendations, and progress is not achieved, or worse, the situation may deteriorate. As a result, the consultant may be called back to the client, sometimes many times, to repeatedly address the same problem due to the client's inaction or badly executed implementation.

Say, for example, that you are an HIM consultant with a long-term contract to monitor HIM operations at a long-term care facility with no credentialed HIM specialist and that you find yourself in the following type of situation: You repeat the same recommendations over and over with no visible results. At some point you will begin to feel uneasy. You may feel that your professional integrity is being threatened because your recommendations are being ignored. Also, you may feel guilt at not living up to your professional obligation to do good for the client because your actions are not influencing changes in behavior.

You may feel added tension because your client's coding errors could expose the client (and possibly you, too) to legal sanctions under Medicare compliance statutes. If you have a middle-level administrator as a primary contact, you may consider talking with a more senior staff member. However, this action could represent disloyalty to your primary client (the person who hired you). However, you are no doubt aware that, no matter who has signed the contract, your ultimate loyalty is to the organization as a whole and that you are obliged to put its overall welfare and the welfare of its patients ahead of any individual loyalties.

Knowing all this, you may still find it difficult to take the proper course of action. Why is no one heeding repeated recommendations? Are the reports even being read? If the client does not value your recommendations, why are your invoices paid and your contracts continued? The answers to these questions are often not easily understood. If you insist on meetings with management, your concerns may not be welcomed, and you risk souring your relationship with the client. The safer course might be to say nothing and simply continue to submit your written reports. However, if future harm is done as a result of continuing problems, you may not feel that you did all you could have done to rectify the problems; worse, you may be held accountable by management and others for not having been more assertive in raising awareness about the situation.

Conflicts of Interest

In addition to professional expertise, a consultant brings another important asset to an engagement—objectivity. When hired to diagnose a problem or to assist with the evaluation of a product or service, the consultant is there to assemble and analyze factual data and provide expertise on what will best meet the client's needs. If the consultant has entered into business relationships or has other current interests in potential vendors, objectivity may be compromised. Currently, many consulting firms are diversifying their services. As a result, the consultant or the firm may itself offer the product or service being evaluated. In these cases, consideration should be given to the duty to objectivity before accepting a consulting engagement. Any potential conflicts of interests should be disclosed to the client. If fully disclosed and understood by the client, these relationships may not hinder the consultant's ability to render an objective recommendation.

The Collaborative Role

Scenario 22-A at the beginning of this chapter illustrates some common dilemmas faced by HIM consultants who are in a collaborative role with a client. The consultant who assumes a collaborative role enters the relationship with the client with the notion that problems can be resolved most effectively by joining the consultant's specialized knowledge with the client's skills and knowledge of the organization. In this relationship, problem solving becomes a joint undertaking. Consultants do not solve problems for their clients. Rather, they apply their skills and expertise to help their clients solve their own problems. The distinction is significant. The key assumption underlying the collaborative role is that the client is actively involved in data gathering and analysis, in setting goals and developing action plans, and, finally, in sharing responsibility for success or failure.

In many ways, collaboration can be a more effective relationship for both the consultant and the client. By becoming a member of the team, the consultant can establish a helping relationship designed to broaden the client's competence and support sustained solutions and internal growth. The client becomes more empowered in this type of relationship than when dealing with the consultant as an expert. However, problems can arise in collaborative relationships.

In a collaborative relationship, the consultant and the client become interdependent, sharing responsibility for the success of the project. Issues of roles, responsibility, and control can be ambiguous. Decision making will be based more on consensus building. Within this context, the consultant must still act primarily by influencing others, because no line authority exists. This may be more difficult if the consultant is viewed more as an equal than as an expert. The consultant may feel that his or her integrity is being threatened if the client team does not accept the consultant's input. Also, the team may develop an agenda or action plan that conflicts with the consultant's view as to what is right or what will work. If these conflicts are significant, they may be at odds with the consultant's professional or personal values. As a result, the consultant may find it difficult to discuss his or her concerns with other members of the team, because the consultant is not a full-time member of the staff.

If you are a consultant, you can work through such dilemmas in three ways. First, you should not forget to honor your own right to professional autonomy. Even though you are working at the pleasure of the client, your professional principles are important and should not be abandoned to meet a client's expectations. In fact, you owe your best judgment as a duty to the client, and you must be willing to speak out when necessary. At the same time, you must remain aware of the team's culture and dynamics and respect the values and perspectives of the other members of the team.

If open and honest communication is fostered, more facts will be revealed and better decisions may be reached through an amalgamation of ideas and perspectives. Keep in mind that disagreements and debate are to

be expected and are important ingredients in crafting effective solutions to difficult problems. Actions that may sabotage the integrity of the team or any individual member should be avoided. In the end, you must weigh all relevant factors and put forth your best effort to work successfully with the client. If, after doing so, you feel that you cannot be effective or cannot endorse the direction the team is taking, you must have the courage to discuss this problem with the client and, if necessary, to withdraw from the engagement in a professional and respectful manner.

Scapegoating

Consultants often encounter a special problem when working in a collaborative role with a client. Consider what happens when the hiring party says, "I need your expertise to work with me to solve a problem. I have done my own examination and analysis, but I would like your opinion as an informed, objective party. Once I have your input, we will work together to design an action plan." On the face of it, this seems like a reasonable engagement objective.

The problem arises when your diagnosis of the problem does not match the client's assessment. As a result, the client tries to persuade you to change your evaluation to more closely match the client's. In effect, the client has already made up his or her mind about the situation and may be using you as a "scapegoat" to confirm the client's opinion. In this case, the client is not open to your input, let alone willing to rely on your judgment. This can place you in a delicate position, made more difficult because you are not likely to identify this situation until well into the engagement's progress.

Despite uncomfortable feelings, you may have no choice but to continue. However, being used as a scapegoat violates an individual's personal integrity and professional autonomy, and, over time, the strategy usually becomes transparent to others. However, you should not rush to judgment, confusing the client's honest disagreement with your conclusions with attempts at scapegoating you. Scapegoating is often used when difficult decisions need to be made that will negatively affect other people, such as staff downsizing. These situations bring considerations of fairness and justice to others. Scapegoating is generally a no-win relationship for the consultant and the client, but it is often difficult for the situation to be openly discussed and categorized as such.

Special Opportunities for the Consultant to Act as Moral Voice

As a consultant, you have special opportunities to exercise moral leadership. As a professional, you are relied upon as a trusted advisor and agent of change. With this can come a mantle of authority and leadership, often augmented by opportunities to write and speak on subjects within your scope of expertise. Every engagement offers a platform for sharing what you know and for teaching others, including HIM colleagues and members of other healthcare disciplines. Success can bring both financial rewards and professional acclaim.

Yet, with these opportunities come responsibilities. First, you must be self-aware and clear about your personal beliefs and value structure. Second, you must be knowledgeable about your professional values and be able to articulate these to others in a variety of situations. You must strive to continue to become a better professional and to use the power conferred on you wisely and with respect for the rights of others. You must be able to act authentically—in harmony with your own values—even as you work on behalf of your client interests. It is a delicate and difficult balance requiring honesty, vigilance, and sometimes courage. Actions may involve personal and professional risks and may require standing alone in the midst of misunderstanding and substantial resistance to change.

However, working with diligence and care, you can play a leadership role in affecting how health care is delivered in the twenty-first century. You can be a special voice of moral authority as society tackles the increasingly complex issues of managing health information. At stake are approaches that honor the values and traditions of the HIM profession and serve the best interests of patients, providers, and the many other stakeholders who value the quality, protection, and appropriate use of patient information.

Let us return to Val's dilemma (Scenario 22-A) with her client that opened this chapter. What function-based ethical issues is Val facing in her role as consultant? What values should she consider before deciding what to do? She has competing values of truth-telling versus loyalty to her client. Do you see a clear course of action? Referring back to the discussion of business ethics, do you see competing constituencies to be considered? The competing constituencies are facility, patients, and accreditation body. What duties does Val owe to each group? Or, is this situation better analyzed by weighing the consequences of each potential course of action? What risks does Val face if she pursues the issue with Dr. Harper? Does this situation offer her an opportunity to act as a voice for truth and honest reporting? Is this important within the larger context of the goals of the organization? The principles of her professional practice?

Relationship-Based Issues for the Independent Contractor

In contrast to function-based ethical issues, relationship-based issues refer to ethical concerns arising from the relationship between the independent contractor and the primary recipient of the HIM services, namely, the client. These issues can arise regardless of the role or service being performed. As described earlier in the chapter, the HIM professional may work as an independent contractor, practicing the HIM profession under contractual arrangements with clients. Independent contractors may be found providing consulting services, managing HIM departments, performing coding or transcription services, coordinating release of information, or conducting many other typical and emerging duties.

The independent contractor is distinguished from the traditional HIM professional by the unique relationship that exists between the provider and the recipient of HIM services. That relationship is one of business partners rather than one of employee–employer. Products and services are bought and sold. The nature and terms of the services to be provided are articulated in a written contract, which must be negotiated for each engagement. Often the patient, whose interests the profession holds as primary concern, is a secondary, unmentioned customer in the professional service contract. Competition among service providers to win contracts can be intense. Client relationships must be developed, nurtured, and sometimes terminated. Expectations and behaviors can be influenced by market forces and financial goals, which may conflict with personal and professional values. As a result, principles of business ethics play an important role in guiding business transactions. Often, the independent contractor will have contracts with multiple clients simultaneously.

The contractor–client relationship rests on a foundation of trust. Whether the contract calls for consultative or other HIM services, the client measures the value of the service relationship in terms of the quality of the service and the trustworthiness of the service provider. The client trusts the contractor to be competent and to use expertise, judgment, and conscientious effort in pursuit of the client's best interest.

Because the primary and arguably only real asset of a service organization is its reputation, maintaining client trust is key to the contractor's success. Therefore, the contractor must be self-aware and skillful at independent, ethical deliberation. Vigilance is key, because the contractor relies primarily on individual resources and self-motivation. Developing support networks among colleagues is helpful, but this can be difficult to do in a competitive business environment. Self-improvement is as necessary as self-awareness. Every situation carries lessons to be learned, and greater understanding should develop as experience is gathered. If vigilant, the contractor will be better equipped to respond effectively, efficiently, and with care to each new ethical situation. Over time, practiced attention to what works best will not only prepare the HIM entrepreneur for ethical leadership in the profession, but also be an essential ingredient for business and professional success.

Following are special ethical challenges that emerge for the independent contractor as a result of the business relationship between an independent service provider and the client. They include psychosocial issues, practical problems, and rights and responsibilities in the independent contractor–client relationship.

▪ Social Isolation

One aspect of the contractor–client relationship is the independent nature of the individual providing service. The independent contractor works from outside the client organization, as a partner in providing service. Often working alone or as the head of a service firm, the contractor must bring to the engagement the wisdom and resources needed when confronted with ethical challenges. Although resources from the client, such as mission statements, policy manuals, and deliberations of ethics committees, may be available to guide decision making, these may not be readily shared with the independent contractor or they may in fact conflict with the contractor's values and positions.

Additionally, the employee's social support network of peers and senior advisors is not readily available to the independent contractor. This network is often more valuable than the organization's formal sources of moral guidance. Peers and mentors with shared values and experiences can provide the comfort and guidance not available in manuals or mission statements. When this support is missing, the independent contractor may feel isolated and lonely in the midst of situations involving unclear or conflicting values. Like independent contractors, intrapreneurs can experience this isolation if, for example, they are involved in an unpopular effort to pioneer organizational changes.

To deal effectively with these situations, independent contractors must rely heavily on solid internal values and professional integrity when ethical dilemmas arise in the workplace. As head of a service firm employing other service providers, the contractor may be called upon to set the tone and provide guidance for an entire organization. The goal of integrity is to enable you to act on your own convictions in a meaningful way for your own life. At the same time, it acknowledges that at times conflicting ideas must be internally negotiated and brought together as a whole.

The key to safely navigating turbulent ethical issues as an independent contractor is to have a strong personal value system, sometimes referred to as an "inner rudder." An inner rudder is a reliable internal guidance mechanism built on a clear understanding of your values, an ability to identify when they are at risk of being compromised, and the an-

alytical skills and wisdom to steer through circumstances in a way that honors your values and respects other stakeholders. Clear personal values are necessary for a reliable inner rudder, as well as an understanding of current professional ethical standards and historic traditions. When confronted with a complex or troubling situation, ethicists and leadership experts emphasize the importance of honoring emotional responses, "gut feelings," or "hunches" as alerts and guides to action. The discomfort of physical tension, stomach aches, or other symptoms of anxiety or anger are often reliable signs that your values may be compromised or may conflict with others. Although emotional reactions should not be used to replace rational analysis, strongly felt reactions should not be ignored and should be weighed with the facts before deciding on a course of action.

Independent contractors must be particularly attuned to these emotional or intuitive signals, because the judgments of coworkers or superiors cannot be relied on to guide their thinking. Often, they must act on these feelings quickly to address problems with business relationships or to solve challenges presented by clients. Protracted fact gathering, analysis, and deliberation are not always possible.

Scenario 22-B: Negotiating Contracts

Kathy Watson is the president of HIM Coders, Inc., a professional service firm specializing in providing medical coding services to hospitals and other healthcare providers. Kathy has just concluded a contract negotiation for a new project to alleviate a coding backlog for a loyal hospital client for whom Kathy's firm has provided a large volume of service over the years. Because of the quality of the work done in the past, the client has not subjected the contract to a formal bidding process but rather has come directly to Kathy to determine if her firm can handle the project. As the deal is about to be closed, Wanda Matthews, HIM director for the hospital, casually asks Kathy whether her firm's fees are the best available for coding services. Kathy knows for a fact that her fees are 10% higher than those of one of her competitors for essentially the same service. Although Kathy knows her fees are reasonable, and although she prides herself on the quality of her coding services, she has no concrete evidence to differentiate her services from the other firm's on the basis of quality.

Questions

1. What should Kathy say in response to Wanda's question? Should she reveal what she knows about the other firm's fees? Should she admit that her fees are higher? If she does admit to having higher fees, should she try to justify the price difference by emphasizing the quality of her services over those of her competition?

2. What ethical reasoning should guide Kathy's decision?

A completed ethical decision-making matrix for the scenario is provided at the end of the chapter.

▪ Negotiating Contracts

The two most important issues to spell out in a professional service contract are (1) who the client is and (2) the nature of the work product to be delivered. Establishing the fees for service runs a distant third in importance. At first glance, answering these questions may seem simple and straightforward. However, this is often not the case, particularly with consulting and other professional service engagements.

Nevertheless, these issues must be clearly articulated to establish a stable and workable contract. First, establishing the identity of the client or customer for the engagement is not always easy. Many projects have multiple clients. The individual who calls the contractor and signs the contract may be the primary client, but others in the organization may also have an interest in and expectations for the consultant's services.

It is important to identify and meet with all interested parties as part of the contracting phase. Otherwise, it will be impossible to establish the answer to the second question: What are the project's work products or deliverables? Project deliverables should be concrete and stated in terms that are clear and measurable. Sometimes significant effort is required when writing contract terms to reach consensus on the description of the project objectives and the standards to be used to measure the project's success. When negotiating a contract, the contractor has a duty to be honest about the services the firm is capable of providing. It may be tempting to exaggerate abilities or promise stellar outcomes to get a contract signed, but the practice is unethical and will set the project up for failure. If the client's expectations do not match the firm's skills or abilities, the contractor should attempt to negotiate toward common ground. If negotiations reach an impasse, the contractor has a responsibility to him- or herself and to the client to acknowledge that fact and withdraw from consideration.

Setting professional service fees is also the product of negotiation. The contractor has an obligation to price services fairly in accordance with their value and with current market conditions. As demonstrated in Scenario 22-B, negotiating professional service fees can be a delicate matter that requires honesty, fairness, and flexibility on the part of the contractor as well as the potential client.

Scenario 22-C: Unrealistic Client Expectations

Beth Abernathy is an independent medical coder who has a contract to provide coding services to County General Hospital. After several months of work, Beth is audited by a private coding auditing firm, along with the rest of the employed coding staff. When the results of the audit are presented, Beth learns that County General is revising its coding policies, including one policy that calls for aggressive interpretation of bacterial pneumonia based on clinical findings only. Because there is pressure to reduce the hospital's accounts receivable days, all of the coders are being told to make their own judgments based on clinical findings, complete the case for billing, and forward any questionable cases to physicians for later review. The coders are told not to worry—if the physician reviewers disagree with the coder's interpretation, they will have the case rebilled for a lower DRG rate.

This new policy conflicts with Beth's expertise about current coding guidelines regarding interpreting clinical findings without supporting physician documentation. She also knows that rebilling cases for lower DRG rates can expose the organization to government audits.

Questions

1. What are the ethical issues involved here?

2. What are Beth's options and some likely consequences?

3. What course of action would you suggest and why?

A completed ethical decision-making matrix for the scenario is provided at the end of the chapter.

In Scenario 22-C, Beth faces a dilemma because the client's rules for behavior now conflict with her standards of professional practice. Beth's role as an independent contractor places her in a particularly vulnerable position.

If Beth were an employee rather than a contractor, could she more comfortably comply with the new coding policy unless it clearly violated standards of ethical coding? Could she also be assured of protection from personal liability under the hospital's liability insurance? In this case, a regulatory or ethical violation is not clear-cut. However, if a compliance issue is identified on audit, Beth could be held personally accountable for her contribution to inappropriate coding and billing.

As a result, Beth is faced with reconciling her own beliefs and values about proper coding and her fear of personal liability with the wishes of her client. She could challenge the private auditor's recommendations and the new coding policy and attempt to have

the new policy reversed. But her role as an independent contractor is to code, not to provide advice on coding policy. That is what the auditor was hired to do. Further, as an independent coder, her views may carry little weight. If she is unsuccessful in her attempt to have the policy changed, she may alienate the client and risk losing the contract. If she defies the new policy, she may likewise be found to be in breach of her contract and terminated. But if she complies with the policy and ignores her discomfort, she may be plagued by internal distress because of the conflict with her own values and principles. Worse yet, if auditors from the Office of the Inspector General or some other government agency find the practice to be unethical or illegal in the future, she is not likely to be protected, and she may be found personally liable for fraudulent coding practices.

Another option would be to report the practice to the authorities and potentially expose the client. This course of action could be justified by the argument that the primary interest to be served is justice in the form of proper billing. But becoming a whistle-blower, while potentially lucrative (because whistle-blowers are often entitled to a portion of the dollars recovered in prosecutions involving fraud and abuse, e.g., in billing government programs such as Medicare and Medicaid, and these payouts can be substantial), is a risky course of action with career-limiting potential.

Scenario 22-D: Discovering Sensitive Information about a Client, Competitor, or Colleague

Brian Winter, founder and part-owner of Just-In-Time Coding Services, is preparing for a meeting with his business partner to discuss an important new business opportunity. Just-In-Time is one of two finalists for a long-term outsourcing contract being offered by Blue Horizons Healthcare, the region's largest integrated delivery system. Brian and his partner need to discuss their strategy for tomorrow's business meeting with Jim Foster, Horizons' CFO, and Liz Raymond, the corporate HIM director. To date, only Brian has been in discussions with Liz Raymond while he prepared the initial proposal. Brian knows Liz well and has worked with her on several committees of their regional and state HIM associations.

Just-In-Time Coding Services is in its tenth year of operation. Brian and his partner have worked hard to build the firm into a successful business. The firm has enjoyed financial success by building a loyal clientele based on the expectation of high-quality services. It has grown slowly, but steadily, in size. Despite the firm's moderate size, Brian knows that they were offered the opportunity to bid on this contract because of Brian's relationship with Liz and the firm's solid reputation for quality and reliable service.

The Blue Horizons business would represent a significant contract—potentially increasing revenues by 20 percent, by Brian's estimate. It would also, however, require recruiting at least eight new coders, positions that Brian knows will not be easy to fill.

Brian also knows some things about the other finalist vying for the contract. Uniworld, Inc., is a large, national coding service that has grown even larger over the past few years, mostly through acquisitions of local and regional services. Brian has himself had several discussions with Uniworld management about their interest in acquiring Just-In-Time. Brian also suspects that Uniworld is planning to offer deep discounts during final negotiations—discounts that will be difficult for Brian's firm to match.

Brian knows a few other things about the competition that trouble him. Recently, he learned from a trusted source at another Uniworld client that the hospital recently underwent a painful coding compliance audit and was slapped with a multi-million-dollar fine for coding improprieties. Coding at that hospital is 100% outsourced to Uniworld, and, worse yet, a Uniworld coder is rumored to have been the whistle-blower who initiated the coding audit. Brian's source revealed that once the settlement between the hospital and the government is finalized, the hospital is likely to pursue legal action against Uniworld for its coding performance and will be seeking substantial monetary damages. This news is currently confidential under a gag order imposed by the government, but, according to Brian's source, it should become public knowledge within the next 60 to 90 days.

Up to this point, Brian has shared this information with no one—not with Liz or even with his partner. He wonders whether he should tell anyone what he knows. He also wonders how aggressively he should pursue the business with Blue Horizons, given the obvious advantages Uniworld has over his firm. On the other hand, it would give him great satisfaction to win this business from a large conglomerate. It could also be a financial boon for Just-In-Time. Further, he is troubled by the allegations he has heard against Uniworld. He feels a loyalty to Liz and does not believe she is aware of the trouble in the other city. She fought hard for approval to outsource coding, and he would not want to see her badly served by Uniworld.

Brian knows his partner will probably defer to his judgment on how to approach the final negotiations. He just wishes he knew what to recommend as their best course of action. As he checks the clock, he sees that it is 3:45 PM. His partner will be back in the office in 15 minutes for their meeting.

Questions

1. Does Brian have a clear course of action?

2. What ethical issues should Brian ponder before advising his business partner? In addition to these issues, are there general standards of business ethics that should inform his decision? Should his personal values enter into his business strategy?

3. What strategies would you suggest for the upcoming business meeting with Blue Horizons? Which course of action will best serve his loyalty to his own firm? To its employees? To his business partner? To his colleague and potential client?

A completed ethical decision-making matrix for the scenario is provided at the end of the chapter.

• Learning Sensitive Information about a Client, Competitor, or Colleague

While in the course of providing service to a client, an independent contractor will often have access to a large volume of information about staff, patients, and the client's business practices. Much of that information will be confidential. Of course, any information about patients should be treated as confidential in accordance with HIM professional standards. Secure handling and disposition of patient health information should be addressed in the independent contractor's Business Associate Agreement with the client, as required by HIPAA. But what about information, factual and circumstantial, related to activities of the client staff? About the client's organizational plans and operating performance?

Suppose, for example, that an independent contractor has been hired for a long-term engagement to reorganize the client's HIM department. Large amounts of information have come into the contractor's possession about personnel, physicians, business strategies, and audit results. Independent contractors have an obligation of loyalty to keep all information about the client confidential. This is especially important because contractors often serve multiple clients simultaneously, some of whom may be in direct competition for patients and market share. If information is leaked from one client to another, they could rightly or wrongly be blamed, resulting in damage to their professional reputation. A different dilemma may arise if they learn of potentially damaging information about a staff member.

Great care should also be taken in the handling of this information. Whereas an employee could go in confidence to a superior or support group to discuss such an ethical situation, such resources may not be readily available to an independent contractor. Loyalty to the organization may conflict with loyalty to a colleague. In any case, prudence should guide the handling of sensitive information until as much factual information as possible is known about a particular situation.

A similar ethical dilemma can arise when information is uncovered about a competitor, as in Scenario 22-D. Business is competitive by nature, and knowing as much as possible about competitors and their products is important to succeed in the marketplace. However, when potentially damaging information is uncovered about a competitor or its practices, careful consideration is needed before that information is revealed to other competitors or to clients. Divulging incomplete or erroneous information may result in legal action by the injured party. More importantly, bad-mouthing competitors can be seen as a distasteful tactic and can damage the firm's reputation among business prospects as well as professional colleagues. However, in some cases, the firm may feel a duty to disclose knowledge if it is confident as to the truthfulness of the information in its possession and if the business practice or other situation has the potential of causing harm to clients, patients, the profession, or society as a whole.

▪ Managing Client Relationships

Relationships with clients are like living organisms. A client relationship is in a state of constant change and requires ongoing nurture and attention. Circumstances, priorities, and individuals change. The independent contractor, in addition to performing good work, must focus on protecting and developing client relationships. This includes asking for and receiving feedback on client satisfaction, dealing with problems when they arise, and looking for ways to improve the relationship. Underpinning all these activities is the need to continually work to strengthen the bond of trust between the contractor and the client.

The most powerful tool for building a clientele is a solid reputation of trust with each individual client. Authentic behavior builds trust. Quickly and honestly resolving errors or failures builds trust. Trust cannot be bought and sold; it must be earned over and over again by consistent behavior. Turnover is common in client organizations. As new players come on board, new trust relationships must be built. It is an ongoing effort.

Sometimes, despite the independent contractor's best efforts, a relationship with a client deteriorates or a project is unsuccessful, and the relationship is terminated. This situation is never pleasant, but it is rarely a surprise. Generally, the independent contractor is aware of clues well in advance of the contract termination that things are not going well. The confident professional will confront these clues head on in an effort to rectify the situation. However, sometimes this is not possible. In fact, there are times when the independent contractor should consider provoking the event. If, for instance, expectations have changed or the contractor has lost some capacity to provide services as promised, the independent contractor may consider voluntarily withdrawing from the engagement in fairness to the client. This is not an easy decision, because, in addition to facing the prospect of lost revenue, the independent contractor may be genuinely concerned about the impact on the client of terminating service.

Leaving the client without resources could do more harm than good. However, behaving with honesty and authenticity, particularly in the face of service failures, is a powerful tool for building relationships and sustaining client trust. Authentic behavior means that independent contractors communicate what they are really experiencing as they work with the client during both good and bad times of the relationship.

▪ Rights of the Independent Contractor

Another important element in the contractor–client relationship is that, in addition to the client, the independent contractor also has rights. This can be easily forgotten in the desire to serve clients and build business.

Among other things, the independent contractor has a need for acceptance and inclusion by the client, as well as validation that what the independent contractor has to offer is valuable to the client. In addition, as a professional, an independent contractor has a right to professional autonomy. The independent contractor's individual values and professional principles are part of the service provided and should not be subjugated to client wishes. Also, independent contractors have a right to have their intellectual property and proprietary secrets kept confidential by the client. Techniques and methods of performing work are important assets to the independent contractor, as is any staff brought in to work on the client's project. Finally, the independent contractor has a right to have its business interests protected. This means that changes to scope of work, issues with service quality, intentions related to renewing or terminating service, and so on should be communicated honestly to the independent contractor and on a timely basis to allow for redress or reaction without endangering the independent contractor's business or reputation.

The independent contractor is entitled, in the interest of fairness, to have these needs met. The independent contractor should be skillful in articulating these needs as terms of the service contract and in verbal communications with the client. These communications are important for setting expectations early on in the relationship as well as later if threats are perceived or other issues arise.

CONCLUSION

Entrepreneurship is a growing trend among HIM professionals. Entrepreneurs share common traits such as creativity, competitiveness, and commitment to excellence. Entrepreneurs are skilled at identifying and capitalizing on opportunities for change. The HIM entrepreneur can work independently (as an independent contractor) or from within an organization (as an intrapreneur). Regardless of the work setting, the HIM entrepreneur occupies a special role as change agent, identifying needs for new or improved HIM services and developing innovative approaches to address unmet needs.

To expand future career options, the HIM professional should understand the traits and skills that distinguish entrepreneurs and learn to utilize entrepreneurial opportunities as they occur. In addition, HIM professionals must understand the special ethical challenges that may be faced by those who choose an entrepreneurial path. Among these challenges are issues related to maintaining business relationships, as well as special ethical dilemmas encountered by consultants and independent contractors. Increasingly complex practice issues, competitive pressures, and accelerated industry changes will continue to confront the HIM entrepreneur in the future. A clear understanding of one's personal values, coupled with knowledge of ethical principles and current professional practice standards, is needed to analyze and respond to ethical dilemmas. Key ethical values such as fairness, integrity, and trust provide the entrepreneur with guides for ethical decision making.

The entrepreneur's path is often unpaved and strewn with obstacles. And in a world of increasing complexity and accelerated change, a strong moral compass is essential to survival. Despite difficult challenges, entrepreneurship offers HIM professionals unique opportunities for growth, challenge, and professional rewards. HIM entrepreneurs also possess a special opportunity to exercise moral leadership both within and outside traditional healthcare organizations.

By working on the front lines of change, the entrepreneur can identify new challenges, influence ethical dialogue, and lead other healthcare professionals and the public to a future where healthcare delivery and information management decisions are shaped by thoughtful decision making and careful and caring ethical actions.

Key Terms

- Business ethics
- Consultant
- Contract
- Due care
- Independent contractor (IC)
- Intrapreneur

Chapter Summary

- Entrepreneurship is a growing trend among HIM professionals. Entrepreneurs often act as agents of change for their clients or customers. Intrapreneurs are traditional employees with an entrepreneurial spirit, acting as internal champions of change. Most HIM entrepreneurs work as consultants or independent contractors.

- Business ethics are the foundation of the entrepreneur's ethical framework. Ethical principles create valid business contracts. Advertising should be responsible as well as effective. Profits are a means rather than an end in business activity. Society needs business, and business needs ethics to survive.

- The HIM entrepreneur faces unique ethical challenges. Some ethical issues are based on functions performed by HIM consultants. Acting in the role of an "expert" requires care and a commitment to truthfulness and integrity. Delivering a difficult message to a client can create tension between ethical values. Conflicts or potential conflicts of interest should be disclosed. Collaborating with clients carries special conflicts and potential ethical dilemmas. Ethical challenges arise when the consultant is used as a "scapegoat" by a client. The consultant has a special opportunity to exercise moral leadership to improve HIM practices.

- Other ethical issues arise from the independent contractor–client relationship. The independent contractor may lack the social support network available to the traditional employee, leading to feelings of personal isolation. Negotiating professional service contracts involves special ethical considerations. Situations in which client expectations are unrealistic or are in conflict with the contractor's values create an ethical dilemma. Sensitive information uncovered about a client or a competitor must be handled with care. The independent contractor has rights as well as responsibilities for ethical treatment that must be articulated to the client in the terms of the service contract and in verbal communications.

References

American Health Information Management Association [AHIMA]. (2003). *eHIM—a vision of the eHIM future.* Chicago: Author.

American Health Information Management Association [AHIMA]. (2004). *AHIMA code of ethics.* Chicago: Author.

Glauser, M. J. (1998). *Glorious accidents: How everyday Americans create thriving companies.* Salt Lake City, UT: Shadow Mountain.

McLean, B., & Elkind, P. (2003). *The smartest guys in the room: The amazing rise and scandalous fall of Enron.* New York: Penguin.

Solomon, R. C. (1997). *It's good business: Ethics and free enterprise for the new millennium.* Totowa, NJ: Rowman & Littlefield.

Stein, J. (Ed.). (1975). *Random House dictionary of the English language* (Unabridged edition). New York: Random House.

Surowiecki, J. (2004). *The wisdom of crowds: Why the many are smarter than the few and how collective wisdom shapes business, economies, societies, and nations.* New York: Doubleday.

Timmons, J., Smollen, L. E., & Dingee, A. L. M. (1990). *New venture creation: Entrepreneurship in the 1990s,* 3d ed. Homewood, IL: Richard D. Irwin.

Velasquez, M. G. (2002). *Business ethics: Concepts and cases,* 5th ed. Upper Saddle River, NJ: Prentice Hall.

Additional Resources

Barrow, C. (1993). *The essence of small business.* Upper Saddle River, NJ: Prentice Hall.

Baty, G. (1990). *Entrepreneurship for the nineties.* Upper Saddle River, NJ: Prentice Hall.

Block, P. (1981). *Flawless consulting.* San Francisco: Jossey-Bass Pfeiffer.

Covey, S. R. (1992). *Principle-centered leadership.* New York: Simon & Schuster.

Goleman, D. (1998). *Working with emotional intelligence.* New York: Bantam.

Hawken, P. (1998). *Growing a business.* New York: Simon & Schuster.

Purtillo, R. (1999). *Ethical dimensions in the health professions,* 3d ed. Philadelphia: W.B. Saunders.

The ethical decision-making matrix is a tool to help you organize complex, ethical problems; however, there is no simple fill-in-the-box approach to ethical decision making. The objective is to follow each step of the process and not move from the question directly to what should be done or how to prevent it next time. If you skip steps, you will not fully understand all of the values and options for action. Also, the matrix provided for each scenario in this book is not the only way to examine the problem. You can make an equally compelling ethical argument for a different decision—just be sure to follow all the steps of the matrix.

SCENARIO 22-A: COMPETING CONSTITUENCIES

Steps	Information	
1. What is the ethical question?	Should Val continue to work on the project?	
2. What are the facts?	**KNOWN**	**TO BE GATHERED**
	• Larry plans to use inaccurate information for the JCAHO survey. • Larry has asked Val to participate in their preparations for the survey.	• Would Val's participation in the survey make her guilty of fraud? • If Val withdrew her agreement to participate, would she still be obligated to report the company's tactics? • What are the customary practices in such cases? • What is the likely impact on self and family of discontinuing work with this company?
3. What are the values? Examine the shared and competing values, obligations, and interests of the stakeholders (i.e., patient, HIM professional, healthcare practitioner(s), administrators, society, and other advocates) involved in order to fully understand the complexity of the ethical problem(s).	**Patient:** Values accurate medical records; values well-being of treatment facility. **HIM professional:** Truth, integrity, accuracy (tell the truth regarding the accuracy of the records); protect personal and professional integrity; fairness (follow the rules and obey the law); avoid harm (compliance with the company's deceptive practices could result in loss of future business); disclosing the company's practices could result in loss of employment. **Administrators:** Benefit patients by providing high-quality care; promote welfare of facility. **Society:** Promote full compliance with JCAHO guidelines.	

4. What are my options?	• Accept Larry's directive and continue work on the project. • Refuse to work on the project.	
5. What should I do?	Refuse to work on the project.	
6. What justifies my choice?	**JUSTIFIED**	**NOT JUSTIFIED**
	• Obligation to tell the truth. • Preserve professional integrity. • Follow rules equally for all. • Respect the guidelines of the JCAHO. • Demonstrate loyalty to client, unless asked to push legal boundaries.	• Continue work on the project. • Make special exception to the rules to preserve good relationship with the client. • Compromise professional integrity. • Knowingly violate JCAHO guidelines.
7. How can I prevent this ethical problem?	• Determine if system changes are needed. • Discuss standards and the values that support them with colleagues. • Learn more about ethical issues surrounding client–entrepreneur relationships. • Evaluate institutional integrity at initial contract interview and subsequently as ethical problems arise.	

The ethical decision-making matrix is a tool to help you organize complex, ethical problems; however, there is no simple fill-in-the-box approach to ethical decision making. The objective is to follow each step of the process and not move from the question directly to what should be done or how to prevent it next time. If you skip steps, you will not fully understand all of the values and options for action. Also, the matrix provided for each scenario in this book is not the only way to examine the problem. You can make an equally compelling ethical argument for a different decision—just be sure to follow all the steps of the matrix.

SCENARIO 22-B: NEGOTIATING CONTRACTS

Steps	Information	
1. What is the ethical question?	Should Kathy tell Wanda the truth, as she knows it?	
2. What are the facts?	**KNOWN**	**TO BE GATHERED**
	• Kathy's company has worked with the client in the past. • Kathy has prepared a contract for new services for the client. • Wanda has asked Kathy if her fees are the best available for coding services. • Kathy knows that her fees are 10% higher than those of one of her competitors.	• How do Kathy's fees compare to those of her competitors? • What will be the consequences if Kathy lies and Wanda later finds out that her fees are higher than the other competitors? • What are the customary practices in such cases? • What are the likely consequences of losing the contract for this job?
3. What are the values? Examine the shared and competing values, obligations, and interests of the stakeholders (i.e., patient, HIM professional, healthcare practitioner(s), administrators, society, and other advocates) involved in order to fully understand the complexity of the ethical problem(s).	**Client:** Values high-quality coding services; values competitive pricing; values honesty. **HIM professional:** Truth and integrity (honesty with client); fairness (give client all relevant information to make an informed choice); personal values (promote welfare of self, family, and company by protecting relationships with client). **Society:** Values quality of coding services.	

4. What are my options?	• Lie to Wanda about the prices charged by competitors. • Tell Wanda the truth about Kathy's company's prices compared to those of competitors.	
5. What should I do?	Tell Wanda the truth about Kathy's company's prices compared to those of competitors.	
6. What justifies my choice?	**JUSTIFIED**	**NOT JUSTIFIED**
	• Obligation to be honest with the client. • Protect professional integrity.	• Lie to Wanda about the prices charged by competitors. • Jeopardize professional integrity. • Jeopardize relationship with client.
7. How can I prevent this ethical problem?	• Determine if system/pricing changes are needed. • Discuss pricing standards and the data that support them with colleagues. • Learn more about standard coding prices throughout the market. • Evaluate clients' values at contract stage and subsequently thereafter as projects progress.	

The ethical decision-making matrix is a tool to help you organize complex, ethical problems; however, there is no simple fill-in-the-box approach to ethical decision making. The objective is to follow each step of the process and not move from the question directly to what should be done or how to prevent it next time. If you skip steps, you will not fully understand all of the values and options for action. Also, the matrix provided for each scenario in this book is not the only way to examine the problem. You can make an equally compelling ethical argument for a different decision—just be sure to follow all the steps of the matrix.

SCENARIO 22-C: UNREALISTIC CLIENT EXPECTATIONS

Steps	Information	
1. What is the ethical question?	What should Beth do?	
2. What are the facts?	**KNOWN**	**TO BE GATHERED**
	• Beth is an independent medical coder. • Beth has been instructed to use her own best judgment to code, then physicians will rebill for lower DRG rates if they disagree with the coding.	• Would billing cases for lower DRG rates put the organization at significant risk for government audits? • Is following these instructions unethical? • Would Beth be guilty of fraud if she follows these procedures? • What are the customary practices in such cases? • What consequences would Beth face for discontinuing her contract? • Does the contract include binding obligations? • What is the likely impact on self and family of discontinuing the contract?
3. What are the values? Examine the shared and competing values, obligations, and interests of the stakeholders (i.e., patient, HIM professional, healthcare practitioner(s), administrators, society, and other advocates) involved in order to fully understand the complexity of the ethical problem(s).	**Patient:** Values accuracy of medical record. **HIM professional:** Truth, integrity, accuracy (code accurately and reliably rather than to maximize speed); fairness (follow the rules and obey the law); loyalty to client; avoid harm (inaccurate documentation may harm the patient, lack of reimbursement could harm patients and healthcare workers through damage to the facility); personal values (promote welfare of self and family by avoiding loss of client). **Healthcare professionals:** Promote welfare of patients through accurate documentation for future care; truth-telling; fairness in following rules equally for all. **Administrators:** Benefit patients and keep from harm; promote welfare of facility; maximize reimbursement without compromising truth-telling; control healthcare costs; fairness in applying rules for all. **Society:** Control costs; promote fair and just allocation of resources; follow rules of coding equally for all.	

4. What are my options?	• Agree to go along with the instructions. • Do not agree to go along with the instructions.
5. What should I do?	Tell employer that she cannot follow the instructions to code without supporting physician documentation.

6. What justifies my choice?	**JUSTIFIED**	**NOT JUSTIFIED**
	• Obligation to tell the truth. • Support accuracy of the medical record. • Preserve professional integrity. • Follow rules equally for all. • Respect the law. • Demonstrate loyalty to client, unless asked to push legal boundaries.	• Agree to go along with the in-structions. • Tell a lie. • Make special exceptions to the rules to maximize speed of reimbursement. • Not fair to those who follow rules. • Miscoding undermines the entire system. • Miscoding increases costs in the long run. Miscoding could subject the organization to government audits.

7. How can I prevent this ethical problem?	• Determine if system changes are needed. • Discuss standards and the values that support them with colleagues and clients. • Learn more about ethical issues surrounding coding. • Evaluate organizational integrity at contract stage and subsequently as ethical problems arise.

The ethical decision-making matrix is a tool to help you organize complex, ethical problems; however, there is no simple fill-in-the-box approach to ethical decision making. The objective is to follow each step of the process and not move from the question directly to what should be done or how to prevent it next time. If you skip steps, you will not fully understand all of the values and options for action. Also, the matrix provided for each scenario in this book is not the only way to examine the problem. You can make an equally compelling ethical argument for a different decision—just be sure to follow all the steps of the matrix.

SCENARIO 22-D: DISCOVERING SENSITIVE INFORMATION ABOUT A CLIENT, COMPETITOR, OR COLLEAGUE

Steps	Information	
1. What is the ethical question?	What should Brian do?	
2. What are the facts?	**KNOWN**	**TO BE GATHERED**
	• Just-In-Time is up for a contract that could bring significant income. • Just-In-Time would have difficulty hiring enough qualified coders to handle the contract. • Brian has learned that their biggest competitor for the contract, Uniworld, is under investigation for suspect coding practices, but there is a gag order on the case. • The meeting to discuss the contract is in 15 minutes.	• What are the consequences for violating a gag order? • Would Liz's respect for Brian and his company be affected by Brian violating a gag order? • Could Liz's company be harmed if they select Uniworld? • Is the information about Uniworld's litigation definitely true? • How would Just-In-Time be affected if they do not win the contract? • What are the customary practices in such cases?
3. What are the values? Examine the shared and competing values, obligations, and interests of the stakeholders (i.e., patient, HIM professional, healthcare practitioner(s), administrators, society, and other advocates) involved in order to fully understand the complexity of the ethical problem(s).	**Just-In-Time/HIM professionals:** Value steady income; value maintenance of high standards and reputation for quality. **Blue Horizons Healthcare:** Values high-quality coding. **Uniworld:** Could launch litigation against Just-In-Time if information released is not true or violates gag order. **Society:** Financial loss of miscoding could drive up costs at Blue Horizons.	

4. What are my options?	• Do not disclose information about Uniworld to Blue Horizons. • Warn Blue Horizons about the litigation in which Uniworld is allegedly involved.	
5. What should I do?	Refuse to disclose information about Uniworld to Blue Horizons Healthcare.	
6. What justifies my choice?	**JUSTIFIED**	**NOT JUSTIFIED**
	• Obligation to obey gag order. • Protect professional integrity. • Protect Just-In-Time from possible litigation from Uniworld.	• Warn Blue Horizons about alleged Uniworld litigation. • Break the gag order and the law. • Jeopardize professional integrity and relationship with client. • Expose Just-In-Time to litigation brought by Uniworld.
7. How can I prevent this ethical problem?	• Determine if system changes are needed. • Discuss values and the standards that support them with colleagues. • Discuss ethical and legal issues surrounding information learned about competitor.	

VENDOR MANAGEMENT

Keith Olenik, MA, RHIA, CHP

Learning Objectives

After completing this chapter, the reader should be able to:

- Identify ethical challenges and key issues that influence the interactions between vendors and health information management (HIM) professionals.
- Define skills needed to assist in vendor selection and relationship management.
- Understand the risks, benefits, and ethical issues that routinely surface in the request for proposal (RFP) and contract negotiation processes.

Abstract

Vendors perform important roles in their relationship with health information management (HIM) professionals. Both the vendor and the HIM professional may contribute to the success or failure of these crucial business relationships. In order to communicate effectively with vendors, HIM professionals must recognize common ethical dilemmas. This chapter will describe skills needed to communicate with vendors as well as how to select vendors, manage vendor relationships, create requests for proposals (RFPs), and negotiate contracts.

Scenario 23-A: Vendor Request

Regional Medical Center has been using the National Dictation Company's dictation and transcription system for over 15 years. An upgrade to National's new technology platform was accomplished four years ago, after considering several other vendors during the selection process. The new system has been operating as expected, and there are no plans to make any changes to this application at the present time.

A salesperson from a company that competes directly with the National Dictation Company has recently made numerous attempts to contact the HIM director at Regional Medical Center. The salesperson wants to provide a quote for a replacement for the current dictation and transcription system. The HIM director has repeatedly declined to schedule a meeting with this salesperson. The salesperson sends a letter to the CEO of Regional Medical Center stating that the HIM director is exhibiting unfair business tactics by not meeting with him to discuss the option of a new dictation and transcription system.

Questions

1. What should the HIM director do when she is informed by the CEO of the salesperson's action?

2. What does this action say about the salesperson and his company?

A completed ethical decision-making matrix for the scenario is provided at the end of the chapter.

VENDOR RELATIONS

A vendor is "one that sells," and a customer is "one that buys goods or services"(Steinmetz & Downling, 1997). The definitions of these two terms make it sound simple. Somebody sells something and somebody buys something. The reality of this relationship is infinitely more complex, and it can be frustrating. A vendor relationship is an agreement between an organization that has a need with specific requirements and a vendor who provides components, experience, expertise, judgment, wisdom, management, and/or leadership to fulfill those needs and requirements.

What about the relationship between vendors and healthcare organizations? Vendor relationships in the health information management (HIM) environment are not the same as buying a meal in a restaurant. Although a customer may repeatedly return to a restaurant, each meal is a time-specific event. Relationships with vendors, by definition, occur over a continuum. Vendors aim to sell, and healthcare organizations try to control costs—goals that seem inherently at odds. Today's best partnerships are no longer merely contractual, but are based on the premise that the vendor and the organization have joined together for mutual benefit.

In a true partnership between a vendor and a customer, the two organizations optimize resources, focus on their individual core competencies, and end up together in a much better place than either one could have gotten to without the other. To move the vendor–customer relationship into the realm of a partnership, both the vendor and the healthcare organization must invest the necessary time to learn as much as possible about each other. Healthcare organizations expect their vendors to understand their business, but the healthcare organizations must also know the vendor and understand what that company's goals are. When it comes to relationships, both parties must understand that this symbiotic relationship is much like a friendship. If they do not discuss problems or if they fail to communicate with each other, chances are the relationship will not last.

It is also important to understand the vendor's strategy of forward momentum while ensuring that the vendor's strategy is in alignment with the organization's. For example, a vendor may currently offer scheduling, billing, and patient education software, but may plan to specialize in only one of these applications in the future. If the buyer is not aware of this strategy, two of the applications it purchased may need to be replaced (in an emergency situation) due to lack of vendor support.

Sales Ethics

The competitive salesperson in Scenario 23-A was willing to sacrifice integrity and reputation to obtain business from the organization. Although we do not know exactly what motivated the salesperson's desperate action, job performance is one potential factor. The salesperson may have been at risk of losing his job unless new business was obtained. Questionable sales tactics may have been requested by the salesperson's direct supervisor. Regardless, the action was extremely unethical and will probably create a long-lasting negative effect that will prohibit the organization from doing business with the vendor in the future.

The HIM director felt that she was being ethical by not responding, because the organization had no plans or desire to investigate an alternative product and she did not want the vendor to waste time and resources unfairly. However, ignoring the vendor without explanation is not a professional way to behave. Most people get paid for doing a day's work, regardless of the quantity of the work for a given day, whereas salespeople are paid for results of their work. If you were asked to list the stereotypical characteristics of salespeople, the first thing you might say is that they are motivated by money.

The stereotypical image of a salesperson might further be described as someone who is greedy, pushy, aggressive, and deceitful. However, one study (Gitomer, 2000) outlining characteristics that separated high-performing salespeople from low-performing ones indicated a different set of characteristics. According to Gitomer (2000), good salespeople:

- Believe in the company, the product, and themselves
- Have an ability to maintain price integrity
- Demonstrate personal values and ethics
- Exhibit an ability to generate profit and loyal customers
- Have a desire to help others get what they want, rather than merely selling something just for the love of money

An ethical salesperson can be successful with their company and the customer. The following is a list of qualities that salespeople could use as a guide (Kahle, 2001):

- They correct any misunderstandings.
- They walk away from short-term gains in return for long-term gains.
- They do what they say they are going to do.
- They demonstrate social responsibility.
- They recognize others who assist them.
- They do not speak badly of the competition.
- They do not misrepresent information.

A *Business Horizons* (2003) study found that customers increasingly base their buying decision on whether they believe a company is ethical. Companies that take the "high road" will make lifelong customers. It is the salesperson who acts as the company's primary communication tool for the ethical behavior and integrity of the vendor organization.

Scenario 23-B: Vendors as Friends

Karen used to be the HIM director at Lakeside General Hospital before going to work for Genesis, an information technology vendor that provided the health information system (HIS) software at the facility. She has retained several friendships with people she used to work for at the hospital and socializes with them on a frequent basis. The hospital is currently in the process of selecting an electronic health record system, and Genesis is one of the companies being considered. Jane is the new HIM director and is a key member of Lakeside's selection committee; she is also Karen's friend.

Karen has been asked to be a key member of the vendor's sales team due to her knowledge of the organization. It is common knowledge at Lakeside the Karen and Jane are friends. Jane and Karen have discussed the potential issue with this situation and have agreed to not share any information about the project outside their defined roles.

Questions

1. Should either Jane or Karen have asked to be excluded from the project?

2. Is it appropriate for Karen to use previous information about the organization to her new employer's advantage?

A completed ethical decision-making matrix for the scenario is provided at the end of the chapter.

It is only natural to develop friendships while working with vendors over a prolonged period of time. Establishing boundaries with these types of relationships is extremely important. HIM professionals are seen as valuable employees to vendors within the healthcare community. As with any job, a person is hired for his or her knowledge and experience. It is to the company's advantage to hire people who can provide firsthand knowledge of what customers want and need.

If both parties demonstrate professional values and act in an ethical way, their information exchange outside the working relationship will not be compromised. However, the two individuals could choose to use their relationship for personal gain by inappropri-ately sharing information to obtain a lower purchase price or guarantee receipt of the business. It will be up to each individual to decide how much information can be shared. In the scenario, Karen and Jane discussed the potential issue and established professional, ethical boundaries.

The two women could have had discussions with their superiors to ensure that neither one would compromise the vendor-selection process. Genesis may have been viewed to have an advantage, but any of the other vendors could have hired someone with more intimate knowledge of an organization. Past experience is one of the primary factors considered by any hiring organization. A former employee is entitled to use his or her past experience as a means to obtain a new job and should be expected to use that information to the advantage of the new employer.

Scenario 23-C: Gifts

Carol is the HIM director at Central Medical Center. The Center has been outsourcing the release-of-information process for several years to a local release-of-information vendor. Carol has not been happy with the quality of service lately and has decided to consider using another vendor to provide this service. A request for proposal (RFP) is sent out to several release-of-information companies.

Prior to signing the contract, the new company offers to fly both Carol and her release-of-information manager, Mike, out to visit the company's corporate office in California to meet with some of the key players who will be involved in the account. Due to the lengthy travel distance, the company offers to have the two stay over the weekend and enjoy some of the local sights.

Questions

1. Should Carol accept the offer to visit the corporate office?

2. Is it appropriate for Carol and Mike to spend the weekend at the vendor's expense?

3. Would the decision to visit the office be viewed differently if it had been before the final selection?

A completed ethical decision-making matrix for the scenario is provided at the end of the chapter.

A discussion about vendors and ethics would be incomplete without the topic of gifts. Where does the vendor draw the line between good business practice and unnecessary expense? Where does the buyer draw the line between undue influence and the receipt of gifts that are valuable or needed? In Scenario 23-C, the vendor offered to fly the two hospital employees to its corporate office to meet with key members of the team that would be handling the release-of-information function.

Oftentimes, it is not clear whether a gift should be accepted. Consider the same scenario, but say that the offer of the trip is made at the beginning of the process rather than after the final decision.

- Would it have been appropriate to go on the trip and then not choose the vendor?
- Would the trip have been a deciding factor in choosing the vendor?

Some states have laws that regulate gift transactions. For example, New York state law dictates that, under most circumstances, executives at publicly funded institutions cannot accept gifts or coverage for expenses worth more than $75. Those who do accept such gifts can be fired and face fines for up to $10,000 per violation, as well as misdemeanor criminal charges. The New York State Ethics Commission evaluates potential problems with accepting gifts and hospitality from technology vendors beyond what's allowed by state laws (McDougall, 2003).

Business ethics has become increasingly complex in the public arena because of various corporate scandals and billion-dollar bankruptcies that have occurred over the past couple of years. Business ethics can be defined as the branch of ethics that examines ethical rules and principles within a commercial context; the various moral or ethical problems that can arise in a business setting; and any special duties or obligations that apply to persons who are engaged in commerce (Beauchamp & Bowie, 1993; Hoffman & Frederick, 1995; Velasquez, 2001). Business scandals have raised issues regarding the lack of appropriate checks and balances that would ensure communication about company activity among corporate executives, stockholders, and employees. Lawyers have been working to restore trust to the investment community and the employees of companies such as Enron, Tyco, and WorldCom by creating legislation that will prevent future incidents (Vickers, 2002).

In light of the scandals many ask how such ethical lapses can occur:

- Did the owners of these companies have no conscience?
- Did they fail to consider the impact of their unethical business decisions on others?
- Did they take actions merely to make a profit at any cost and then rationalize the decision?

As a result of these corporate scandals, many corporations have established formal ethics programs to ensure that they do not incur similar problems. In the post–Enron era, many healthcare executives are beginning to question the seemingly innocent perks that are meant to help vendors and customers develop relationships (McDougall, 2003). One of the most common perks is the business lunch or dinner. Depending on the location or size of the group, the associated dollars spent can be considerable compared to how much of the conversation was business versus personal during the meal.

Every company should have a written policy outlining the limits on the types of gifts or gratuities an employee is allowed to receive. This type of information is usually part of a conflicts of interest policy. Such a policy should also include statements on reasonable and reciprocal entertainment, in keeping with social and business customs. Every employee who has the potential to interact with vendors should be educated on the policy.

Employees should discuss with their superiors any business meals or trips that are paid for by vendors. The following questions should be considered when deciding whether such perks are ethical: Is the gift or gratuity reasonable? Will it obligate the employee to the vendor? It is often difficult to determine when the line between ethical and unethical has been crossed. Professional values are importa nt, because no policy will address every possible situation. The bottom line is that under no circumstances should a gift or expense payment influence a business decision.

Prevention of Ethical Problems

The organization should investigate the potential vendor's ethics program. Every vendor will not have a formal program documenting its actions and ethics, but most will have mission statements, codes of ethics, policy and personnel manuals, training manuals, and a complaint process that can be reviewed. All of the questions asked as part of the ethical decision-making matrix can be applied to the vendor-selection process. See Appendix 23-A for a sample "gifts" policy.

Scenario 23-D: Preferred Vendors

County Medical Center has decided to investigate its options for a new encoder. It is going to send out a request for proposal (RFP) as required by the county to select the new coding software. Sue, the HIM director, has only been at the facility for six months; she used the encoder from Atlantis at her last facility. She has also participated in a similar review and selection process for an encoder at her previous job, and she is familiar with the various software programs available.

Sue believes that the encoder software chosen should be able to produce reports. She considers the Atlantis product to be superior based on comparisons she has made in the past. She also has an established working relationship with the vendor representative from Atlantis. Although Sue isn't the only person involved in the vendor-selection process, she has already made up her mind about which product she is going to pick, even before the RFP is sent out. Sue is also actively soliciting support from other people on the selection committee to go with her choice. Sue's preferred vendor submitted the RFP after the due date.

Questions

1. Is it appropriate for Sue to have made up her mind on the final selection before the RFP is sent out?

2. Should Sue be attempting to influence other members of the selection committee before they have reviewed any of the responses?

A completed ethical decision-making matrix for the scenario is provided at the end of the chapter.

REQUESTS FOR PROPOSALS

A **request for proposal,** or **RFP,** is a formal document detailing the functional requirements of a project that is provided to a group of vendors who are being asked to provide a service or product. This type of document is most appropriate for high-dollar or high-risk projects that will involve the acquisition or use of hardware and software. It can also be beneficial when selecting an outsourcing vendor for transcription, coding, release of information, or other HIM operations. The responses to the RFP should provide the vendor-selection committee with information that will assist them in making a decision about which vendors to consider in the final selection process (Carpenter, 1998; Hamilton, 2003; Little, 2002).

The typical RFP has four main components: introduction, directions, standard text, and statement of work. In some cases, a fifth component, social responsibility, may be included (Boatright, 2003).

Introduction

The introduction section of the RFP typically specifies when the proposal is due, who the contact person will be, and gives time esti-

mates. It should include a statement that RFPs received after the deadline will not be considered. It is important that no exceptions be made to this date to be fair to those vendors who submit their proposal on time. Each member of the vendor-selection team should receive a copy of the RFP, so the vendor should be asked to provide the required number of original documents to facilitate the review process.

It is recommended that one person within the organization be identified as the contact person for the vendor to ask questions of or request clarification. The use of a single contact person will ensure that consistent responses are provided. The selection of the contact person is important, because that person will establish the first impression between the vendor and the customer.

Making sure that all questions are answered by the healthcare organization's identified contact ensures consistency and also prevents a vendor from obtaining additional information through other resources that may give it an unfair advantage. This requirement must be supported by all employees who might have contact with the vendors involved in the process. If any points of clarification are provided to one vendor, all vendors need to be notified, especially if the clarification changes the RFP.

The group developing and sending out the RFP must be very reasonable about its time estimates as to how long it will take vendors to respond. It is extremely important to stick with the stated due date and not give any one company the advantage of extra time to submit a response.

Directions

This section of the RFP explains what the vendors should include in the proposal and how the RFPs will be evaluated. All required forms should be provided to the vendors at the beginning of the selection process. Forms will ensure consistency among the different proposals. A pricing form is one example of a form that will ensure consistency in how information is submitted and reviewed. It will also eliminate any potential confusion that would occur when comparing prices submitted in a variety of formats and categories.

The use of the specific criteria that will be used to evaluate the vendors should be documented and could include the following. These criteria can be organized in the order of importance, as decided upon by the organization:

- Compliance with the RFP requirements
- Vendor's experience with similar projects
- Skill set and educational background of the vendor's team
- Length of time in business
- Reference checks, including results of site visits, if applicable
- Compatibility of the vendor's team with the customer's team
- Total estimated cost of the project and all related items

A rating system should be created so that the reviewers can be objective when evaluating the proposals. If a rating system is applied to the criteria just listed, it must be adhered to for all vendors. Making an exception for one vendor that failed to complete one section of the RFP may seem like a reasonable action, but it could compromise the integrity of the vendor-selection process. The rating of the criteria should also be made as objectively as possible to eliminate any personal biases that could be made by members of the team who may favor one vendor over another.

Some organizations may ask the vendors to make formal presentations before or after the RFPs have been reviewed and the list of potential vendors has been narrowed. The timing of these presentations is up to the facility seeking the RFP. The expectations for this presentation, outlining in detail what the vendor will be required to present, should be documented, including a statement that the vendor will be responsible for all expenses related to the presentation.

A list of formal references for similar clients or projects should be requested from each vendor. Reference checks can be conducted before, during, or after the selection process. Ideally, reference checks should be done prior to the selection process to obtain an accurate assessment of the vendor's abilities to produce the product or service. The vendor should supply the following information about each reference it provides:

- Name of the organization
- Location
- Facility size
- Contact person
- Telephone number
- Length of association

Members of the selection team may also use personal references from peers or professional colleagues. Such references are oftentimes more valuable than those that are preselected by the vendor. Careful consideration must be made as to how this information is incorporated into the evaluation process and communicated to all members of the selection team. Confidentiality is of the utmost importance.

Standard Text

This section of the RFP may include general information about the organization, such as the type of facility, pertinent statistics, annual revenues, strategic goals, and mission.

Expectations of warranties should be outlined, including exact terms or general requirements. Maintenance expectations should also be documented and then compared to the options presented by the vendor. These elements can all be negotiated upon final vendor selection. The deadline for the review of all proposals and a decision date should be stated.

Statement of Work

This is the most important part of the RFP. This section should outline the problem the customer is trying to solve or the specific objectives related to the product or service that is to be acquired. The statement of work should include the following:

- A list of detailed requirements for the required hardware and software.
- A project plan, including a time line or estimated completion date for the project.
- The organization's training requirements should be outlined.

Some vendors may be hesitant to provide an extensive amount of detailed information under this section if the information could be considered intellectual property. Every member of the organization's RFP selection committee has an obligation to keep all of the information submitted by the vendor confidential. However, most vendors understand that recommendations from each vendor's response may be included in the final project plan.

Social Responsibility

In addition to the four common sections of an RFP, a fifth category evaluating the vendors' social responsibility may be included. **Social responsibility** is the selection of a vendor based on ethical standards or judgments or social desirability rather than profits (Boatright, 2003). The following are corporate activities that demonstrate social responsibility:

- Choosing to operate on an ethical level that is higher than what the law requires
- Making contributions to civic and charitable organizations and nonprofit institutions
- Providing benefits for employees and improving the quality of life in the workplace beyond economic and legal requirements
- Taking advantage of an economic opportunity that is judged to be less profitable but more socially desirable than some alternatives
- Using corporate resources to operate a program that addresses some major social problem

The weight given to social responsibility will depend on the sophistication of the vendor and the importance of the service it is going to provide. If the relationship with the vendor is going to be long term, such as in an outsourcing situation, the social responsibility of the vendor will be important, because the company will be an extension of the organization. At a minimum, an organization should have policies outlining how it handles issues of an ethical nature. A question about the vendor's process of handling billing discrepancies is a good example of a policy that should be reviewed in the RFP process.

Ethical Considerations for the RFP Process

Information contained in an RFP should be considered confidential and should not be shared with competing vendors. However, it may be difficult not to incorporate portions of various proposals into the final project plan.

It is unethical to show favoritism to one vendor. Any information shared with one vendor should be shared will all vendors. At no time during the selection and evaluation process should specific pricing information from one vendor be shared with another. It is appropriate to provide ranges and indicate in general where a particular vendor's proposal has fallen within the range of all proposals. However, telling a vendor that the total price on their proposal was the highest when it was not is inappropriate. A better way to get the vendor to reduce its price is to say that the price was higher than what you had anticipated, if, in fact, that is a true statement.

The RFP should be created without any particular vendor in mind. The RFP should not be tailored to a particular vendor. If it is, this would lead to an unfair outcome. If vendors discover that one vendor is being favored, they will most likely rescind their submissions, which will reduce the organization's bargaining power. Responding to RFPs is a time-consuming process for the vendor. A valid RFP process should not be entered into with any preconceived ideas as to the expected outcome. It is unfair to the vendors if the organization does not intend to evaluate the RFPs but is required by organizational policy or some type of state law to go through a selection process. An organization can stand to gain a poor reputation if it does not use the RFP process appropriately.

Scenario 23-E: Negotiating

Oceanview Hospital has been considering proposals for a new cancer registry software program. The review process included several members from the hospital's cancer committee. An amount of $150,000 has been budgeted for this project. Two companies have been selected as finalists. Davis Enterprises is offering a more robust initial training package with annual updates at a slightly higher price than The Smith Company.

A comparison of the prices submitted from the two companies is as follows:

Item	Davis	Smith
Software	$75,000	$50,000
Installation	$15,000	$12,500
Training	$30,000 (100 hours)	$25,000 (75 hours)
Total	**$120,000**	**$107,500**
Annual Maintenance	$16,000	$10,000

Meetings are set up with both companies to answer questions and to determine who is going to be selected. During both meetings, the representative from each company asks if there is anything that needs to be added to its offerings and how its price compares to the other offers. Steve from purchasing leads the discussion during the first meeting with Davis Enterprises. He states that the quote was higher than they had anticipated and asks the representative if Davis can do better on the total price. In the Smith meeting, Steve says the hospital might be willing to accept the offer if Smith can increase the training hours to 150.

Questions

1. How much information should be provided to the vendors on their proposals' shortcomings?

2. Does the committee have an obligation to tell each vendor if its price is either the highest or the lowest?

A completed ethical decision-making matrix for the scenario is provided at the end of the chapter.

NEGOTIATION

Negotiation, the process of bargaining with another individual, is definitely as much an art as a skill. If this skill is not practiced on a regular basis, the results can be disastrous. Organizations should involve someone with experience and knowledge during the negotiation stage of the vendor-selection process to either lead the negotiations or to provide expert guidance. Everyone involved in the vendor-selection process should have an understanding of basic negotiating practices. The negotiating approach of the salesperson or company will also offer insight into the company's values and ethics.

AHIMA's Code of Ethics (2004) requires all HIM professionals to be aware of the profession's ethical principles and to practice in a manner consistent with them by acting honestly and responsibly. Most ethical codes do not specifically provide guidelines on how much information should be shared or withheld during the negotiation phase. Although lying is never considered appropriate, certain types of communication may stretch the truth or exclude information that would alter perceptions and decisions. For the vendor to retain its reputation, it should be open and honest during the negotiation phase as well. A survey of individuals involved in negotiating identified two distinct styles and the characteristics of the people who used them (Schneider, 2002). The two distinct styles—problem solving and adversarial—and the characteristics

of people who use each style are listed in Table 23–1.

Although these two styles share some of the same qualities, the problem solvers were viewed as more effective negotiators. The organization cannot control what type of negotiator it will deal with, but it can at least anticipate the salesperson's style based on the characteristics he or she displays during the sales process.

In the traditional view of negotiating, one party wins and the other party loses. If both sides are more focused on the negotiating tactics rather than on achieving a common goal of meeting the needs of both sides, someone is definitely going to lose. However, negotiation should be more about deciding how the two parties will deal with each other and meet their shared and different needs; this concept of negotiation is referred to as "principled negotiation" or a "win-win situation" (Fisher & Ury, 1991).

Table 23–1 Negotiation Styles

Problem Solving	Adversarial
Ethical	Egotistical
Experienced	Demanding
Personable	Ambitious
Trustworthy	Forceful
Realistic	Stubborn
Confident	Experienced
Perceptive	Confident
Self-controlled	Bluffer

The following is a brief description of some of the more common negotiating techniques (Dawson, 1999):

- **Ask for more than you expect to get.** This technique is pretty self-explanatory. It is a common negotiating principle. Sometimes you might get what you ask for.
- **Bracketing.** This is the next step after you have established what you are willing to take or offer for the product. A simple example is as follows: Say that the buyer offers $100 million for the product; the seller is willing to take $150 million and starts the bidding at $200 million. The final outcome in this type of situation will usually be somewhere in the middle, around $150 million.
- **Never say yes to the first offer or counteroffer.** The motivation behind this technique is that if you accept the first offer, the other party is going think it could have done better or that something is wrong. The other party will think that they should have asked for more or less, depending on its role in the negotiation. The other party might also think that it missed some piece of information that led you to your original request or offer. This tactic is more about helping the other person feel good about the final price.
- **Flinching.** This is the physical response to an offer to let the other person know you are shocked by the stated price. The primary purpose is to let the other party know that the original price is unacceptable and adjustments or concessions will need to be made.
- **Concentrate on the issues.** The key to this technique is to not get thrown off by the actions of the other person. One of the parties in this situation may be legitimately upset, but the other party needs to remain calm and not take it personally. The goal here is to bring the conversation back to something that can be agreed upon and get the negotiation back on track.

- **The vise.** This style involves one simple statement, "You will have to do better than that." After making this statement, the key is to not say anything else and wait for the other party to either accept the offer or make some type of concession. This is also known as the "silent close" in the world of sales. Be prepared though for the counter response of "How much better than that do I have to do?"

In Scenario 23-E, Steve chose not to specifically address the questions asked by both vendors, but instead attempted to gain the upper hand by making demands. Depending on the attitude or style of the vendor, this approach may or may not produce the desired end result. Regardless of the approach, Steve had no responsibility to discuss where either vendor was related to pricing with the other vendor. The organization will have greater bargaining power if it leads each vendor to believe that its price was the highest. This is not unethical unless a response includes a blatant lie.

No matter what types of negotiation techniques or styles are used, the end result is always one of four situations:

- Two winning parties
- Winning salesperson, losing customer
- Winning customer, losing salesperson
- Two losing parties

Although some salespeople might think that the second situation is the best way to increase sales, smart negotiators will try to end up with the first situation. To ensure successful negotiations, keep in mind the following four key points (Fisher & Ury, 1991):

- Include several issues in your negotiations so if you need to concede on one point, you will have more control over the others.
- Realize that two people are not negotiating for the same thing. The needs of both parties are different, and flexibility will be required.

- Don't be greedy, because one side will end up feeling bad.
- Go above and beyond what was agreed upon at the end of the negotiation, because this will lead to positive future interactions.

ENHANCEMENT OF VENDOR RELATIONSHIPS

The rise of outsourcing has expanded the number and depth of vendor relationships. Increases in the use and implementation of complex enterprise computer applications mean that relationships with a vendor can last for years. It is in the organization's best interest to enhance its relationships with its vendors. The following are some ways that vendor–organization relationships can be enhanced (Murray, 2001):

- Consider becoming a reference account for the vendor. This would entail allowing prospective customers to observe how the vendor's product or service functions in your environment. It may take some time and effort to prepare the information that will be presented about your experiences, both good and bad, with the vendor. This is a good tactic to position your organization at the head of the queue with respect to vendor recognition and face time.
- Leverage your organization's experience in a case study. This is a highly effective way of getting increased visibility within your vendor's support ranks. Organizations that interact more with the vendor have the opportunity to provide suggestions on enhancements.
- Be willing to share any measurable statistics on productivity improvements, customer satisfaction, or efficiency gains in an effort to solidify a good working relationship. This same information can be used during the site visit.
- Provide both good and bad feedback about the vendor's products and services. Vendors appreciate customers

who are willing to do this. The organization will also receive prompt responses to any issues that may emerge. Constant and steady communication through reports, conference calls, and face-to-face meetings are key to maintaining the relationship.

- Review with skepticism any vendor that is always uncomfortable or unwilling to say no to your requests. This may be a sign of other issues that have yet to be uncovered.

ETHICAL BEHAVIOR

Healthcare organizations and vendors are both subject to a myriad of laws, rules, and regulations. Both parties are also required to implement corporate compliance programs. However, implementation of these programs and following the law does not necessarily guarantee ethical behavior. Executives who ignore ethics run the risk of personal and corporate liability in an increasingly tough legal environment (Paine, 1994).

To create an environment that promotes exemplary behavior, an organization needs a comprehensive approach that goes beyond the punitive compliance program. This is where the organization's mission and values come into play. And to be truly effective, there must be a connection with each employee's values and sense of personal ethics. True success involves a collaborative approach of both organizational and personal ethics. The organization's culture must promote an atmosphere of expected behavior, attitudes, and values.

Hallmarks of an effective ethics program include the following (Paine, 1994):

- Guiding values and commitments that make sense are clearly communicated.
- Company leaders are personally committed, credible, and willing to take action on the values they espouse.
- Espoused values are integrated into the normal channels of management

decision making and are reflected in the organization's critical activities.

- Company systems and structures support and reinforce the company's values.
- Managers throughout the company have the decision-making skills, knowledge, and competencies needed to make ethically sound decisions on a day-to-day basis.

Success in achieving an environment that promotes ethically responsible behavior requires more than just the creation of a program and the provision of education. Inclusion of the defined values in decision making and demonstration of the expected behaviors will be the measure of a truly successful business ethics program.

CONCLUSION

Interactions with vendors can be extremely positive when developed and maintained with mutually agreed upon goals and objectives that are based on ethical business practices. HIM professionals must educate themselves on these concepts and become comfortable working with vendors as the entire healthcare industry adopts and implements improvements for the information system, such as coding software, tracking systems, and the electronic health record (EHR). These systems will require the collaboration of HIM professionals and vendors in order to solve the complex problems that are presented. Following established RFP protocols can lead to successfully negotiated partnerships. Utilization of the theories and suggestions for the selection and management of vendors can result in successful outcomes. Failure to negotiate ethical contracts that are followed could increase costs and delay the implementation of needed changes in the information system.

Key Terms

- Business ethics
- Negotiation
- Request for proposal (RFP)
- Social responsibility

Chapter Summary

- Interaction with vendors within the HIM profession will increase as more and more facilities implement technology to improve processes. As HIM operations become more sophisticated, the number of opportunities to interact with vendors providing a variety of consulting and outsourcing services will increase.
- HIM professionals are assuming roles as vendors, because the healthcare community realizes the value of their education, knowledge, and experience. However, working as a vendor brings with it a different set of ethical dilemmas and requirements.
- Selection of the best vendor to provide either a product or service is critical, especially if the relationship is going to be long term, as in the case of an outsourcing relationship. Limited funds require that the best possible decision be made and mistakes that the organization cannot afford be avoided.
- The request for proposal (RFP) document provides a template that can be followed to outline requirements for a service, evaluate potential vendors, and ultimately make a logical and fair decision. This tool is widely used in the vendor community and offers a framework to simplify an often difficult and confusing process.
- Negotiation is a skill that must be learned and practiced to ensure success. An understanding of the basic styles and principles of negotiating can be beneficial to the HIM

professional, even if he or she is not the primary communicator with the vendor during the period of the selection process.

- Social responsibility is a concept that can be investigated to differentiate one vendor from another when product offerings are viewed to be equal. Sharing the organization's values and ethics with the vendor is just as important as the product or service requirements. Taking the time up front to determine if there are shared values and ethics can eliminate or reduce future issues.
- Managing the relationship with a vendor is just as important as selecting the best vendor. If the right decision has been made, the incidence of ethical dilemmas will be minimal or nonexistent. Unfortunately, issues will arise as the vendor–organization relationship develops and unanticipated situations are encountered. Excellent communication on both sides will be key to improving and enhancing the relationship.

References

American Health Information Management Association. (2004). *AHIMA code of ethics.* Chicago: Author.

Beauchamp, T. L., & Bowie, N. E. (1993). *Ethical theory and business,* 4th ed. Englewood Cliffs, NJ: Prentice Hall.

Boatright, J. (2003). *Ethics and the conduct of business.* Upper Saddle River, NJ: Pearson Education, Inc.

Carpenter, J. (1998). Writing an effective request for proposal (RFP). Practice Brief. *Journal of AHIMA.* Retrieved January 27, 2004, from http://library.ahima.org/xpedio/groups/public/documents/ahima/pub_bok1_000065.html.

Dawson, R. (1999). *Secrets of power negotiating for salespeople.* Franklin Lakes, NJ: Career Press.

Fisher, R., & Ury, W. (1991). *Getting to yes, negotiating agreement without giving in.* New York: Penguin Books.

Gitomer, J. (2001). Specific characteristics are what make top sales people tops. *American City Business Journals.* Retrieved August 31, 2004, from http://houston.bcentral.com/houston/stories/2001/07/02/smallb2.html.

Hamilton, M. (2003). *TechRepublic Solutions: Tips for submitting winning government RFPs.* Retrieved August 30, 2004, from http://techrepublic.com.com/5102-06329-5068110.html.

Hoffman, W. M., & Frederick, R. E. (Eds). (1995). *Business ethics: Readings and cases in corporate morality.* New York: McGraw-Hill.

Kahle, D. (2001). The ten commandments for the ethical salesperson. Retrieved August 31, 2004, from http://www.davekahle.com/chap16.htm.

Lanser, E. (2002). Managing your vendor relationships. *Healthcare Executive, 17,* 52–53.

Little, M. (2002). Finding and responding to RFPs: Tips for IT consultants. Retrieved August 30, 2004, from http://techrepublic.com/5102-6330-1039248.html.

McDougall, P. (2003). Where's the line? Retrieved August 13, 2004, from http://www.informationweek.com/story/showArticle.jhtml?articleID = 9400016.

Murray, K. (2001). Managing your vendor. Retrieved January 27, 2004, from http://www.nwc.com/1208/1208ws22.html.

Organ, D. (2003). Business ethics 101. *Business Horizons, 46,* 1–2.

Paine, L. (1994). Managing for organizational integrity. *Harvard Business Review on Corporate Ethics,* pp. 85–112. Boston: Harvard Business School Publishing.

Schneider, A. (2002). Shattering negotiation myths: Empirical evidence on the effectiveness of negotiation style, *Harvard Negotiation Law Review, 143(7),* 185–189.

Steinmetz, S., & Dowling, J. (Eds.). (1997). *Random House Webster's College Dictionary.* New York: Random House.

Velasquez, M. G. (2001). *Business ethics: Concepts and cases,* 5th ed. Englewood Cliffs, NJ: Prentice Hall.

Vickers, M. (2002). *The betrayed investor.* Retrieved November 2, 2004, from http://www.businessweek.com/magazine/content/02-08/bs771001.html.

Appendix 23-A Sample Gifts Policy

Policy Subject: Gifts   **Approved by:** President/CEO

Date:

PURPOSE: The purpose of this policy is to guide and direct those serving (name of organization):

- To fulfill their fiduciary responsibilities and exercise stewardship in ways that promote and protect the best interests of (name of organization); and

- To avoid situations that create a conflict, or the appearance of a conflict, between interests of an individual associated with (name of organization).

This policy is intended to supplement but not replace any applicable state laws governing conflicts of interest applicable to nonprofit charitable corporations. It applies to all interested and affected persons, as more specifically defined below, in a position to exercise substantial influence over the affairs of (name of organization) and who have direct or indirect financial interests in (name of organization).

POLICY: Interested and affected persons, as defined herein, shall carry out their respective responsibilities in a manner that serves the best interests of (name of organization) and shall avoid conflicts of interest. To the extent an actual or potential conflict of interest arises, interested and affected persons shall disclose the actual or potential conflict of interest in accordance with the procedures of (name of organization).

Further, interested and affected persons shall not accept gifts, directly or indirectly; entertainment; or other compensation from outside concerns when such acceptance, considered individually or in the aggregate, could influence or appear to influence their decisions or action on behalf of (name of organization).

DEFINITIONS: Interested Persons. Any board member, who has direct or indirect financial interest, as defined below, is an interested person.

Affected Persons. Any (name of organization) executive, department head, management-level employee with hiring and/or contracting authority, employed or contracted physician, purchasing agent/buyer, and any other healthcare professional who has direct or indirect financial interest, as defined below, is an affected person.

Financial Interest. A person has financial interest in (name of organization) if the person has, directly or indirectly, through business, investment, or immediate family:

a. an ownership or investment in any entity with which (name of organization) has a transaction arrangement, except investment in publicly traded securities, or

b. a compensation arrangement with (name of organization) or with any entity or individual with which (name of organization) has a transaction or arrangement, or

c. a potential ownership or investment interest in/or compensation arrangement with, any entity or individual with which (name of organization) is negotiating a transaction or arrangement, except investments in publicly traded securities.

Compensation includes direct and indirect remuneration, as well as gifts or favors that are over $100 in value. Gifts, gratuities, entertainment, and travel provided by any outside individual or entity to an employee or agent who is acting on behalf of (name of organization) shall not exceed $100 annually. In certain circumstances, such items may also be inappropriate even if less than $100 annually (e.g., such items are provided by outside entities that are doing, or are seeking to do, business with or are a competitor of [name of organization] in circumstances where it may be inferred that such action was intended to influence or possibly could influence such individual in the performance of their duties).

The ethical decision-making matrix is a tool to help you organize complex, ethical problems; however, there is no simple fill-in-the-box approach to ethical decision making. The objective is to follow each step of the process and not move from the question directly to what should be done or how to prevent it next time. If you skip steps, you will not fully understand all of the values and options for action. Also, the matrix provided for each scenario in this book is not the only way to examine the problem. You can make an equally compelling ethical argument for a different decision—just be sure to follow all the steps of the matrix.

SCENARIO 23-A: VENDOR REQUEST

Steps	Information	
1. What is the ethical question?	Should the HIM director meet with the vendor, based on the request to the CEO?	
2. What are the facts?	**KNOWN**	**TO BE GATHERED**
	• Transcription system is operating as expected. • There are no plans to change the transcription system. • The competitor wants to provide a quote and meet with the HIM director, who refuses. • Vendor contacts CEO to complain about "unfair business tactics."	• Did the vendor violate principles of integrity and reputation? • What is the vendor's motivation? • Should the HIM director have ignored the vendor? • What is the historical relationship between the HIM director and the vendor, if any? • What is the vendor's reputation?
3. What are the values? Examine the shared and competing values, obligations, and interests of the stakeholders (i.e., patient, HIM professional, healthcare practitioner(s), administrators, society, and other advocates) involved in order to fully understand the complexity of the ethical problem(s).	**HIM professional:** Support the organization's practices and procedures; do not give special deals or show preferences for some vendors; act with integrity for all business relationships; follow appropriate chain of command. **Vendor:** Meet performance standards for establishing new contracts; act with integrity. **Administrators:** Managers follow established policies and procedures when dealing with vendors; desire for most efficient software applications at most reasonable cost; fairness. **Society:** Ethical business practices; reasonable costs to support the information system.	

4. What are my options?	• Meet with vendor, based on the request to the CEO. • Don't give the vendor special privileges.	
5. What should I do?	Don't give the vendor special privileges.	
6. What justifies my choice?	**JUSTIFIED**	**NOT JUSTIFIED**
	• Treat all vendors equally and fairly. • Follow organizational policies and procedures.	• Give some vendors special deals to avoid conflicts with the CEO. • Violate policies and procedures.
7. How can I prevent this ethical problem?	Make sure that all vendors are aware of business plans that clarify procedures for accepting proposals for services.	

The ethical decision-making matrix is a tool to help you organize complex, ethical problems; however, there is no simple fill-in-the-box approach to ethical decision making. The objective is to follow each step of the process and not move from the question directly to what should be done or how to prevent it next time. If you skip steps, you will not fully understand all of the values and options for action. Also, the matrix provided for each scenario in this book is not the only way to examine the problem. You can make an equally compelling ethical argument for a different decision—just be sure to follow all the steps of the matrix.

SCENARIO 23-B: VENDORS AS FRIENDS

Steps	Information	
1. What is the ethical question?	Should Karen or Jane ask to be excluded from the project because of their friendship?	
2. What are the facts?	**KNOWN**	**TO BE GATHERED**
	• Hospital is currently selecting an EHR system. • Jane, the HIM director, is friends with Karen, who used to be the HIM director and who is now working for the vendor submitting a proposal.	• Should one or both of the friends be excluded from the decision-making process? If so, who should be excluded? • Can the vendor use information that is known from Karen's previous employment at the hospital? • Will the vendor violate principles of integrity and reputation if this information is used?
3. What are the values? Examine the shared and competing values, obligations, and interests of the stakeholders (i.e., patient, HIM professional, health-care practitioner(s), administrators, society, and other advocates) involved in order to fully understand the complexity of the ethical problem(s).	**HIM professional:** Support organization's practices and procedures; do not give special deals or show preference for some vendors; act with integrity for all business relationships; follow appropriate chain of command. **Vendor:** Meet performance standards for establishing new contracts; act with integrity. **Administrators:** Managers follow established policies and procedures when dealing with vendors; desire for most efficient software applications at most reasonable cost; fairness; establish boundaries for friendships that exist in a professional environment. **Society:** Ethical business practices.	

4. What are my options?	• Allow both Karen and Jane to stay on the project. • Remove one or both of them from the project.	
5. What should I do?	Allow both Karen and Jane to stay on the project.	
6. What justifies my choice?	**JUSTIFIED**	**NOT JUSTIFIED**
	• Disclose boundaries of relationship and biases/values that could affect decision making. • Build relationships that support the knowledge and experience of both the vendor and the HIM director.	• Assume inappropriate behaviors without justification.
7. How can I prevent this ethical problem?	Facility employees must disclose friendships, prior working relationships, and/or personal relationships with vendors, prior to proposal process.	

The ethical decision-making matrix is a tool to help you organize complex, ethical problems; however, there is no simple fill-in-the-box approach to ethical decision making. The objective is to follow each step of the process and not move from the question directly to what should be done or how to prevent it next time. If you skip steps, you will not fully understand all of the values and options for action. Also, the matrix provided for each scenario in this book is not the only way to examine the problem. You can make an equally compelling ethical argument for a different decision—just be sure to follow all the steps of the matrix.

SCENARIO 23-C: GIFTS

Steps	Information	
1. What is the ethical question?	Should Carol and Mike accept the vendor's offer to visit the corporate office in California prior to making the decision to contract with the vendor for services?	
2. What are the facts?	**KNOWN**	**TO BE GATHERED**
	• Carol is unhappy with current vendor providing ROI services. • RFP has been sent, and one vendor offers a trip to California (weekend for sight-seeing included) for Carol and the ROI manager.	• What are the organization's practices for accepting gifts from vendors? • Is it appropriate to accept this gift? • What are the implications of accepting the gift and not choosing the vendor? • Will the trip/gift influence the decision-making process? • Who will make the decision? • What are the state laws regarding gifts from vendors?
3. What are the values? Examine the shared and competing values, obligations, and interests of the stakeholders (i.e., patient, HIM professional, healthcare practitioner(s), administrators, society, and other advocates) involved in order to fully understand the complexity of the ethical problem(s).	**HIM professional:** Support the organizational practice and procedures; do not give special deals or show preferences for some vendors; act with integrity for all business relationships; follow appropriate chain of command. **Vendor:** Meet performance standards for establishing new contracts; act with integrity. **Administrators:** Managers follow established policies and procedures when dealing with vendors; desire for most efficient software applications at most reasonable cost; fairness; establish boundaries for friendships that exist in a professional environment. **Society:** Ethical business practices.	

4. What are my options?	• Accept the vendor gift. • Do not accept the gift.	
5. What should I do?	Do not accept the gift.	
6. What justifies my choice?	**JUSTIFIED**	**NOT JUSTIFIED**
	Refuse a gift that could influence the decision-making process.	Allow one vendor to offer gifts, especially one that includes some sight-seeing.
7. How can I prevent this ethical problem?	• Establish clear "gifts" policy so that vendors and facility managers are aware of the rules and follow them. • Make sure that one vendor is not given preference over another.	

The ethical decision-making matrix is a tool to help you organize complex, ethical problems; however, there is no simple fill-in-the-box approach to ethical decision making. The objective is to follow each step of the process and not move from the question directly to what should be done or how to prevent it next time. If you skip steps, you will not fully understand all of the values and options for action. Also, the matrix provided for each scenario in this book is not the only way to examine the problem. You can make an equally compelling ethical argument for a different decision—just be sure to follow all the steps of the matrix.

SCENARIO 23-D: PREFERRED VENDORS

Steps	Information	
1. What is the ethical question?	Should Sue decide on a vendor, prior to the completion of the RFP process?	
2. What are the facts?	**KNOWN**	**TO BE GATHERED**
	• An RFP is going to be sent out for a new encoder. • Sue, the HIM director, wants the vendor she used at her last position. • Sue actively solicits support from others making the decision. • Sue's preferred vendor was late in submitting the RFP.	• What are the policies and procedures for dealing with vendors that have a prior history with members of the group deciding on what RFP to accept? • Should members of the group disclose this information? • Is soliciting of a preferred vendor allowed? Under what circumstances? • Should Sue exert influence prior to the review of all RFPs? • Should any proposal be accepted that is submitted past the due date?
3. What are the values? Examine the shared and competing values, obligations, and interests of the stakeholders (i.e., patient, HIM professional, healthcare practitioner(s), administrators, society, and other advocates) involved in order to fully understand the complexity of the ethical problem(s).	**HIM professional:** Support the organizational practice and procedures; do not give special deals or show preferences for some vendors; act with integrity for all business relationships; follow appropriate chain of command. **Vendor:** Meet performance standards for establishing new contracts; act with integrity. **Administrators:** Managers follow established policies and procedures when dealing with vendors; desire for most efficient software applications at most reasonable cost; fairness; establish boundaries for prior business relationships that exist in a professional environment. **Society:** Ethical business practices.	

4. What are my options?	• Sue should be allowed to decide on a vendor outside of the context of the RFP process. • Sue should not be able to decide on a vendor outside of the context of the RFP process.	
5. What should I do?	Do not allow Sue to make the decision about a vendor outside of the context of the RFP process.	
6. What justifies my choice?	**JUSTIFIED**	**NOT JUSTIFIED**
	• All RFP information must be considered confidential and considered in the context of the complete process of submission and evaluation. • Comparative information must be the same for all vendors.	• Some vendors should not be allowed exclusions or be allowed to skip steps in the RFP process. • Favoritism must not be allowed. • Inappropriate influencing of decision making is not appropriate. • Deciding on vendors prior to the RFP process is not appropriate.
7. How can I prevent this ethical problem?	• Establish consistent policies and procedures for RFPs that do not allow special deals with some vendors and that do not allow some decision makers to influence the process based on personal preferences. • Make sure that one vendor is not given preference over another.	

The ethical decision-making matrix is a tool to help you organize complex, ethical problems; however, there is no simple fill-in-the-box approach to ethical decision making. The objective is to follow each step of the process and not move from the question directly to what should be done or how to prevent it next time. If you skip steps, you will not fully understand all of the values and options for action. Also, the matrix provided for each scenario in this book is not the only way to examine the problem. You can make an equally compelling ethical argument for a different decision—just be sure to follow all the steps of the matrix.

SCENARIO 23-E: NEGOTIATING

Steps	Information	
1. What is the ethical question?	Should Steve give vendors information about competitive bids so that they can improve their RFP proposal?	
2. What are the facts?	**KNOWN**	**TO BE GATHERED**
	• Two RFPs have different proposals for software, installation, and training. • Steve meets individually with the vendors and informs them they are higher than the competitor and asks if they can improve their proposal.	• What are the policies and procedures for dealing with vendors, in terms of giving them information about the competition? • Should new proposals be allowed, based on the information?
3. What are the values? Examine the shared and competing values, obligations, and interests of the stakeholders (i.e., patient, HIM professional, healthcare practitioner(s), administrators, society, and other advocates) involved in order to fully understand the complexity of the ethical problem(s).	**HIM professional:** Support the organization's practices and procedures; do not give special deals or show preferences for some vendors; act with integrity for all business relationships; follow appropriate chain of command. **Vendor:** Meet standards when dealing with RFPs; act with integrity. **Administrators:** Managers follow established policies and procedures when dealing with vendors; desire for most efficient software applications at most reasonable cost; fairness; establish boundaries for appropriate business practices. **Society:** Ethical business practices.	

4. What are my options?	• Steve should give vendors information about competitive bids so that they can improve their RFP proposals. • Steve should not give vendors information about competitive bids so that they can improve their RFP proposals.	
5. What should I do?	Steve should not give information to vendors.	
6. What justifies my choice?	**JUSTIFIED**	**NOT JUSTIFIED**
	• All RFP information must be considered confidential and considered in the context of the complete process of submission and evaluation. • Information should not be given about a competitor's RFP. • Comparative information must be the same for all vendors.	• Meeting separately with vendors to give them information that would improve the RFP. • Giving information regarding competitors' proposals.
7. How can I prevent this ethical problem?	• Establish consistent policies and procedures for RFPs. • Make sure that all negotiations are conducted by experienced staff.	

ADVOCACY

Susan Helbig, MA, RHIA

Learning Objectives

After completing this chapter, the reader should be able to:

- Understand the general concept of advocacy and applications for health information management (HIM) practice, including advocacy for patients, peers, staff, and self.
- Identify difficult advocacy situations and reasons why there is tension among the different courses of action that can be taken.
- Consider ways in which personal and professional goals can be attained through advocacy.
- Identify precepts for HIM advocacy.

ABSTRACT

Advocacy is ethics in action—choosing to take a stand for and speak out for the rights or needs of a person, group, organization, or community. Health information management (HIM) professionals have many opportunities to advocate for patients, peers, the staff they supervise, the organization for which they work, themselves, and the larger community and society in which they live. Advocacy involves tensions and risks, but it can also produce benefits both personally and professionally.

Scenario 24-A: Violating the Privacy of a Prominent Citizen

Noreen M., the wife of Jack M., who is a candidate in the city's mayoral election race, is admitted to a hospital during the night. The next morning, a newspaper story contains very specific details about Noreen's condition; some of the details describe sensitive information. Upon reading the newspaper article, Janie, the hospital's health information management (HIM) director, concludes that someone has accessed Noreen's medical record, the hospital's computerized information system, or both.

Questions

1. What is the best course of action for Janie to take?

2. Should Janie consider herself an advocate for Noreen and her health information? What kind of trust was implied when Janie accepted the position of HIM director?

3. What are the causes and effects of actions taken or not taken regarding this patient's sensitive health information, which is now part of a newspaper story?

A completed ethical decision-making matrix for the scenario is provided at the end of the chapter.

ADVOCACY: THE CHOICE OF ETHICS IN ACTION

The word **advocate** is both a noun and a verb derived from the Latin *advocare,* which means "to summon from." As a noun, an *advocate* is someone who pleads the cause of another and defends or maintains a cause or proposal. Synonyms include *champion, proponent,* and *supporter.* As a verb, *to advocate* means "to side with or uphold." Related verbs include *justify, vindicate, advance, forward, and promote* (American Heritage Dictionary, 1996). To advocate for a person or group is to take a stand and speak out for their rights or needs to someone or some entity that can make a difference. Today's HIM professionals have the opportunity to become advocates for patients, peers, the staff they supervise, the organization in which they work, the larger community and society,

and themselves. They have the opportunity and responsibility to do the following:

- Speak out, because they are highly educated, committed HIM experts and because their knowledge and skills are needed wherever patient information is collected, processed, or disseminated.

- Collaborate with peers and colleagues so that their shared values and collective voice become a force for sustaining the principles of professional practice during the current period of rapid changes in information technology (IT).

- Support and encourage their health information staffs that carry out the intellectual, technical, and administrative processes that support and maintain the health information infrastructure.

- Challenge the organizations in which they serve to be proactive in designing and lobbying for public policy that exemplifies their professional standards regarding privacy, security, and confidentiality of individual and collective patient information.

- Volunteer their special expertise within their professional organizations, local communities, and the society at large.

Advocacy is always a choice. HIM professionals will be challenged many times during their professional careers by difficult ethical issues, and they will have a choice as to whether to advocate for a person or a cause. They may have myriad opportunities to advocate not only for individual and collective patients, but also for staff, peers, the organization, the community, and even themselves. Being an effective advocate means choosing to champion the tenets of the HIM code of ethics in a visible, truthful, and intentional posture. It means choosing to educate, empower, and inspire others through one's own behaviors regarding ethical matters. To do this, HIM professionals must be able to communicate ethical **values** and principles regarding health information to others in the workplace and the community and to patients themselves. It means choosing to take a stand to defend a cause that may not always be popular in the workplace. Effective HIM advocates are those who:

- Can deal with issues as they actually are rather than as what they want them to be
- Are courageous when telling the truth about an issue without blame or judgment
- Have compassion, respect, and concern for the character qualities, rights, and dignity of all individuals
- Are responsible for their own experiences and right use of power when dealing with conflicts
- Are clear about their own personal and professional values and clearly communicate them when writing or speaking
- Are committed to ongoing learning not only about professional issues, but also about themselves and their relationship to others and the world
- Make conscious agreements and keep them to the best of their ability

- Comply with all laws, regulations, and standards governing HIM
- Promote and protect the privacy, confidentiality, and security of medical records and health information
- Promote high standards for health information practice

This is not to say that advocacy is always easy to practice. Often it is not. If, however, HIM professionals do not take a stand on those issues and values that are core to HIM practice, who will?

ADVOCATING FOR PATIENTS

Patient advocacy and health information advocacy have been part of healthcare practice ever since the Greek physician Hippocrates formulated a set of guiding principles known as the Hippocratic Oath. In one part of the oath, the physician pledges to refrain from causing hurt or harm and never to divulge information learned either during treatment or from the patient (Privacy Protection Study Commission, 1977).

The patient advocate may be a member of the family who speaks to the head social worker in a skilled nursing facility and asks that the social worker assist her mother in helping her to understand and complete her insurance forms. Or, the advocate may be a member of a group such as an AIDS action committee that is promoting special protection for sensitive information at the state legislative level. Or, the advocate may be a patient representative employee charged with resolving patient complaints. Or, the advocate may be the facility's Privacy Officer who is charged with investigating and acting on information privacy complaints.

The Patient's Bill of Rights

In HIM practice, advocating for patients means speaking up for patient rights regarding such issues as privacy, confidentiality, and security of health records; informed consent;

patient review of health records; and disclosures of information. Often, advocacy for a specific patient ends up highlighting larger issues of organizational practices that affect many patients, resulting in reform on a larger scale.

The creation of a **patient's bill of rights** is an example of general patient advocacy. This document is most often a set of statements that acknowledges the rights of patients during healthcare events. Some organizations include a patient's bill of rights in their documentation. The Joint Commission on the Accreditation of Healthcare Organizations (JCAHO) includes patient rights and organizational ethics as part of its hospital accreditation standards. The overview to this section states that the goal of the patient rights and organization ethics function is to help improve patient outcomes by respecting each patient's rights and conducting business relationships with patients and the public in an ethical manner (JCAHO, 2005). Those organizations that expect to be or are accredited by the JCAHO are required to formulate their own patient rights policies.

The bill of rights for most organizations contains statements that pertain directly to the HIM practice domains just mentioned: privacy, confidentiality, and security of health information; informed consent; review of one's own medical record; and disclosure of information.

Health Information: Individual Patient and Collective Patients Stories

Health information means different things to different people depending on the context in which it is being used or discussed. Original health information—information created during an interaction between a patient and a healthcare professional—has a life cycle of its own and often goes through many permutations before it is filed and complete. Oftentimes, such information is used even beyond the individual's death. How one person's information is handled is a microcosm of how all patient information is handled.

During the course of a lifetime, a person's medical records are created and maintained in many different settings, for example, hospitals, doctors' offices, schools, the military, and so on. Each of these medical records contains health information that describes parts of an individual patient's story as seen through the eyes of different health professionals. The chapters in the stories of an individual patient are unique to that patient; they are personal and private. Hopefully, the patient has trusted his or her doctor, nurse, and other health professionals enough to be honest in telling about his or her pain, concerns, intimate personal and family facts, hopes, and fears. The health professional has listened to the patient, read his or her history, ordered tests, asked colleagues for expert consultation, and pondered this information to come up with diagnoses, plans, reassurances, more questions, and proposed actions so that the patient can become healthier. In response, the patient agrees to undergo surgery, change one's diet, take medication, and so forth. Various healthcare professionals document what they think and what they do. And they name the patient's condition with a diagnosis.

The individual patient's story does not simply reside in a medical record, if indeed it ever did. The story is used for many other valid purposes that the patient may or may not know about. The individual stories are gathered to generate **collective patient stories.**

The collective patient stories ultimately belong to our society, our nation, and our world. These stories are produced by applying coding, indexing, and grouping technologies coupled with computer and human analyses to provide new information and knowledge to improve the health care of the world's citizens. The collective stories are used to identify epidemics, monitor the health/disease continuum of various populations, choose which research to fund, and allocate monetary and staffing resources. The collective stories have improved health care in this country and will continue to do so. The term *collective patient stories* emphasizes that these are stories about groups of people and are not merely *aggregate information,* a phrase that depersonalizes the patient information.

Patients need advocates with respect to protection of their individual and collective stories as long as the record exists. Sometimes it is relatively easy to be a patient information advocate; at other times, it is difficult and challenging and involves choices on the part of the HIM professional. But the stories contained in manual and electronic medical records are the stories of people with problems, people like you and me. We cannot forget this.

In Scenario 24-A, Janie has a choice. She may choose to take a stand to honor and respect Noreen's right to privacy, confidentiality, and security of health information. After all, the hospital includes these rights in its mission statement, and HIM professional values and ethics speak to the need to protect clinical information. Noreen is the wife of a public figure, however, and Janie may wonder if the public has a right to this information. Maybe she should just stay quiet and say nothing. To take no action, however, would mean that Janie would not be honoring her professional ethics.

Janie can decide to search out who caused the violation of Noreen's privacy, even if taking that action may not be appreciated. She can decide to involve others to determine appropriate action in this specific instance and to create a greater consciousness of patient rights for the future. The following continuation of the scenario indicates one possible outcome.

That morning, Janie goes to the IT department and requests an immediate access report listing all persons who have accessed electronic information on the candidate's wife since her admission. She also calls the hospital administrator to alert him to the security and confidentiality breach.

While returning to her office, Janie encounters the chairman of the medical record committee, who asks her if she has seen the aforementioned article in the newspaper that morning. The chairman says that someone who was not on the patient's care team asked him a question that morning that would have required information from the computer system to ask. Janie is able to tell the chairman that she has already requested an access report. The IT department does not, however, immediately release the report to her. When she finally reads it, she finds that 173 people have accessed the patient's information since admission. Not all of the 173 persons had an authorized, valid reason for access. Some are from the HIM department, some are care providers, and some are from administration. As a result of this incident, employees are disciplined, access policies are revised, and clear consequences for unauthorized access are promulgated within that hospital. Janie brings the confidentiality breach to the hospital's ethics committee as an agenda item. Her presentation underscores the need to treat privacy, security, and confidentiality of patient information as a core subject area for this committee and a core competency for all the hospital's employees and clinicians. Summaries of the ethics committee minutes are always sent to the hospital board for review and discussion. The board learns that Mr. and Mrs. M. could have filed a suit against the hospital for this unfortunate incident.

Scenario 24-A illustrates the expanding awareness among HIM professionals of the role that they play as patient advocates. Patients place their trust in the hospital to keep information on their medical problems confidential and secure. It does not matter whether the breach occurs with a public figure or a private citizen. Trust extends to anyone receiving care. It is the responsibility of the HIM professional to consciously and continually expand the awareness of the sacredness of this trust among everyone within the organization where he or she works. It means educating IT professionals about the need for security; making sure human resources understands the gravity of an employee confidentiality statement and the consequences involved in breaking policy; and reviewing all contracts in which individual health information is part of a transaction to ensure that there is intent and language to protect the patient and the healthcare organization and that the contract provides for sanctions if this extended trust is broken. It means being proactive and looking for breaches so that processes can be fixed and people can be educated.

Scenario 24-B: Compassion in Action for an Alcoholic Peer

Steve is an HIM administrative director in a multihospital organization. At a state-level professional meeting, several of Steve's colleagues, including Patty, Connie, Jack, and MaryBeth, observe him drinking three cocktails at lunch; later they see him getting drunk in the hotel bar. When these same colleagues meet for breakfast, Steve becomes a topic of conversation. It soon becomes obvious that the drinking is a pattern that has been noticed for some time. Patty, who works for Steve, makes derisive comments about his drinking while at work. Connie, a recovering alcoholic, asks Patty about his behavior at work. Connie, drawing on her own experience and what she has learned as a lay alcohol counselor, tells the group that there is a high likelihood that Steve has become an alcoholic. Jack says that it's Steve's life and they should let him do what he wants with it. Patty doesn't think Steve would listen to anyone. The questions Connie brings up show that Steve's professional work is suffering.

Questions

1. What are the ethical issues in this situation? What responsibility do Steve's peers have?
2. What course of action might they take?
3. What options do they have?

A completed ethical decision-making matrix for the scenario is provided at the end of the chapter.

ADVOCATING FOR PEERS

Professional organizations are the HIM practitioner's base community of peers and persons who are concerned with the same body of issues. Members of these organizations are joined in a **collective consciousness** because they understand the technical language of their field and because they know their field's challenges, frustrations, and joys and why their expertise is needed (if not always welcomed) in the current healthcare information environment. They thrive, in part, because they have a collective consciousness about who they are and what their purpose and mission are in the healthcare field. But do they stand up for each other in times of great pressure? Do they extend themselves to assist a colleague when it is uncomfortable for them or when a situation reveals too much about themselves? It is time to look at the concept of peer advocacy and to begin to take action when needed.

But what does peer advocacy entail? Peer advocacy means:

- Upholding competent professional practice
- Refraining from damaging the professional reputation of a peer by not taking part in gossip or destructive conversation
- Choosing to intervene on a personal and professional level when observable behavior appears compromised by illness or other impairment
- Choosing to champion a peer for elected professional office by citing accomplishments and qualities
- Being a sounding board for colleagues for difficult or ethical work problems
- Promoting a formal peer intervention process to one's professional organization
- Sharing information with peers and being available to give of one's expertise
- Practicing active compassion by acknowledging colleagues' humanity and professional skills as well as possible impairments
- Telling the truth to a colleague even when it is a difficult thing to do

Several courses of action are possible in Scenario 24-B. One is that Steve's colleagues take no action to address his worsening job performance. If they do nothing, and the organization, unalerted to the problem, also does nothing, the HIM department may deteriorate, and Steve may become increasingly incompetent until he leaves the field and his expertise is no longer available to health information practice. The following continuation of the scenario indicates a different possible outcome.

As the group's discussion continues, MaryBeth says she feels there should be some way to help Steve deal with his obvious problem.

Connie says that Steve won't do anything until he bottoms out. Jack says that the group doesn't have a right to interfere. MaryBeth says Steve is not only hurting himself, but is also placing his staff and organization in jeopardy. She says the group has a right and an obligation to intervene. Connie adds that part of being an alcoholic is thinking that no one else cares. She says that if enough compassionate people could be found who care for Steve, they could actually talk with him as a group and let him know that they care and are concerned. Connie continues and says that there is always the chance that he would hear what they have to say and take steps to help himself. Patty says she would like the group to talk to Steve but that she wants no part of it.

MaryBeth says it is important that only those who are sincerely compassionate and can support Steve be part of the intervention group. Connie agrees and says it will serve no purpose to talk about Steve and this conversation in a negative way outside the group. Connie tries to secure agreement not to gossip and to communicate only to those colleagues who would have compassion to want to assist Steve. An intervention by colleagues is arranged in concert with the organization.

Complex ethical issues are involved in whether it is a right or an obligation for someone to intervene in what seems to be a private matter. Drinking or abusing other substances on the job, however, brings the question of right or obligation into a different arena. HIM professionals have an ethical responsibility to confront an impaired colleague to protect their organization and staff, the public at large, and the HIM profession from potential jeopardy by the actions (or nonactions) of an impaired colleague.

Not taking action may serve an unethical person who may want Steve's job and who is just waiting and hoping for Steve to get fired. Ethical action, however, serves Steve, his peers, the staff, and the organization.

Scenario 24-C: Cockroaches in the HIM Department

Jackie, a new HIM manager, observes that water always seems to appear on the floor in the department's lunch area and that insects make their appearance with regularity. She and Don, the facilities manager, determine that the root cause lies within the physical facility itself. Housekeeping and HIM staff also contribute to the problem. Housekeeping does not clean the area every day, and because of the long-term nature of the problem, the area cannot be adequately cleaned even if it is cleaned every day. The HIM staff is discouraged and exacerbates the problem with poor habits in the lunch area. Don is unwilling to spend unbudgeted resources to correct the problem. Jerry, the housekeeping manager, blames the HIM staff and Don. HIM staff members are too discouraged to do anything except complain. The cockroaches like the status quo.

Questions

1. How might Jackie take action on this problem?

2. What are the ethical issues here?

A completed ethical decision-making matrix for the scenario is provided at the end of the chapter.

ADVOCATING FOR STAFF

The following continuation of Scenario 24-C depicts one possible outcome. Jackie chooses to fight this battle, even though this is a relatively minor battle among the many from which she could choose, most of which have a more direct bearing on actual HIM work processes. In her role as advocate for her staff, she lets her administrator, Rob, know about the problem. She invites her administrator to have lunch with her in the HIM lunch area and suggests to the chairman of the medical record committee that he hold the committee's meetings in the area as well. The cockroaches appear during both of these events. Jackie also talks with Joyce, the employee health nurse, about possible health problems. As a result of Jackie's advocacy, space for a new, separate lunch area is found and constructed, and the new lunchroom remains clean and tidy.

When managers of health information and/or related departments in organizations champion HIM staff needs, the result is a better HIM function. Advocacy in supervision and management includes:

- Finding and maintaining adequate work environments
- Advancing fair market compensation
- Developing humane work processes
- Proposing ongoing education, upgrading of skills, and advancement tracks
- Listening with compassion to employees' personal problems
- Creating an atmosphere where staff are respected and treated with respect both within the organization and by the organization's consumers

Being a staff advocate is not easy in this day of shrinking healthcare resources. As stated in the opening chapter, however, our foremothers believed that courage was a quality needed in the HIM professional.

The ethical issue in this scenario is that staff members deserve and have a right to a clean, healthy work environment. Jackie could have chosen to focus on a coding or record availability issue rather than an employee issue. Her choice was to deal with how an organization treats its employees rather than attempting to placate the employees by using excuses and staying on even terms with the other involved departments. A manager advocating for staff will endeavor to correct problems like this one even though the manager's efforts may cause tension: in this case, tension between Jackie and her administrator, Rob, and between Jackie and other department managers, Don and Jerry.

Such a small thing as creating a clean, bright space for staff members to eat lunch sets up pride and respect for the HIM staff.

Pride and self-respect are the basis for ethical action. HIM staff members who are treated with respect are more likely to treat their tasks, customers, and each other with respect and compassion while getting the work done.

There is a curious phenomenon in the helping professions: People who do good works are not often treated as well as those who work in a purely business sector. This is an attitude that pervades health care as well as other helping professions and that has kept wages and working conditions at a lower standard than that of the marketplace. Although it is perhaps true that doing good works is its own reward, there is no ethical reason to punish people in the helping professions.

Scenario 24-D: Unfair Treatment of Part-time Workers

A busy county hospital with a plethora of outpatient clinics uses a large, ever-changing complement of temporary workers to augment its permanent staff for ongoing departmental work. The definition of "temporary" in this workplace means that workers are not allowed to work more than 1,000 hours per year. They earn no benefits, are not represented by a union, and cannot work in the system again until at least one year has lapsed since their separation from the hospital.

Rick is the manager of the HIM department, which is currently computerizing its manual records system. It is a large, traditional department with 125 full-time employees and includes the usual HIM functions: inpatient, outpatient, emergency department record processing; release of information; tumor registry; coding; analysis; transcription; and birth certificates. Until computerization of the hospital's medical records began, the department had no computers except for one PC in the director's office.

The need to become proficient in the use of computers in general and in the HIM functions specifically has placed a huge stress on the staff. Whereas in the past permanent staff could more or less train temporary staff on a continual basis, it is becoming impossible for permanent staff to learn new skills, train new staff, and still keep the department running smoothly. In fact, the department is not running smoothly. The collective intelligence of the department is suffering because there never seems to be a gain in knowledge and skill due to the constant influx of temporary workers. Permanent staff turnover, however, is very low.

Rick realizes that there is something fundamentally unfair about the treatment of the part-time workers. He analyzes his overall staffing statistics to see if there are other detrimental effects arising from the part-time worker policies. He finds that the department has had 53 temporary workers come through its doors during the last 12 months! He believes the department would function at a higher level if there were far fewer temporary employees performing daily work. He also believes that the ongoing computer learning would go much faster and would be retained better if the department were made up primarily of permanent staff. He realizes it will cost the hospital more money in the short term, but he believes it will be worthwhile in the long run. He also notices in the local newspaper that other temporary county employees are suing the county for what they believe is discrimination about their temporary status.

Questions

1. What are the ethical considerations here?

2. What should Rick do?

A completed ethical decision-making matrix for the scenario is provided at the end of the chapter.

Scenario 24-D raises several ethical considerations. Is it fair that temporary staff are paid less and denied benefits even though they are performing the same work as permanent staff and are required to adhere to the same standards? Is it fair for permanent staff to have an increased training workload and stress while attempting to fulfill their everyday tasks, especially at a time when they are also required to learn new computer skills and cope with rapid change in work processes and increased expectations from their director? The other ethical consideration is that it is possible that laws are being compromised.

Rick can discuss the problem and his beliefs with his supervisor, his human resources representative, and the medical records committee chairman. The following continuation of the scenario indicates a possible outcome.

When Rick brings the situation to the attention of those who could make a differ-

ence, he is initially greeted with mixed reactions. The current practice of hiring temporary workers is not a popular subject with the administration. The human resources recognizes that the current situation may not hold up in court. The medical records committee chairman is horrified that the hospital has temporary employees who do not have health benefits and may fall into the same category of patients that the hospital's mission targets.

A careful analysis by the legal and human resources departments leads to a decision by the hospital's administration to change all but three temporary positions to permanent positions. Thus, Rick's view and the local political climate prevail. When the transition to permanent staff is completed, the improved staff morale increases long-term learning and retention and improves the department's services to its customers. Ethical considerations concerning staff often point the way to improved outcomes as well as improved working conditions.

Scenario 24-E: Small Print on a Consent Form

Rita, the assistant HIM director, is a member of the hospital-wide forms committee. This month, Ann, the risk manager, brings a new general consent form to the committee for approval. The consent form was generated and approved by the risk management committee. Neither Rita nor her director is a member of this committee. Part of the consent form directs patients to authorize disclosure of information to their insurance carrier and for general hospital operations. The portion pertaining to general hospital operations is a list of what patient information will be disclosed for hospital operations. It is printed in much smaller print than the rest of the form and is difficult to read. Rita points this out to the committee and says that it is almost as if the hospital doesn't want patients to know that their information may be used for all these other purposes. She thinks the print should be the same size as the rest of the form. Ann reddens slightly and says that there is so much information that there is not enough room on the form to use the same size print. She also points out that all of the disclosure purposes are posted on the admissions department wall. Brian, the materials manager, seems to agree with Ann, and says that they don't want to pay for printing a two-page form.

Questions

1. What are the ethical issues here?
2. How important is it for Rita to pursue this matter?

A completed ethical decision-making matrix for the scenario is provided at the end of the chapter.

ADVOCATING FOR THE HEALTHCARE ORGANIZATION

Loyalty to the organization in which we practice has long been valued in the HIM profession. It often means raising issues dealing with HIM practice that may not be obvious to other members of the healthcare team at first glance. HIM expertise, after all, is the reason the organization needs HIM professionals. Although emerging technologies often bring new ethical dilemmas to the forefront of HIM practice, it is often more long-standing issues that tax the advocacy strength of HIM practitioners.

In Scenario 24-E, the signed form is a legal contract between the patient and the hospital. In some states, laws specify that contracts be legible and that the typeface be consistent within the body of the form. Patients are often under duress when coming to receive health care and can be in a state of shock. The HIM professional has a responsibility to both the patient and the organization to develop a form (contract) that is readable, understandable, and legal and that promotes the interest of the institution as well as that of the patient. This is a small but potentially very important stand for both ethical and practical reasons. It is unethical to deliberately design forms to obfuscate an issue. The use of such a form may create an unenforceable contract and put the organization at risk for lawsuits and negative publicity.

One possible outcome for Scenario 24-E would be if Rita decides to take on an advocacy role for both the organization and the patients. She might point out that it is the hospital's obligation to communicate clearly to patients and that informed consent needs to be truly informed. If patients signing the form cannot read what they are consenting to, it is not informed consent. Rita can stand her ground and emphasize the patient's right to be respected as a thinking person who can make decisions.

Scenario 24-F: The Data Warehouse Wants to Sell Patient Information

Kristin is both the HIM director and the privacy officer for her hospital. A large data warehouse company has approached the small hospital for which she works with a proposal to store and manage all of the hospital's clinical information using Web-enabled technology. The hospital's medical record system is completely computerized. During negotiations, Kristin discovers that the data warehouse company has another business avenue in which it sells aggregate information derived from the data repositories of its various clients. This is not illegal, because data warehouses are not yet covered under federal or state law. Kristin's hospital, like all others, publicly posts the various uses of its patient information so that patients and possible patients know about it. As Kristin discusses this further with the data warehouse company, she discovers that the company does not have clear criteria for the types of entities that are entitled to buy this information.

The data warehouse company is offering a substantial incentive to Kristin's hospital for every patient information sale it makes. There is no economically feasible way to monitor the security provisions that are written into the potential contract and business associate agreement. The administration believes that staff can be cut by 15% through the use of the data warehouse, an outcome that is attractive to both the administration and the hospital board. Kristin is under pressure to sign off on her part of the contract. At this point in time, the committee believes that the records will be electronically transferred to the vendor six weeks after a patient is discharged as an inpatient and two weeks after a clinic visit. Kristin is a member of the committee that is researching the feasibility of changing the health information operations paradigm. This committee will make a recommendation to the administration as to whether to go forward with the proposal. The committee is led by the chief information officer and also includes the director of IT, the associate medical director for informatics, and the HIM systems project manager. It is a daunting project for all involved.

Questions

1. What are the ethical issues involved in this case?

2. What should Kristin do?

A completed ethical decision-making matrix for the scenario is provided at the end of the chapter.

ADVOCATING FOR THE LARGER COMMUNITY AND SOCIETY

By being active in our profession, we can influence our leaders to take a more public, proactive stand on those issues that most affect society. Considering the inroads that computerization of all personal information is making in the beginning of the twenty-first century, it is even more imperative that we become active advocates for patient privacy.

Situations similar to the one described in Scenario 24-F will test the mettle of HIM practitioners in the coming years. Patient information is being rapidly computerized for storage, transmission, data mining, disclosure, marketing, and other collateral uses beyond the original purpose of patient care.

Furthermore, significant resources are being directed at the emerging Web-enabled medical record. It is easy to see the ethical dilemmas. The laws have not been able to keep up with the changes in technology. And, too often, the resources needed to develop technology to ensure privacy, security, and confidentiality are scarce. The public is only now becoming aware of the gaping holes in computer and Internet security at the system and applications levels.

Technology can create a challenging situation for ethical HIM practice. As HIM professionals, we may be forced to take ethical stands without the full protection of the law. We need to organize individually and collectively within our work environments and within the larger political environment. We need to act as public advocates, educating and influencing our politicians and lawmakers to create laws and sanctions that will truly protect the individual and collective patient stories. We need to communicate to all the various media regarding issues that the public needs to know about.

We need a national forum where we can discuss privacy issues, not only in terms of our professional concerns but also in terms of concerns about our own individual privacy. We, too, are patients and members of the public. Unless we can make patient information privacy, security, and confidentiality a national topic, we will ourselves be increasingly without legal protection when we take ethical stands or we will find ourselves compromising our values and ethics. Appendix 24-A is an example of how an organization can take an advocacy position for society. It is a health information initiative proposed by a state medical record organization at the 1986 national meeting of the American Medical Record Association's House of Delegates.

In Scenario 24-F, one would have to find extraordinary, creative ways of using the company's services while protecting the individual and collective patient stories. This would require collaborating closely with information technologists in the hospital to find technical solutions and engaging the support of the risk manager, the physicians, and other clinicians to develop policies and work processes that would support the privacy and confidentiality of individual patient information.

ADVOCATING FOR ONE'S SELF

To be an advocate for yourself means being clear about your personal and professional values and being willing to share your expertise with others by choosing responsible communication to articulate your values in writing and in speaking. How do you learn to do this? Workshops, books, and articles in HIM journals and other publications are available on personal growth, communication skills, and ethics. Expanding your commitment to continuing self-education will assist you in developing the knowledge and skills to advocate for yourself in situations in which difficult ethical situations may arise. By learning new skills that are grounded in a solid set of values and self-awareness, you can become an articulate advocate for yourself and the values that you hold.

In the process of advocating for other people/patients, staff, the organization, society, you will inevitably gain something yourself. Being active in professional organizations and sharing your HIM expertise in volunteer work in the organizations or in the public arena of politics and the media is a way to advocate for both yourself and the HIM profession.

CONCLUSION

Issues that affect patients, the peers you work with, the staff you supervise, the organization you work for, yourself, and the community and society in which you live are all subject to ethical considerations. Everything from the smallest detail on a form to the overall system that manages the information flow and maintains the privacy, security, and confidentiality of that information can and must be perceived from an ethical perspective. Ethical decisions translate into the opportunity for advocacy. Advocacy is the visible mechanism through which the HIM professional teaches, upholds, defends, and promotes the values and obligations of the HIM field. Choosing to be conscious and aware of ethical issues that arise in health care, staying informed, and informing others is the basic platform for advocacy. Truly, ethical behavior related to the HIM field begins with you.

Key Terms

- Advocacy
- Advocate
- Collective consciousness
- Collective patient stories
- Patient's bill of rights
- Values

Chapter Summary

- Advocacy is the choice one makes to take a stand for and speak out for the rights or needs of a person, group, organization, or community to someone or some entity so that the HIM professional can make a difference.
- HIM professionals have many opportunities to advocate for patients, peers, the staff they supervise, the organization for which they work, themselves, and the larger community and society in which they live.
- Advocating for patients means speaking up for patient rights regarding such issues as privacy, confidentiality, and security of health records; informed consent; patient review of health records; and disclosures of information.
- Advocating for peers involves such actions as intervening personally and professionally when their performance becomes compromised by impairment, promoting a formal peer intervention process, refraining from gossip, and being a sounding board for colleagues with difficult and/or ethical work problems.
- Advocating for staff involves such actions as intervening to improve their working conditions or pay, promoting their ongoing education and skill upgrading, and proposing advancement tracks.
- Advocating for the organization means drawing attention to organizational practices that are unethical or potentially illegal or that work against the organization's interests, reputation, and stated aims.
- Advocating for the larger community and society involves observing what policies are needed on local, state, regional, and national levels and educating the public and promoting public forums on health information issues and legislation.
- Advocating for oneself involves articulating one's personal and professional values and beliefs; it also involves the commitment to the ongoing self-examination that clarifies these values and the ongoing learning that makes communication effective.
- Advocacy can create tensions and risks. But it also can produce many benefits, and gains achieved in one area of advocacy often prove to be gains for other areas as well. Advocacy for organizations or the larger community can achieve gains for patients. Advocacy for staff can achieve gains for the organization and for patients by improving staff morale. Advocacy in any of these areas can achieve gains for the self by honing communication and leadership skills and making work more fulfilling.

References

American Heritage dictionary of the English language. (1996). 3d ed. Boston: Houghton Mifflin.

Arrien, A. (1993). *The four fold way: Walking the paths of the warrior, teacher, healer, and visionary.* New York: HarperCollins Publisher.

Joint Commission on Accreditation of Healthcare Organizations [JCAHO]. (2005). 2006 hospital accreditation standards. Retrieved October 5, 2005, from http://www.jcaho.org/news + room/press + kits/ems/06_hap_accred_stds.pdf.

Privacy Protection Study Commission. (1977). *Personal privacy in an information society.* Washington, DC: U.S. Government Printing Office.

Appendix 24-A Example of Organizational Engagement in Societal Advocacy

Proposed Initiative Presented by the Washington State Medical Record Association at the 1986 National Meeting of the American Medical Record Association, Denver, Colorado

WHEREAS, the citizens of the United States need to know about their rights of privacy and confidentiality concerning their own health care information and the controls or lack of controls over this information, and

WHEREAS, the right to personal privacy may infringe upon the common good of our country, and

WHEREAS, there is a lack of uniform law supporting patients' right to privacy and confidentiality except in drug and alcohol and psychiatric treatment, and

WHEREAS, our increasingly sophisticated computer technology simplifies access to individually identifiable health information, which can be combined with other individual-specific data from census, insurance and credit reports, etc.,

the AMERICAN MEDICAL RECORD ASSOCIATION, as a concerned body of health information specialists, strives to act as a PATIENT INFORMATION ADVOCATE TO:

- EDUCATE THE PUBLIC about their right to privacy and access to private health information by others,
- SUPPORT THE PASSAGE of the UNIFORM HEALTH INFORMATION ACT in all fifty states and territories,
- CREATE THE POSSIBILITY OF PUBLIC FORUMS where citizens, elected officials and others can discuss concerns around the right to privacy and the common good.

We, the Washington State Medical Record Association, believe this initiative is a leading action, which can thrust our profession into the 1990s and provide a service to our country.

Source: Courtesy of Washington State Medical Record Association.

Appendix 24-B Precepts of Effective HIM Advocacy

Health information management (HIM) professionals are committed to the possibility of choosing ethical action whenever issues arise. In choosing to act on an ethical issue, the HIM professional is committed to the following principles:

- Recognizing opportunities and responsibilities to act for
  1. The patient
  2. Peers
  3. Staff
  4. The organization
  5. The larger community and society
  6. The self
- Practicing the values of the HIM founding leaders and finding new applications for those values in today's climate of rapid technological innovation
- Exploring personal and professional beliefs in order to become clear about one's own personal and professional values
- Paying attention to and respecting the importance of one's uncomfortable physical and emotional sensations as potential signals that one is involved in an ethical issue
- Taking responsibility to explore issues in depth
- Respecting and having compassion for the character qualities, rights, and dignity of all persons
- Choosing to use responsible communication to support a cause
- Reaching out to others for support and supporting others when needed
- Collaborating with colleagues to create a collective advocacy voice
- Engaging in lifelong learning with the aim of developing knowledge and skills to master advocacy challenges and sharing those skills with others

The following are questions to ask yourself in preparation for advocacy. Are you willing to:

- Explore your own beliefs and feelings about HIM values in the workplace?
- Learn about responsible communication?
- Identify patterns and reactions in your personal and professional life so that you can make ethical decisions?
- Gather data and identify patterns that support the positions for which you choose to advocate?
- See the correlation between advocating for staff and patients and advocating for yourself as a human being and as an HIM professional?

The ethical decision-making matrix is a tool to help you organize complex, ethical problems; however, there is no simple fill-in-the-box approach to ethical decision making. The objective is to follow each step of the process and not move from the question directly to what should be done or how to prevent it next time. If you skip steps, you will not fully understand all of the values and options for action. Also, the matrix provided for each scenario in this book is not the only way to examine the problem. You can make an equally compelling ethical argument for a different decision—just be sure to follow all the steps of the matrix.

SCENARIO 24-A: VIOLATING THE PRIVACY OF A PROMINENT CITIZEN

Steps	Information	
1. What is the ethical question?	What should Janie do?	
2. What are the facts?	**KNOWN**	**TO BE GATHERED**
	• Noreen was admitted to the hospital during the night. • A story appeared in the paper the next morning that included information that could have come from the hospital's computerized health information system.	• Is the hospital the only possible source of the information? • What are the consequences for the hospital of a security breach? • Could Janie be held liable if she does nothing and the security breach happens again? • What are the customary practices in such cases? • What is the likely impact on self and family of changing jobs?
3. What are the values? Examine the shared and competing values, obligations, and interests of the stakeholders (i.e., patient, HIM professional, healthcare practitioner(s), administrators, society, and other advocates) involved in order to fully understand the complexity of the ethical problem(s).	**Patient:** Entrusts personal information for safeguarding to organization. **HIM professional:** Integrity (preserve confidentiality of medical records and computer information system); avoid harm (patient and/or family could be harmed by information obtained in the security breach); personal values (protect welfare of self and family by avoiding loss of job); tell the truth. **Healthcare professionals:** Value confidentiality of the medical record. **Administrators:** Promote welfare of facility; benefit patients and keep from harm. **Society:** Keep medical records and computer information systems secure.	

4. What are my options?	• Do nothing about the apparent security breach. • Launch an investigation into the apparent security breach. • Determine if national, state, or professional organization or Steve's organization have mechanisms in place to address ethical professional conduct.	
5. What should I do?	Launch an investigation into the security breach, to determine if the hospital is the source of the information.	
6. What justifies my choice?	**JUSTIFIED**	**NOT JUSTIFIED**
	• Obligation to protect confidentiality of the medical record. • Obligation to ensure the security of the computer information system. • Protect professional integrity. • Tell the truth.	• Do nothing about the apparent security breach. • Jeopardize security of the computer information system. • Jeopardize confidentiality of the medical record. • Jeopardize professional integrity.
7. How can I prevent this ethical problem?	• Determine if system changes are needed. • Discuss standards and the values that support them with colleagues. • Out patient advocacy issues. • Evaluate institutional integrity at job interview and subsequently as ethical problems arise.	

The ethical decision-making matrix is a tool to help you organize complex, ethical problems; however, there is no simple fill-in-the-box approach to ethical decision making. The objective is to follow each step of the process and not move from the question directly to what should be done or how to prevent it next time. If you skip steps, you will not fully understand all of the values and options for action. Also, the matrix provided for each scenario in this book is not the only way to examine the problem. You can make an equally compelling ethical argument for a different decision—just be sure to follow all the steps of the matrix.

SCENARIO 24-B: COMPASSION IN ACTION FOR AN ALCOHOLIC PEER

Steps	Information	
1. What is the ethical question?	What should Steve's peers do?	
2. What are the facts?	**KNOWN**	**TO BE GATHERED**
	• Steve is the HIM administrator in a multihospital organization. • Several of Steve's colleagues have seen him drink heavily. • Connie feels that Steve may be an alcoholic. • Steve's professional work is suffering, potentially as a result of his drinking.	• Is Steve's work negatively affected by his drinking? • Does Steve have a drinking problem? • Has anyone ever approached Steve about his problem? • Has anyone ever reported Steve's behavior to his superiors? • What could be the consequences of reporting Steve's behavior to his superiors? • What are the customary practices in such cases? • What is the likely impact on self and family of changing jobs?
3. What are the values? Examine the shared and competing values, obligations, and interests of the stakeholders (i.e., patient, HIM professional, healthcare practitioner(s), administrators, society, and other advocates) involved in order to fully understand the complexity of the ethical problem(s).	**Patient:** Value appropriate health care and medical records. **HIM professional:** Truth and integrity (acknowledge Steve's problems and the damage they could cause to patients and fellow staff); loyalty to employer and to supervisor; avoid harm (allowing Steve to continue this behavior could cause harm to patients, staff, and himself). **Supervisor/Steve:** Perform his job to the best of his ability. **Society:** Protect the HIM system; protect patient care.	

4. What are my options?	• Do nothing and hope that Steve straightens out or is fired. • Report Steve to his superiors. • Approach Steve and discuss concern for his welfare, as well as that of fellow staff and patients.	
5. What should I do?	Approach Steve and discuss his behavior and concerns for his welfare, as well as that of fellow staff and patients.	
6. What justifies my choice?	**JUSTIFIED**	**NOT JUSTIFIED**
	• Obligation to keep patients from harm. • Loyalty to employer/supervisor. • Truth-telling. • Protect professional integrity.	• Do nothing and hope Steve straightens out or is fired. • Do nothing to keep Steve from harm. • Do not protect patients. • Jeopardize professional integrity.
7. How can I prevent this ethical problem?	• Determine if system changes are needed. • Discuss standards and the values that support them with colleagues. • Learn more about issues surrounding peer advocacy.	

The ethical decision-making matrix is a tool to help you organize complex, ethical problems; however, there is no simple fill-in-the-box approach to ethical decision making. The objective is to follow each step of the process and not move from the question directly to what should be done or how to prevent it next time. If you skip steps, you will not fully understand all of the values and options for action. Also, the matrix provided for each scenario in this book is not the only way to examine the problem. You can make an equally compelling ethical argument for a different decision—just be sure to follow all the steps of the matrix.

SCENARIO 24-C: COCKROACHES IN THE HIM DEPARTMENT

Steps	Information	
1. What is the ethical question?	Should Jackie be an advocate for the staff?	
2. What are the facts?	**KNOWN**	**TO BE GATHERED**
	• There is a problem within the physical facility that causes water and bugs to appear in the HIM department's lunch area. • The facilities manager is unwilling to spend unbudgeted resources to fix the problem. • Housekeeping staff do not clean the area every day. • HIM staff have poor habits in the lunch area.	• Would Jackie's intervention be likely to help the situation? • What are the customary practices in such cases? • What are the potential safety and health repercussions of leaving the situation as is? • What is the likely impact on self and family of changing jobs?
3. What are the values? Examine the shared and competing values, obligations, and interests of the stakeholders (i.e., patient, HIM professional, healthcare practitioner(s), administrators, society, and other advocates) involved in order to fully understand the complexity of the ethical problem(s).	**HIM staff:** Want a clean, safe place to eat their lunches. **HIM professional:** Values loyalty and motivation of HIM staff; integrity and avoid harm (obligation to advocate for health and safety of staff); personal values (promote welfare of self and family by avoiding loss/change of job). **Facilities manager:** Values job security; values loyalty, motivation, and welfare of staff.	

4. What are my options?	• Do nothing about the situation. • Take steps to remedy the situation.	
5. What should I do?	Be an advocate for staff and take steps to remedy the situation.	
6. What justifies my choice?	**JUSTIFIED**	**NOT JUSTIFIED**
	• Obligation to protect health and welfare of staff. • Preserve professional integrity. • Demonstrate loyalty to employer and staff.	• Do nothing about the situation. • Ignore health and welfare of staff. • Risk discontentment among staff. • Jeopardize professional integrity.
7. How can I prevent this ethical problem?	• Determine if system changes are needed. • Discuss standards and the values that support them with colleagues. • Learn more about issues surrounding peer conflict and their resolution.	

The ethical decision-making matrix is a tool to help you organize complex, ethical problems; however, there is no simple fill-in-the-box approach to ethical decision making. The objective is to follow each step of the process and not move from the question directly to what should be done or how to prevent it next time. If you skip steps, you will not fully understand all of the values and options for action. Also, the matrix provided for each scenario in this book is not the only way to examine the problem. You can make an equally compelling ethical argument for a different decision—just be sure to follow all the steps of the matrix.

SCENARIO 24-D: UNFAIR TREATMENT OF PART-TIME WORKERS

Steps	Information	
1. What is the ethical question?	What should Rick do?	
2. What are the facts?	**KNOWN**	**TO BE GATHERED**
	• The HIM department has used 53 temporary workers in the last 12 months. • The HIM department is in the process of switching to a computerized record system. • Educating new staff so that they can learn the new computer systems and keeping the department running smoothly are proving difficult for the HIM staff.	• What is the likelihood that the hospital will hire additional permanent staff for the HIM department? • Is the treatment of part-time staff unethical? • Are there organizational policies, state and/or federal laws about the rights of part-time workers? • Are there other ways in which the use of part-time staff negatively impacts the function of the HIM department? • What are the customary practices in such cases? • What does Rick's boss expect him to do? • What is the likely impact on self and family of changing jobs?
3. What are the values? Examine the shared and competing values, obligations, and interests of the stakeholders (i.e., patient, HIM professional, healthcare practitioner(s), administrators, society, and other advocates) involved in order to fully understand the complexity of the ethical problem(s).	**Patient:** Values accurate documentation. **HIM professional:** Integrity, truth, accuracy (operate the department in as efficient and effective a manner as possible); be honest about the problems caused by using so many temporary workers; fairness (follow the rules and obey the law); loyalty to employer; avoid harm (inaccurate documentation could harm patients; trouble with reimbursement and other HIM operations could jeopardize welfare of facility). **Healthcare professionals:** Benefit patients by providing appropriate care; value accurate medical records and welfare of facility. **Administrators:** Benefit patients and keep from harm; maximize HIM department efficiency without compromising accuracy; control budgetary costs. **Society:** Control costs; promote fair and just allocation of resources.	

4. What are my options?	• Try to continue operating the department under current conditions. • Approach administrator about problems running the department under current conditions.	
5. What should I do?	Approach administrator about problems running the department under current conditions. Advocate for staff.	
6. What justifies my choice?	**JUSTIFIED**	**NOT JUSTIFIED**
	• Obligation to tell the truth. • Obligation to protect patient health and accuracy of medical records. • Protect professional integrity. • Demonstrate loyalty to employer, unless asked to push legal and ethical boundaries. • Improve department accuracy and efficiency.	• Try to continue operating the department under current conditions. • Jeopardize patient care and accuracy of medical records. • Treat temporary workers unfairly. • Jeopardize professional integrity. • Jeopardize staff morale.
7. How can I prevent this ethical problem?	• Determine if system changes are needed. • Discuss standards and the values that support them with colleagues. • Learn more about issues surrounding benefits and rights of temporary workers.	

The ethical decision-making matrix is a tool to help you organize complex, ethical problems; however, there is no simple fill-in-the-box approach to ethical decision making. The objective is to follow each step of the process and not move from the question directly to what should be done or how to prevent it next time. If you skip steps, you will not fully understand all of the values and options for action. Also, the matrix provided for each scenario in this book is not the only way to examine the problem. You can make an equally compelling ethical argument for a different decision—just be sure to follow all the steps of the matrix.

SCENARIO 24-E: SMALL PRINT ON A CONSENT FORM

Steps	Information	
1. What is the ethical question?	What should Rita do?	
2. What are the facts?	**KNOWN**	**TO BE GATHERED**
	• The proposed new general consent form includes information in type smaller than that in the rest of the document. • The materials manager and the risk manager do not want the form to run to two pages.	• What is the state law regarding the legibility of and typeface contained in contracts? • What would be the impact of using a two-page form? • What is the potential impact on patients of using the proposed form? • What are the customary practices in such cases? • What does Rita's boss or supervisor expect her to do? • What is the likely impact on self and family of changing jobs?
3. What are the values? Examine the shared and competing values, obligations, and interests of the stakeholders (i.e., patient, HIM professional, healthcare practitioner(s), administrators, society, and other advocates) involved in order to fully understand the complexity of the ethical problem(s).	**Patient:** Has a right to informed consent. **HIM professional:** Truth and integrity (protect patient interest by ensuring legibility of the form); fairness (follow the rules and obey the law); avoid harm (patients could be harmed by signing a form that is not legible; use of the form could put the hospital in jeopardy of litigation); personal values (protect welfare of self and family by avoiding loss of job). **Materials manager:** Protect financial welfare of facility without compromising patient rights. **Society:** Protect informed consent laws.	

4. What are my options?	• Approve the form. • Advocate for patients and hospital and do not approve the form.	
5. What should I do?	Advocate for patients and hospital and do not approve use of the form.	
6. What justifies my choice?	**JUSTIFIED**	**NOT JUSTIFIED**
	• Obligation to protect health and well-being of patients. • Obligation to protect welfare of the hospital. • Preserve professional integrity.	• Approve the form. • Ignore patients' right to informed consent. • Jeopardize welfare of the hospital. • Jeopardize professional integrity.
7. How can I prevent this ethical problem?	• Determine if system changes are needed. • Learn more about issues surrounding patient advocacy. • Discuss standards and the values that support them with colleagues. • Evaluate institutional integrity at job interview and subsequently as ethical problems arise.	

The ethical decision-making matrix is a tool to help you organize complex, ethical problems; however, there is no simple fill-in-the-box approach to ethical decision making. The objective is to follow each step of the process and not move from the question directly to what should be done or how to prevent it next time. If you skip steps, you will not fully understand all of the values and options for action. Also, the matrix provided for each scenario in this book is not the only way to examine the problem. You can make an equally compelling ethical argument for a different decision—just be sure to follow all the steps of the matrix.

SCENARIO 24-F: THE DATA WAREHOUSE WANTS TO SELL PATIENT INFORMATION

Steps	Information	
1. What is the ethical question?	Should Kristin recommend moving forward with the proposal?	
2. What are the facts?	**KNOWN**	**TO BE GATHERED**
	• The data warehouse company has a line of business in which it sells information from its clients' data repositories. • The company does not have clear criteria for the kind of entities that are entitled to buy the information.	• Would the hospital be able to establish a clear set of guidelines for the sale of information from its database? • Could patient interests be harmed by the sale of information from the database? • What are the opinions of the other members of the team? • Could Kristin be held liable if patient confidentiality is violated? • What are the customary practices in such cases? • What does her boss expect her to do? • What is the likely impact on self and family of changing jobs?
3. What are the values? Examine the shared and competing values, obligations, and interests of the stakeholders (i.e., patient, HIM professional, healthcare practitioner(s), administrators, society, and other advocates) involved in order to fully understand the complexity of the ethical problem(s).	**Patient:** Values confidentiality of medical information. **HIM professional:** Truth, integrity (protect patient confidentiality); loyalty to employer; avoid harm (sharing of information could harm patients); personal values (promote welfare of self and family by avoiding loss of job). **Administrators:** Promote welfare of facility. **Society:** Protect confidentiality of medical records.	

4. What are my options?	• Recommend that the hospital move forward with the proposal. • Recommend that the hospital insist that the company institute policies establishing clear criteria for the kind of entities entitled to purchase information.	
5. What should I do?	Recommend that the hospital insist that the company institute policies establishing clear criteria for the kind of entities entitled to purchase information.	
6. What justifies my choice?	**JUSTIFIED**	**NOT JUSTIFIED**
	• Obligation to protect patient confidentiality. • Obligation to protect security of computerized medical record system. • Protect professional integrity.	• Recommend that the hospital move forward with the proposal. • Jeopardize patient confidentiality. • Jeopardize security of the computerized medical system. • Jeopardize professional integrity.
7. How can I prevent this ethical problem?	• Determine if system changes are needed. • Discuss standards and the values that support them with colleagues. • Learn more about confidentiality and security issues surrounding computerized data systems. • Evaluate institutional integrity at job interview and subsequently as ethical problems arise.	

GLOSSARY

Abuse: Incidents or practices of physicians or suppliers of equipment that, although not usually considered fraudulent, are inconsistent with accepted sound medical, business, or fiscal practices.

Adoptee: The term currently used to refer to an individual who has been adopted. The growing sense of openness around adoption has led to the increased use of this term as a designation for self-identification. The history of adoption, which focused on creating families "just like" families created through birth, had little need for this term of identification. Laws referred to "the adopted child," but once adopted children grew up, they were simply considered to be the sons and daughters of the adopting parents. Now, adult adoptees are increasingly using this term to identify themselves.

Adoption: The legal creation of a family in which the rights and responsibilities of one parent or both parents are terminated and those same rights and responsibilities given to another parent or set of parents.

Adoption triad: The three prime participant roles in an adoption: adoptee, birth parents, and adoptive parents. Advocates argue that triad members have a unique relationship to one another that should receive special consideration with regard to sharing of information and access to one another.

Adoptive parent: The adult who becomes the legal parent of an individual (usually a child) who was not born to him or her. The adoptive parent may be a stepparent or relative or may have no prior formal relationship to the parents of the adoptee.

Advocacy: The act of pleading or arguing in favor of something such as a cause, idea, policy; active support.

Advocate: Someone who pleads the cause of another and defends or maintains a cause or proposal. *To advocate* means to side with or uphold.

AHIMA Code of Ethics: A set of values, principles, and professional standards for HIM professionals that addresses obligations to patients and the health care team, the public interest, the employer, the professional association, and the HIM professional him- or herself.

Alert and reminder features: Features of a software system that use information in the EHR to help providers remember important facts, provide information (alerts), and remind them to take action. These systems use "rules" developed by providers that are compared to the information in the EHR to generate reminders and alerts.

Analysis of principles: An approach to ethics based on core ethical principles. Beauchamp and Childress (1994) identified four core ethical principles: respect for autonomy (self-determination); nonmaleficence (not harming); beneficence (promoting good), and justice (fairness).

Analysis of rights: An ethical approach based on consideration of whether an action affirms or violates basic human rights.

Antikickback statute: Statute that makes it illegal to offer, pay, solicit, or receive anything of value for inducing referrals to a federal health care program.

Antireferral statutes: Statutes that prohibit a physician from making referrals for Medicare-covered services to entities with which the referring physician has a financial relationship. Also known as Stark I and II.

Application skills: The set of skills required to apply research, statistical, computer, or information systems theory to actual day-to-day practice.

Appropriateness: The extent to which a particular procedure, treatment, test, or service is clearly indicated, is not excessive, is adequate in quantity, and is provided in the setting best suited to the needs of the patient.

Audit: Retrospective review and analysis of findings.

Audit trail (audit log): Ongoing record of events of accessing patient information. It tends to include the identity of the person accessing the information as well as the time of access, the name of the patient whose records were accessed, the medical record or billing number, and the type of patient data accessed.

Authenticate: Verify or identify access privileges.

Biological father: The term used to describe the man who genetically fathered an adoptee.

Biological mother: The woman who is genetically the mother of an adoptee. This may be a more technically correct term for the *birth mother,* but it has been criticized for being too clinical for the social context.

Biometric authentication: A measurement or observation of a human being for the purpose of uniquely identifying that person.

Biometrics: The combination of access control and human attributes, such as fingerprints or eye retinal patterns; biological characteristics that cannot be stolen, faked, or lost; *see biometric authentication.*

Birth father: Like the term for mothers, this is generally used to identify the father who is biologically the parent of the adoptee.

Birth mother: Currently the favored term for the woman who gave birth to the adoptee. Adoptive parents have advocated for use of this term as more socially sensitive than such terms as either *natural mother* or *real mother,* which might suggest that adoptive parents were not "real" parents or were "unnatural" parents.

Blanket authorization: A one-time form that patients sign consenting to the release of "any and all" information to Medicare or any insurance company.

Business associate (BA): A person or organization, not a member of a covered entity's workforce, that performs functions or activities on behalf of or to a covered entity and involves the use or disclosure of individually identifiable health information.

Business ethics: Business ethics can be defined as the branch of ethics that examines ethical rules and principles within a commercial context; the various moral or ethical problems that can arise in a business setting; and any special duties or obligations that apply to persons who are engaged in commerce.

Case management: A process whereby people with specific health care needs are identified and a plan that efficiently utilizes health care resources is formulated and implemented to achieve optimum patient outcome in the most cost-effective manner.

Certificate of confidentiality: A federal certificate that protects researchers legally from having to disclose information about research participants as a result of a subpoena or court order. It is granted sparingly for projects involving information of a sensitive nature that, if released, could harm participants and can be useful for protecting genetics research data.

Certification: A process whereby a peer group judges the entry-level qualifications on an individual.

Chronic illness: An illness that is persistent over time, that cannot be cured, that usually involves one or more organ systems, that produces symptoms on a regular basis, and that typically worsens progressively, often leading to significant disability and, ultimately, to death.

Clinical data repository: A database designed to aggregate and store patient-specific clinical data that have been captured via other information systems within the health care facility, such as the laboratory, radiology, or medical record systems.

Clinical information system: Computerized systems, also called clinical systems, that have been used for collecting data relevant to the health status of an individual and to health care processes—for example, in order entry, results reporting, or case management. The system(s) included offer technical tools for clinical users. Increasingly, these tools have been linked and integrated to form more comprehensive information systems in the clinical environment. Individually, clinical information systems provide the building blocks for a fully operational EHR system; in their most expansive form, clinical information systems become EHR systems.

Closed adoption: A legal adoption in which identifying information about the adoptive and birth families is not shared. Adoptive and birth families do not know the identities of each other and do not establish or maintain contact over time.

Collaborative decision making: An approach to decision making that brings together all stakeholders in the outcome of a project to contribute their input not only on what they want and why but on how conflicts between different party's wants may be resolved.

Collective intelligence: The sum of the contributions of former HIM professionals and our present-day HIM leaders, thinkers, and practitioners—their knowledge, skills, and values.

Collective patient stories: Aggregate data on patients (such as their DRG and APC classifications) taken from medical records for purposes such as research, public health, funding, and organizational quality improvement.

Common Rule: The regulatory framework for the protection of individuals who participate in research; used by federal agencies that conduct, support, or regulate research. It deals with issues such as the rights of research participants, informed consent, institutional review boards (IRBs), and several other matters.

Communitarianism: A theory that argues that ethical decisions must be based on consideration of social norms, protection of the common good, a fostering of cooperative virtues, and a vision of the "good society."

Compliance guidances: Documents published by the Office of the Inspector General to enable hospitals, home health care, nursing homes, third-party billing companies, and physician practices to establish compliance programs.

Compliance program: A program that is intended to foster the prevention of fraudulent activities in an organization by the development of internal controls.

Comprehensive Alcohol Abuse and Alcoholism Prevention, Treatment and Rehabilitation Act: Legislation that protects the confidentiality of the identity, diagnosis, prognosis, or treatment of any patient for alcohol abuse.

Computer-based patient record (CPR): An electronic patient record that resides in a system specifically designed to support users by providing accessibility to complete and accurate data, alerts, reminders, clinical decision support systems, links to medical knowledge, and other aids.

Confidentiality: The responsibility for limiting disclosure of private matters. It includes the responsibility to use, disclose, or release such information only with the knowledge and consent of the individual.

Consultant: Someone hired to apply special expertise to a situation in order to solve a problem or accomplish a defined objective.

Contract: A codified set of mutual expectations that creates special rights and duties between people and carries the weight of law.

Corporate Integrity Agreement: An agreement between a health care provider and the Office of the Inspector General, imposed in response to provider violations of the False Claims Act, and stipulating that the provider must meet certain government-imposed requirements (such as annual government audits) to ensure ongoing compliance.

Covered entities (CEs): Health plans, health care clearinghouses, and health care providers who perform certain transmissions of health information in electronic form; are required to comply with the HIPAA privacy rule.

Credentialing: A generic term referring to either licensing or certification. A governmental agency, peer group, or credentials committee can evaluate the "credentials" of an individual and delineate privileges to practice within a given institution.

Data integrity: The entire set of characteristics associated with data quality. These include data content, including currency (whether data are up to date or current), relevance to the decision-making purpose, and accuracy (whether data are correct); scope (comprehensiveness); level of detail; composition (issues involved in database structure and the definition of entities and attributes); consistency, including both semantic consistency (consistency in the definitions of data elements, such as "patient number," across entity types, such as "patient" and "encounter") and structural consistency (consistency in the business rules that define the relationships among data elements); and reaction to change, which concerns how data elements are updated, deleted, or added to a database.

Data mart: A small, single-subject data warehouse. The difference between a data warehouse and a data mart is the scope of the problem being addressed. The data mart is generally confined to a department or other business unit within the organization.

Data resource manager: A person who uses technical tools, such as computer-based health record systems, data repositories, and data warehouses, to ensure that the organization's information systems meet the needs of those who provide and manage patient services along the continuum of care and that the organization's data resources are secure, accessible, accurate, and reliable.

Data security: Physical and electronic protection of integrity, availability, and confidentiality of computer-based information and the resources used to enter, store, process, and communicate it. The means to control access and protect information from accidental or intentional disclosure.

Data stewardship: The obligation to protect data integrity and security; *see data integrity*; *see stewardship*.

Data warehouse: A read-only clinical database that is specially designed for ease of data analysis and query processing for decision support.

Database: A collection of related data designed to meet the information needs of its users.

De-identified information: Health information that does not identify an individual and from which there is no reasonable basis to believe the person can be identified.

Deontological theories: Ethical theories that are based on the calculation of duties rather than consequences.

Digital certificate: Electronic credential that establishes one's identity.

Disclose: Access, release, transfer, or otherwise divulge health information to any internal or external user.

Doctor's office quality information technology (DOQ-IT): A project that encourages the adoption and effective use of information technology by physicians' offices to improve quality and safety for Medicare beneficiaries and other Americans by promoting great availability of high quality affordable technology.

Due care: In the ethics of contracts, a special moral duty recognized for the party providing the product or service stipulated in the contract. This duty obligates the seller to take special care to ensure that the customer's interests are not harmed by the products or services offered. Based on the recognition that customers must rely on the greater expertise of the seller about the product being sold, it obliges the seller to deliver a product or service that lives up to the expressed and implied claims about it and to prevent the buyer and others from being injured by that product or service.

Duty to warn: The obligation, mandated by law in many states, to release confidential information on a patient when it is necessary to warn a person who is in imminent danger from that patient.

E-health: The use of the Internet to conduct health-related and health care-related transactions, especially business transactions. E-health includes, but is not limited to, communication between physicians and patients via e-mail, consumers' placement of their personal health records on the Web, health care providers' allowing consumers access to their health records via the Internet, sites that furnish information on diseases and treatment modalities, and the purchase of health-related products and services over the Internet.

EHR Standards: Expectations or requirements for the electronic health record, such as for datasets that have been established by agencies, such as, the Department of Health and Human Services (DHHS), Health Level 7, or the American Society for Testing and Materials (ASTM).

Electronic health information management (e-HIM™): Process by which electronic (digital) health records are created or received and preserved for legal purposes.

Electronic health record (EHR): Any information relating to the past, present, or future physical/mental health or condition of an individual that resides in electronic system(s) used to capture, transmit, receive, store, retrieve, link, and manipulate multimedia data for the primary purpose of providing health care and health-related services.

Electronic medical record (EMR): A patient record within an enterprise-wide electronic system that identifies all patient information, can make all enterprise-wide patient information available to all caregivers, has common workstations to be used by all caregivers, and has a security system to protect patient information.

Enterprise master patient index (EMPI): a merged list all the Master Patient Indexes that make up the Integrated Delivery System.

Epidemiology: The discipline that is concerned with the distribution and determinants of health and disease in populations. Determinants of health encompass behavioral, environmental, biological, and socioeconomic factors that affect the ability of individuals and communities to attain health. The following are examples of each of these types of factors: smoking (behavioral), poor sanitation (environmental), a genetic predisposition to breast cancer (biological), and racism (socioeconomic).

Ethical issue: An issue that involves the core values of practice.

Ethical theory: An organizing structure that helps us identify important language and key concepts in ethics and that provides for systematic reflection and dialogue.

Ethics: The formal process of intentionally and critically analyzing, with respect to clarity and consistency, the basis for one's moral judgments.

Ethics of care: An ethical approach based on what action best supports the relationships of the parties involved.

External disclosure: The release, transfer, or otherwise divulging of confidential information beyond the boundaries of the provider health care organization or other entity that collected the data.

False Claims Act (FCA): A statute that prohibits knowingly presenting false or fraudulent claims to the government.

Federal Drug Abuse Prevention, Treatment, and Rehabilitation Act: Legislation that protects the confidentiality of the identity, diagnosis, prognosis, or treatment of any patient for drug abuse.

Felony-reporting statute: State statutes that dictate the conditions under which a person who knows about a felon-level crime must report it to law enforcement authorities.

Firewall: Hardware or software or a combination of both used to control accesses to or from a protected network.

Fraud: An intentional deception or misrepresentation that an individual knows to be false or does not believe to be true and that he or she nevertheless makes, knowing that the deception could result in some unauthorized benefit to the person who commits the act.

Full disclosure in adoption: A term that is increasingly being used in the practice of adoption. It refers to the gathering and sharing of relevant background information—social, medical, and mental health—with the adopting parents. There are no uniform guidelines for what constitutes full disclosure. However, adoptive parents do bring lawsuits against adoption agencies and others who arrange adoptions for failing to disclose what they consider to be necessary information about the adoptee.

Genetic information: Information about genes, gene products, or inherited characteristics that may derive from the individual or a family member.

Genetic test: The analysis of human DNA, RNA, chromosomes, proteins, or certain metabolites in order to detect disease-related genotypes or mutations. Tests for metabo-lites fall within the definition of genetic tests when an excess or deficiency of the metabolites indicates the presence of a mutation or mutations.

Genetic testing: Performing genetic tests to alert to a heightened risk of some health problems and the need to screen for these risks frequently and thoroughly and to take more preventive measures; concerns about privacy of genetic information, in relationship to genetic research and potential discrimination in employment or insurance.

Guidelines: Systematically developed statements to assist practitioner and patient decisions about appropriate health care for specific clinical circumstances.

Hacker: A person who accesses computers without authorization for malicious purposes.

Health information exchange (HIE): The ability to mobilize clinical information and permit authorized access across multiple providers and locations; seamless exchange of information that enables improvements in quality, safety, and efficiency.

Health information management (HIM) professional: A professional who is responsible for designing and maintaining the system that facilitates the collection, use, and dissemination of health and medical information.

Health Insurance Portability and Accountability Act of 1996 (HIPAA): Statute that establishes national standards for privacy and security of health information. It requires that health care plans, providers, and clearinghouses adopt standards or safeguards to ensure the integrity and confidentiality of health information and protect against threats to the security or integrity of the information and against unauthorized uses of the information.

Health literacy: The capacity to obtain, interpret, and understand basic health information and services and the competence to use such information and services to enhance health.

Health maintenance organization (HMO): Prepaid medical plan that provides and manages health care services to its members for a fixed premium price.

HIPAA Privacy Rule: Establishes guidelines for the application of sophisticated technologies for controlling access to personal health information, including the identification and authentication of individuals authorized to access information and establishing audit trails of those accessing and/or modifying information, and different levels of access (Final Privacy Rule, 2003, http://www.hhs.gov/ocr/hipaa/).

Hospice care: Care that is entirely palliative in intent and that is delivered in a holistic fashion by an interdisciplinary team to relieve the suffering of individuals with terminal illness who have elected to forego further curative or remitting treatments. Hospice care may be provided in a home or institutional setting.

Incidence rate: The rate of development of a disease or health condition in a group over a defined period of time. To calculate an incidence rate, one looks at the number of new cases occurring within a population that is at risk for getting the disease over a specified period of time:

> Incidence rate = No. of new cases of a disease over a specified period of time/ Population at risk

For example, the incidence rate for AIDS cases in Cook County, Illinois, during 1990 was 25.3 cases per 100,000 (IPLAN Data System 2000).

Indemnity (or fee-for-service) insurance: Plan in which physicians, hospitals, and other providers of care are paid for each procedure, medication, piece of equipment, and supply item used in delivering patient care.

Independent contractor (IC): An HIM professional who provides consulting services or traditional HIM services such as data classification and analysis, transcription, release of information, and health record management under contractual arrangements with clients. Unlike HIM employees, who are compensated through a payroll system according to an established wage rate and benefit plan, ICs are paid as an expense under negotiated contract terms.

Independent practice association (IPA): An HMO model in which the HMO contracts with individual physicians and small-group practices to provide care to the HMO enrollees in the individual physician offices. The physicians see their own patients as well as the HMO patients.

Index case: The initial infected individual that started an outbreak. For example, health authorities will investigate college students living on campus to find the index case of a meningitis outbreak.

Individually identifiable health information: Information, including health data, that identifies an individual or is specific enough so that an individual can be identified from it.

Informed consent: Assurance that when individuals give consent to participate in research or to release information, they have explained to them, and clearly understand, their rights as research subjects and the consequences, benefits, and risks that participation or release of information will involve.

Institutional review boards (IRBs): Advisory boards composed of physicians, scientific colleagues, ethicists, and concerned nonscientists (frequently administrators and private citizens) that have been set up by federal legislation to oversee research on human subjects and to ensure protection of those subjects from research abuses.

Integrated delivery system (IDS): Multiple health care facilities, such as, hospitals, outpatient clinics, rehabilitation facilities, hospice or other health care facilities, which coordinate patient services.

Integrity: Data quality; *see data integrity.*

Intrapreneur: An internal entrepreneur: someone who is working as an employee in a traditional organization but is focused on creating innovative products, services, and work methods. Intrapreneurs often work independently or in loosely organized teams and are involved in rethinking current products, services, and organizational structures.

Legal father: This term refers to the man who is considered by law to be the father of a child, even though not the biological father. The specific definition for this varies by state but is frequently the man married to the birth mother at the time of the adoptee's birth or for some period of time prior to the birth. In some jurisdictions, the legal father is named, or has been named automatically, as the father of the adoptee. His rights need to be terminated for an adoption to proceed.

License: A permit usually provided by a government agency, either federal or state, to practice a specific aspect of patient care.

Licensure: The process by which an agency of government grants permission to persons meeting predetermined qualifications to engage in a given occupation and/or use a particular title.

Managed care: A system that (1) integrates health care delivery and health insurance; (2) features network-based arrangements with physicians, hospitals, and other health care professionals; (3) provides a defined set of health care services to enrollees; (4) has criteria and a process for selecting and monitoring health care providers; (5) has systems to gather, monitor, and measure data on health service utilization, physician referral patterns, and other quality and performance measures; (6) has incentives or requirements for members to use providers and procedures associated with the plan; (7) has incentives for providers to encourage the appropriate use of resources; and (8) has activities aimed at improving the health status of members.

Master patient index (MPI): A master list of all the facility's (or IDS's) patients, along with demographic information such as gender, date of birth, social security number, medical record number or other patient ID, address, race and ethnicity, admission and discharge dates, encounter types, and disposition (i.e., intended care setting following discharge). Some optional additional elements are emergency contacts, allergies/reactions, and problem lists.

Minimum necessary: A requirement of the HIPAA privacy rule whereby a covered entity is required to limit the use, disclosure, and request for PHI to the amount needed to accomplish the intended purpose of the use, disclosure, or request.

Moral awareness: Is a concept used to refer to the individual's ability to recognize a situation as having a moral implication. Organizations that allow managers to freely question policies and discuss areas of tension are better prepared to raise the moral awareness of their employees and managers.

Moral muteness: The manager's inability to discuss situations in terms of morality; some managers have an amoral philosophy except when situations have high moral intensity, such as fraud and abuse.

Natural father: Similar to the term *natural mother,* but specifically referring to the biological father.

Natural mother: This is an older term used to describe the "birth" or "biological" mother. Adoptive parents objected to the term on the grounds that it implied that the adoptive mother was "unnatural."

Negotiation: The process of bargaining with another individual, is definitely as much an art as a skill.

Notice of Privacy Practices: A document that covered entities must provide to individuals, notifying them of the uses and disclosures of protected health information that the covered entity may make; the individual's rights; and the covered entity's legal duties relating to protected health information.

Obligatory actions: Actions that are expected or demanded by ordinary moral standards. Obligatory actions must be determined in reference to the norms of an appropriate group; thus, HIM professionals are held to a higher minimum standard of conduct than the layperson when it comes to protecting the accuracy and privacy of medical information.

Office of the National Coordinator for Health Information Technology (ONCHIT): Organized in the Department of Health and Human Services (DHHS) to provide leadership for the development and nationwide implementation of an interoperable health information technology infrastructure to improve the quality and efficiency of health care and the ability of consumers to manage their care and safety.

Open adoption: An adoption in which there is some degree of relationship between the adoptive parents and the birth parents. This may or may not be legally sanctioned or legally binding, but it refers to adoptions where the individuals involved know each other and may maintain some relationship over time. The degree of "openness" varies greatly from one situation to another.

Outcome: The expected, desired, or actual result of health care services.

Palliative care: Care that focuses on the relief of the physical, psychological, emotional, and spiritual discomfort that accompanies illness. Palliative care may be provided in any setting and is not limited to individuals with terminal illness.

Patient safety: The protection of health care recipients from being harmed by the effects of health care services.

Patient's bill of rights: A set of statements that acknowledges the rights of patients during health care events.

Peer review: Evaluation or review of the performance of colleagues by professionals with similar types and degrees of expertise (e.g., the evaluation of one physician's practice by another physician or of one nurse's practice by another nurse).

Per diem: Payment method by which the provider (usually a hospital) is paid for each day a patient is in the facility regardless of the amount of services rendered.

Per member/per month (PM/PM): Defined payment to a provider for each patient for each month, whether the provider provides services to the patient or not.

Performance measurement: Regular collection and reporting of data to track work produced and results achieved; refers to the process of data collection and reporting, not to the individual measures that data are gathered for.

Point of service (POS): Usually an addition to an HMO product. It allows the member to go outside the HMO for services, but at a copay that varies in size with the level of benefit sought. The copay can be substantial.

Preferred provider organization (PPO): Networks of physicians, hospitals, and other health care providers that provide for services under a negotiated fee. PPOs do not bear risk for those to whom they render service. The risk is borne by the insurance company that sponsors the product, by the self-insured employer, or by the third-party administrator. PPOs usually contract for services such as quality assurance and utilization management.

Prevalence: The number of existing cases of a disease or health condition in a defined population at a specific point (or specific duration) in time. To calculate the prevalence rate of a disease one divides the number of persons with the disease by the total population of the defined group.

Prevalence rate = No. of existing cases of a disease at a point (or period) in time/Total population

For example, between 1988 and 1991, 21.9 million women in the United States 18 years of age or older were hypertensive, or 22 percent of that population (Burt et al. 1995).

Prima facie argument: An argument or principle that is presumed to be true unless there is sufficient argument or evidence offered to rebut the presumption. As used in this book, the term implies that an ethical principle is sound and rational, but is not irrefutable and may be controverted with persuasive argument to the contrary.

Privacy: The right of an individual to be let alone. It includes freedom from intrusion or observation into one's private affairs and the right to maintain control over certain personal and health information.

Profession: An occupation that requires its members to undergo extensive and specific education to master a complex body of knowledge and to have the ability to apply that knowledge; that makes a valued contribution to society through its services; that allows its members a significant degree of autonomy in making decisions and exercising judgment; and that is regulated by a set of behavioral standards commonly called a code of ethics or conduct.

Project management: The coordination of activities, tools, and techniques needed to assure that a project can be completed to meet timeline, budgetary, and quality standards requirements.

Protected health information (PHI): Individually identifiable health information held or transmitted by a covered entity that relates to an individual's past, present, or future physical or mental health care, condition, or payment for services; confidential information that is private and to which access is restricted; federal and state statutes and regulations that protect information, including the patient's personal health information that is collected within health care facilities.

Public interest and benefit activities: Twelve situations, provided by HIPAA, whereby a covered entity may disclose protected health information without an individual's authorization.

Putative or presumptive father: These and similar terms such as *alleged father* refer to the man who is possibly the biological father of a child. He may be named by the mother as the father but not be the legal parent. The terms also identify that he is not confirmed to be the father, and paternity may be confirmed by DNA testing of more than one presumptive father. The man who is presumed to be the father; recent advances in DNA testing have made it possible to identify the biological father but the social and legal issues remain.

Quality: The degree to which a product or service meets requirements and expectations.

Quality improvement: A system in which individuals in the organization look for ways to do things better, usually based on understanding and control of variation. Sometimes referred to as continuous performance improvement.

Quality management (QM): A system by which a health care organization measures, assesses, and improves the quality of health care services. Sometimes referred to as *quality program*, *performance improvement program*, or *performance management program*.

***Qui tam* statutes:** "Whistle-blower" statutes that permit private individuals to bring lawsuits under the False Claims Act, alleging individual's or organizations' fraudulent behavior against the government.

Rationalization: Occurs when the employee seeks to justify the reason for unethical behaviors.

Regional health information organizations (RHIOs): A framework for strategic action to achieve nationwide linkage of health care information systems that will allow patients, physicians, hospitals, public health agencies and other authorized users to share clinical information in real-time under stringent security and privacy protections.

Reportable diseases and conditions: Diseases for which regular, frequent, and timely information on individual cases is considered necessary for the prevention and control of that disease; such as, tuberculosis or syphilis; sometimes referred to as notifiable diseases.

Request for proposal (RFP): Document that provides a template that can be followed to outline requirements for a service, evaluate potential vendors, and ultimately make a logical and fair decision; tool is widely used in the vendor community and offers a framework to simplify an often difficult and confusing process.

Requests: Protected health information asked for by a covered entity.

Resource management: Planning, organizing, directing, and controlling of the health care product in a cost-effective manner while maintaining quality of patient care and contributing to the overall goals of the organization.

Risk analysis: Identifies the risks, vulnerabilities, and threats to the organization's assets, including information systems, applications, physical plant, and equipment.

Risk management: The investigation and analysis of the frequency of causes of adverse incidents that injure patients, visitors, and staff and the development of measures to minimize risk and redesign systems to protect the financial assets of the organization against the consequences and the costs of risks.

Robust computer systems: Systems that prove trustworthy under varying circumstances.

Safe harbors: Categories that have been defined by the Department of Health and Human Services for practices that technically violate either the antireferral or the antikickback statutes but have been exempted from penalty because they are unlikely to bring harm to the federal health care programs.

SAS: The SAS System, a product of the SAS Insitute, is an integrated suite of software for enterprise-wide information delivery built around the four data-driven tasks common to virtually any application—data access, data management, data analysis, and data presentation. Applications of the SAS System include executive information systems; data entry, retrieval, and management; report writing and graphics; statistical and mathematical analysis; business planning, forecasting, and decision support; operations research and project management; statistical quality improvement; computer performance evaluation; and applications development.

Scope of practice: In the health professions, the professional activities that a health professional is authorized to perform under the laws of the state in which the health professional is licensed.

Security: *See data security.*

Security audits: The systematic review of an organization's information systems activity vulnerabilities and threats; *see threat*; *see vulnerability*.

Serious illness: An illness with the potential to significantly impair a person's functioning, lead to terminal illness, or cause death. Many serious illnesses can be cured, such as appendicitis. Others, such as myocardial infarction, can be treated so as to not lead to terminal illness or to cause death.

Smart card: Credit-type card embedded with a computer chip that stores information and incorporates security features. Smart cards are used in ATMs and pay phones and may be used at computer workstations to obtain IT-based services.

Social responsibility: A concept that can be investigated to differentiate one vendor from another when product offerings are viewed to be equal; sharing the organization's values and ethics with the vendor is just as important as the product or service requirements; shared values and ethics can eliminate or reduce future issues.

Socialization: Is a process in which employees learn the norms and acceptable behaviors of the group. The process of socialization is very powerful because it has an impact on the employee as an individual and exists long after the employee leaves the organization.

Software development life cycle: A process with four stages—planning, selection, implementation, and maintenance.

SPSS (Statistical Package for the Social Sciences): Data management and analysis software produced by SPSS, Inc. that can perform a variety of data analysis and presentation functions, including statistical analyses and graphical.

Stakeholder: Someone who will be affected by the decision to be made; any entity that has a genuine interest in the pursuit or outcome of a specific goal, regardless of the role or relationship to the enterprise.

Standards of Ethical Coding: A code of conduct developed by the American Health Information Management Association to provide a basis for ethical decision making in coding practice.

Stark I and II: See *antireferral statutes.*

Stewardship: Custodial responsibilities for ensuring data quality and security.

Supererogatory actions: Actions that are optional in terms of the moral minimum but are morally meritorious and praiseworthy: that is, actions that exceed what is expected or demanded by common morality. Such actions are often thought of as the moral ideal.

Surveillance: The systematic collection of data pertaining to the occurrence of specific diseases and health events, the analysis and interpretation of these data, and the dissemination of the results within government, to the public, and to other interested parties.

Telehealth: Use of electronic information and telecommunications technologies to support long-distance clinical health care, patient and professional health-related education, and public health and health administration.

Telemedicine: The use of medical information, whether in textual data, text, sound, still video, or motion video, exchanged from one site to another via electronic communications for the care and education of the patient or health care provider and for the purpose of improving patient care. Telemedicine includes the examination and treatment of patients through the participation of a consultant at a distant location. It is increasingly available in locations where health services may be limited.

Terminal illness: An illness that limits life expectancy. Many ethical dilemmas arise over the use of this term; for instance, when should a chronic illness be considered terminal and when is treatment futile?

Threat: A material, environmental or human factor which can be taken advantage of or takes advantage to harm the information system, such as, a staff member (threat) whose the access privileges were not terminated at the time she resigned (vulnerability).

Treatment, payment, and operations (TPO): Functions performed by a covered entity for which certain HIPAA privacy rule requirements are removed or relaxed.

Unbundling: Billing separately for each component of a procedure instead of using the proper code for the entire procedure because fees for the separate procedures result in a higher reimbursement.

Upcoding: Billing for a higher level of service than rendered in order to receive a higher reimbursement.

Use and disclosure: Two mechanisms, limited by the HIPAA privacy rule, by which protected health information may be handled. *Use* refers to the legitimacy and degree of access by those within a covered entity. *Disclosure* refers to the release of protected health information to a recipient external to the covered entity.

Utilitarianism: A theory that argues that ethical decisions must be based on a criterion of efficiency and consideration for what is good for the greatest number. The theory assumes that for most decisions the aggregate result of individuals acting in their own best interest will usually result in "the greatest good for the greatest number." The theory is focused on individual rights and liberties rather than interests that are enjoyed and shared at the community level.

Value: A principle, standard, or quality considered worthwhile or desirable.

Virtue-based ethics: An ethical approach that emphasizes how the action expresses and shapes the character of the person who performs it.

Vision 2006: A description of emerging roles for HIM professionals, set forth by AHIMA (1999).

Visual integration tools: New tools being developed for accessing, extracting, and integrating patient-specific information from disparate clinical information systems and presenting it visually to the user.

Voluntary disclosure protocol: A procedure that providers may follow to self-disclose claims presented to the government that are found to be mistaken or fraudulent.

Vulnerability: Any gap in policies and procedures or in technical and physical safeguards.

Wrongful adoption: A term being applied to adoptions in which the terms of the adoption are challenged due to the misrepresentation or withholding of crucial facts. In most cases, the adoptive parents bring suit against an adoption agency or the individual who arranged an adoption. The most common charges are that important medical or mental health history was kept from the adopting parents so that they now have a child with problems when they expected to have a healthy child.

INDEX

A

Absenteeism, 500, 510–511, 518–519
Abuse
  definition, 70, 101
  health information technology and, 410
  PHI disclosure issues, 367
Academy of Distinguished Entrepreneurs, 533
Access. *See also* E-health
  to data, 183, 186–187, 285
  EHR systems and, 292
  health information technology and, 410
  to healthcare documentation, 7–8
  HEDIS and, 238
  to the Internet, 390–391
  linking EHR systems and, 296–297
  managed care and, 237
  by MCOs, 241–243
  to patient records, 54, 243–244
  to protected information, 57–59
  security and, 364
Accuracy, of data, 11–12
Action plans, business ethics, 111–112
Administration, 116–118. *See also* Hospital
  administration; Management
Admissions, verification of, 465, 473–475,
  488–489
Adoptees, 442, 458–459
Adoption
  definition, 442
  historical issues, 442–443
  information relating to, 439–461
  terminology of, 445–446
  trends in, 444–445
Adoption triad, 442
Adoptive parents, 442, 447–451
Advance Beneficiary Notice, 108
Advance care planning, 262–267, 272–273
Advancement of Telehealth (OAT), 406
Adverse Pregnancy Outcomes Reporting System
  (APORS), 201

Advertising, ethical, 537–538
Advocacy
  for change, 13
  choice of, 597
  defined, 596–597
  effective, 611
  ethical issues, 595–623
  for healthcare organizations, 605
  for patients, 620–621
  for peers, 614–615
  resources for, 220–221
  role of HIM professionals, 219–223
  for self, 607
  societal, 606–607, 610
  for staff, 603–604, 616–619
Age/aging, information issues, 258–259
Agency for Healthcare Research and Quality
  (AHRQ), 406, 407
Aggregate information, 599
AHIMA (American Health Information
  Management Association), 145
  on advocacy, 219
  Codes of Ethics, 10–15, 23–24, 25–32, 218
  e-health phenomenon and, 384
  on electronic health information management
    (eHIM™), 404, 405
  ethics survey, 148
  HIM professionals and, 14–15
  HL7 standards and, 285
  Mission Statement, 23
  national conference scenario, 507–508
  on patient privacy, 56
  Policy and Government Regulations, 220–221
  Recommendations to Ensure Privacy and
    Quality of Personal Health Information on
    the Internet, 393
  Standards of Ethical Coding, 103
  support for HIPAA, 61
  survey, 150
  Vision initiative, 177

Aid to Families with Dependent Children (AFDC), 501
Alcohol abuse, 463–495, 600, 614–615
Alert features, EHR systems, 283
Alignment, MCOs, 246
Alleged fathers, 446
Alliance to End Discrimination, 200, 211
Alternative and complementary medicine, 388
American Academy of Pediatrics, 313
American Association of Medical Librarians (AAMRL), 9–10
American College of Pathologists (CAP), 407
American College of Surgeons, 9
American Hospital Association (AHA), 71, 105
American Medical Association (AMA)
    Council on Ethical and Judicial Affairs, 425
    CPT Assistant, 105, 113
    CPT codes and, 104
    on encryption of messages, 316–317
    on pain management, 265
American Medical Record Association, 20–21, 22, 609, 610
American Society for Healthcare Risk Management (ASHRM), 145
American Society for Quality (ASQ), 145, 151
American Society for Testing and Materials (ASTM), 310, 333
Analogy, arguments from, 42
Analysis of principles, 40
Analysis of rights, 40
Antikickback statutes, 75
Antireferral statutes, 75–76
Archives, EHRs and, 282
Arrest warrants, 464, 480–481
Artificial insemination, 452
Association of Record Librarians of North America, 9
Attorneys, communications with, 471. See also Legal counsel
Audit logs, 315–316
Audit trails, 315–316
Audits
    by case managers, 245–246
    coding accuracy studies, 108
    EHRs and, 298–300
    ethical dilemmas, 5
    outcomes, 149, 170–173
    processes for, 80
    providing information to, 58
    violations, 13–14
Authenticity, security and, 311
Authority, of HIM position, 13

Authorizations
    blanket, 59–60, 108
    elements of, 190
    legibility of, 605
    from patients, 56–57
    for public interest and benefit activities, 466–467
    umbrella releases, 390
    written, 189–190
Autonomy
    cultural influences, 259
    ethical principle of, 211
    evolution of, 259
    informed consent and, 242
    respect for, 40, 241, 447
    treatment choices and, 261
Availability, security and, 311

B
Babson College, 533
Bad news, scenario, 268
Behavioral health information
    admissions, 473–475
    confessions of crimes, 471–472
    ethical challenges in treatment of, 465–478
    protection of, 468
Behavioral information, 463–495
Behavioral Risk Factor Surveillance System (BRFSS), 210
Beneficence, 189
    ethical principle of, 212–214, 218
    respect for, 40
    treatment goals and, 261–263
Beneficiary Incentive Program, 78
Benefit activities, disclosure standards, 78
Benefit design, managed care, 236
Benefits, utility and, 213–214
Bentham, Jeremy, 38
Biases, exposing, 42
Billing activities
    coding choices and, 104
    coding on abstracts, 106
    EHR systems and, 288
    ethical coding, 108
    health information technology and, 410
    HIPAA and, 101–102
    patient protection and, 151
Bioethicist's toolbox, 41–42
Biological fathers, 446, 453
Biological mothers, 446
Biometrics, 315
Bioterrorism, 221–223

Birth fathers, 446
Birth mothers, 446, 450–451, 460–461
Black's Law Dictionary, 71
Blanket authorizations, 59–60, 108
Bonus arrangements, 246
Bracketing, defined, 578
Brailer, David, 384
Brigham and Women's Hospital—Partners
    Healthcare, 285
Brown, June Gibbs, 74
Bureau of the Census, U. S., 210
Business associates (BAs)
    agreements, 50, 292
    disclosure to, 58–59
    PHI disclosure issues, 368
Business ethics, 111–112, 535–540, 539–540,
    571–572. *See also specific issues*
Business Horizons, 569

C

Capitation, 236, 246
Care Management Performance pilot program,
    410
Career management, 534–353
Caregivers
    e-health technology and, 381–401
    PHI disclosure issues, 368
Carpal tunnel syndrome, 425
Case management, 236, 245–246
Center for Health Workforce Studies, 177
Centers for Disease Control and Prevention
    (CDC), 208, 475
Centers for Medicare and Medicaid Services
    (CMS), 389
    reporting fraud to, 101
    resources, 220
    on systems interoperability, 406
Central-line infections, 143–144, 158–165
Certificates of confidentiality, 432–433
Certification, 103–104, 151
Certification Commission for Healthcare
    Information Technology (CCHIT), 408
Certified Coding Associates (CCAs), 103
Certified Coding Specialists (CCS), 103
Certified Coding—Physician based (CCS-P), 103
Chadwick, Edwin, 202
Chain-of-trust concept, 78
Changes
    advocacy for, 13
    environmental, 533
    in organizational cultures, 16, 17
Channeling, defined, 236

Chief Compliance Officers (CCOs), 80
Chief Executive Officers (CEOs), 147–148
Chief Financial Officers (CFOs), 94–95, 332
Chiefs of Staff, 331–332
Child custody cases, 429
Children's protective services (CPS), 477,
    494–495
Chronic Care Improvement Program, 389
Chronic illnesses
    provision of care in, 259
    treatment goals and, 261
Clergy, disclosure issues, 368
Clients
    expectations of, 550–551, 562–563
    relationships with, 552–554
Clinical care process, 291
Clinical data repository (CDR), 343, 349–350,
    358–359
Clinical decision support systems (CDSSs), 309,
    403
Clinical information systems, 281, 376–377
Clinical judgments, 12
Clinical Laboratory Improvement Amendments of
    1988 (CLIA), 428
Clinical validity, defined, 428
Clinton, William, 189, 430
Closed adoptions, 442
Coalition for Responsible Reporting, 200,
    212–213, 213
Cockroach scenario, 602–603, 616–617
Coders, pressures on, 100
Codes, billing edits and, 104
Codes of Conduct
    for health websites, 397–398
    HIM professional, 9–10
Codes of Ethics
    AHIMA, 10–15, 23–24, 25–32
    American Medical Record Association, 20–21,
        22
    for health websites, 397–398
    inconsistencies in, 146–147
    limitations of, 511
    practice of Medical Record Science, 19
    professional, 3–32
    professional associations, 145
Coding. *See also* Miscoding
    accuracy studies, 108
    AHIMA standards applied to, 104–109
    complications, 105
    deontological approach to, 103
    ethical approaches, 102–104
    ethical dilemmas, 97–137

Coding—*continued*
　future of, 122
　guidelines, 120–121
　health information technology and, 410
　inappropriate employer instructions, 134–135
　incomplete documentation and, 94–95
　integrity of, 71, 106–107
　level of service and, 98
　physician suggested, 104
　reimbursement and, 8
　specificity, 120–121
　of symptoms, 105
　turnaround times, 84
　upcoding patterns, 78
　Coding Clinic for ICD-9-CM, 71, 105, 113
Coding compliance plans, 120
Coding procedures, 80
Cognitive function, 263
Collaboration
　consultants and, 545–546
　ethical decision-making and, 16
　interdisciplinary, 12
Collective consciousness, 600
Collective patient stories, 598–599
Commission on Accreditation for Health
　　Informatics and Information Management
　　Education (CAHIM), 151
Committees, protection of, 12
Common Rule, 432
Communication skills, 194, 385
Communitarianism, 215–216
Communities, advocacy for, 606–607
Community health information networks (CHINs),
　409
Community health management information
　　systems (CHMIS), 409
Comorbid conditions, 106
Compensation, levels of, 13
Competence, issues of, 237. *See also* Certification;
　Credentialing
Competitive analysis, 186
Complaints, 61, 80
Compliance committees, 80
Compliance guidance documents, 79
Compliance officers, 43
Compliance programs, 79–81
Complications
　codes for, 105
　postoperative, 107
　retrospective documentation, 106
Comprehensive Alcohol Abuse and Alcoholism
　　Act, 464

Comprehensiveness of data, 368
Compromises, negotiation of, 42
Computer-Based Patient Record Institute (CPRI),
　287
Computer-based patient records, 344–345
Computerized physician order entry (CPOE), 239
Computers, privacy and, 288
Confidentiality
　agreements, 296
　AHIMA Code on, 11
　certificates of, 432–433
　consumer concerns about, 308
　contractors and, 552–553, 564–565
　of data, 182
　definition, 53, 427
　duty and, 220
　"duty to warn" and, 470
　EHR systems and, 285–286, 287, 293
　ethical dilemmas, 4, 5
　health information technology and, 410
　information systems and, 246–247
　linking EHR systems and, 298
　privacy and, 51–65
　research and, 191
　security and, 311
　substance abuse and, 464–465
*Confidentiality, Privacy, Access and Data Security
　　Principles for Health Information, Including
　　Computer-based Patient Records* (ASTM), 290
Conflict avoidance, 110, 113, 128–129
Conflict resolution, 34
Conflicts of interest
　competing constituencies, 530–532, 558–559
　consultants and, 545
　e-health information and, 392
　loyalties and, 242
　managed care plans and, 246
Connecting for Health, 282, 388, 409
Consent-for-treatment, 59–60
Consent forms, 604–605
Consequences, exposing, 42
Consistency of data, 368
Consolidated Health Informatics Initiative (CHI),
　405, 406
Consolidated Health Initiative (CHI), 333
Constituencies, competing, 530–532
Consultants
　advice ignored, 544–545
　conflicts of interest, 545
　definition of, 542
　EHR development, 330–331
　function-based issues for, 542

as a moral voice, 547
    scapegoating, 546–547
Consumers. *See also* Patients
    e-health technology and, 381–401
    managed care and, 235
Contact tracing and notification, 208–209
Continuing education, 14, 15, 108
Continuity of care records (CCRs), 408
Contractors
    client relationships, 552–554
    confidentiality issues, 552–554, 564–565
    expectation management by, 550–551,
        562–563
    social isolation of, 548–550
    trust of, 554
Contracts
    definition, 536–537
    negotiation of, 549–550, 550–553, 560–561
    with vendors, 568–573
Cooley, Thomas, 427
Cooperating Parties, 120–121
Cooperation, interdisciplinary, 12
Core competencies, 103–104
Coroners, 367
Corporate ethics, 536
Corporate Integrity Agreement (CIA), 74
Corporate responsibility, 539
Corrective actions, 80
Court orders, 468
Covered entities (CEs)
    chain-of-trust concept, 78
    HIPAA, 55
    personal health information use by, 185
    sending information to, 59
CPT Assistant, 105, 113
CPT (Current Procedural Terminology), 104, 105
Credentialing, 103–104, 237–238, 241
Crimes, 467, 471–472, 484–485
Cultural influences, 259
Currency of data, 369

D

Data
    access to, 186–187
    acquisition of, 182–186
    analysis of, 240
    audit trails, 315–316
    collection of, 183, 194, 370
    confidentiality of, 182
    definition clarity, 369
    deidentification, 187
    integrity of, 181–182, 184, 298, 302–303

    limited sets of, 58
    need to know and, 312–314
    research access to, 350–352, 360–361
    research records, 427–428
    sample policy on, 183
    secondary sources, 192
    validity of, 410
Data analysts, 193–194
Data marts, 343
Data mining, 344
Data processing policies, 183
Data quality
    characteristics of, 369
    data editing and, 291–292
    EHR systems and, 288
    health information technology and, 410
    issues, 368–375
    linking EHR systems and, 298
Data reporting, 11–12, 186
Data resource management, 341–361
Data resource managers, 342
Data stewardship, 181–182
Data warehouses, 343, 344, 606, 622–623
Databases, 183, 342
Dates, authorization process, 56
De George, Richard, 539
De-identification of data, 187
De-identified information, 56, 168, 368, 387
Death, right to, 40
Death notices, 467
Decision making
    advance care planning and, 254–265
    collaborative approach to, 334–335
    cost-benefits analysis and, 213–214
    documentation of, 6
    duty and, 210–211
    EHR systems and, 289
    ethical, 33–50, 148–149
    human resources-related, 501–506
    leadership failures and, 511–514
    process of, 35–38
    rational, 217–219
    values and, 15
Decision-making matrices, 50
Decision support analysts, 178, 344
Decision support specialists (DSSs), 175–198
Dementia, 266
Deontological theories, 39, 103
Department of Health and Human Services
        (DHHS), 61, 71, 333, 385, 465
Department of Health Care Fraud and Abuse
        Control, 71

Department of Justice (DOJ), 71
Deselection of physicians, 238
Designated health services, 76
Diagnoses
    code assignments, 104
    confirmation of, 80
    selection of, 105
Diagnostic-related groups (DRGs), 235
Digital-divide, 390
Disaster relief, 368
Discharge summaries, 83–84
Disciplinary guidelines, 80
Disclosure
    of adoption information, 440–441
    authorization for, 190
    criteria, 367–368
    of genetic information, 425–427
    information security and, 310
    law enforcement and, 467
    minimum necessary, 476–477
    obligation of, 432–433
    online health consumers and, 392–393
    patient authorization process, 56
    prisoners with AIDS, 475, 490–491
    purposes of, 56
    societal benefits of, 313
    use and, 57
    wrongful, 77, 473–474
Discrimination, 428–429
Disease registries, 204–205
Distributive justice, 214–216
"Do no harm" principle, 212
Do not resuscitate (DNR) orders, 262–263,
        264–265
Doctor's Office Quality—Information Technology
        (DOQ-IT), 407–408
Documentation
    billed procedures and, 88–89
    clarification of, 106
    discovering misrepresentation, 109–110,
        126–127
    of discussions, 43
    DRG assignment and, 46–47
    of employee performance, 513–514
    ethical dilemmas, 4–5
    fraudulent practices, 82–83
    integrity of, 71
    retrospective, 6–7, 48–49, 82–83, 92–93
    review of, 13
    templates, 108–109
    trends, 6–7
Domestic Security Enhancement Act of 2003, 221
Domestic violence, 367

Downsizing, 532
DRGs (Diagnosis-related groups)
    assignment of, 34, 37, 115–116
    documentation, 46–47
    validation of, 108
Drug Enforcement Agency (DEA), 265
Due care, defined, 536–537
Duty, decision-making and, 39
Duty to warn, 470

E

E-health technology, 381–401. *See also* Electronic
        health information management (e-HIM)
    changing healthcare system and, 386–387
    definition, 384
    e-HIM and, 403–419
    ethical issues, 390–393
    health literacy and, 391
    HIM professionals and, 389–390
    national policy and, 388–389
    potential, 385–386
    quality issues, 392–393
    risks, 385
    security issues, 316–317
    unique identifiers for individuals, 394
E-mail
    advantages, 385
    EHRs and, 298–300
    privacy issues, 60
    security issues, 316–317
Economic credentialing, 238, 241
Education
    EHR materials, 285
    employee programs, 80
    healthcare documentation and, 6
    of medical staff, 107
Efficiency principle, 214
Egg donation, 452, 453
eHealth Initiative (eHI), 408
Electronic health information management
        (eHIM), 404, 405, 411–412, 534. *See also*
        E-health technology
Electronic health record (EHR) systems, 6, 239, 240
    changes through, 309
    chief financial officer criteria, 332
    competing interests, 338–339
    computerized patient records and, 344–345
    CPR user requirements, 284
    criteria, 331–334
    decision making and, 289
    description, 281–285
    ethical issues, 279–305, 286–300
    future of, 285–286

health care organizations and, 286
implementation, 289–291, 329
infrastructure, 293
institutional values and, 289
linking of, 293–297, 304–305
management of, 404
planning, 330
problems, 292
security, 386
unique identifiers for individuals, 394
Electronic mail, 285
Ellis, Gary, 192
Emotional remedies, 388
Employees
anonymous hotlines, 511
curiosity of, 308, 322–323
disclosure of PHI, 367–368
documentation of performance, 513–514
feedback to, 514
long-term, 513–514
monitoring systems, 185–186
orientation, 508–510
part-time, 603–604, 618–619
retention rates, 501
terminations, 510–511, 514–525
Employers
duty to, 216–217, 218, 228–229
genetic testing and, 425–426
health care options and, 244
HIM code of ethics and, 12–13
inappropriate instructions from, 116–118, 134–135
professional ethics and, 152
use of genetic information, 428
Employment, use of healthcare information, 7
End of life care, 257–275
Entrepreneurs, characteristics of, 533–534
Entrepreneurship, 529–565, 540–542
Epidemiology, 203–204
Equity, 259–261, 382–383, 398–399, 509–510
Ethic of care, 40–41, 537
Ethical conflicts, analysis of, 218–219
Ethical decision-making matrix, 50
Ethical reasoning, 38–42
Ethical sensitivity. *See* Moral awareness
Ethics
approach to issues, 34
definition, 33, 34
dilemmas for HIM professionals, 4–5
HIM entrepreneurship and, 540–542
resources, 43–44
teaching of, 35
theories, 38, 39

Ethics committees, 15–16, 43, 265
Ethics in Patient Referral Act, 75
Evidence-based medicine, 238, 411
Evidence-based Medicine (Sackett), 239
Expectation management, 550–551, 562–563
Experts, 542–543
Expiration dates, 56
Eye donation, 367

F

Facilities fees, 101
Facility directories, 368, 473–474. *See also* Master patient index (MPI)
Facts, decision-making and, 36
Fairness, 40, 447
False claims, 101–102
False Claims Act, 71–72
Families
adoption information, 440–441
bad news scenarios, 268
communication with, 52, 64–65
genetic information and, 426
genetic information used by, 429
patient wishes and, 263
providing information to, 58
Family practice specialties, 239, 368
Faxes, privacy issues, 60
Federal Bureau of Investigation (FBI), 71
Federal Drug Abuse Prevention, Treatment, and Rehabilitation Act, 464
Federal Privacy Act of 1974, 429–430
Federal Register, 220, 309
Federal Sentencing Guidelines, 79
Felony-reporting statutes, 471
Fiduciary obligations, 79–80, 246
Fiduciary relationships, 241–242
"Fill-in" codes, 106
Financial reimbursement, 6
Firing. *See* Termination of employment
Flinching, defined, 578
Form design, 604–605, 620–621
Frailty, information issues, 258–259
Fraud
definition, 70, 101
documentation practices, 82–83
health information technology and, 410
reporting to CMS, 101
Voluntary Disclosure Protocols, 73–75
Fraud and Abuse Control Program, 78
Fraudulent activity, 121–122
Friends, 52, 64–65, 368
Full disclosure, defined, 446

Fund-raising, 367
Funeral directors, 367

G

"Gag rules," 241
Gaucher's disease, 426
General Accounting Office (GAO), U.S., 71, 407
General ethics, defined, 535
Genetic information, 423–437
    discrimination and, 428–429
    ethical dilemmas, 5
    federal legislative protections, 429–430
    issues, 424–426
    misuse of, 428–429
    privacy of, 436–437
    state legislative protections, 430–431
Genetic testing, 424–425, 429
Genetics and Public Policy Center, 425
Gifts, 570–571, 582–583, 588–589
Gilligan, Carol, 503–504, 506
Global infections, 221–223
Global packages, 101
Goals, nonmoral, 41
Golden-rule analysis, 39
Government, disclosure issues, 367
"Great Sanitary Movement," 202–205
Guidelines
    deviation from, 151
    for health websites, 397–398

H

Hand-wringing, 42
Happiness, 38–39, 40
HCA—The Healthcare Company, 148
Health care
    promotion of, 11
    right to, 40
Health Care Compliance Association, 152
Health Care Fraud and Abuse Control Program, 101
Health Care Information and Management Systems Society (HIMSS), 282
Health department activities, 204
Health information. *See also* Patient information; Protected health information (PHI)
    accepting money for, 81–82, 90–91
    for adoptees, 444–445
    authorization for use, 185, 190
    commercial interest in, 389–390
    concepts in security of, 310
    de-identified, 56
    expanded use of, 292
    life cycle of, 598

patient authorization process, 56
project planning, 331–335
protection of, 53, 55–56
release of, 54
requests for, 54
timely management of, 71
Health information exchange (HIE), 409
Health Information Management (HIM) Director, 333–334
Health Information Management (HIM) professionals
    AM activities, 140–144
    compliance with legislation, 433
    e-health and, 389–390
    effective advocacy by, 611
    entrepreneurship among, 532–534
    ethical dilemmas for, 4–5, 447
    HIPAA roles for, 79
    managed care and, 231–255, 240
    in MCOs, 244–246
    in provider organizations, 245–246, 254–255
    required skills for, 373
    roles of, 8–9, 404–405
    as stakeholders, 36–37
Health information systems
    ethical, 15–16
    history of, 5–8
Health information technology (HIT)
    e-health phenomenon and, 387
    ethical challenges, 409–412
    national plan for, 388
    product certification, 408
    public sector, 405–408
Health insurance. *See* Insurance companies; Managed care
Health Insurance Portability and Accountability Act (HIPAA), 51, 181
    Administrative Simplification Standards, 77–79
    AHIMA support for, 61
    billing activities and, 102
    business associate agreements, 292
    data access and, 365
    data resource management and, 342
    e-health and, 394
    EHR systems and, 287
    enforcement programs, 78
    false claims penalties, 78–79
    fraud investigations and, 71
    genetic information and, 426, 429–430
    goals of, 76–79
    health information technology and, 410
    Privacy Rule, 310–312, 386, 394, 464, 476–477
    privacy standards, 78, 185, 187

on public interest and benefit activities, 466–467, 469–470

requests for information and, 54

sanctions, 312

security matrix, 314

security standards, 77–78

on sexually-transmitted diseases, 475–476

state confidentiality statutes and, 430

Title 1, 55

Health Level-7 EHR Functional Model, 285, 335, 406–407

Health literacy, 391

Health maintenance organizations (HMOs), 233, 234. *See also* Managed care

Health on the Net, 397

Health Plan Employer Data and Information Set (HEDIS), 238

Health Plan Report Card, 238

Health Resources and Services Administration (HRSA), 406

Healthcare continuum, 261

Healthcare documentation. *See also* Health information
    access to, 7–8
    release of, 7–8
    uses of, 6–7

Healthcare Fraud and Abuse Data Collection Program, 78

Healthcare Information and Management Systems Society (HIMSS), 408

Healthcare providers, 58

Healthcare systems, trends, 6

Herbal medications, 388

Hereditary nonpolyposis colorectal cancer (HNPCC), 425

"Hierarchy of lying," 537

Hippocratic Oath, 597

HIV/AIDS
    discrimination issues, 212
    prisoners with, 475, 490–491
    reporting, 200, 226–227

HL7. *See* Health Level-7 EHR Functional Model

Home health care, 143–144, 158–161, 266

Honesty, requirement for, 14

Hospice care, 262

Hospital administration
    confirming discussions with, 43
    HIM professional's obligations to, 37
    instructions from, 116–118

Hospitalization, verification of, 465

Hospitals
    HIM professionals in, 245–246
    managed care and, 235

Hotlines, anonymous, 511

Hull, Eleanor F., 140, 153

Human Genome Project, 424

Human resource management, 500–506, 508–510

Human rights, 40

Human subject research, 187–192, 432

Huntington disease, 425, 426

I

ICD-9-CM (International Classification of Diseases, 9th revision, clinical modification), 104

Identifiers, removal of, 56, 168, 187, 368, 387

Identity, questions of, 453

Illinois Department of Public Health, 210

Illinois Health Care Cost Containment Council, 210

Illinois State Cancer Registry, 210

Immunization registries, 318–319

Implications, exposing, 42

Incentives
    managed care plans and, 246
    pay programs, 104, 108

Incidence, defined, 208

Inconsistencies, exposing, 42

Indemnity (fee-for-service) plans, 233, 234

Independent contractors (ICs), 532–533, 547–555

Independent practice associations (IPAs), 234

Individually identifiable health information, 59

Individuals, respect for, 211

Industrial espionage, 186

Information. *See* Health information

Information exchange, 403–419

Information security officers (ISOs), 308, 310

Information systems, 311, 315. *See also* Health information systems

Information technology, 387, 403–419. *See also* Health information technology (HIT)

Information technology specialist, 332–333

Informed consent, 189, 242, 319

Initiative, 194

Institute of Medicine (IOM), 282, 406

Institutional Review Boards (IRBs)
    protocol submission to, 181, 191
    research and, 431, 432
    walls of protection, 189

Institutional values, 289

Insurance companies
    attitudes toward, 107
    claims information, 245
    coded diagnoses and, 8
    diagnosis codes and, 106

Insurance companies—*continued*
    employers and, 244
    ethical dilemmas, 4
    genetic information and, 429
    professional-client relationships and, 242
    use of healthcare information, 7
Integrated delivery systems (IDSs), 238–239,
        363–379, 409
Integrated health systems (IHSs), 239
Integrity. *See also* Corporate Integrity Agreement
        (CIA)
    of data reported, 11–12
    issues, 43
    security and, 311
    value of, 540
Interdisciplinary cooperation, 12
Internal business audits, 58
Internet. *See also* World Wide Web
    AHIMA recommendations, 393
    consumer access to, 7
    digital-divide, 390
    e-health and, 384
    information access and, 308
    privacy protections and, 391–392
    quality of information, 400–401
    security issues, 316–317
Interoperatibility, 387, 405–408
Intranets, information access and, 308
Intrapreneurs, 534–535
Introspection, moral, 42

J

JCAHO. *See* Joint Commission on the
        Accreditation of Health Care Organizations
Job abandonment, 510–511
Joint Commission on the Accreditation of Health
        Care Organizations (JCAHO), 43–44
    incomplete medical records, 147–148
    on pain management, 265
    on patient rights, 598
    record reviews, 83
    retrospective documentation and, 92–93
Journal of the American Medical Association, 263
Judgment calls, 511–514
Judicial proceedings, 367, 429
Juengst, Eric, 41–42
Justice, 40, 189, 214–216, 218, 447
Justification, ethical reasoning and, 38–42

K

Kant, Immanuel, 211, 212
Kickbacks, 75

"Knowingly," defined, 71
Kohlberg, Lawrence, 502–503, 504–506

L

Language
    form design and, 604–605
    health literacy and, 391
    legible, 620–621
    of rights, 40
    standardization of vocabulary, 407
Laptops, security of, 316, 318, 326–327
Lateness, 500, 518–519
Law enforcement
    disclosure to, 467
    PHI disclosure issues, 367
    public safety and, 469–471
    requests from, 468–469
Laws
    compliance with, 12–13
    decision-making and, 35–36
Leadership, failure of, 511–514
Legal counsel, 468, 470, 471. *See also* Attorneys
Legal fathers, 446
Legal liability, 43
Legislative Information Service, 220
Level of service, coding and, 98, 124–125
Liberty, right to, 40
Library of Congress, 220
Licensure
    confirmation of, 146, 162–165
    definition, 144
    QM activities and, 149
    state laws, 144–145
Life, right to, 40
Life spans, lengthening, 386–387
Lifelong learning, 14
Living Wills. *See* Advance care planning
Loyalty, to employers, 12
Lying, hierarchy of, 537

M

Mail fraud, 76
Managed care
    access to care, 237
    access to patient information, 241–243
    characteristics of, 234
    choice of plans, 232–233
    description, 233–234
    growth of, 234–235
    HIM professionals and, 231–255
    ownership of, 233
    payment systems, 246

pricing, 235–236
strategies, 235–240
Managed care organizations (MCOs)
choice of plans, 250–251
conflicts of interest and, 242–243
HIM professionals in, 244–246
Management, issues facing, 499–527
Managers, obligations of, 511–514
Mandatory reporting laws, 205–207
Marketing, 6, 367
Master patient index (MPI)
core elements, 371
description, 281–282, 370–371
enterprise-wide, 371–372
inconsistencies, 372–373, 378–379
Material witnesses, 467
Medical examiners, 367
Medical information. *See* Health information
Medical necessity, 101
Medical Record Science, 19
Medical records. *See also* Health information;
Patient information; Protected health
information
access to, 222
alterations to, 80
case management audits of, 245–246
contents of, 282
electronic, 283
inaccurate entries, 151
incomplete, 104, 147–148, 166–170
paper-based, 388
patient stories, 598–599
release of, 7–8
researcher access to, 191–192, 431–432
retrospective completion, 83–84
in retrospective studies, 192
review, 83, 120
state confidentiality statutes, 430
unlocated, 106
workers' compensation requests, 492–493
Medically unnecessary items, 78
Medicare, utilization review, 140
Medicare Health Support Program, 389
Medicare Integrity Program, 78
Medicare Modernization Act of 2003, 389
Medicare Prescription Drug, Improvement, and
Modernization Act of 2003, 407, 410
Medicare Support Program, 389
Mental health records, 222–223, 463–495
Mill, John Stuart, 38, 211, 212
Mine Safety and Health Administration, 476
"Mini security rule," 310

"Minimum necessary" requirement, 57
Miscoding
conflict avoidance and, 110, 113, 128–129
discovery of, 114–115, 130–131
Misrepresentation, in documentation, 109–110
Missing persons, 467
Monitoring
of employees, 185–186
processes for, 80
Moral awareness, 500–507
Moral development, 500–506
Moral distress, 42–43
Moral intensity. *See* Moral awareness
Moral introspection, 42
Moral justification, 189
Moral maxims, 41
Moral muteness, 514
Moral principles, 41
Morality, defined, 34
Multimedia tools, 281
Myers, Grace Whiting, 9, 10
MyHealth*e*Vet, 389

N

National Alliance for Health Information
Technology, 408
National Association of County and City Health
Officials (NACCHO), 204
National Association of Healthcare Quality, 145
National Cancer Registrars' Association (NCRA),
145
National Commission for the Protection of
Human Subjects in Research, 432
National Committee on Quality Assurance
(NCQA), 238, 388
National Committee on Vital and Health Statistics
(NCVHS), 384, 405–406
National Coverage Decisions, 105
National Electronic Telecommunications System
for Surveillance (NETSS), 207
National Health Information Infrastructure (NHII),
384, 405
National Health Information Technology
Coordinator, 345
National Hospice and Palliative Care
Organization, 263
National Institutes of Health (NIH), 192
National Practitioner Data Bank, 78
National Society of Professional Engineers
(NSPE), 151–152
Natural fathers, 446
Natural mothers, 446

"Need to know" criteria, 7, 57, 310, 312–314
Neglect, PHI disclosure issues, 367
Negotiation
    of compromises, 42
    of contracts, 549–550, 550–553, 560–561
    management of, 576–579, 592–593
    styles of, 577
Nonconfidential information, 368
Nonmaleficence, 40, 211–212, 447
Notice of Health Information Practices, 296, 298
Notice of Privacy Practices, 57, 60
Notifiable diseases, 205
Notification laws, 203
Nurses, communications with, 472
Nurse's aides, communications with, 472, 486–487

O

Obligatory action, concept of, 219
Occupational Safety and Health Administration
    (OSHA), 476
Office for Protection from Research Risks, 432
Office of Civil Rights (OCR), 61
Office of Protection from Research Risks, 192
Office of the Inspector General (OIG), 70, 73–74,
    79, 80, 81, 122
Office of the National Coordinator for Health
    Information Technology (ONCHIT), 406
Omnibus Budget Reconciliation Act (OBRA), 75
Open adoptions, 444
Opioid use, 265
Organ donation, 367, 450–451
Organizational cultures
    change in, 16, 17
    socialization and, 509
    values, 147–148
Organizations, advocacy for, 605
Outcomes research, 387
Outpatient office visits, 105, 106
Outsourcing, 410, 532
Over-the-counter medications, 388
Oversight groups, 367. See also specific
    organizations

P

Pain management, 265
Palliative care, 265–266, 274–275
Palliative care specialization, 266
Paradigm cases, 42
Parental rights, 452
Partnerships, management of, 318–319
"Passing the buck," 42
Passwords, 348, 356–357

Paternalism, 213
Patient information. See also Health information;
    Medical records
    access to, 241–243, 243–244
    administrative level access, 313
    aggregate, 283
    analysis of, 240
    authorization from patients, 56–57
    "bad news," 258
    continuity of, 237
    historical, 237
    protection of, 55–56
    provided by physician practices, 252–253
    reporting QM issues, 151
Patient interest, 288–289
Patient notification
    informed consent and, 319
    linking EHR systems and, 298
Patient privacy. See Privacy
Patient records. See also Medical records
    access to, 54
    EHR systems and, 289–290
    integrity of, 280–281, 289–290
    Privacy Rule and, 394
Patient rights, 61
Patient satisfaction, 187, 238, 283
Patient support, 345
Patients
    access to data, 285
    advocacy for, 596, 597–600, 620–621
    authorization from, 56–57
    E-health technology and, 381–401
    empowerment of, 389 (see also E-health)
    expectation of privacy, 60–61
    financial liability, 106–107
    identity of, 465
    as stakeholders, 36
Patient's Bill of Rights, 597–598
Peers
    advocacy for, 596–597, 600–601, 614–615
    bringing honor to, 14
    review by, 140
Pennsylvania Department of Health authorities,
    209
Per diem, defined, 235
Per member per month (PM/PM), 236
Performance-based judgments, 511–514,
    526–527
Performance data, inaccurate, 156–157
Personal career management, 534–535
Personal digital assistants (PDAs), 316
Personal effectiveness, 194

Personal Health Dimension, 384
Personal health records (PHRs), 388. *See also* Health information; Medical records
Personal identity, 53–54
Personal Responsibility and Work Opportunity Reconciliation Act (PRWORA), 501
Physician-patient relationships, 241–242
Physician practices, 252–253
Physicians
   advocacy by, 243
   biases, 259–261
   consultation with, 120
   contracts with MCOs, 237
   deselection by MCOs, 238
   information provided by, 243
   managed care and, 235
   MCO contracts with, 241
   privileged communications with, 471
   questions to, 106
   satisfaction of, 283
   withholds and, 236
   working relationships with, 121
Physicians' Electronic Health Record Coalition (PEHRC), 408–409
Picture archive communication (PAC) systems, 309
Point-of-service (POS) plans, 233, 234
Policies
   about gifts, 572
   on coding, 107–108
   compliance guidelines, 79–80
   compliance with, 12–13
   on gifts, 582–583
   for health websites, 397–398
   IRB and, 189
   linking EHR systems and, 294–296
   for security, 312
Postoperative complications, 107
Power of Attorney for Health Care. *See* Advance care planning
Practice guidelines, 236, 238, 239
Practice procedures, 106
Precedents, arguments from, 41
Precision, defined, 369
Preexisting conditions, 107
Preferred provider organizations (PPOs), 233, 234
Preferred vendors, 590–591
Prescriptions, review of, 285
Preservation of information, 11
President's Advisory Commission on Consumer Protection and Quality in the Health Care Industry, 220

President's Information Technology Advisory Committee (PITAC), 406
Prevalence, defined, 208
Preventive care, 239–240
Prima facie arguments, 214
Primary care physicians (CPCs), 237, 239, 309
Principle diagnoses, 105, 120
Principles of Biomedical Ethics (Beauchamp and Childress), 40
Prison system, 367, 475, 490–491
Privacy
   adoption issues and, 452–453
   children's protective services (CPS), 494–495
   committee deliberations, 12
   computers and, 288
   confidentiality and, 51–65
   consumer concerns about, 308
   de-identification of data, 187
   definition, 53, 427
   duty to protect, 220
   EHR systems and, 286–288
   in electronic environments, 60–61
   equity and, 382–383, 398–399
   ethical challenges, 5, 61–62
   of genetic information, 436–437
   HIPAA rule, 54–59, 426, 429–430, 476–477
   HIPAA standards, 78, 185
   information security and, 310
   information systems and, 246–247
   of medical information, 427
   online, 391–392, 400–401
   penalties for violations of, 77
   prisoners with AIDS, 475, 490–491
   protection of, 10, 11, 12–13, 220, 612–613
   public safety *versus,* 482–483
   Recommendations to Ensure Privacy and Quality of Personal Health Information on the Internet, 393
   research and, 191
   of research records, 427–428, 431–432
   right to know and, 210–217
   safety of citizens *versus,* 469
   security related to, 310–312
   unique identifiers and, 394
   verification of admissions, 488–489
Privacy Act of 1974, 54
Privacy Rule, HIPAA, 426, 429–430, 476–477
Private health information. *See* Health information; Protected health information (PHI)
Privileged communications, 471, 472, 484–487
Procedure, appeals to, 42

Procedures, CPT codes, 105
Professional associations, 14–15. *See also specific associations*
Professionals, characteristics of, 8–9
Profit motives, 538–539
Progress notes, 107
Project design, 194
Project management, 335, 574–576
Protected health information (PHI), 55–56. *See also* Health information; Medical records
    access to, 55–59
    definition, 311, 365
    electronic (e-PHI), 308
    flow of, 366
    health information technology and, 411
    patient access to, 60
    security of, 307–327
Provider numbers, 109
Provider organizations, 246–247, 254–255
Psychiatrists, 470–471, 471, 484–485
Public, duty to, 216–217, 228–229
Public health
    ethical challenges, 210–219
    evolution of, 202–205
    interventions and, 202
    local health department activities, 204
    overview, 201–202
    PHI disclosure issues, 367
    responsibilities of HIM professionals, 199–229
Public Health Service Act, 432
Public interest, 13–14, 58, 78
Public interest and benefit activities, 466, 469–470
Public safety, 469–471, 482–483
Putative fathers, 446

Q
Quality
    audits, 5, 13–14, 149, 170–173
    commitment to, 148
    e-Health information, 392–393
    online protections for, 400–401
Quality management
    ethical commitment to, 146
    ethical conduct, 151–152
    ethical questions, 149–160
    ethical standards affecting, 144–148
    HIM professionals and, 139, 140–144, 143
    importance of measures, 239
    inaccurate performance data, 156–157
    people involved in, 151

Quality of care
    healthcare documentation and, 6
    HEDIS and, 238
    managed care and, 237–240
Qui Tam Statutes, 72–73

R
Rationalization, 509
Rawls, John, 215
Reciprocity, ethical argument of, 219
References, authoritative, 105
Regents of University of California, Tarasoff v., 470
Regional health information organization (RHIO), 407
Registries
    data sharing with, 313
    in EHR environment, 283
    organization, 318–319
Regulations, compliance with, 12–13
Reimbursement
    appropriateness of, 106
    coding and, 8
    False Claims Act, 71–72
    under false pretenses, 108
    providing information to, 58
    retrospective documentation and, 48–49
Relators, definition, 73
Relevance of data, 369
Religious traditions, 39
Reminder features, 283
Reportable diseases, 205, 217–219
"Reportable diseases and conditions" statutes, 205
Reporting
    aggregate patient data, 283
    clinical judgments and, 12
    ethical dilemmas, 4–5
    of fraud, 108
    fraudulent activity, 121–122
    HIV/AIDS status, 200, 226–227
    mandatory, 203
    obligations, 472
    patient protection and, 151
    quality issues, 143
    registries, 283
    of violations, 13–14
Reports, presentation of, 194
Requests
    for information, 54
    from law enforcement, 468–469
Requests for proposals (RFPS)
    directions, 574

ethical considerations, 575–576
social responsibility, 575
standard text, 574–575
statement of work, 575
vendors and, 584–585
Research
access to data, 191–192, 350–352, 360–361, 431–432
Common Rule, 432
confidentiality and, 191
design, 194
healthcare documentation and, 6
human subject, 187–192, 432
IRBs and, 431, 432
on outcomes, 387
participation in, 14
PHI disclosure issues, 367
privacy and, 191, 431–432
protocol submission to IRBs, 191
records, 427–428, 431–432
retrospective studies, 192
secondary sources, 192
skill and knowledge inventory, 193–194
subject selection, 189
Research Analysts, 178–179
Research Data Analysts, 179
Research resource-based relative value systems (RBRVSs), 235
Research specialists (RSs), 175–198
Resources
allocation of, 246
ethics, 43–44
Respect for persons, 189
Retrospective documentation
to avoid suspension, 92–93
comorbid conditions, 106
complications, 106
retyping progress notes, 107
scenario, 82–83
Retrospective studies, 192
Review processes, 54–55, 526–527
"Right to know," 210–217
Rights, analysis of, 40
Risk assessment
coding procedures, 80
data security, 317–318
software use, 118–119, 136–137
Role modeling, 16

S

Sackett, D. L., 239
"Safe Harbor" categories, 76, 410

Safety. *See also* Security
of citizens, 469
cockroach scenario, 602–603, 616–617
health information technology and, 410
professional ethics and, 144–146
Sales ethics, 569–572
Salespeople, 569
Sanches, Linda, 61
SAS software, 177–178
Scale development, 176–177
Scapegoating, 546–547
Scheduling, EHRs and, 285
Science Panel on Interactive Communication and Health, 392
Secure Sockets Layer, 316
Security. *See also* Safety
access to data and, 364
audit trails, 315–316
baseline, 312–319
biometrics and, 315
data integrity and, 302–303
definitions for, 311
EHR systems and, 287, 290–291
failure to log off, 324–325
of health information, 11, 307–327
health information technology and, 410
incidents, 311
information security programs, 309
information systems and, 246–247
integrity of patient records, 280–281
linking EHR systems and, 297
password, 348, 356–357
privacy-related, 310–312
sanctions, 312
of sensitive information, 552–554
Security officials, 308
Self-advocacy, 607
Self-care, 388
Self-determination. *See* Autonomy
Self-reporting, 73–75
Sentencing Commission Guidelines, U.S., 79–80
Sequencing rules, 120
Serious illnesses, 259, 263
Service contracts, 410
Services, AHIMA Code on, 11
Sexual information, 463–495
Sexually-transmitted diseases (STDs), 208–209, 475–476
Shared traditions, 41
Shattuck, Lemuel, 202
Sickle cell anemia, 425
Siegler, Mark, 243–244

Sign-in sheets, 58
Signatures, 56, 190
Social inequality, 215
Social information, 11
Social norms, 511–514
Social responsibility, 575
Socialization, 509
Societal morality, 535
Society
    obligations to, 37
    reciprocal duty owed to, 219
Software
    decision support, 118–119, 136–137, 177–178
    development, 329–339
    erasing, 316
    health plan requirements and, 109
    implementation, 329–339
Southern Institute for Business and Professional
    Ethics, 147
Sperm donation, 452, 453
Spiritual remedies, 388
SPSS (Statistical Package for the Social Sciences)
    software, 177–178
Staff
    advocacy for, 596–597, 602–603, 616–617
    part-time, 603–604, 618–619
Stages of moral development, 502–503, 504–506
Stakeholders, 36
Standardization, 387, 407
Standards
    basis of, 34
    of conduct, 79–80
    reporting violations of, 13–14
Standards of Ethical Coding, 103
Stark, Pete, 75
Stark I, 75–76
Stark II, 75–76
State confidentiality statutes, 430–431
State of Delaware Department for Children, Youth
    and Their Families, 148
State of Illinois Project for Local Assessment of
    Needs (IPLAN), 209
Subject selection, 189
Subpoenas, 468
Substance abuse, 463–495
Supererogatory action, 219
Superior knowledge, duty and, 219–220
Surveillance, 204, 208
Surveys
    design of, 176–177, 198
    response biases, 176–177
Symptoms, coding of, 105

T

Tarasoff v. Regents of University of California, 470
Tavistock Group, 146, 147, 151
Telehealth, 406
Telemedicine, 285
Temporary Assistance for Needy Families (TANF)
    program, 501–502
Terminal, meaning of, 263–264
Terminal illnesses, 259
Termination of employment, 510–511, 514–525
Terrorism, 221–223, 222
The Computer Based Patient Record—An Essential
    Technology for Health Care, 344
A Theory of Justice (Rawls), 215
Third-party liability cases, 429
Threats, security, 317
Tissue donation, 367
Tools, lack of, 115–116, 132–133
Transcendental arguments, 42
A Treatise on the Law of Torts (Cooley), 427
Treatment
    choices, 260, 270–271
    goals, 261
    payment and healthcare (TPO) options, 57
Trend data, 285
Trust
    of clients, 554
    ethics and, 34
    in hospitals, 599–600
Truth, 537–538, 543–544
Tuskegee Syphilis Experiment, 189
Tyler and Company, 152

U

UCR (usual, customary, and reasonable) pricing,
    235
Umbrella releases, 390
Unbundling, description of, 100–101
Unethical practices, response to, 13
Uniform Hospital Discharge Data Set, 120
Unique identifiers, 394
Upcoding, 100
URAC standards, 393
USA PATRIOT Act of 2001, 221
Use and disclosure, 57
User IDs, 290–291, 314–315. See also
    De-identification of data; Identifiers, removal
    of; Security
Utilitarianism, 38–39, 102–103, 214
Utility principle, 213
Utilization, 238
Utilization review (UR) programs, 140, 236

V

V-codes, 105
Validity, clinical, 428
Value of persons, 39
Values
  advocacy and, 597
  codes of ethics and, 3–32
  decision-making processes and, 15
  institutional, 38
  organizational, 147–148
  personal convictions, 148
  potential conflicts, 34
  professional, 145–147
Vendors
  EHR systems and, 293–297
  ethical behavior, 579–580
  friendship with, 570, 586–587
  gifts from, 570–571
  management of, 567–593
  negotiations with, 576–579
  preferred, 572–573, 590–591
  relations with, 568–573, 579
  requests, 568, 584–585
  sales ethics, 569–572
Veterans Administration (VA), 389
Veteran's Health Administration, 265

Videos, EHRs and, 285
Virtual private networks (VPNs), 308, 316
Virtue-based ethics, 41
The vise, defined, 578
Vision 2006, 15
Visual integration tools, 344, 345
Voluntary Chronic Care Improvement Program,
  410
Voluntary disclosure protocols, 73–75
Volunteering, 14, 533
Vulnerabilities, security, 317

W

Walker Information, 152
Walls of protection, 189
Welfare worker employees, 501
Whistleblowers, 80
Wire fraud, 76
Wireless networks, 308, 316
"Withholds," defined, 236
Workers' compensation, 367, 476,
  492–493
Workstations, 311, 316
World Health Organization, 265
World Wide Web, 384. *See also* Internet
Wrongful adoptions, 446